AF719517

Innovations in Diagnosis and Therapy of Neurodegenerative Diseases

Innovations in Diagnosis and Therapy of Neurodegenerative Diseases

Edited by Anna Roberts

STATES
ACADEMIC PRESS
www.statesacademicpress.com

States Academic Press,
109 South 5th Street,
Brooklyn, NY 11249, USA

Visit us on the World Wide Web at:
www.statesacademicpress.com

© States Academic Press, 2022

This book contains information obtained from authentic and highly regarded sources. Copyright for all individual chapters remain with the respective authors as indicated. All chapters are published with permission under the Creative Commons Attribution License or equivalent. A wide variety of references are listed. Permission and sources are indicated; for detailed attributions, please refer to the permissions page and list of contributors. Reasonable efforts have been made to publish reliable data and information, but the authors, editors and publisher cannot assume any responsibility for the validity of all materials or the consequences of their use.

ISBN: 978-1-63989-290-7

Trademark Notice: Registered trademark of products or corporate names are used only for explanation and identification without intent to infringe.

Cataloging-in-Publication Data

Innovations in diagnosis and therapy of neurodegenerative diseases / edited by Anna Roberts.
p. cm.
Includes bibliographical references and index.
ISBN 978-1-63989-290-7
1. Nervous system--Degeneration. 2. Nervous system--Degeneration--Diagnosis.
3. Nervous system--Degeneration--Treatment. I. Roberts, Anna.
RC348 .I56 2022
616.804 75--dc23

Table of Contents

Preface

Neurodegenerative disease occurs when the nerve cells of the brain and peripheral nervous system lose their function over time and eventually die. Currently, there are no cures that can permanently cure or slow down the progression of these diseases. The risk of developing neurodegenerative diseases increases dramatically with age. Parkinson's and Alzheimer's disease are the two most common neurodegenerative diseases. The risk factor for neurodegenerative diseases is a combination of environmental and genetic factors. A person might have a gene that can make them more susceptible to a particular neurodegenerative disease. But the time and severity of the disease depends on the environmental exposures throughout life. This book presents the complex subject of neurodegenerative diseases in the most comprehensible and easy to understand language. It is compiled in such a manner, that it will provide in-depth knowledge about the innovations in diagnosis and therapy of these diseases. This book will provide comprehensive knowledge to the readers.

Significant researches are present in this book. Intensive efforts have been employed by authors to make this book an outstanding discourse. This book contains the enlightening chapters which have been written on the basis of significant researches done by the experts.

Finally, I would also like to thank all the members involved in this book for being a team and meeting all the deadlines for the submission of their respective works. I would also like to thank my friends and family for being supportive in my efforts.

Editor

1

Impairment of Long-Term Plasticity of Cerebellar Purkinje Cells Eliminates the Effect of Anodal Direct Current Stimulation on Vestibulo-Ocular Reflex Habituation

*Suman Das[1,2,3], Marcella Spoor[2], Tafadzwa M. Sibindi[2], Peter Holland[1,2], Martijn Schonewille[2], Chris I. De Zeeuw[2,4], Maarten A. Frens[2,5] and Opher Donchin[1,2]**

[1] Department of Biomedical Engineering and Zlotowski Center for Neuroscience, Ben Gurion University of the Negev, Be'er Sheva, Israel, [2] Department of Neuroscience, Erasmus Medical Center, Rotterdam, Netherlands, [3] Department of Integrative Neurophysiology, Center for Neurogenomics and Cognitive Research, Vrije Universiteit Amsterdam, Amsterdam, Netherlands, [4] Netherlands Institute for Neuroscience, Amsterdam, Netherlands, [5] Faculty of Social and Behavioral Sciences, Erasmus University College, Erasmus University, Rotterdam, Netherlands

Edited by:
Luca Berdondini,
Fondazione Istituto Italiano di Technologia, Italy

Reviewed by:
Stefano Vassanelli,
University of Padua, Italy
Enrique Claverol,
Universitat Politecnica de Catalunya, Spain

***Correspondence:**
Opher Donchin
donchin@bgu.ac.il

Anodal direct current stimulation (DCS) of the cerebellum facilitates adaptation tasks, but the mechanism underlying this effect is poorly understood. We have evaluated whether the effects of DCS effects depend on plasticity of cerebellar Purkinje cells (PCs). Here, we have successfully developed a mouse model of cerebellar DCS, allowing us to present the first demonstration of cerebellar DCS driven behavioral changes in rodents. We have utilized a simple gain down vestibulo-ocular reflex (VOR) adaptation paradigm, that stabilizes a visual image on the retina during brief head movements, as behavioral tool. Our results provide evidence that anodal stimulation has an acute post-stimulation effect on baseline gain reduction of VOR (VOR gain in sham, anodal and cathodal groups are 0.75 ± 0.12, 0.68 ± 0.1, and 0.78 ± 0.05, respectively). Moreover, this anodal induced decrease in VOR gain is directly dependent on the PP2B medicated synaptic long-term potentiation (LTP) and intrinsic plasticity pathways of PCs.

Keywords: tDCS, LTP, purkinje cell, vor, cerebellum

INTRODUCTION

Transcranial direct current stimulation (tDCS) modulates cerebellar dependent motor learning tasks (Jayaram et al., 2012; Hardwick and Celnik, 2014; Herzfeld et al., 2014; Avila et al., 2015) by applying a weak constant electrical current (amplitude <2 mA) through scalp electrodes. This technique allows us to stimulate the target region by the positive (anodal) or negative (cathodal) current (Das et al., 2016). Data collected in humans suggests that polarity specific effects of tDCS may be obtained by changing cerebellar cortical excitability (Galea et al., 2009). However, the mechanism behind tDCS dependent modulation of motor learning is unclear (Das et al., 2016). To optimally use tDCS in various cerebellar dependent motor learning disorders, a better understanding of mechanisms is vital (Ivry and Spencer, 2004; Xu-Wilson et al., 2009; Bastian, 2011; Hardwick and Celnik, 2014; Benussi et al., 2015).

Various animal models of DCS (direct current stimulation that is not transcranial) serve in exploration of the mechanism of tDCS (Creutzfeldt et al., 1962; Bindman et al., 1964; Purpura and Mcmurtry, 1965). In these models, a small part of the skull is removed at the site of stimulation in order to reduce the inter-subject variability of transcranial-conductance.

Our current study aims to explore the mechanism of action of DCS on cerebellar learning. To probe polarity specific effects of DCS on cerebellar learning, we employed a gain-down vestibulo-ocular reflex (VOR) adaptation task. The VOR aims to compensate for head movement by making an eye movement in the opposite direction, in order to stabilize the image on the retina (Probst et al., 1986). This compensatory eye movement can be adapted based on mismatched visual input, a process that requires the cerebellum (Kawato and Gomi, 1992). Here we presented a sinusoidal optokinetic stimulation by using a 360° virtual environment and vestibular stimulus by using a turntable in phase, resulting in a decrease of the response to the same vestibular stimulus in the dark (Tempia et al., 1991). The turntable mimics the head movement while the movement direction of the virtual environment demands orientation specific compensation of the eye movement (similar to the natural environment).

The gain-down adaptation of the VOR (Tiliket et al., 1993) may depend partly on both the cerebellar flocculus and the downstream vestibular nuclei (VN) (Lisberger and Fuchs, 1974; Ito, 1982). To test the importance of Purkinje cell (PC) plasticity in polarity-specific DCS modulation, we investigated L7-PP2B mice, lacking postsynaptic and intrinsic plasticity of PC (Schonewille et al., 2010). Our prediction is that at least some DCS effects (caused either by anodal or cathodal stimulation) would be compromised in this mutant because DCS has an extensive modulatory role on PC dendrites (Chan and Nicholson, 1986; Chan et al., 1988).

A rodent model of DCS has been validated in cortical spreading depression (Liebetanz et al., 2006a) and epilepsy (Liebetanz et al., 2006b). Anodal stimulation of frontal cortex enhances the Blood-oxygen-level dependent (BOLD) signal, an indication of higher neuronal activity (Takano et al., 2011). Furthermore, DCS alters neocortical plasticity not only by altering pre-synaptic sensitivity (Márquez-Ruiz et al., 2012) but also by promoting brain-derived neurotrophic factor (BDNF) dependent long-term potentiation (LTP) (Fritsch et al., 2010). As the plasticity mechanisms of the cerebellar cortex are different from those in neocortex (Hansel, 2005; Lamont and Weber, 2012) there is ample justification for an animal model of cerebellar DCS. Moreover, the cerebellum is ideal to identify the mechanism(s) of DCS because—(i) the structure of rodent cerebellum is clear and accessible, (ii) the plasticity mechanisms are well studied, and (iii) there is a wide range of mutant mouse models available to test which pathways are functionally relevant (De Zeeuw et al., 2011). Therefore, the present study focuses not only on developing an animal model of cerebellar DCS but also utilizes one of the most important mutant mouse models to unravel the role of PC plasticity in mediating DCS effects on VOR adaptation.

METHODS

Summary of Methodology

C57BL/6 (wild type, $N = 24$) and L7-PP2B (LTP deficient mutants, $N = 22$) mice were implanted with a DCS-implant for administration of DCS over the cerebellum. DCS was applied to separate groups of mice as anodal, cathodal or sham-stimulation. Eye movements were recorded using an infrared-sensitive CCD camera during horizontal VOR gain-down adaptation learning. In testing sessions, the eye response to vestibular stimulation, i.e., the motion of the table, (amplitude of 5° at 1 Hz frequency) in the dark was recorded. In training sessions, vestibular and visual stimulation (amplitude of 5° at 1 Hz frequency) were coupled so as to cause reduction of the VOR gain. Two baseline test sessions were followed by 10 min of DC stimulation and then by an additional baseline test session. There were then 5 training sessions of 5 min each, each followed by a test session. We subsequently compared the reduction of VOR gain in the different stimulation groups and across strains.

Experimental Paradigm

Mice were habituated to the experimental apparatus for a minimum of 2 days to reduce the novelty-induced anxiety and restrain-stress after they recovered from the surgery.

Each experiment consisted of 8 test (T) and 5 training (Tr) sessions. The duration of each test session was 1 min, and the duration of each training session was 5 min. In test sessions, a sinusoidal vestibular stimulation which was generated by moving the table with a 5° amplitude at 1 Hz frequency, was applied in the dark. Eye movements were recorded simultaneously. In training sessions, in phase vestibular and optokinetic sinusoidal stimuli (5° amplitude at 1 Hz frequency) were given (**Figure 1A**), in order to reduce the VOR gain. Eye movements were continuously recorded.

Every experiment was initiated by two baseline measurements of VOR (T1 and T2). Then the mice were randomly divided into 3 groups, and received anodal, cathodal or sham DC stimulation. The current amplitude was ramped up over 30 s to 113.2 μA and kept constant for 10 min (positive polarity for the anodal group, negative polarity for the cathodal group). For the sham group, amplitude was then immediately ramped down (over 30 s) while for the anodal and cathodal groups current was maintained for 10 min of stimulation. After the stimulation, another session of testing (T3) was conducted and then gain-down adaptation learning training was initiated. A testing session was conducted to calculate the learning rate after every training session (**Figure 1A**).

Experimental Procedure

Animals

C57BL/6 ($N = 24$) mice were acquired from Charles River laboratories, Inc. (Wilmington, MA, USA). L7-PP2B mutants ($N = 22$) were bred in Erasmus MC, Rotterdam. Mouse lines used in this study have been described previously (Schonewille et al., 2010). Three to four mice were caged together in temperature-regulated (22 ± 1°C) housing with a 12:12 light-day

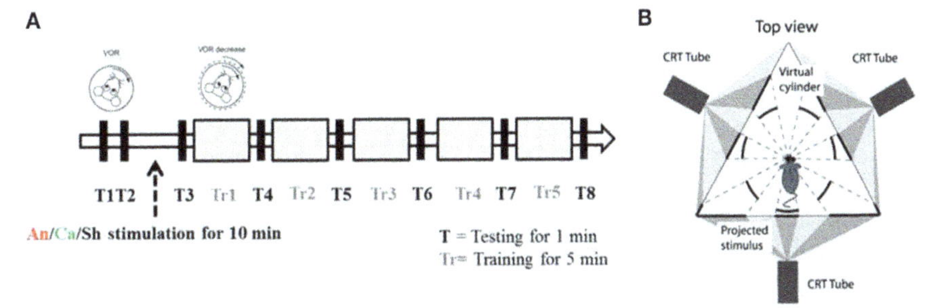

FIGURE 1 | Experimental paradigm and set up **(A)** Schematic diagram of the experimental paradigm. *T* represents a testing session during which the animal is exposed to VOR in the dark by moving the turntable in a sinusoidal manner (5° amplitude at 1 Hz). *Tr* represents the training session during which the animal is presented with a sinusoidal visual cue which is in phase with the table movement. After two testing sessions (*T1* and *T2*) the animals were randomly assigned to the anodal (*An*), cathodal (*Ca*) or sham (*Sh*) stimulation group. **(B)** Schematic diagram of the experimental apparatus. Top down view describes the position of the mouse in relation to the virtual environment created by three projectors.

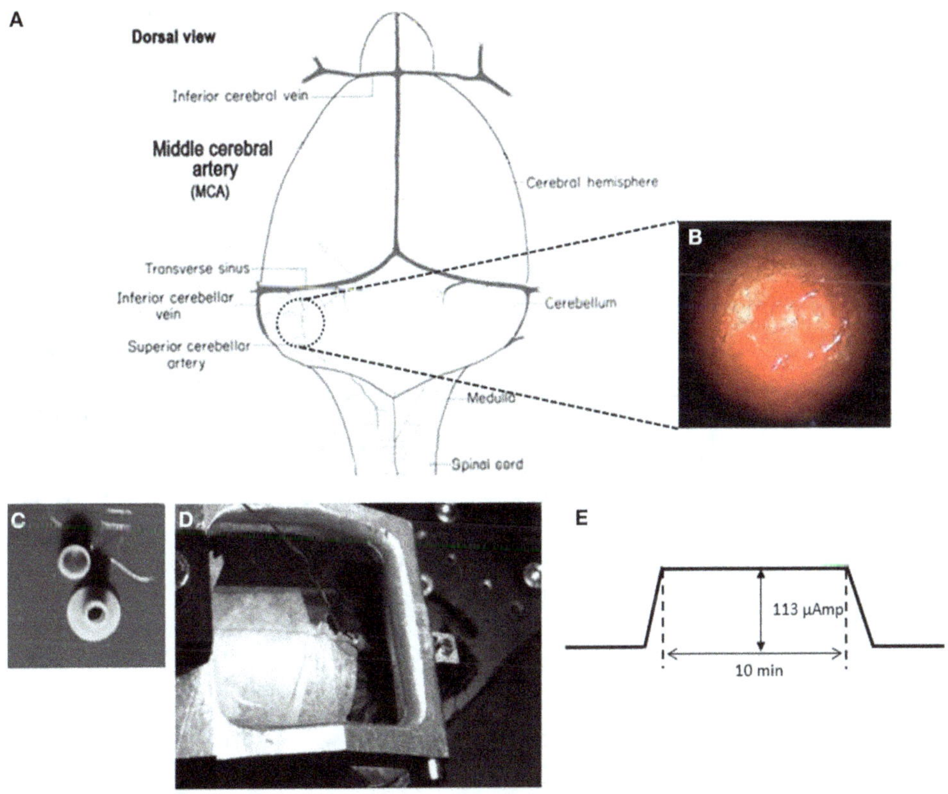

FIGURE 2 | DCS location and procedure **(A)** Schematic representation of craniotomy for placement of implant over the cerebellum of a mouse brain. **(B)** Craniotomy. Anatomical location for the DCS-implant placement. **(C)** DCS implant. The DCS chamber serves as a bridge between the stimulating electrode and the brain. Above the chamber is the cap that serves to protect the brain from infection. **(D)** Stimulating the mouse cerebellum. The DCS chamber is filled with saline (0.9% NaCl) solution. A silver wire that touches the saline solution but not the dura directly is connected to the current generator (SUI-91, Isolated current source). During stimulation the mouse is awake but head restrained. **(E)** Stimulation paradigm. DCS is ramped up to 113 μAmp. The current is maintained at its peak value for 10 min. After the stimulation the current is ramped down.

cycle. Behavioral experiments were performed in the light cycle. Food and water was provided *ad libitum*. All experiments were reviewed and approved by the Erasmus animal ethics committee and conducted in accordance with Animal Welfare Committee of the Erasmus University and the European Communities Council Directive (86/609/EEC).

Surgery

Mice, aged 10–12 weeks, were handled for 2 days before the surgery to reduce the effect of handling-induced stress. The surgical procedure was performed under sterile conditions. Isoflurane (5% induction, 1.5% in 0.5 L/min O_2, and 0.2 L/min air) was administered as an anesthetic drug while body temperature was regulated around 36.5 ± 0.5° via a feedback-controlled heating pad. Breathing profile was continuously monitored. After shaving the head, a 1 cm long mid-sagittal incision was given. The bone was etched (37.5% phosphoric acid, Kerr, CA, USA) and a primer (Optibond, Kerr, CA, USA) was applied. To immobilize the animal during eye tracking, a pedestal containing two M1.4 nuts was glued to the skull using dental acrylic (Charisma, Flowline, Hereaus Kulzer GmBH, Germany).

In order to place a DCS implant, a circular craniectomy (approximately 2 mm in diameter) on the left occipital bone was performed after careful removal of the neck-muscles (vertical and horizontal) (**Figures 2A,B**). The placement was on the center of the left parietal bone (by keeping the superior cerebellar artery at the center of the implant). A lubricating ointment (Duratears, Alcon Nederland BV, NL) was applied epidurally to protect the exposed area of brain from drying. The DCS implant (**Figure 2C**) was placed identically in all animals using an anatomical marker (**Figures 2A,B**) and then glued to the skull using cyanoacrylate gel (Plastic One Inc., VA, USA).

The mice were given an analgesic (0.1 ml/mg of body weight Buprenorphine/Temgesic) and placed under an infrared heating lamp until the animals started to move. Mice were allowed at least 4–5 days to recover before recordings were performed.

Apparatus

Visual and Vestibular Stimulation

Mice were head-fixed in a restrainer, which was fixed onto the center of a turntable, placed at the center of an isolateral triangle made by three projector-screens. A panoramic virtual reality display with 360° field of view was created by projecting monochrome green dots on to those screens (**Figure 1B**). Horizontal rotation of the turntable was driven by a servomotor (Mavilor-DC motor 80, Infranor, Spain). Visual stimuli and movement of the turntable were under control of in-house software written in C++. Training and testing sessions were evoked by rotating the dots and/or the turntable sinusoidally. During each session, stimuli were ramped up to their peak velocity in 5 s for a smooth transition from static to dynamic state. They were also ramped down at the end.

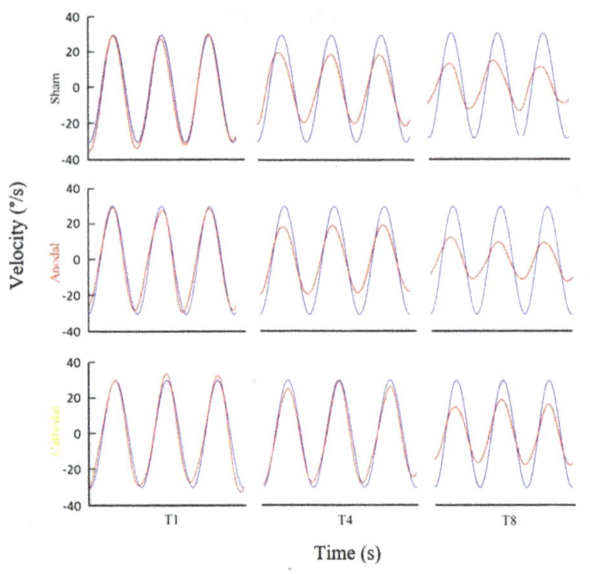

FIGURE 3 | Examples of eye movement in different stimulation conditions. Examples of filtered eye velocity illustrate results from mice that exhibited a decrease in the VOR after training with sham (top panels), anodal (middle panels) and cathodal (bottom panels) stimulation. Blue is vestibular stimulus and red is eye amplitude (solid red line is filtered eye-velocity, dotted red line fitted sine wave). Eye-trace of each stimulus condition has been presented during pre-training (T1), after first-training (T4) and after final-training (T8) in the left, middle and right panels, respectively.

Eye Movement Recordings

Eye movements were recorded with an infrared video system (ETL-200 with marker tracking modifications; ISCAN, Burlington, MA). The camera and lens were mounted under the table surface to reduce hindrance of the mouse vision. A hot mirror which was transparent to visible light and reflective to infrared light was used. The eye was illuminated with three infrared LEDs. The camera, mirror and LEDs were all mounted on an arm that could rotate about the vertical axis over a range of 26.12° (peak to peak). Eye movement recordings and calibration procedures were similar to those described by Stahl et al. (2000). Images of the eye were captured at 120 Hz with an infrared-sensitive CCD camera. The eye image contained a bright corneal reflection and a dark pupil reflection. The image was focused by manipulating the offset and the gain of the detectors through the ISCAN software. From this image, x and y positions of each of the three markers were recorded in real time giving their location on a 512 × 256-pixel grid, with a resolution of one-third pixel horizontally and one-tenth pixel vertically (van Alphen et al., 2010). These x and y translational positions of eye on the grid were converted into the angular rotation of the eyeball by the ISCAN system (resolution of 0.2° over a ±25° horizontal and ±20° vertical range using the pupil/corneal reflection difference). The horizontal and vertical pupil position data from the ISCAN were output as ±5 VDC signals. A delay of 30 ms in the eye movement signal was introduced by the video system. Furthermore, this output signal was low-pass filtered with a cutoff frequency of 300 Hz (Cyberamp 380; Axon Instruments, CA, USA), sampled at 1 kHz and stored for offline analysis.

Direct Current Stimulation

A low amplitude (113 μA) of continuous DCS was applied using a constant current stimulator (SUI-91, Isolated current source, Cygnus Technology Inc., NC, USA; range = 0.1 μA–10 mA). This intensity corresponded to a current density of 3.6 mA/cm^2 (Liebetanz et al., 2009). Currents were applied to the epidural surface of the cerebellar cortex through a circular DCS implant with a defined contact area (2 mm inner diameter). Prior to stimulation, the electrode was filled with saline solution (0.9% NaCl). A silver wire electrode connected to the stimulation device was attached to the DCS implant such that the tip of the silver wire touched the top level of the saline solution but did not touch the

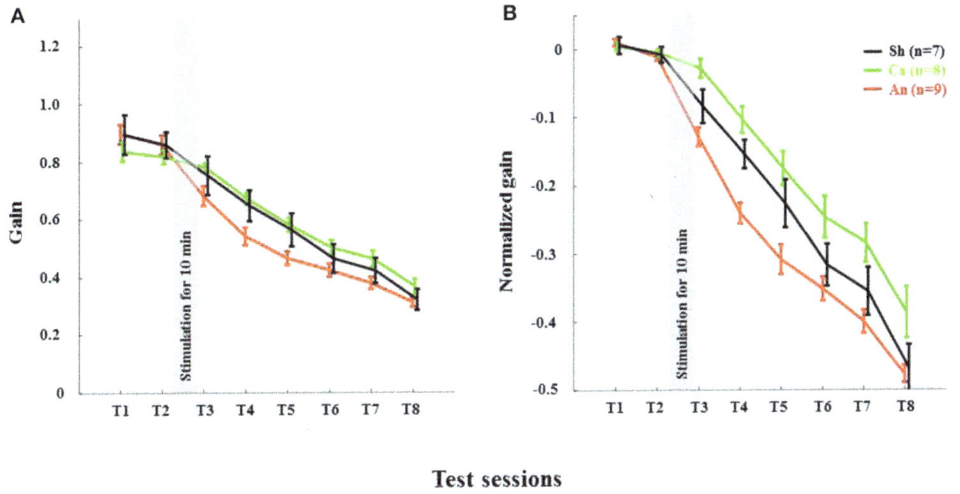

FIGURE 4 | Anodal stimulation reduces VOR gain acutely in wild type C57BL/6 mice. **(A)** Time course of gain reduction due to adaptation: Changes in mean VOR gain during VOR-decrease training. The VOR was tested pre- and post-training by measuring the eye movement response to the vestibular stimulus. **(B)** Time course of normalized gain reduction due to adaptation: Trial-to-trial changes in mean normalized VOR gain during VOR-decrease training. Black, Green and Red lines are for sham, cathodal and anodal stimulation conditions, respectively. The gray bar indicates the stimulation period. Error bars represent SEM.

brain directly. This circular active electrode (**Figure 2C**) was chosen to create a symmetric current density without any edge effects (Ambrus et al., 2011). A disposable foam electrode (Kendall Medi-Trace mini resting ECG electrode, Davis medical products Inc., CA, USA), was placed onto the ventral thorax of the animal to complete the circuit. The entire circuit was connected through a multimeter to check online current amplitude. Mice were awake during DCS to prevent possible interactions between DCS effects and anesthetic drugs. In addition, mice were introduced to the adaptation task right after the stimulation to quantify acute effects of stimulation. To avoid stimulation break effects (Liebetanz et al., 2009), the current intensity was ramped up and down gradually over 30 s.

Data Analysis

Custom routines written in MATLAB (The MathWorks Inc., Natick, MA, USA) were designed and employed for automated offline data analysis. The position signal was shifted 30 ms back in time to correct for the camera delay. A median filter (width 50 ms) with a low-pass cutoff of 10 Hz was applied to smooth the position data before transforming to velocity domain by a Savitski-Golay differentiating filter (frequency 50 Hz with a 3° polynomial). Rapid eye movements were detected and removed via a velocity threshold (150°/s). Then a 3 Hz FIR Butterworth low pass filter of 50 ms width was applied.

The processed data was divided into non-overlapping epochs of 2 s (corresponding to two cycles of the stimulus). Amplitude data was obtained by fitting sine waves to the eye movement data in custom-made Matlab curve fitting routines using the least-squares method. Median amplitude values of the eye movement were calculated from the fitted sine waves. Gain was calculated for,

$$G_T = \frac{E_{Tn}}{S} \quad \begin{aligned} &E = \text{fit eye amplitude of a testing session, } n = 1 \text{ through } 8,\\ &S = \text{stimulus amplitude,} \end{aligned} \tag{1}$$

each testing session as the ratio between the fit eye velocity amplitude and stimulus velocity amplitude (***S***).

Mice were excluded when the absolute difference between baseline gains (G_{T1}–G_{T2}) was > 0.2. The baseline gain (***G_B***) was set as the mean of gains in G_{T1} and G_{T2}. Normalized gain (***G_N***) was also calculated for every test session.

$$G_N = \frac{G_B - G}{G_B + G} \tag{2}$$

Statistical Analysis

Statistical analysis of the data was performed using SPSS 20.0 (SPSS, Chicago, IL). A three way mixed-ANOVA with repeated measures was used to compare interaction and group effects, as the data showed a normal distribution. Significance levels were set to 0.05. Later on, a Bonferroni corrected *post-hoc* analysis was applied to find intra-/inter-group interactions. Values are represented here as mean ± SEM.

RESULTS

Degree of Adaptation at the End of Training Session

The VOR gain-down adaptation paradigm caused a gradual reduction in VOR-amplitude in all mice (**Figures 3–6**). Initially, the amplitude of the eye movement was similar to the stimulus amplitude; i.e., the gain at T1 for C57BL/6 and L7-PP2B mice was 0.88 ± 0.03 and 1.03 ± 0.03, respectively (**Figures 4, 6**). The

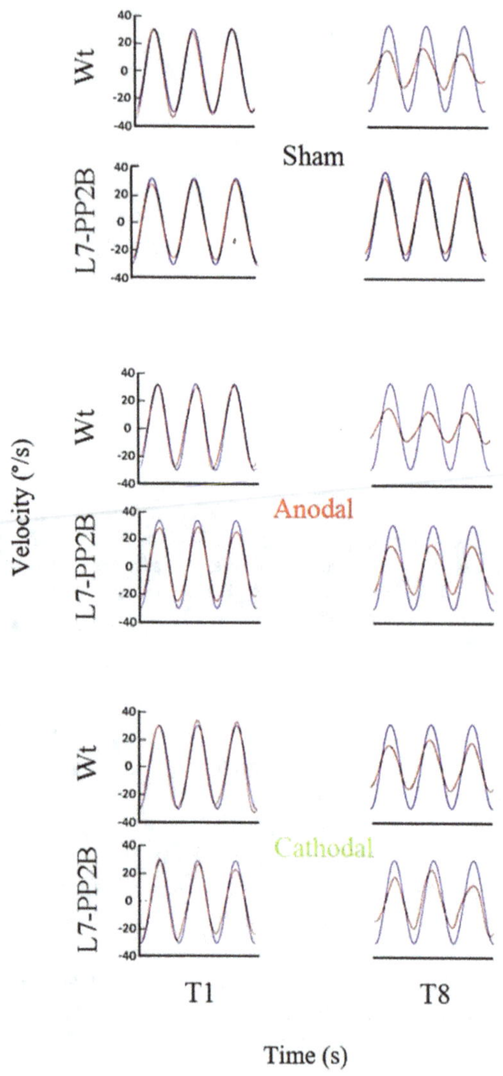

FIGURE 5 | Eye amplitude show clear deficit in learning of L7-PP2B mice in all three stimulus conditions. Example filtered eye velocity traces illustrate typical results from mice of both genetic backgrounds before (T1) and after (T8) adaptation. Blue is vestibular stimulus and red is eye velocity (solid red line is filtered eye-signal, dotted red line is the fitted sine wave). Eye amplitude decreases from pre- to post-training sessions (T1 and T8, respectively) in wild type mice. In contrast, L7-PP2B undergoes little change between T1 and T8 sessions.

baseline VOR gain in L7-PP2B of more than 1 indicated that the eye amplitude overshot the head amplitude in these mice. After being subjected for 25 min to the gain-down training, the amplitude of VOR at T8 was reduced for both C57BL/6 (raw T8 gain = 0.33 ± 0.03) and L7-PP2B (raw T8 gain = 0.70 ± 0.03) group. In our multivariate ANOVA on the non-normalized data, the main effect of training over the time course was highly significant, $F_{(7, 34)} = 46.20$, $p < 0.001$. However, comparison of the sham stimulation data showed that the degree of adaptation was significantly higher in C57BL/6 than L7-PP2B mice, $F_{(5, 40)} = 14.94$, $p < 0.001$.

Reduction of Gain in C57BL/6 and L7-PP2B Mice

The reduction in gain made across the eight test sessions was strongly dependent upon the genetic composition of mice, $F_{(7, 38)} = 4.98$, $p < 0.001$. We sought to find out at which steps the gain was maximally reduced between C57BL/6 and L7-PP2B mice. To do that, we checked the gain difference between two successive test sessions and then compared that across the mouse types. The tests of within-subjects contrasts illustrated that the gain reduction from T5 to T6 [$F_{(5, 40)} = 2.48$, $p < 0.05$] and from T7 to T8 [$F_{(5, 40)} = 2.66$, $p < 0.05$] was significantly greater for C57BL mice compared to the L7-PP2B mice.

Effects of DCS on VOR Adaptation

ANOVA further indicated that DCS polarity had a significant modulatory role on the gain reduction, $F_{(14, 70)} = 2.07$, $p < 0.05$, suggesting that the amplitude of gain decrease across the eight tests (from T1 to T8) was dependent upon stimulus polarity. Moreover, the gain decrease across eight test sessions yielded a significant interaction between stimulus polarity and genetic background of the mice (C57BL/6 and L7-PP2B mice, [$F_{(7, 35)} = 2.52$, $p < 0.05$]. In the following sections, we discuss how the modulatory role of DCS was altered depending on the mouse type.

Anodal Stimulation Reduced VOR Gain in C57BL/6 Acutely

The anodal stimulation triggered faster initial VOR gain reduction compared to the cathodal stimulation [$F_{(2, 21)} = 9.56$, $p < 0.001$, **Figure 4A**] in wild type mice. There was a significant post-stimulation reduction of gain at T3 (pre-training reduction of gain) in the anodal group compared to the cathodal group. The contrast analysis, T2 vs. T3, comparing the raw gain at T2 with that made in T3, was statistically significant [$F_{(2, 21)} = 6.01$, $p < 0.01$]. Interestingly, the anodal, sham and cathodal groups finished at the same degree of adaptation (T8), although the anodal group showed significant initial reduction in VOR gain.

Next, we normalized the gain of every mouse to its own baseline to provide a comparable measure of gain for all animals. Normalized gain (**Figure 4B**) depicted a clear polarity-dependent divergence. The initial post-stimulation period showed that the cathodal stimulation significantly decelerated gain reduction compared to the anodal stimulation. The reduction of gain in the sham condition—as expected—remained between the rate in the anodal and the cathodal conditions (**Figure 4B**).

Deletion of PP2B in PC Abolished Anodal Effect

Anodal stimulation lost its modulatory role when potentiation was eliminated from PCs (**Figures 6A,B**). Anodal stimulation failed to improve learning in L7-PP2B mice (T8 gain = 0.74 ± 0.04), compared to the sham group (T8 gain = 0.65 ± 0.08; **Figure 5**). Moreover, anodal stimulation could not reduce the baseline gain in these mutants (T2 gain = 1.06 ± 0.04, T3 gain = 0.99 ± 0.04). The large error bars in the sham condition is due to low sampling numbers ($N = 3$). Moreover, we think that chronic mutation (deletion of LTP in PCs) leads to the adoption of various adaptation mechanisms in the network. Therefore, when an external current stimulus was applied the network showed varied responses to cope with the situation. This could be the cause for finding a large variability in the stimulation groups.

An hour long sinusoidal oscillatory stimulus led to decrease in VOR gain (approximately to 28%) across various species (Tempia et al., 1991; Dow and Anastasio, 1998; Clément et al., 2002). The cause of this VOR gain reduction in rodents has been pointed out as habituation rather than learning (Tempia et al., 1991). Therefore, we think that the gain reduction (27 ± 2%) in L7-PP2B mice (similar to Schonewille et al., 2010) across all three stimulation-conditions is due to the habituation.

DISCUSSION

Our study demonstrates three major findings of the polarity specific effects of DCS on VOR gain-down adaptation. First, anodal stimulation of cerebellar cortex decreases VOR gain acutely compared to the cathodal stimulation condition in C57BL/6 control mice. Second, despite differences in initial post-stimulation reduction in gain amplitude, the final gain reduction is similar in the anodal and the cathodal stimulation groups of C57BL/6 control mice. Third, our data, remarkably, shows when potentiation of the PCs is genetically ablated in L7-PP2B mice, anodal stimulation no longer led to VOR gain reduction. Hence, our interpretation is that anodal stimulation driven VOR gain reduction depends on a PP2B-dependent PC potentiation pathway, either at the upstream dendritic level or at the downstream axonal level where PCs innervate VN neurons (Schonewille et al., 2010).

We found that anodal stimulation of the cerebellum decreases VOR gain acutely (**Figures 4A,B**), though we don't see an effect on adaptation-rate like in other studies (Jayaram et al., 2012; Herzfeld et al., 2014; Zuchowski et al., 2014; Avila et al., 2015). We see that VOR gain is reduced prior to the training. Perhaps anodal stimulation induced an acute increase in inhibition by enhancing PC activity. Indeed, others have also reported that artificial activation of PCs may contribute to the induction of VOR gain-down adaptation (Nguyen-Vu et al., 2013). Moreover, a low amplitude external electric field (EEF) is sufficient to modulate PC activity (Chan and Nicholson, 1986; Chan et al., 1988). Together these results suggest that anodal DCS may induce higher PC activity, which in turn could lead to inhibition of its downstream structures.

The possibility that the effects of DCS on plasticity are in part secondary effects on downstream structures comports with there being at least two sites of VOR plasticity (Hansel, 2005): one in the floccular region of cerebellar cortex and one in the VN (Gao et al., 2012). Physiological studies would be necessary to elucidate the relative effects, and these studies would need to include direct measurements from both regions.

We also found that the total gain reduction was similar in the anodal and the cathodal stimulation conditions although the gain reduction at the early phase is clearly different (**Figure 4A**). In our study, training and testing are assessed post DCS, whereas most of the reports available today are based on stimulation applied during learning. For instance, anodal stimulation facilitates learning in locomotor (Jayaram et al., 2012), force field (Herzfeld et al., 2014), and saccade (Avila et al., 2015) adaptation as well as eye-blink conditioning tasks (Zuchowski et al., 2014), while cathodal stimulation hinders

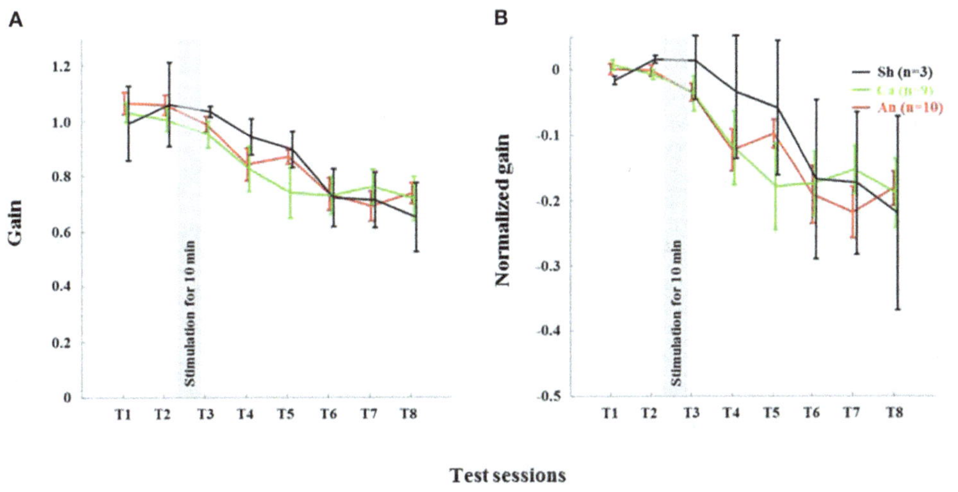

FIGURE 6 | Genetic ablation of PC plasticity in L7-PP2B mice abolishes effects of anodal stimulation on gain-down adaptation. **(A)** Plot of gain during gain-down adaptation: Changes in VOR gain during VOR-decrease training in L7-PP2B mice. The VOR was tested pre- and post-training by measuring the eye movement response to the vestibular stimulus. **(B)** Plot of normalized gain throughout the course of the behavioral paradigm: Changes in VOR gain during VOR-decrease training. Black, Green and Red lines are for sham, cathodal and anodal stimulation conditions, respectively. The gray bar indicates the stimulation period. Error bars represent SEM, because of large SEM we do not find any significant difference between the groups.

leaning in all these tasks. Surprisingly, the post-stimulation deadaptation curve (Jayaram et al., 2012; Herzfeld et al., 2014) or extinction rate (Zuchowski et al., 2014) shows no difference across various stimulation groups. The later finding is notable because irrespective of altered rate and total amount of learning, polarity has no effect on post-stimulation de-adaptation/ learning processes. In our study, we find that DCS has no post-stimulation effect on the learning phase. Therefore, our study clearly depicts both anodal and cathodal stimulation have short-lasting effects on the habituation phase of the gain-down VOR adaptation task. The de-adaptation experiment (like other studies) is redundant, as we have done all the adaptation training sessions in the post-stimulation period. To discover the actual cause, similar experiments should be performed with a gain increase VOR adaptation paradigm (Gao et al., 2012).

L7-PP2B mice often showed more than one gain during baseline measurements (**Figure 6A**). Possibly, the eye overshoots the head-position as we have used higher sinusoidal velocity (amplitude of 5° at 1 Hz frequency). We think that sensory signals coming from the parallel fibers fail to excite PC sharply, as there is no LTP in L7-PP2B mice. Therefore, when the high velocity head-movement stops, PCs could not generate sharp inhibition on the VN to stop the eye-movement. A sub-optimal PC inhibition may have caused facilitation of the eye movement in the absence of the head-movement.

We propose three, non-exclusive, possibilities that may explain reduced sensitivity to anodal stimulation in the L7-PP2B mutants: (i) PCs in the mutants may receive more background inhibition; (ii) plasticity at the PC-VN synapses may be essential for VOR gain-down adaptation (De Zeeuw and Ten Brinke, 2015; See CSHP book by Kandel); and/or (iii) plasticity of synapses on PCs in mutants may be saturated, preventing adaptation. The first point reflects the possibility that anodal stimulation may cause inhibition rather than excitation of PCs when there is no LTP or intrinsic plasticity at PCs. Anodal stimulation driven subthreshold depolarization may augment GABA release from molecular layer interneurons (MLI) (Christie et al., 2011; Stagg and Nitsche, 2011) and thereby increase inhibition onto PCs. The second possibility is that anodal DCS has a direct impact on PC-VN plasticity and thereby directly regulates the adaptation process. Loss of PC LTP may retard the effects of anodal stimulation on these synapses. The third reason could be that loss of LTP makes the circuit unresponsive to the pairing of the sensory stimulus with the motor response, as intrinsic plasticity of PCs is also erratic in these mutants (Schonewille et al., 2010). The PP2B transgene may disrupt normal signaling through the PCs or the homeostasis of the network (Lamont and Weber, 2012). This can corrupt the instructive signals sent by PCs to downstream sites like the VN.

Cathodal stimulation induced inhibition of adaptation in L7-PP2B mutants is significantly stronger compared to C57BL/6 mice but similar to the sham group of L7-PP2B mice (**Figures 5, 6B**). It is evident that this cathodal suppression is a by-product of the mutation of potentiation at the PCs, as these mice fail to learn cerebellar tasks (Schonewille et al., 2010). In addition, we need to examine to what extent long-term depression (LTD) at PF-PC pathway plays a role following cathodal stimulation.

In conclusion, we have successfully developed a mouse model of cerebellar DCS, allowing us to present the first demonstration of cerebellar DCS driven behavioral changes in rodents. We used this model in combination with the popular paradigm of VOR adaptation to test the effect of current stimulation on motor adaptation. The results presented here provide evidence that anodal DCS reduces VOR gain acutely, an effect that is disrupted by ablation of PP2B in PCs. This study, also finds support for recent claims that anodal and cathodal stimulation modulate cerebellar dependent adaptation acutely through distinct pathways. Future research must address the neuronal activity following cerebellar stimulation to understand the spatiotemporal aspects of DCS effects.

AUTHOR CONTRIBUTIONS

SD, MSp, MF, and OD conceived and designed the experiments. SD performed the experiments. SD and PH analyzed the data. TS helped in building the experimental set-up. SD, OD, MF, MSc, and CD interpreted the data. SD drafted the manuscript. OD, MSc, MF, TS, and PH performed a critical review of the manuscript. CD and MSc were responsible for mutant verification. All the authors read and approved the final version of the manuscript.

REFERENCES

Ambrus, G. G., Antal, A., and Paulus, W. (2011). Comparing cutaneous perception induced by electrical stimulation using rectangular and round shaped electrodes. *Clin. Neurophysiol.* 122, 803–807. doi: 10.1016/j.clinph.2010.08.023

Avila, E., van der Geest, J. N., Kengne Kamga, S., Verhage, M. C., Donchin, O., and Frens, M. A. (2015). Cerebellar transcranial direct current stimulation effects on saccade adaptation. *Neural Plast.* 2015:968970. doi: 10.1155/2015/968970

Bastian, A. J. (2011). Moving, sensing and learning with cerebellar damage. *Curr. Opin. Neurobiol.* 21, 596–601. doi: 10.1016/j.conb.2011.06.007

Benussi, A., Koch, G., Cotelli, M., Padovani, A., and Borroni, B. (2015). Cerebellar transcranial direct current stimulation in patients with ataxia: a double-blind, randomized, sham-controlled study. *Mov. Disord.* 30, 1701–1705. doi: 10.1002/mds.26356

Bindman, L. J., Lippold, O. C. J., and Redfearn, J. W. T. (1964). The action of brief polarizing currents on the cerebral cortex of the rat (1) during current flow and (2) in the production of long-lasting after-effects. *J. Physiol.* 172, 369–382. doi: 10.1113/jphysiol.1964.sp007425

Chan, C. Y., Hounsgaard, J., and Nicholson, C. (1988). Effects of electric fields on transmembrane potential and excitability of turtle cerebellar Purkinje cells *in vitro*. *J. Physiol.* 402, 751–771. doi: 10.1113/jphysiol.1988.sp017232

Chan, C. Y., and Nicholson, C. (1986). Modulation by applied electric fields of Purkinje and stellate cell activity in the isolated turtle cerebellum. *J. Physiol.* 371, 89–114. doi: 10.1113/jphysiol.1986.sp015963

Christie, J. M., Chiu, D. N., and Jahr, C. E. (2011). Ca^{2+}-dependent enhancement of release by subthreshold somatic depolarization. *Nat. Neurosci.* 14, 62–68. doi: 10.1038/nn.2718

Clément, G., Flandrin, J.-M., and Courjon, J.-H. (2002). Comparison between habituation of the cat vestibulo-ocular reflex by velocity steps and sinusoidal vestibular stimulation in the dark. *Exp. Brain Res.* 142, 259–267. doi: 10.1007/s00221-001-0930-7

Creutzfeldt, O. D., Fromm, G. H., and Kapp, H. (1962). Influence of transcortical d-c currents on cortical neuronal activity. *Exp. Neurol.* 5, 436–452. doi: 10.1016/0014-4886(62)90056-0

Das, S., Holland, P., Frens, M. A., and Donchin, O. (2016). Impact of transcranial direct current stimulation (tDCS) on neuronal functions. *Front. Neurosci.* 10:550. doi: 10.3389/fnins.2016.00550

De Zeeuw, C. I., Hoebeek, F. E., Bosman, L. W. J., Schonewille, M., Witter, L., and Koekkoek, S. K. (2011). Spatiotemporal firing patterns in the cerebellum. *Nat. Rev. Neurosci.* 12, 327–344. doi: 10.1038/nrn3011

De Zeeuw, C. I., and Ten Brinke, M. M. (2015). Motor learning and the cerebellum. *Cold Spring Harb. Perspect. Biol.* 7:a021683. doi: 10.1101/cshperspect.a021683

Dow, E. R., and Anastasio, T. J. (1998). Analysis and neural network modeling of the nonlinear correlates of habituation in the vestibulo-ocular reflex. *J. Comput. Neurosci.* 5, 171–190. doi: 10.1023/A:1008818016900

Fritsch, B., Reis, J., Martinowich, K., Schambra, H. M., Ji, Y., Cohen, L. G., et al. (2010). Direct current stimulation promotes BDNF-dependent synaptic plasticity: potential implications for motor learning. *Neuron* 66, 198–204. doi: 10.1016/j.neuron.2010.03.035

Galea, J. M., Jayaram, G., Ajagbe, L., and Celnik, P. (2009). Modulation of cerebellar excitability by polarity-specific noninvasive direct current stimulation. *J. Neurosci.* 29, 9115–9122. doi: 10.1523/JNEUROSCI.2184-09.2009

Gao, Z., van Beugen, B. J., and De Zeeuw, C. I. (2012). Distributed synergistic plasticity and cerebellar learning. *Nat. Rev. Neurosci.* 13, 619–635. doi: 10.1038/nrn3312

Hansel, C. (2005). When the B-team runs plasticity: GluR2 receptor trafficking in cerebellar long-term potentiation. *Proc. Natl. Acad. Sci. U.S.A.* 102, 18245–18246. doi: 10.1073/pnas.0509686102

Hardwick, R. M., and Celnik, P. A. (2014). Cerebellar direct current stimulation enhances motor learning in older adults. *Neurobiol. Aging* 35, 2217–2221. doi: 10.1016/j.neurobiolaging.2014.03.030

Herzfeld, D. J., Pastor, D., Haith, A. M., Rossetti, Y., Shadmehr, R., and O'Shea, J. (2014). Contributions of the cerebellum and the motor cortex to acquisition and retention of motor memories. *Neuroimage* 98, 147–158. doi: 10.1016/j.neuroimage.2014.04.076

Ito, M. (1982). Cerebellar control of the vestibulo-ocular reflex–around the flocculus hypothesis. *Annu. Rev. Neurosci.* 5, 275–296. doi: 10.1146/annurev.ne.05.030182.001423

Ivry, R. B., and Spencer, R. M. C. (2004). The neural representation of time. *Curr. Opin. Neurobiol.* 14, 225–232. doi: 10.1016/j.conb.2004.03.013

Jayaram, G., Tang, B., Pallegadda, R., Vasudevan, E. V. L., Celnik, P., and Bastian, A. (2012). Modulating locomotor adaptation with cerebellar stimulation. *J. Neurophysiol.* 107, 2950–2957. doi: 10.1152/jn.00645.2011

Kawato, M., and Gomi, H. (1992). The cerebellum and VOR/OKR learning models. *Trends Neurosci.* 15, 445–453. doi: 10.1016/0166-2236(92)90008-V

Lamont, M. G., and Weber, J. T. (2012). The role of calcium in synaptic plasticity and motor learning in the cerebellar cortex. *Neurosci. Biobehav. Rev.* 36, 1153–1162. doi: 10.1016/j.neubiorev.2012.01.005

Liebetanz, D., Fregni, F., Monte-Silva, K. K., Oliveira, M. B., Amâncio-dos-Santos, A., Nitsche, M. A., et al. (2006a). After-effects of transcranial direct current stimulation (tDCS) on cortical spreading depression. *Neurosci. Lett.* 398, 85–90. doi: 10.1016/j.neulet.2005.12.058

Liebetanz, D., Klinker, F., Hering, D., Koch, R., Nitsche, M. A., Potschka, H., et al. (2006b). Anticonvulsant effects of transcranial direct-current stimulation (tDCS) in the rat cortical ramp model of focal epilepsy. *Epilepsia* 47, 1216–1224. doi: 10.1111/j.1528-1167.2006.00539.x

Liebetanz, D., Koch, R., Mayenfels, S., König, F., Paulus, W., and Nitsche, M. A. (2009). Safety limits of cathodal transcranial direct current stimulation in rats. *Clin. Neurophysiol.* 120, 1161–1167. doi: 10.1016/j.clinph.2009.01.022

Lisberger, S. G., and Fuchs, A. F. (1974). Response of flocculus Purkinje cells to adequate vestibular stimulation in the alert monkey: fixation vs. compensatory eye movements. *Brain Res.* 69, 347–353. doi: 10.1016/0006-8993(74)90013-4

Márquez-Ruiz, J., Leal-Campanario, R., Sánchez-Campusano, R., Molaee-Ardekani, B., Wendling, F., Miranda, P. C., et al. (2012). Transcranial direct-current stimulation modulates synaptic mechanisms involved in associative learning in behaving rabbits. *Proc. Natl. Acad. Sci. U.S.A.* 109, 6710–6715. doi: 10.1073/pnas.1121147109

Nguyen-Vu, T. D. B., Kimpo, R. R., Rinaldi, J. M., Kohli, A., Zeng, H., Deisseroth, K., et al. (2013). Cerebellar Purkinje cell activity drives motor learning. *Nat. Neurosci.* 16, 1734–1736. doi: 10.1038/nn.3576

Probst, T., Brandt, T., and Degner, D. (1986). Object-motion detection affected by concurrent self-motion perception: psychophysics of a new phenomenon. *Behav. Brain Res.* 22, 1–11. doi: 10.1016/0166-4328(86)90076-8

Purpura, D. P., and Mcmurtry, J. G. (1965). Intracellular activities and evoked potential changes during polarization of motor cortex. *J. Neurophysiol.* 28, 166–185.

Schonewille, M., Belmeguenai, A., Koekkoek, S. K., Houtman, S. H., Boele, H. J., van Beugen, B. J., et al. (2010). Purkinje cell-specific knockout of the protein phosphatase PP2B impairs potentiation and cerebellar motor learning. *Neuron* 67, 618–628. doi: 10.1016/j.neuron.2010.07.009

Stagg, C. J., and Nitsche, M. A. (2011). Physiological basis of transcranial direct current stimulation. *Neuroscientist* 17, 37–53. doi: 10.1177/1073858410386614

Stahl, J. S., van Alphen, A. M., and De Zeeuw, C. I. (2000). A comparison of video and magnetic search coil recordings of mouse eye movements. *J. Neurosci. Methods* 99, 101–110. doi: 10.1016/S0165-0270(00)00218-1

Takano, Y., Yokawa, T., Masuda, A., Niimi, J., Tanaka, S., and Hironaka, N. (2011). A rat model for measuring the effectiveness of transcranial direct current stimulation using fMRI. *Neurosci. Lett.* 491, 40–43. doi: 10.1016/j.neulet.2011.01.004

Tempia, F., Dieringer, N., and Strata, P. (1991). Adaptation and habituation of the vestibulo-ocular reflex in intact and inferior olive-lesioned rats. *Exp. Brain Res.* 86, 568–578. doi: 10.1007/BF00230530

Tiliket, C., Shelhamer, M., Tan, H. S., and Zee, D. S. (1993). Adaptation of the vestibulo-ocular reflex with the head in different orientations and positions relative to the axis of body rotation. *J. Vestib. Res.* 3, 181–195.

van Alphen, B., Winkelman, B. H. J., and Frens, M. A. (2010). Three-dimensional optokinetic eye movements in the C57BL/6J mouse. *Invest. Ophthalmol. Vis. Sci.* 51, 623–630. doi: 10.1167/iovs.09-4072

Xu-Wilson, M., Chen-Harris, H., Zee, D. S., and Shadmehr, R. (2009). Cerebellar contributions to adaptive control of saccades in humans. *J. Neurosci.* 29, 12930–12939. doi: 10.1523/JNEUROSCI.3115-09.2009

Zuchowski, M. L., Timmann, D., and Gerwig, M. (2014). Acquisition of conditioned eyeblink responses is modulated by cerebellar tDCS. *Brain Stimul.* 7, 525–531. doi: 10.1016/j.brs.2014.03.010

2

Prenatal Exposure to Arsenic Impairs Behavioral Flexibility and Cortical Structure in Mice

Kyaw H. Aung[1,2], *Chaw Kyi-Tha-Thu*[1], *Kazuhiro Sano*[3], *Kazuaki Nakamura*[2], *Akito Tanoue*[2], *Keiko Nohara*[3], *Masaki Kakeyama*[4], *Chiharu Tohyama*[5], *Shinji Tsukahara*[1] *and Fumihiko Maekawa*[3]*

[1] Division of Life Science, Saitama University, Saitama, Japan, [2] Department of Pharmacology, National Research Institute for Child Health and Development, Setagaya, Japan, [3] Molecular Toxicology Section, National Institute for Environmental Studies, Tsukuba, Japan, [4] Faculty of Human Sciences, Waseda University, Tokorozawa, Japan, [5] Faculty of Medicine, University of Tsukuba, Tsukuba, Japan

Edited by:
Riccarda Granata,
University of Turin, Italy

Reviewed by:
Maria E. Gonsebatt,
Universidad Nacional Autónoma de México, Mexico
Andrea Allan,
University of New Mexico, USA

***Correspondence:**
Fumihiko Maekawa
fmaekawa@nies.go.jp

Exposure to arsenic from well water in developing countries is suspected to cause developmental neurotoxicity. Although, it has been demonstrated that exposure to sodium arsenite ($NaAsO_2$) suppresses neurite outgrowth of cortical neurons *in vitro*, it is largely unknown how developmental exposure to $NaAsO_2$ impairs higher brain function and affects cortical histology. Here, we investigated the effect of prenatal $NaAsO_2$ exposure on the behavior of mice in adulthood, and evaluated histological changes in the prelimbic cortex (PrL), which is a part of the medial prefrontal cortex that is critically involved in cognition. Drinking water with or without $NaAsO_2$ (85 ppm) was provided to pregnant C3H mice from gestational days 8 to 18, and offspring of both sexes were subjected to cognitive behavioral analyses at 60 weeks of age. The brains of female offspring were subsequently harvested and used for morphometrical analyses. We found that both male and female mice prenatally exposed to $NaAsO_2$ displayed an impaired adaptation to repetitive reversal tasks. In morphometrical analyses of Nissl- or Golgi-stained tissue sections, we found that $NaAsO_2$ exposure was associated with a significant increase in the number of pyramidal neurons in layers V and VI of the PrL, but not other layers of the PrL. More strikingly, prenatal $NaAsO_2$ exposure was associated with a significant decrease in neurite length but not dendrite spine density in all layers of the PrL. Taken together, our results indicate that prenatal exposure to $NaAsO_2$ leads to behavioral inflexibility in adulthood and cortical disarrangement in the PrL might contribute to this behavioral impairment.

Keywords: sodium arsenite, developmental neurotoxicity, behavioral impairment, neurite outgrowth, prelimbic cortex

INTRODUCTION

The developing brain is vulnerable to disruption by environmental factors including toxic chemical exposure. Environmental exposures may therefore account for an increase in the prevalence of neurodevelopmental and neuropsychiatric disorders including autism spectrum disorders, attention deficit hyperactivity disorders (ADHD), and learning disabilities (Grandjean and Landrigan, 2006, 2014). Recent studies suggest that *in utero* and lactational exposure to toxic chemicals affects the development of the brain. For example, exposure to inorganic lead, methylmercury, and polychlorinated biphenyls during gestation and early childhood are associated with the prevalence of mental retardation, cerebral palsy, and ADHD in children (Grandjean and Landrigan, 2006; Bisen-Hersh et al., 2014). These studies indicate that early life environmental exposures play a role in the etiology of neurodevelopmental disorders.

It has been long suspected that arsenic exposure can lead to developmental neurotoxicity. More than 200 million people worldwide have been estimated to be chronically exposed to arsenic in drinking water at concentrations above the World Health Organization (WHO) recommended safety limit of 10 μg/L (WHO, 2008). A large number of epidemiological studies have demonstrated that chronic exposure to arsenic produces peripheral neuropathies and decreases cognitive performance in children such as lowered memory and intelligence quotient scores on standardized tests (Rocha-Amador et al., 2007; Rosado et al., 2007; Wasserman et al., 2007), which are indicative of higher brain function deficits. Additionally, follow-up studies on victims of arsenic poisoning from the Morinaga formula incident in Japan revealed an association between oral exposure to arsenic during infancy and various brain disorders, including mental retardation and epilepsy (Dakeishi et al., 2006). These studies suggest that early life arsenic exposure can affect higher brain function later in life. This notion is supported by some studies in animal models. For example, exposure to low level arsenic in maternal drinking water throughout gestational and lactational period increased indices of anxiety in mouse offspring during a novel object exploration task (Martinez-Finley et al., 2009). Moreover, few behavioral deficits such as an increase in pivoting, a type of abnormal gait behavior, was observed in younger mouse offspring following a short period of gestational exposure to arsenic (Colomina et al., 1996).

Arsenic exposure could produce behavioral changes through effects on the developing brain directly since arsenic freely crosses the fetus-placenta and blood-brain barrier in human (Willhite and Ferm, 1984; Hirner and Rettenmeier, 2010). *In vitro* and *in vivo* experimental models have been used to elucidate how arsenic exposure impairs higher brain function. A previous study showed that sodium arsenite ($NaAsO_2$) exposure produces both apoptotic and necrotic cell death in developing brain cells in rat (Chattopadhyay et al., 2002). Our *in vitro* studies have shown that $NaAsO_2$ exposure induces apoptotic cell death and inhibits neuritogenesis (Koike-Kuroda et al., 2010; Aung et al., 2013). The inhibitory effect of $NaAsO_2$ on neuritogenesis is in part result from alterations in cytoskeletal components (Aung et al., 2013) and the downregulation of AMPA receptors, which are known to regulate the expression of cytoskeletal proteins (Maekawa et al., 2013). In animal studies, embryonic arsenic exposure produces neural tube defects, increase neuronal apoptosis, disrupt neural outgrowth, and reduce overall head size in both mouse and zebrafish models (Chaineau et al., 1990; Li et al., 2009). Further, it has been reported that arsenic exposure in rats from gestation throughout lactation and development until the age of 4 month alters morphology of nerve fibers and axon in the corpus striatum (Rios et al., 2009). These studies indicate that structural changes of brain such as neural network formation might contribute to the impairment of higher brain function following early life exposure to $NaAsO_2$. However, the precise mechanism by which developmental arsenic exposure produces impairments in higher brain function remains largely unknown.

Executive function such as planning, goal-directed action, and behavioral flexibility are core units of higher brain function, and impairment of these functions has been observed in a variety of neurodevelopmental disorders (Valencia et al., 1992; Kipp, 2005; Hill and Bird, 2006). To evaluate these executive processes in mice, a model of behavioral flexibility was recently established using the IntelliCage system, which is a fully automated behavioral testing apparatus for mice under group-housing conditions (Endo et al., 2011, 2012). This testing apparatus allows for the comprehensive and reproducible evaluation of behavioral flexibility. In humans, the brain areas responsible for executive function of goal-directed actions and behavioral flexibility are located in the medial prefrontal cortex (Yan et al., 2015). Several studies have shown that the prelimbic cortex (PrL), a part of the medial prefrontal cortex, is critically involved in a variety of cognitive and executive processes (Dalley et al., 2004; Marquis et al., 2007; Ragozzino, 2007). It has been also reported that the PrL is affected by exposure to chemicals, such as methylmercury, lead, and dioxin, and that exposure-associated impairments in the PrL are associated with decreased executive function in rodents (Ferraro et al., 2009; Tomasini et al., 2012). Accordingly, we decided to investigate the structure of the PrL as a possible target of arsenic-induced brain impairment.

In the present study, we used a fully automated behavioral analysis system to investigate the effects of prenatal $NaAsO_2$ exposure on murine behavioral flexibility in adulthood, and then analyzed the morphology of neuronal cells in these animals in order to determine how early life $NaAsO_2$ exposure produces neurotoxicity.

MATERIALS AND METHODS

Animals and $NaAsO_2$ Exposure

Pregnant C3H mice were purchased from JAPAN SLC (Shizuoka, Japan) and housed on a 12-h light/dark cycle at a temperature of 24 ± 1°C with free access to water and food. From gestational days 8–18, pregnant females were given *ad libitum* access to regular water or water containing 85 parts per million (ppm) $NaAsO_2$ (equivalent to 85 mg/L). To examine the water consumption of pregnant dams, the weight of water bottle for each dam was measured before and after providing *ad libitum* access to water. Pregnant dams tolerated the dose of $NaAsO_2$ at 85 ppm, and no obvious effects on maternal toxicity or teratogenicity were observed.

The pups were weaned at post-natal day 21 and housed under the same conditions as the dams. The number and sex of pups born from dams were then measured. At 60 weeks of age, control and $NaAsO_2$-exposed offspring were prepared for behavioral flexibility testing using the IntelliCage system (TSE Systems GmbH, Bad Homburg, Germany). Mice were randomly selected per dams (number of dams: control = 6 and $NaAsO_2$ = 9) to minimize the litter effects. After selecting mice, they were lightly anesthetized with diethyl ether and subcutaneously implanted with a glass-covered transponder. Each transponder had a unique ID code for radiation frequency identification (RFID) for use with the IntelliCage system. Males and females were separately tested using different IntelliCage apparatuses. The control and $NaAsO_2$-exposed groups includes 9 mice per group for females and 6 or 10 mice per group for males. All procedures were approved by the Institutional Animal Care and Use Committee of the National Institute for Environmental Studies (NIES) and conducted strictly in accordance with NIES guidelines.

Intellicage Apparatus

The IntelliCage is a computer-based, fully-automated testing apparatus that can be used to monitor the spontaneous and cognitive behaviors of group-housed RFID-tagged mice in a large home cage (**Figure 1A**). Briefly, a large standard plastic cage ($55 \times 37.5 \times 20.5\ cm^3$) was equipped with four triangular operant learning chambers (hereafter referred to as corners) ($15 \times 15 \times 21\ cm^3$) that fit into each corner of the cage. RFID readers and other sensors allowed the simultaneous monitoring of up to 16 transponder-tagged mice living in the same cage. Mice were allowed to enter each corner (hereafter referred to as a "corner visit") through a short, narrow tunnel that functioned as an RFID antenna. Only one mouse was able to enter a given corner at any one time due to the limited size of the tunnel. In the inner space of each corner was equipped with two nose poke holes that were monitored via an infrared beam-break response detector. Nose poke behavior triggered to open a motorized gate access to a water bottle nipple. For each behavioral event (corner visit, nose poke, and licking), mouse ID and corner ID were automatically recorded through the RFID readers, infrared sensors, and lickometers.

Intellicage Test Procedures

Acclimation

The control and $NaAsO_2$-exposed male or female mice at 67 weeks of age were separately introduced to IntelliCage apparatuses on the same day. The number of mice in each IntelliCage apparatus was counterbalanced within groups. Acclimation and behavioral tests were then conducted according to test procedures. In acclimation phase 1 (3 days), the motorized gates controlling access to water bottle nipples were kept open in all 4 corners; thus, mice were allowed to drink water in each corner *ad libitum*. In acclimation phase 2 (1 day), the mice were trained to perform the nose poke task. Initially, all motorized gates were closed and mice were only given access to water bottle nipples after a nose poke event. The gate remained open for 4 sec following each nose poke, and water was available through the nose poke task for 24 h. In acclimation phase 3 (5 days), mice were only given the opportunity to gain access to water through the nose poke task for a 3-h period (19:00–22:00) per day. During acclimation phase, four female mice (one from control group and three from $NaAsO_2$-exposed group) were not able to learn how to access water drinkable corners, and such mice were not used in the following behavioral tasks.

Behavioral Sequencing Task

The behavioral flexibility test, also referred to as the behavioral sequencing task, was composed of an acquisition phase and a serial reversal task phase. The acquisition phase consisted of 11 or 21 sessions of the behavioral sequencing task (**Figure 1B**) and the serial reversal task phase consisted of repetitions of a reversal task (Rev. 1−11, **Figure 1C**). Water-deprived mice had 4 sec of access to water as a reward when they visited designated corners during a daily 3-h test session (19:00−22:00; **Figure 1D**). A total of 67 sessions for male mice and 83 sessions for female mice were conducted. In each session, mice were rewarded continuously if they alternated visits between two particular diagonally opposed corners (**Figure 1C**). The diagonal pair of corners was either active or inactive in a mutually exclusive manner, meaning that there was always one active reward corner, one inactive reward corner, and two never-rewarded corners. Mice were able to open the gate in an active corner by nose poke, and the gate remained open for 4 s to permit drinking. After the reward period, the corner instantly became inactive, and this signal was synchronized with the activation of the diagonally opposed corner. The alteration of corner assignments was controlled for each mouse independently by the IntelliCage software. Thus, the mice had to alternate between two diagonally opposed reward corners in order to acquire rewards continuously. A visit to either of the two never-rewarded corners was regarded as a discrimination error. The number of discrimination errors within the first 100 visits in each session provided a discrimination error rate that was used to analyze inter-session learning performance.

Histological Staining

After the last session of behavioral experiments, the same female mice were immediately sacrificed for morphometrical analysis of neuronal cells, while male mice were used for gene expression analyses (not described in this study). Mice were deeply anesthetized with sodium pentobarbital (60 mg/kg) and brains were harvested for analysis. Brains were histologically processed using the FD Rapid GolgiStain Kit (FD NeuroTechnologies, Ellicot City, MD, USA). Briefly, brains were rinsed with distilled water, immersed in 5 mL of equal parts Solution A and Solution B at room temperature, and stored for 2 weeks in the dark. Storage solution was replaced with fresh solution on the second day. Tissues were next immersed in Solution C at 4°C for at least 48 h. Solution C was replaced with fresh solution on the second day. Samples were then quickly frozen at −70°C and stored at −20°C until use. Coronal brain sections (60 μm) were cut using a cryostat (Leica CM1900; Leica Microsystems, Wetzlar, Germany), where the temperature of chamber and specimen head were set to −22°C and −23°C, respectively. Brain sections were mounted on gelatin-coated glass slides and allowed to dry at room temperature. Sections were then stained with a solution of 1 part Solution D, 1 part Solution E, and 2 parts distilled water for 10 min at room temperature. Golgi-stained brain sections were rinsed in distilled water twice for 4 min each and counterstained with 0.1% Cresyl Fast Violet solution. The Golgi- and Cresyl Fast Violet-stained sections were used for stereological analysis. The group average number of neurons and glial cells, length of

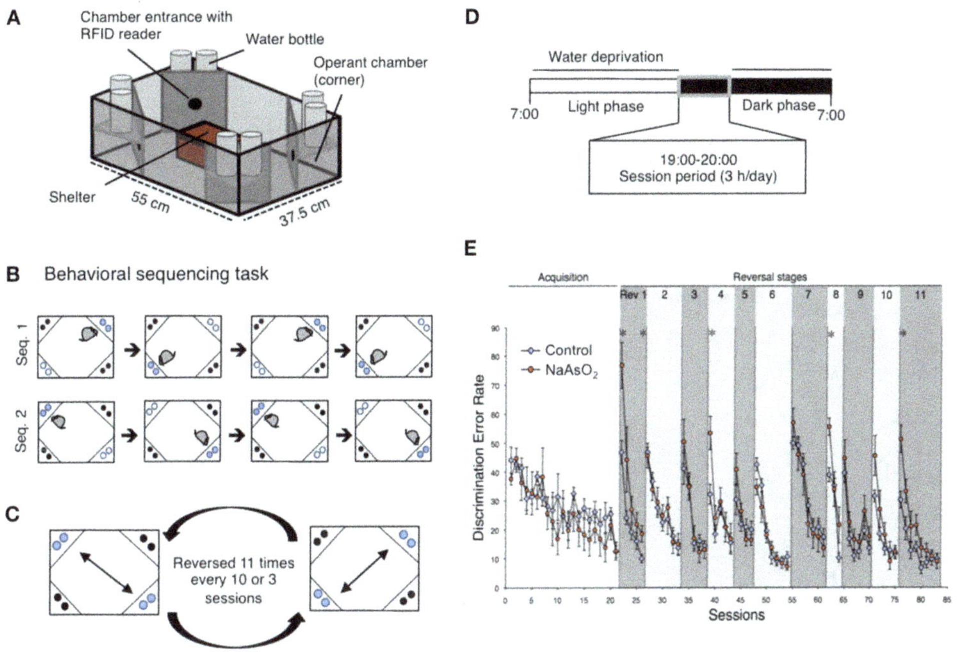

FIGURE 1 | Impaired behavioral flexibility in adult mice born to dams that were administered $NaAsO_2$ during gestation. (A) Overview of an IntelliCage apparatus. **(B)** Behavioral sequencing task. Mice were allowed to make an access to water as a reward for 4 s during their visits at an active reward corner (blue circle). The location of the active reward corner was automatically alternated to a diagonally opposed corner each time the mouse received a reward. Therefore, mice obtained rewards continuously by acquiring a behavioral sequence (alternating between the two reward corners). A visit to a never-rewarded corner (black circle) was counted as a discrimination error. **(C)** Serial reversal task. For each mouse, the assigned spatial patterns of the rewarded corners (sequence 1 or sequence 2) were reversed 11 times every 3 or 8 sessions. **(D)** Timeline of the experiment for each day. **(E)** Learning performance of control or $NaAsO_2$-exposed female mice in the behavioral flexibility test. Discrimination error rates (the number of discrimination errors in the first 100 corner visits of a session) are expressed as mean ± SEM (control group $n = 8$, $NaAsO_2$-exposed group $n = 6$). An asterisk indicates a statistical difference ($p < 0.05$) from the control group.

neurites, and density of dendritic spines were calculated from five or seven brains of mice, which was randomly selected and blind from behavioral data, for control and $NaAsO_2$-exposed group, respectively.

Stereological Analysis of the Length of Neurites and the Number of Neuronal Cells

The length of neurites and the number of neurons and glial cells in the PrL were measured using StereoInvestigator software (MicroBrightField (MBF) Bioscience, Williston, VT., USA) and a light microscope (DM5000B; Leica Microsystems) connected to a CCD camera. The boundaries between the PrL and the infralimbic cortex (IL) and between the PrL and the dorsal anterior cingulate (ACd) were determined by observing differences in cell size and density in the cortical layers of Cresyl Fast Violet-stained brain sections (Van De Werd et al., 2010). The rostrocaudal level of the PrL was determined by referring to an atlas of the mouse brain (Franklin and Paxinos, 2008; **Figure 2A**).

The length of neurites on Golgi-stained neurons in the left PrL was measured using the Space Ball probe utility of the Stereo Investigator software. The contours of the PrL in each brain section were drawn using a 5X objective lens magnification according to the criteria mentioned above. We set grid sizes of 150 × 200 μm, and used a sphere with a 40-μm radius and a highest top guard zone of 2.5 μm for the quantification of neurite length. The intersectional points between Golgi-stained neurites and the spherical line (**Figure 3B**) were counted in three consecutive sections of the PrL using a 100X oil immersion objective lens magnification, and the number of intersection points was used to compute the estimated length of Golgi-stained neurite in the selected region of the PrL for each mice (Mouton et al., 2002). The estimated length of Golgi-stained neurite was then normalized by dividing it by the estimated volume of the selected region in each animal. The coefficient of error (Gundersen, $m = 1$) for the estimation of neurite length was 0.05–0.09 for each animal.

The optical fractionator method was used to measure the number of Cresyl Fast Violet-stained neurons (pyramidal and non-pyramidal neurons) and glial cells in three different cortical layers (layer II–III, V, and VI) of the left PrL in accordance with the system work flow of the Stereo Investigator software. Since cortical layer IV is completely disappeared in the mice PrL (Van De Werd et al., 2010), it was not included in this analysis. The cortical layer boundaries were distinguished based on differences in cell size and density in Cresyl Fast Violet-stained brain sections (**Figure 2B**). The contours for layers II–III, V, and VI were drawn in each section using a 5X objective lens magnification and a frame size of 30 × 30 μm within the grid size of 150 × 150 μm. The height of the optical dissector was 40 μm and the top guard zone was 2.5 μm. Cell numbers were counted manually

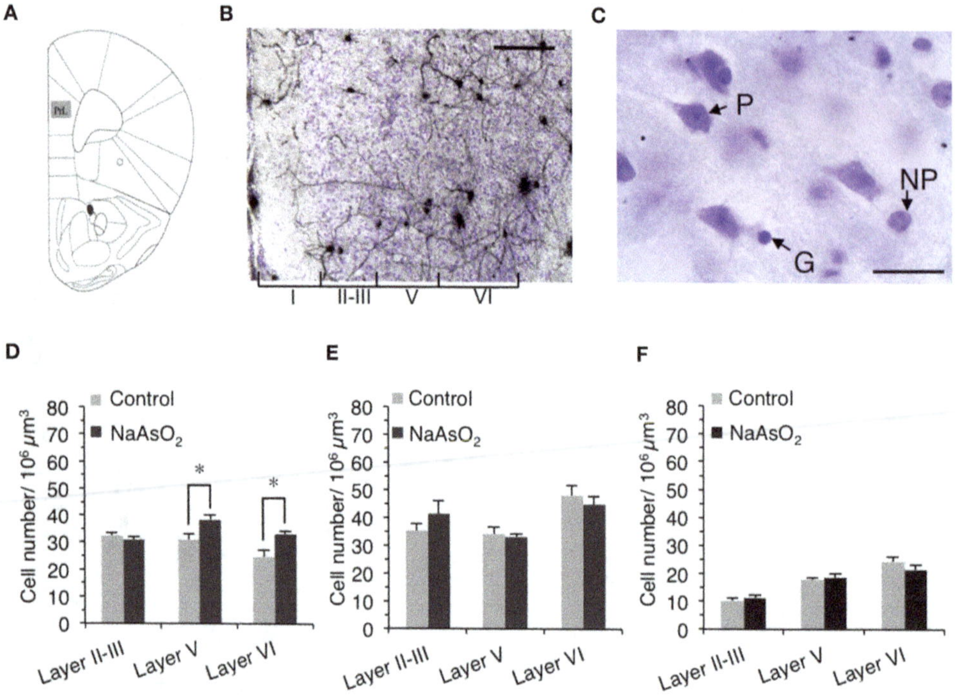

FIGURE 2 | Alteration in the number of neuronal cells in the PrL of adult female mice born to dams that were administered $NaAsO_2$. (A) Illustration of the region of interest, the PrL, adapted from a mouse brain atlas (Franklin and Paxinos, 2008). **(B)** Representative photomicrograph of the PrL in Golgi- and Cresyl Fast Violet-stained coronal brain sections. The Greek numbered (I–VI) regions indicate the cortical layers of the PrL. Scale bar = 20 μm. **(C)** Photomicrographs of the PrL at high magnification showing a Cresyl Fast Violet-stained pyramidal neuron (P), a non-pyramidal neuron (NP), and a glial cell (G). The length of scale bar indicates 5 μm. The number of pyramidal neurons **(D)**, non-pyramidal neurons **(E)**, and glial cells **(F)** in the PrL. Values are expressed as mean ± SEM (control group $n = 7$, $NaAsO_2$-exposedgroups $n = 5$). An asterisk indicates $p < 0.05$ vs. the control group.

using a 100X oil immersion objective lens magnification. The setting for cell counting was sufficient to generate a coefficient of error (Gundersen, $m = 1$) of 0.05–0.06. The estimated number of pyramidal neurons, non-pyramidal neurons, and glial cells in each layer of the PrL was normalized by dividing each number by the estimated volume of its respective layer. The morphological criteria used to identify neuronal and glial cells observed in Cresyl Fast Violet-stained brain sections have been previously reported (Tsukahara et al., 2011). To distinguish pyramidal neurons from non-pyramidal neurons, the following criteria were used: (1) the cell bodies of pyramidal neurons exhibited a characteristic triangular shape with a single large apical dendrite extending vertically toward the pial surface, (2) non-pyramidal neurons were identified by the absence of the preceding criteria and exhibited a relatively smaller cell body size than that of pyramidal neurons (**Figure 2C**).

Imaging and Analysis of Dendritic Spine Morphology

The dendritic segments of Golgi-stained pyramidal neurons were used in morphometrical analyses. Sequential z-series images of dendritic segments were taken every 0.4 μm with an oil immersion lens (Plan Apo VC 100X, Numerical Aperture 1.40, Oil; Nikon, Tokyo, Japan) and a BioRevo 9000 microscope (Keyence Co., Osaka, Japan). The applied zoom factor (1.5X) provided images with 0.14 μm/pixel resolution. Images were then deconvoluted using Keyence BZ II Analyzer software (Keyence) and constructed into three-dimensional images using ImageJ software (National Institutes of Health, Bethesda, MD, USA) for analyses of dendritic spine morphology. The density and head diameter of dendritic spines were analyzed using Spiso-3D automated dendritic spine analysis software, which has an equivalent capacity to Neurolucida (MBF Bioscience, USA) (Mukai et al., 2011). The primary basilar dendritic segments of Golgi-stained pyramidal neurons, lying between 10 and 100 μm from the soma, were used to analyze the morphology of dendritic spines. For each cortical layer (layer II–III, V, or VI), 30–45 dendritic segments were analyzed per experimental group. Spine density was calculated from the number of spines existing on the total length of 40–100 μm dendritic segments. To examine spine morphological changes in response to prenatal $NaAsO_2$ exposure, the diameter of the spine head was classified into three categories: (1) small-head spines with a diameter of 0.2–0.4 μm, (2) middle-head spines with a diameter of 0.4–0.5 μm, and (3) large-head spines with a diameter of 0.5–1 μm.

Statistical Analysis

Changes in mouse behavioral flexibility were analyzed using the non-parametric Mann Whitney U-test with R software (The R Foundation for Statistical Computing, Vienna, Austria) because the sample size of each group for each session was relatively small and it didn't follow a normal distribution. Morphometrical and other general assessments (including body weight, number of pups, and water intake) were analyzed with the parametric Student's unpaired *t*-test with Welch's correction with Prism software (GraphPad Software, La Jolla, CA, USA). Statistical differences were evaluated between the control and $NaAsO_2$-exposed groups. $P \leq 0.05$ were considered to be statistically significant.

RESULTS

Maternal and Embryonic Toxicity

No dams were found to develop significant abnormalities in general health parameters including the body weight gain of the dams during pregnancy (Figure S1) and maternal death. In addition, there were no differences in the number of live pups between the control and $NaAsO_2$-exposed groups (Figure S2).

Basal Activity Levels of Offspring

No toxic effects of prenatal $NaAsO_2$ exposure on body weight gain and blood glucose level of offspring were observed (Figure S3). In addition, there were no apparent differences in most of basal activity indices of the offspring in the acclimation phase of the behavioral flexibility test were observed between the two groups, except significant increase in duration of nose poke in $NaAsO_2$-exposed female mice (Tables S1, S2).

Impaired Behavioral Flexibility in $NaAsO_2$-Exposed Mice

Behavioral flexibility was examined by evaluating the number of incorrectly visiting the two never-rewarding corner within the first 100 visits of a given test session (discrimination error rate). In acquisition phase of the behavioral sequencing task, mice were imposed to discriminate rewarded corners from never-rewarded corners with acquirement of shuttling behavior between the two distantly positioned rewarded corners to obtain water continuously (**Figure 1B**). No apparent differences in the acquisition of the behavioral sequencing tasks were observed between the control and $NaAsO_2$-exposed groups of both sexes (**Figure 1E**, Figure S4). However, a delay in acquiring the behavioral sequencing tasks was observed in both the control and $NaAsO_2$-exposed females. While the discrimination error rate of both the control and $NaAsO_2$-exposed males was significantly decreased to approximately 10% by session 11 (Figure S4), the discrimination error rate of both groups of females was decreased to approximately 15% by session 21 (**Figure 1E**). It indicates that female mice took longer time to be able to adapt the behavioral sequencing task than that taken by male mice regardless of prenatal exposure to $NaAsO_2$.

In the subsequent serial reversal task, the discrimination error rate for the control and $NaAsO_2$-exposed groups of both female and male mice was elevated in the first session of each reversal phase (Rev 1–11; **Figure 1E**, Figure S4), indicating that each group of both male and female mice properly acquired the behavioral sequence assigned in the previous phase. However, in $NaAsO_2$-exposed female mice, the discrimination error rate was significantly higher than that of the control mice in the first session of reversals 1, 4, 8, and 11, and in the fifth session of reversal 1 (**Figure 1E**). These results suggest that $NaAsO_2$-exposed female mice are impaired in the initial adaptation process of reversal learning. Nevertheless, the increased discrimination error rate in the first session of reversals was significantly reduced in subsequent reversal phase sessions of both groups of female mice (**Figure 1E**), demonstrating a day-to-day improvement in the adaptive behavior in female mice. In male mice, tendency of overall increases in discrimination error rate between the control and and $NaAO_2$-exposed groups was observed. Significant increases were observed in the second session of reversals 5 and 11 (Figure S4), whereas significant decrease in discrimination error rate was found in first session of Rev 6. These results suggest that $NaAsO_2$-exposed male mice showed impairment in adaptation to reversals, but the degree of impairment in males might not be severe compared to that in females.

Alteration in the Number of Neurons and Glial Cells in the PrL of $NaAsO_2$-Exposed Mice

To determine whether $NaAsO_2$ exposure-related behavioral alterations in mice are associated with changes in brain histology, the number of Cresyl Fast Violet-stained pyramidal neurons, non-pyramidal neurons, and glial cells were measured in three different layers (layer II–III, V, and VI) of the PrL (**Figures 2B,C**). Stereological analysis revealed that the number of pyramidal neurons in layers V and VI but not in layer II–III of the PrL was significantly ($p < 0.05$) increased in the $NaAsO_2$-exposed group as compared to the control group (**Figure 2D**). No significant differences in the number of non-pyramidal neurons and glial cells were observed between the control and *$NaAsO_2$-exposed* groups in any observed layer of the PrL (**Figures 2E,F**).

Alteration of the Morphology of Neurites in the PrL of $NaAsO_2$-Exposed Mice

We next evaluated the morphology of neurites on Golgi-stained neurons in the PrL. A reduction in the length of neurites on Golgi-stained neurons in the PrL was observed in $NaAsO_2$-exposed mice as compared to neurites in the control group (**Figure 3A**). Space Ball probe analysis indicated that $NaAsO_2$ exposure was associated with a significant ($p < 0.05$) decrease in the length of neurites in Golgi-stained neurons of the PrL as compared to the control group (**Figure 3C**).

The Density and Morphology of Dendritic Spines of Pyramidal Neurons in the PrL of $NaAsO_2$-Exposed Mice

The density and head diameter of dendritic spines from Golgi-stained pyramidal neurons were measured in three different cortical layers (layer II–III, V, and VI) of the PrL (**Figure 4A**). The total density of dendritic spines in pyramidal neurons was not significantly different between control mice and $NaAsO_2$-exposed mice in any observed layer of the PrL (**Figure 4B**). Spine head diameters were also not significantly different between the

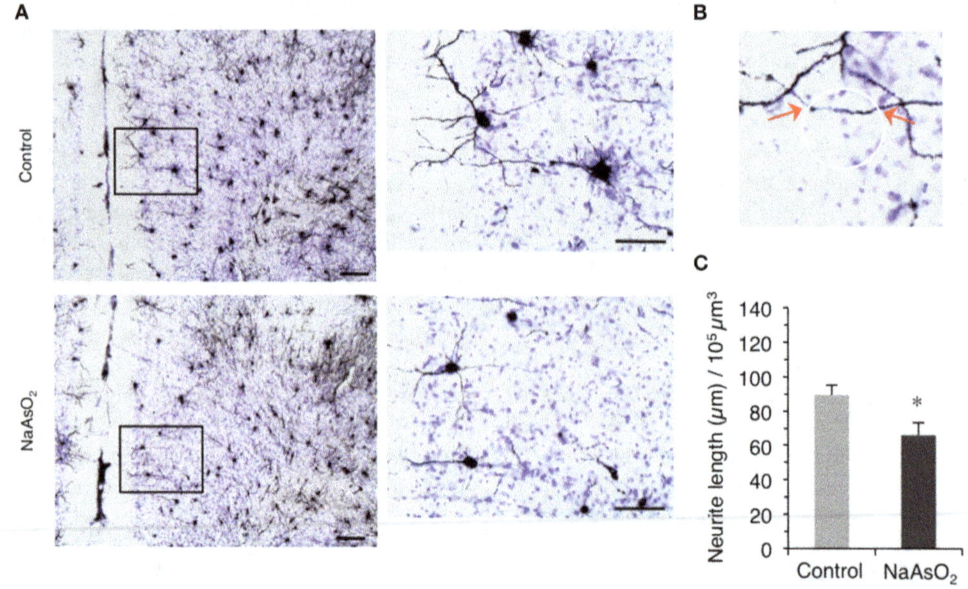

FIGURE 3 | Altered morphology of neurites in the PrL of adult female mice born to dams that were administered $NaAsO_2$ during gestation. (A) Representative photomicrographs of the PrL in Golgi- and Cresyl Fast Violet-stained coronal brain sections from female mice with or without prenatal exposure to $NaAsO_2$. The rectangular area was magnified and shown in the corresponding right panel. Bars = 20 μm (low magnification) and 10 μm (high magnification). **(B)** Demonstrative photomicrograph for the intersection points (indicated by red arrows) between a virtual sphere "Space Ball" (white circle) and Gogli-stained neurite. **(C)** Estimated neurite lengths in Golgi-stained PrL neurons as measured by the Space Ball method. Values (mean ± SEM) were normalized to the estimated volume of the selected PrL region (control group $n = 7$, $NaAsO_2$-exposed group $n = 5$). An asterisk indicates $p < 0.05$ vs. the control group.

control and $NaAsO_2$-exposed groups in any observed layer of the PrL (**Figures 4C–E**).

DISCUSSION

In the present study, we investigated the effect of prenatal $NaAsO_2$ exposure on the behavioral flexibility/reversal learning of adult mice using the IntelliCage system, which is an efficient tool for monitoring multiple aspects of cognitive behavior in a social environment (Endo et al., 2012; Benner et al., 2015). The core finding of our work is that exposure of dams to $NaAsO_2$ produces behavioral inflexibility to reversal learning and abnormal formation of the PrL in adult offspring. These findings suggest that behavioral impairments caused by $NaAsO_2$ exposure are associated with structural changes of brain, particularly in the PrL cortical region.

Here, we provided pregnant female mice with drinking water that contained 85 ppm $NaAsO_2$ during a critical period of embryonic brain development (gestational day 8–18). A series of studies by Colomina et al. evaluated the effect of $NaAsO_2$ exposure on development of nervous system. Exposure to $NaAsO_2$ at 10 mg/kg/day throughout gestational day 15–18 delayed neurodevelopmental indices such as eye opening in female offspring (Colomina et al., 1997). Furthermore, they have shown that single $NaAsO_2$ exposure at 30 mg/kg induces deficit in neuromotor development (Colomina et al., 1996). In accordance with these studies, we considered that providing $NaAsO_2$ about 10 mg/kg to pregnant mice during gestation might induce higher brain function deficits in offspring. It has been reported that mice drink around 5 ml of water daily (Bachmanov et al., 2002). However, our own measurement showed that a 25–35 g pregnant mouse drink about 3.5 ml of water daily when the mouse is provided with $NaAsO_2$-containing water (Figure S5). Based on these estimates, a 25–35 g dam consumes 0.39 mg $NaAsO_2$/day (which is equivalent to 8.5–12 mg/kg/day) when dams are provided with drinking water containing 85 ppm $NaAsO_2$. The selected $NaAsO_2$ dose used in the current study did not produce any obvious maternal toxicity or embryonic toxicity (Figures S1, S2), which is consistent with the previous studies (Rodriguez et al., 2002; Waalkes et al., 2003; Markowski et al., 2012).

Behavioral flexibility describes the ability of an organism to adapt to a changing environment. Behavioral flexibility occurs in many kinds of animal, such as mice, rat, and monkey, and is often assessed using rule-shift learning task paradigms that include a sequencing reversal task. In this study, we assessed the behavioral flexibility of control or $NaAsO_2$-exposed female mice using an altered action-outcome contingency paradigm during inter-sessions, and inter-reversal stages that included a serial reversal task (Endo et al., 2012). In the inter-session analysis, day-to-day improvements in adaptive behavior, as observed in a decreasing trend of discrimination error rate in each reversal phase, were clearly observed not only in control but also arsenite-exposed groups. However, $NaAsO_2$-exposed mice demonstrated a lower degree of achievement in reversal learning than the control group. It may be inferred that the repetition of reversal learning lead to difficultly in re-acquiring reversal learning for the $NaAsO_2$-exposed group. Such effects of arsenic have

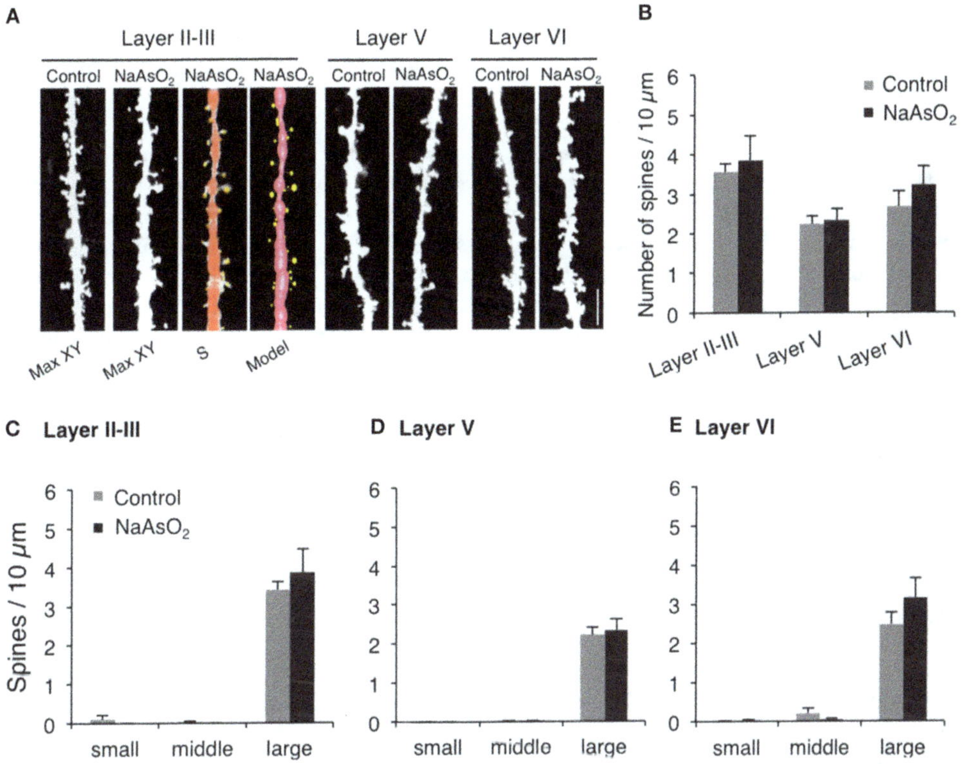

FIGURE 4 | The density and the morphology of dendritic spines in the PrL of adult female mice born from dams exposed to $NaAsO_2$ during gestation. Dendritic spines were analyzed along the primary basilar dendrites of Golgi-stained pyramidal neurons in three different cortical layers (layer II–III, V, and VI) of PrL. **(A)** Representative photomicrographs of dendritic spines with maximal intensity projections onto the XY plane from Z-series images (Max-XY) for the control group (Control) and $NaAsO_2$-exposed group. Photomicrographs analyzed by Spiso-3D (S) and three-dimensional models (Model) are also shown for the analysis of dendritic spines in the layer II–III of the $NaAsO_2$-exposed group. **(B)** Effect of $NaAsO_2$ exposure on the total dendritic spine density of pyramidal neurons in three different cortical layers. Effect of $NaAsO_2$ exposure on the density of three subtypes of dendritic spines, small-head spines (small), middle-head spines (middle), and large-head spines (large), in three cortical layers of the PrL: Layer II–III **(C)**, Layer V **(D)**, and Layer VI **(E)**. The density of dendritic spines is expressed as the number of spines per 10 μm of dendrite. A total 500–1200 spines from 30 to 45 dendritic segments of 30–45 neurons were analyzed for each cortical layer. Values are expressed as mean ± SEM (control group $n = 7$, $NaAsO_2$-exposed group $n = 5$).

been reported in adulthood exposure. A series of studies have demonstrated that arsenic exposure in adult mice produces an increase in the number of errors in an egocentric task (Rodriguez et al., 2001, 2002). Our present findings suggest that $NaAsO_2$ exposure in early life also produces behavioral impairments in learning function in mice. The first session of each reversal stage in the serial reversal-learning task tests the ability of mice to adapt to a changing task, because in this first session, mice must alter their behavioral sequence in order to receive a reward. Mice in the control group adapted to new behavioral sequences after a series of reversals, whereas mice in the $NaAsO_2$-exposed group did not adequately adapt to changing tasks (**Figure 1E**) that was likely indicative of behavioral inflexibility.

We also revealed a possible link between behavioral alterations and structural changes in the PrL cortical region. The PrL is known to be involved in the regulation of cognitive and executive processes (Dalley et al., 2004; Marquis et al., 2007; Ragozzino, 2007). It has been demonstrated that the PrL plays a fundamental role in behavioral flexibility. For example, patients who have the frontal lobe (including PrL) damage show impaired adaptation to changes in reinforcement contingencies in spite of the fact that these patients can acquire novel skills or adopt new rules with relative ease (Owen et al., 1993). It has also demonstrated that either lesion or inactivation of the PrL impairs behavioral flexibility in rodents (Ragozzino et al., 1999). Accordingly, structural changes in the PrL can contribute to the impairment of behavioral flexibility. $NaAsO_2$ is known to produce neurotoxicity by inducing apoptotic cell death (Wong et al., 2005; Keim et al., 2012) and/or cellular necrosis (Chattopadhyay et al., 2002; Yang et al., 2003). Therefore, in the present study, we measured the number of neurons and glial cells in the PrL in order to determine whether cell viability was affected by prenatal $NaAsO_2$ exposure. Contrary to our expectations, these morphometrical analyses revealed that $NaAsO_2$ exposure increased the number of pyramidal neurons in layers V and VI of the PrL (**Figure 2D**). Our previous *in vitro* work showed that a high concentration of $NaAsO_2$ (2 μM) reduced the viability of mouse primary cortical neurons, but that a low concentration of $NaAsO_2$ (0.5 μM) conversely increased cell viability and promoted cellular proliferation (Maekawa et al., 2013). It suggests that the concentration of $NaAsO_2$ (85 ppm) used in the present study reflect the low concentration of $NaAsO_2$ exposure resulting in the increase in the number of pyramidal neurons in the present. On the other hand, the number of non-pyramidal neurons and glial cells was not affected by $NaAsO_2$ exposure in the present study. The difference between the effect of $NaAsO_2$ exposure on pyramidal and non-pyramidal cells (**Figures 2D,E**) could be due to differences in the timing of neurogenesis and neuronal migration. The majority of cerebral cortical neurons are generated during embryonic day 11–17 in mouse (Price and Lotto, 1996; Price et al., 1997), whereas neurogenesis for each cortical layer is not simultaneous and occurs with variable timing (Finlay and Darlington, 1995). Additionally, pyramidal neurons are generated from the ventricular zone and migrate through the cortical layers radially, while interneurons including non-pyramidal neurons are generated from the ganglionic eminence and migrate tangentially (Nadarajah et al., 2003). Therefore, the timing of generation and migration of pyramidal neurons is different from that of non-pyramidal neurons, and these differences may reflect the layer-specific and cell type-specific effects of $NaAsO_2$ on the number of neurons in the PrL observed in the present study. Several studies have already shown that chemical exposures affect neuronal migration by disrupting the inside-out pattern of migration (Kakita et al., 2002; Schreiber et al., 2010). Taken together, the generation and migration of neurons may be at least partially affected by prenatal $NaAsO_2$ exposure, although the mechanisms by which $NaAsO_2$ exposure specifically increases the number of pyramidal neurons in a layer-dependent manner has not yet been identified. Regarding glial cells, morphological or functional changes have been shown to occur at higher $NaAsO_2$ concentrations than those, which affect the morphology of neurons (Wang et al., 2012). Therefore, the observed lack of effect of $NaAsO_2$ exposure on the number of glial cells in this study was expected, and may be due to an insufficient level of prenatal $NaAsO_2$ exposure.

Another critical finding of our study is that behavioral inflexibility is clearly associated with structural changes in PrL neurons. We previously demonstrated that $NaAsO_2$ disrupts neuritogenesis in primary cultured neurons (Maekawa et al., 2013) and neuronal cell lines (Aung et al., 2013), and that inhibition of neuritogenesis by $NaAsO_2$ is caused by alterations in the expression of cytoskeletal genes, tau, tubulin, and neurofilament (Aung et al., 2013), and suppression of glutamate AMPA receptor expression (Maekawa et al., 2013). Thus, inorganic arsenic adversely affects the fate and maturation processes of young neurons, which may lead to abnormal formation of neural circuits. In the present study, we found that the length of neurites in the PrL was significantly lower in the $NaAsO_2$-exposed group, suggesting that prenatal exposure to $NaAsO_2$ has an adverse effect on neuritogenesis. Elongation of the axon and dendrites is an essential event for the formation of basic neuronal circuitry. Impairments in the length and morphology of dendrites in the frontal cortex are involved in the pathogenesis of cognitive deficits and mental retardation (Armstrong et al., 1998). It indicates that the alteration in the morphology of neuron, particularly the PrL neuron, is strongly associated with the pathophysiological states of cognitive and learning dysfunction and that prenatal exposure to $NaAsO_2$ may contribute to the pathogenesis. Additionally, it has been reported that the degree of learning disability is positively correlated with the severity and extent of dendritic abnormalities (Kaufmann and Moser, 2000). Therefore, we subsequently examined the density and morphology of pyramidal neuron dendritic spines in different layers of the PrL. In contrast to the impairment in neurite length, the morphology and the density of dendritic spines in PrL pyramidal neurons were not affected by $NaAsO_2$ exposure. We recently demonstrated in cultured neurons that $NaAsO_2$ specifically alters the gene expression of cytoskeletal proteins including tau, tubulin, and neurofilaments, but does not affect the expression of actin protein (Aung et al., 2013). Since dendritic spines are actin-rich protrusions from dendrites that form the post-synaptic component of a synapse (Hotulainen and Hoogenraad, 2010), our current finding that $NaAsO_2$ exposure did not have an effect on synapse number agrees with our previous study regarding the expression of actin protein. $NaAsO_2$ exposure has however been reported to impair the expression of AMPA and NMDA glutamate receptors (Maekawa et al., 2013; Ramos-Chavez et al., 2015), suggesting that $NaAsO_2$ exposure can affect glutamate transmission. Because glutamate transmission is critically involved in the regulation of synapse formation (Rasse et al., 2005), we cannot exclude the possibility that the exposure to $NaAsO_2$ alters synapse formation in areas other than the PrL. Taken together, the present study highlights the possible association between behavioral impairment in mice caused by prenatal $NaAsO_2$ exposure and morphological alteration of brain, particularly cortical disarrangement in the prelimbic cortex.

On the other hand, the suggested association between the behavioral inflexibility and morphological alteration of the PrL was come from the morphometrical analysis, which was however carried out following the behavioral flexibility test. It has been demonstrated in human subjects that goal-directed learning is strongly associated with increase neural activity in prefrontal cortex (Valentin et al., 2007) and higher neurite density in medial orbitofrontal cortex (Morris et al., 2016). Since the control mice performed better than $NaAsO_2$-exposed mice in this study of behavioral flexibility tasks, we could not deny the possibility of increase neurite length in the PrL of the control mice, which might be outcome of better goal-directed learning in behavioral flexibility tasks. In addition, it is important to note that the reduced maternal water consumption was observed in the group of dams provided with water containing $NaAsO_2$, and the difference between the two groups was about 2 ml per day (Figure S5). It might be due to unpalatability of dams to water containing $NaAsO_2$. Although we did not observe the obvious signs of maternal or embryonic toxicity such as maternal weight (Figure S1) and the number of pups (Figure S2) between the two groups of this study, several studies reported the possibility that maternal dehydration due to reduced water intake during pregnancy was associated with long-term physiologic effects on offspring such as development of brain function and plasma composition (Desai et al., 2005; Ross et al., 2005; Zhang et al., 2011). Therefore, we had to assume that behavioral inflexibility observed in mice prenatally exposed $NaAsO_2$ could be induced by the combinatorial effect of the toxicity of prenatal $NaAsO_2$ exposure and maternal dehydration.

In this study, we used male and female mice at 67 week (15.5 month) of their age in this study of behavioral flexibility tests, which additionally lasted for 10–12 weeks (about 2–3 month). Therefore, the age of mice in the last day of behavioral tests was being 17.5–18.5 month, which could be generally considered as old aged mice. It has been demonstrated that arsenic-induced increase in oxidative stress (such as glutathione level in the blood) was more prominent in young and old rats compared to adults (Jain et al., 2011, 2012). Motor impairments caused by prenatal arsenic exposure were observed in young juvenile mice, but such effects observed in young mice were subsided with advancing age (Markowski et al., 2012). These studies indicate age-dependent effects of arsenic-induced toxicity. Therefore, although we observed $NaAsO_2$-induced behavioral inflexibility in old aged mice in the present study, we need further studies to test the age-dependent effects of prenatal $NaAsO_2$ exposure on behavioral flexibility.

In conclusion, we demonstrate the possibility that *in utero* $NaAsO_2$ exposure leads to behavioral inflexibility to changing tasks in adulthood, and cortical disarrangement in the PrL might contribute to this behavioral impairment. Further studies are required to elucidate how $NaAsO_2$ disrupts neuronal development including axonal and dendritic elongation particularly in prefrontal cortex. Since behavioral inflexibility is observed in children with neurodevelopmental disorders such as autism spectrum disorders, our findings put forth a new perspective on how environmental exposures affect the pathogenesis of neurodevelopmental disorders.

AUTHOR CONTRIBUTIONS

KA designed and performed experiments, analyzed data and wrote the paper; CT, KS performed experiments and analyzed data; KaN, AT, KeN, MK, and CT edited the paper; ST designed experiments and edited the paper; and FM designed experiments, analyzed data and wrote the paper.

ACKNOWLEDGMENTS

This work was supported by JSPS KAKENHI 24590307 to FM, 23310043 to ST, FM, 15K14556 to ST and 24221003 to CT, by the National Institute for Environmental Studies [14309][14013] to FM, and in part by The Grant of National Center for Child Health and Development (25-3) to KN and by the Health Labour Sciences Research Grant from The Ministry of Health Labour and Welfare, Japan to MK.

REFERENCES

Armstrong, D. D., Dunn, K., and Antalffy, B. (1998). Decreased dendritic branching in frontal, motor and limbic cortex in Rett syndrome compared with trisomy 21. *J. Neuropathol. Exp. Neurol.* 57, 1013–1017. doi: 10.1097/00005072-199811000-00003

Aung, K. H., Kurihara, R., Nakashima, S., Maekawa, F., Nohara, K., Kobayashi, T., et al. (2013). Inhibition of neurite outgrowth and alteration of cytoskeletal gene expression by sodium arsenite. *Neurotoxicology* 34, 226–235. doi: 10.1016/j.neuro.2012.09.008

Bachmanov, A. A., Reed, D. R., Beauchamp, G. K., and Tordoff, M. G. (2002). Food intake, water intake, and drinking spout side preference of 28 mouse strains. *Behav. Genet.* 32, 435–443. doi: 10.1023/A:1020884312053

Benner, S., Endo, T., Kakeyama, M., and Tohyama, C. (2015). Environmental insults in early life and submissiveness later in life in mouse models. *Front. Neurosci.* 9:91. doi: 10.3389/fnins.2015.00091

Bisen-Hersh, E. B., Farina, M., Barbosa, F. Jr., Rocha, J. B., and Aschner, M. (2014). Behavioral effects of developmental methylmercury drinking water exposure in rodents. *J. Trace Elem. Med. Biol.* 28, 117–124. doi: 10.1016/j.jtemb.2013.09.008

Chaineau, E., Binet, S., Pol, D., Chatellier, G., and Meininger, V. (1990). Embryotoxic effects of sodium arsenite and sodium arsenate on mouse embryos in culture. *Teratology* 41, 105–112. doi: 10.1002/tera.1420410111

Chattopadhyay, S., Bhaumik, S., Purkayastha, M., Basu, S., Nag Chaudhuri, A., and Das Gupta, S. (2002). Apoptosis and necrosis in developing brain cells due to arsenic toxicity and protection with antioxidants. *Toxicol. Lett.* 136, 65–76. doi: 10.1016/S0378-4274(02)00282-5

Colomina, M. T., Albina, M. L., and Domingo, J. L. (1996). Influence of maternal restraint stress on arsenic-induced pre- and postnatal alterations in mice. *Psychobiology* 24, 227–234.

Colomina, M. T., Albina, M. L., Domingo, J. L., and Corbella, J. (1997). Influence of maternal stress on the effects of prenatal exposure to methylmercury and arsenic on postnatal development and behavior in mice: a preliminary evaluation. *Physiol. Behav.* 61, 455–459. doi: 10.1016/S0031-9384(96)00462-3

Dakeishi, M., Murata, K., and Grandjean, P. (2006). Long-term consequences of arsenic poisoning during infancy due to contaminated milk powder. *Environ. Health* 5, 31. doi: 10.1186/1476-069X-5-31

Dalley, J. W., Cardinal, R. N., and Robbins, T. W. (2004). Prefrontal executive and cognitive functions in rodents: neural and neurochemical substrates. *Neurosci. Biobehav. Rev.* 28, 771–784. doi: 10.1016/j.neubiorev.2004.09.006

Desai, M., Gayle, D., Kallichanda, N., and Ross, M. G. (2005). Gender specificity of programmed plasma hypertonicity and hemoconcentration in adult offspring of water-restricted rat dams. *J. Soc. Gynecol. Investig.* 12, 409–415. doi: 10.1016/j.jsgi.2005.04.007

Endo, T., Kakeyama, M., Uemura, Y., Haijima, A., Okuno, H., Bito, H., et al. (2012). Executive function deficits and social-behavioral abnormality in mice exposed to a low dose of dioxin in utero and via lactation. *PLoS ONE* 7:e50741. doi: 10.1371/journal.pone.0050741

Endo, T., Maekawa, F., Voikar, V., Haijima, A., Uemura, Y., Zhang, Y., et al. (2011). Automated test of behavioral flexibility in mice using a behavioral sequencing task in IntelliCage. *Behav. Brain Res.* 221, 172–181. doi: 10.1016/j.bbr.2011.02.037

Ferraro, L., Tomasini, M. C., Tanganelli, S., Mazza, R., Coluccia, A., Carratu, M. R., et al. (2009). Developmental exposure to methylmercury elicits early cell death in the cerebral cortex and long-term memory deficits in the rat. *Int. J. Dev. Neurosci.* 27, 165–174. doi: 10.1016/j.ijdevneu.2008.11.004

Finlay, B. L., and Darlington, R. B. (1995). Linked regularities in the development and evolution of mammalian brains. *Science* 268, 1578–1584. doi: 10.1126/science.7777856

Franklin, K., and Paxinos, G. (2008). *The Mouse Brain in Stereotaxic Coordinates, Compact, 3rd Edn.* Amsterdam: Elsevier Academic Press.

Grandjean, P., and Landrigan, P. J. (2006). Developmental neurotoxicity of industrial chemicals. *Lancet* 368, 2167–2178. doi: 10.1016/S0140-6736(06)69665-7

Grandjean, P., and Landrigan, P. J. (2014). Neurobehavioural effects of developmental toxicity. *Lancet Neurol.* 13, 330–338. doi: 10.1016/S1474-4422(13)70278-3

Hill, E. L., and Bird, C. M. (2006). Executive processes in Asperger syndrome: patterns of performance in a multiple case series. *Neuropsychologia* 44, 2822–2835. doi: 10.1016/j.neuropsychologia.2006.06.007

Hirner, A. V., and Rettenmeier, A. W. (2010). Methylated metal(loid) species in humans. *Met. Ions Life Sci.* 7, 465–521. doi: 10.1039/9781849730822-00465

Hotulainen, P., and Hoogenraad, C. C. (2010). Actin in dendritic spines: connecting dynamics to function. *J. Cell Biol.* 189, 619–629. doi: 10.1083/jcb.201003008

Jain, A., Flora, G. J., Bhargava, R., and Flora, S. J. (2012). Influence of age on arsenic-induced oxidative stress in rat. *Biol. Trace Elem. Res.* 149, 382–390. doi: 10.1007/s12011-012-9432-7

Jain, A., Yadav, A., Bozhkov, A. I., Padalko, V. I., and Flora, S. J. (2011). Therapeutic efficacy of silymarin and naringenin in reducing arsenic-induced hepatic damage in young rats. *Ecotoxicol. Environ. Saf.* 74, 607–614. doi: 10.1016/j.ecoenv.2010.08.002

Kakita, A., Inenaga, C., Sakamoto, M., and Takahashi, H. (2002). Neuronal migration disturbance and consequent cytoarchitecture in the cerebral cortex following transplacental administration of methylmercury. *Acta Neuropathol.* 104, 409–417. doi: 10.1007/s00401-002-0571-3

Kaufmann, W. E., and Moser, H. W. (2000). Dendritic anomalies in disorders associated with mental retardation. *Cereb. Cortex* 10, 981–991. doi: 10.1093/cercor/10.10.981

Keim, A., Rossler, O. G., Rothhaar, T. L., and Thiel, G. (2012). Arsenite-induced apoptosis of human neuroblastoma cells requires p53 but occurs independently of c-Jun. *Neuroscience* 206, 25–38. doi: 10.1016/j.neuroscience.2012.01.001

Kipp, K. (2005). A developmental perspective on the measurement of cognitive deficits in attention-deficit/hyperactivity disorder. *Biol. Psychiatry* 57, 1256–1260. doi: 10.1016/j.biopsych.2005.03.012

Koike-Kuroda, Y., Kakeyama, M., Fujimaki, H., and Tsukahara, S. (2010). Use of live imaging analysis for evaluation of cytotoxic chemicals that induce apoptotic cell death. *Toxicol. In vitro* 24, 2012–2020. doi: 10.1016/j.tiv.2010.07.022

Li, D., Lu, C., Wang, J., Hu, W., Cao, Z., Sun, D., et al. (2009). Developmental mechanisms of arsenite toxicity in zebrafish (Danio rerio) embryos. *Aquat. Toxicol.* 91, 229–237. doi: 10.1016/j.aquatox.2008.11.007

Maekawa, F., Tsuboi, T., Oya, M., Aung, K. H., Tsukahara, S., Pellerin, L., et al. (2013). Effects of sodium arsenite on neurite outgrowth and glutamate AMPA receptor expression in mouse cortical neurons. *Neurotoxicology* 37, 197–206. doi: 10.1016/j.neuro.2013.05.006

Markowski, V. P., Reeve, E. A., Onos, K., Assadollahzadeh, M., and Mckay, N. (2012). Effects of prenatal exposure to sodium arsenite on motor and food-motivated behaviors from birth to adulthood in C57BL6/J mice. *Neurotoxicol. Teratol.* 34, 221–231. doi: 10.1016/j.ntt.2012.01.001

Marquis, J. P., Killcross, S., and Haddon, J. E. (2007). Inactivation of the prelimbic, but not infralimbic, prefrontal cortex impairs the contextual control of response conflict in rats. *Eur. J. Neurosci.* 25, 559–566. doi: 10.1111/j.1460-9568.2006.05295.x

Martinez-Finley, E. J., Ali, A. M., and Allan, A. M. (2009). Learning deficits in C57BL/6J mice following perinatal arsenic exposure: consequence of lower corticosterone receptor levels? *Pharmacol. Biochem. Behav.* 94, 271–277. doi: 10.1016/j.pbb.2009.09.006

Morris, L. S., Kundu, P., Dowell, N., Mechelmans, D. J., Favre, P., Irvine, M. A., et al. (2016). Fronto-striatal organization: defining functional and microstructural substrates of behavioural flexibility. *Cortex* 74, 118–133. doi: 10.1016/j.cortex.2015.11.004

Mouton, P. R., Gokhale, A. M., Ward, N. L., and West, M. J. (2002). Stereological length estimation using spherical probes. *J. Microsc.* 206, 54–64. doi: 10.1046/j.1365-2818.2002.01006.x

Mukai, H., Hatanaka, Y., Mitsuhashi, K., Hojo, Y., Komatsuzaki, Y., Sato, R., et al. (2011). Automated analysis of spines from confocal laser microscopy images: application to the discrimination of androgen and estrogen effects on spinogenesis. *Cereb. Cortex* 21, 2704–2711. doi: 10.1093/cercor/bhr059

Nadarajah, B., Alifragis, P., Wong, R. O., and Parnavelas, J. G. (2003). Neuronal migration in the developing cerebral cortex: observations based on real-time imaging. *Cereb. Cortex* 13, 607–611. doi: 10.1093/cercor/13.6.607

Owen, A. M., Roberts, A. C., Hodges, J. R., Summers, B. A., Polkey, C. E., and Robbins, T. W. (1993). Contrasting mechanisms of impaired attentional set-shifting in patients with frontal lobe damage or Parkinson's disease. *Brain* 116(Pt 5), 1159–1175. doi: 10.1093/brain/116.5.1159

Price, D. J., Aslam, S., Tasker, L., and Gillies, K. (1997). Fates of the earliest generated cells in the developing murine neocortex. *J. Comp. Neurol.* 377, 414–422.

Price, D. J., and Lotto, R. B. (1996). Influences of the thalamus on the survival of subplate and cortical plate cells in cultured embryonic mouse brain. *J. Neurosci.* 16, 3247–3255.

Ragozzino, M. E. (2007). The contribution of the medial prefrontal cortex, orbitofrontal cortex, and dorsomedial striatum to behavioral flexibility. *Ann. N.Y. Acad. Sci.* 1121, 355–375. doi: 10.1196/annals.1401.013

Ragozzino, M. E., Detrick, S., and Kesner, R. P. (1999). Involvement of the prelimbic-infralimbic areas of the rodent prefrontal cortex in behavioral flexibility for place and response learning. *J. Neurosci.* 19, 4585–4594.

Ramos-Chavez, L. A., Rendon-Lopez, C. R., Zepeda, A., Silva-Adaya, D., Del Razo, L. M., and Gonsebatt, M. E. (2015). Neurological effects of inorganic arsenic exposure: altered cysteine/glutamate transport, NMDA expression and spatial memory impairment. *Front. Cell. Neurosci.* 9:21. doi: 10.3389/fncel.2015.00021

Rasse, T. M., Fouquet, W., Schmid, A., Kittel, R. J., Mertel, S., Sigrist, C. B., et al. (2005). Glutamate receptor dynamics organizing synapse formation *in vivo*. *Nat. Neurosci.* 8, 898–905. doi: 10.1038/nn1484

Rios, R., Zarazua, S., Santoyo, M. E., Sepulveda-Saavedra, J., Romero-Diaz, V., Jimenez, V., et al. (2009). Decreased nitric oxide markers and morphological changes in the brain of arsenic-exposed rats. *Toxicology* 261, 68–75. doi: 10.1016/j.tox.2009.04.055

Rocha-Amador, D., Navarro, M. E., Carrizales, L., Morales, R., and Calderon, J. (2007). Decreased intelligence in children and exposure to fluoride and arsenic in drinking water. *Cad. Saude Publica* 23 (Suppl. 4), S579–S587. doi: 10.1590/s0102-311x2007001600018

Rodriguez, V. M., Carrizales, L., Jimenez-Capdeville, M. E., Dufour, L., and Giordano, M. (2001). The effects of sodium arsenite exposure on behavioral parameters in the rat. *Brain Res. Bull.* 55, 301–308. doi: 10.1016/S0361-9230(01)00477-4

Rodriguez, V. M., Carrizales, L., Mendoza, M. S., Fajardo, O. R., and Giordano, M. (2002). Effects of sodium arsenite exposure on development and behavior in the rat. *Neurotoxicol. Teratol.* 24, 743–750. doi: 10.1016/S0892-0362(02)00313-6

Rosado, J. L., Ronquillo, D., Kordas, K., Rojas, O., Alatorre, J., Lopez, P., et al. (2007). Arsenic exposure and cognitive performance in Mexican schoolchildren. *Environ. Health Perspect.* 115, 1371–1375. doi: 10.1289/ehp.9961

Ross, M. G., Desai, M., Guerra, C., and Wang, S. (2005). Prenatal programming of hypernatremia and hypertension in neonatal lambs. *Am. J. Physiol. Regul. Integr. Comp. Physiol.* 288, R97–R103. doi: 10.1152/ajpregu.00315.2004

Schreiber, T., Gassmann, K., Gotz, C., Hubenthal, U., Moors, M., Krause, G., et al. (2010). Polybrominated diphenyl ethers induce developmental neurotoxicity in a human *in vitro* model: evidence for endocrine disruption. *Environ. Health Perspect.* 118, 572–578. doi: 10.1289/ehp.0901435

Tomasini, M. C., Beggiato, S., Ferraro, L., Tanganelli, S., Marani, L., Lorenzini, L., et al. (2012). Prenatal exposure to 2,3,7,8-tetrachlorodibenzo-p-dioxin produces alterations in cortical neuron development and a long-term dysfunction of glutamate transmission in rat cerebral cortex. *Neurochem. Int.* 61, 759–766. doi: 10.1016/j.neuint.2012.07.004

Tsukahara, S., Tsuda, M. C., Kurihara, R., Kato, Y., Kuroda, Y., Nakata, M., et al. (2011). Effects of aromatase or estrogen receptor gene deletion on masculinization of the principal nucleus of the bed nucleus of the stria terminalis of mice. *Neuroendocrinology* 94, 137–147. doi: 10.1159/000327541

Valencia, E., Gil, A., Zapico, R. M., Garcia Rodriguez, M. C., Pintado, V., Lopez Dupla, M., et al. (1992). [Azidothymidine in the treatment of patients with human immunodeficiency virus infection and persistent generalized adenopathies]. *An. Med. Interna* 9, 531–537.

Valentin, V. V., Dickinson, A., and O'doherty, J. P. (2007). Determining the neural substrates of goal-directed learning in the human brain. *J. Neurosci.* 27, 4019–4026. doi: 10.1523/JNEUROSCI.0564-07.2007

Van De Werd, H. J., Rajkowska, G., Evers, P., and Uylings, H. B. (2010). Cytoarchitectonic and chemoarchitectonic characterization of the prefrontal cortical areas in the mouse. *Brain Struct. Funct.* 214, 339–353. doi: 10.1007/s00429-010-0247-z

Waalkes, M. P., Ward, J. M., Liu, J., and Diwan, B. A. (2003). Transplacental carcinogenicity of inorganic arsenic in the drinking water: induction of hepatic, ovarian, pulmonary, and adrenal tumors in mice. *Toxicol. Appl. Pharmacol.* 186, 7–17. doi: 10.1016/S0041-008X(02)00022-4

Wang, Y., Zhao, F., Liao, Y., Jin, Y., and Sun, G. (2012). Arsenic exposure and glutamate-induced gliotransmitter release from astrocytes. *Neural Regen. Res.* 7, 2439–2445. doi: 10.3969/j.issn.1673-5374.2012.31.005

Wasserman, G. A., Liu, X., Parvez, F., Ahsan, H., Factor-Litvak, P., Kline, J., et al. (2007). Water arsenic exposure and intellectual function in 6-year-old children in Araihazar, Bangladesh. *Environ. Health Perspect.* 115, 285–289. doi: 10.1289/ehp.9501

WHO (2008). "*Guidelines for drinking-water quality, recommendations,*" in *Incorporating 1st and 2nd Addenda. Vol. 1, 3rd Edn* (Geneva: World Health Organization), 306–308b. Available online at: http://www.who.int/water_sanitation_health/dwq/gdwq3/en/index.html

Willhite, C. C., and Ferm, V. H. (1984). Prenatal and developmental toxicology of arsenicals. *Adv. Exp. Med. Biol.* 177, 205–228. doi: 10.1007/978-1-4684-4790-3_9

Wong, H. K., Fricker, M., Wyttenbach, A., Villunger, A., Michalak, E. M., Strasser, A., et al. (2005). Mutually exclusive subsets of BH3-only proteins are activated by the p53 and c-Jun N-terminal kinase/c-Jun signaling pathways during cortical neuron apoptosis induced by arsenite. *Mol. Cell. Biol.* 25, 8732–8747. doi: 10.1128/MCB.25.19.8732-8747.2005

Yan, C., Yang, T., Yu, Q. J., Jin, Z., Cheung, E. F., Liu, X., et al. (2015). Rostral medial prefrontal dysfunctions and consummatory pleasure in schizophrenia: a meta-analysis of functional imaging studies. *Psychiatry Res.* 231, 187–196. doi: 10.1016/j.pscychresns.2015.01.001

Yang, D., Liang, C., Jin, Y., and Wang, D. (2003). [Effect of arsenic toxicity on morphology and viability of enzyme in primary culture of rat hippocampal neurons]. *Wei Sheng Yan Jiu* 32, 309–312.

Zhang, H., Fan, Y., Xia, F., Geng, C., Mao, C., Jiang, S., et al. (2011). Prenatal water deprivation alters brain angiotensin system and dipsogenic changes in the offspring. *Brain Res.* 1382, 128–136. doi: 10.1016/j.brainres.2011.01.031

3

Metal Ion Toxins and Brain Aquaporin-4 Expression

Adriana Ximenes-da-Silva *

Setor de Fisiologia, Instituto de Ciências Biológicas e da Saúde, Universidade Federal de Alagoas, Maceió, Brazil

Edited by:
Fumihiko Maekawa,
National Institute for Environmental Studies, Japan

Reviewed by:
Luc Pellerin,
University of Lausanne, Switzerland
Shinji Tsukahara,
Saitama University, Japan

***Correspondence:**
Adriana Ximenes-da-Silva
ximenes.adri@gmail.com

Metal ions such as iron, zinc, and manganese are essential to metabolic functions, protein synthesis, neurotransmission, and antioxidant neuroprotective mechanisms. Conversely, non-essential metals such as mercury and lead are sources of human intoxication due to occupational activities or environmental contamination. Essential or non-essential metal accumulation in the central nervous system (CNS) results in changes in blood-brain barrier (BBB) permeability, as well as triggering microglia activation and astrocyte reactivity and changing water transport through the cells, which could result in brain swelling. Aquaporin-4 is the main water channel in the CNS, is expressed in astrocyte foot processes in brain capillaries and along the circumventricular epithelium in the ventricles, and has important physiological functions in maintaining brain osmotic homeostasis and supporting brain excitability through regulation of the extracellular space. Some evidence has pointed to a role of AQP4 during metal intoxication in the brain, where it may act in a dual form as a neuroprotector or a mediator of the development of oxidative stress in neurons and astrocytes, resulting in brain swelling and neuronal damage. This mini-review presents the way some metal ions affect changes in AQP4 expression in the CNS and discuss the ways in which water transport in brain cells can be involved in brain damage.

Keywords: aquaporin-4, neurotoxicity, astrocytes, metal ions, oxidative stress, brain edema

INTRODUCTION

Several metals, including zinc, iron, and manganese are important as major or trace elements in cellular biological functions, acting as catalytic cofactors of enzymes (Kress et al., 2002), cellular antioxidants, and neuromodulators (Paoletti et al., 1997). In contrast, metals such as mercury, lead, cadmium, and nickel have no known biological functions. Both essential and non-essential metal ions may lead to brain damage when they accumulate in the central nervous system (CNS).

Non-essential metals are an important cause of human intoxication due to occupational exposure or air, soil, and water contamination, resulting in serious health problems (Valko et al., 2005; Park and Zheng, 2012), including severe hematopoietic, renal, and neurological conditions (Tchounwou et al., 2012). More recently, the role of glial cells in protecting neuronal damage caused by metal ion accumulation in the brain has been studied, showing that astrocytes have a central role in reducing neural excitotoxicity by taking up metals that cross the blood-brain barrier (BBB) (Ni et al., 2011; Noguchi et al., 2013), while microglia release mediators of inflammatory and immune responses when activated by metal ions. As a consequence, oxidative stress is generated in brain cells, and reactive nitrogen and oxygen species (RNOS) contribute to the apoptotic process, leading to neurodegenerative diseases (Yuste et al., 2015).

Metal intoxication often leads to increased water transport through the BBB and astrocytes, which could have important consequences on the expression of aquaporins in the brain. Aquaporins are integral membrane proteins that mediate the bi-directional transport of water through the cells, regulating the osmolarity of the intra- and extracellular medium. Aquaporins possess six membrane-spanning domains and five connecting loops. To date, thirteen main isoforms of aquaporins have been described (AQP0 to AQP12). The isoforms AQP3, 7, 9, and 10 are known as aquaglyceroproteins, which mediate the transport of glycerol, urea, and carbon dioxide in addition to water.

In the CNS, AQP1 is mainly found in the apical membrane of the epithelium of the choroid plexus and in the ependyma and pia (Nielsen et al., 1993), while AQP4 is the main water channel expressed in glial cells (Jung et al., 1994). In astrocytes, AQP4 is localized in the foot processes apposed to brain capillaries and along the circumventricular epithelium in the ventricles (Nielsen et al., 1997). The distribution of AQP4 in astrocyte processes is polarized, and the channels are assembled as orthogonal arrays of particles (OAPs; Yang et al., 1996), which share the same distribution as the inwardly rectifying K^+ channel Kir4.1 (Nagelhus et al., 1999), showing an expressive role for AQP4 in regulating homeostasis of brain osmolarity and excitability via the extracellular clearance of K^+.

Therefore, oxidative stress due to metal intoxication seems to have an important role in brain excitotoxicity and damage, with cells swelling as a consequence or cause of neuronal damage. This mini-review aims to bring an overview of the role of AQP4 during metal intoxication and cellular mechanisms involved in neuroprotection and toxicity of the brain.

EXPOSURE TO NON-ESSENTIAL METALS AND THE ROLE OF ASTROCYTE WATER TRANSPORT IN BRAIN INJURY (TABLE 1, FIGURE 1)

Mercury

Human intoxication due to mercury exposure is associated with occupational activities, including mining and smelting of cinnabar ore, environmental pollution, and consumption of seafood contaminated with mercury. Central nervous system symptoms related to mercury exposure include paresthesia, cerebellar ataxia, and decrease of cognition (Ye et al., 2016).

Elemental mercury is lipid-soluble and crosses the BBB by diffusion. In brain cells, it is oxidized through catalase and peroxidase to inorganic mercury (Hg^+ and Hg^{2+}). Methylmercury (MeHg) is an important source of human intoxication through seafood intake. MeHg is carried through the endothelial cells of the BBB by a neutral L-cysteine amino acid carrier, and is preferentially taken up by astrocytes and microglia. In astrocytes, MeHg promotes RNOS production through decreased availability of cysteine, reducing the antioxidant responses. Moreover, MeHg stimulates arachidonic acid synthesis, which in turn inhibits glutamate uptake by astrocytes, leading to neurotoxicity through ROS production (Ni et al., 2012).

Aquaporins are mercury-sensitive water channels. Most AQPs are inhibited by Hg^{2+}, therefore decreasing cell water permeability (Agre et al., 1998), except for AQP6, which is activated by Hg^{2+} exposure (Yasui et al., 1999). The effects of mercury on cell's water transport were described in an early study in ghost erythrocytes treated with p-chloromercuribenzene sulphonate. In erythrocytes, mercury inhibited ~36% of water diffusion (Benga et al., 1985).

AQP4 has two isoforms (M1 and M23) that have been described as mercurial-insensitive water channels (MIWC), since their osmotic water permeability was not inhibited by mercury compounds (Shi and Verkman, 1996). In cells, the AQP4 monomer is normally oriented with the cysteine residue in loop D facing the intracellular side, preventing mercury binding to the channel and rendering AQP4 mercury-insensitive. However, mutagenic assays directed to the cysteine residues in the rat AQP4M23 isoform in proteoliposomes, in which the cysteine residue in loop D was randomly positioned inside or outside the proteoliposome membrane, demonstrated that when the AQP4M23 Cys178 in loop D faced the outside of proteoliposomes, mercury was efficient in reducing water permeability through AQP4. Covalent binding of mercury to the Cys178 residue might induce conformational changes in the AQP4 monomer, reducing water permeability (Yukutake et al., 2008). One *in vivo* study demonstrated the effects of 14 days of MeHg exposure (1.5 mg Hg/kg/day p.o.) on AQP4 expression in the brain of marmosets. MeHg intoxication increased AQP4 mRNA in the frontal lobe, occipital lobe, and cerebellum, while the AQP4 protein was increased in the occipital lobe and cerebellum (Yamamoto et al., 2012).

Lead

Lead (Pb) intoxication effects in the CNS include lethargy, memory deficits, encephalopathy, and coma. Lead poisoning in humans occurs by breathing dust or swallowing paint, water, or food containing lead. When bound to sulfhydryl groups of hemoglobin, lead reaches brain vessels and crosses the BBB by diffusion or competition with the same carrier system for other metal ions, as iron. Mechanisms of lead intoxication are mainly related to ROS production and disturbed ionic mechanisms, as lead can substitute for bivalent cations as Ca^{+2}, Mg^{+2}, and Fe^{+2}, leading to neurotransmission deficits, impaired subcellular signaling, and oxidative stress (for review, see Needleman, 2004).

Lead intoxication changes BBB permeability as a result of its accumulation in endothelial cells, leading to capillary weakness and brain swelling. Cultured rat astrocytes exposed to lead showed a 40% increase in osmotic water permeability (*Pf*) in AQP4-expressing astrocytes. The lead chelator DMSA (meso-2, 3-dimercaptosuccinic acid) abolished the effects of lead on water permeability, showing that AQP4 in astrocytes is central to cell swelling after lead intoxication (Gunnarson et al., 2005).

Changes in astrocyte water permeability would be caused by the calcium/calmodulin-dependent protein kinase II (CaMKII) pathway; astrocyte exposure to a CaMKII inhibitor abolished the lead effects on water permeability. The AQP4 phosphorylation site for CaMKII is located at the Ser111 residue; when mutated to Ser111Ala, the effect of lead on water permeability was

TABLE 1 | Effects of metal-ions on aquaporin-4 (AQP4) expression in the brain.

Metal Ion	Experimental approach	AQP4 expression	Water permeability	References
Mercury	*in vivo*			
	Rat brain	↑mRNA ↑protein	–	Yukutake et al., 2008
	in vitro			
	Xenopus oocytes	–	↓	Shi and Verkman, 1996
	AQP4 cystein-residue mutants			Yukutake et al., 2008
	AQP4 reconstituted in proteoliposomes	–	↓	
Lead	*in vivo*			
	Rat brain	no changes mRNA	–	Gunnarson et al., 2005
	in vitro			
	Cultured astrocytes	–	↑	Gunnarson et al., 2005
Manganese	*in vitro*			
	cultured astrocytes	↑protein in plasma membrane no changes mRNA	↑	Rao et al., 2010
Zinc	*in vitro*			
	AQP4.M23 proteolipossomes	–	↓	Yukutake et al., 2009
Iron	*in vivo*			
	Rat brain	↑protein	↑	Qing et al., 2009
	in vitro			
	cultured astrocytes	↑protein	–	Wang et al., 2015

↑, Increased; ↓, Decreased.

prevented. Assentoft et al. (2013, 2014) have questioned the effect of Ser111 residue phosphorylation on AQP4's regulation of water permeability. Mutation of the Ser111Ala residue to abolish the potential site of AQP4 phosphorylation and mutation to aspartate (S111D) to mimic serine phosphorylation did not change water permeability in *Xenopus* oocytes. Similarly, primary culture of astrocytes exposed to a cGMP-dependent protein kinase (PKG) activator did not change water permeability, indicating that phosphorylation of AQP4 could not be implicated in cell swelling. Another *in vivo* study in Sprague-Dawley rats did not indicate lead-related changes in AQP4 expression. Ten and fourty day old rats that received lead acetate intraperitoneally or by gavage showed no difference in AQP4 mRNA in the cerebellum and cerebrum at either age, although significantly increased brain lead levels could be detected (Gunnarson et al., 2005).

BIOLOGICALLY-NECESSARY METALS AND THE ROLE OF ASTROCYTE WATER TRANSPORT IN BRAIN INJURY (TABLE 1, FIGURE 1)

Manganese

Manganese is an essential metal and a constituent of metalloproteins and mitochondrial enzymes in oxidative metabolism (Aschner, 2000). Manganese poisoning occurs mainly through occupational exposure of miners, industrial steel workers, or welders to heavy metals. High exposure to manganese results in neurological symptoms, including bradykinesia, dystonia, and gait disturbance. At a cellular level, manganese poisoning will disturb antioxidant defense and water transport in cells, leading to swelling (Erikson et al., 2004). Primary cultures of rat astrocytes treated with manganese showed increased AQP4 proteins in the plasma membrane. This effect was time-dependent, and there was no corresponding increase in mRNA. Conversely, astrocyte cultures transfected with siRNA targeted to AQP4 showed a significant reduction (~86%) of astrocyte swelling mediated by the AQP4 protein when exposed to manganese. The effects of manganese on cell swelling seem to involve mitogen-activated protein kinases (MAPKs) in astrocytes, since inhibition of ERK1/2/3 and p38-MAPK prevented AQP4 protein increases in the plasma membrane (Rao et al., 2010).

Zinc

Zinc is an essential trace element for all cells, involved in various metabolic and signaling pathways as component of regulatory and catalytic proteins (Mizuno and Kawahara, 2013). In the brain, zinc is mostly bound to proteins and has important modulatory functions in glutamatergic synapses (Tamano and Takeda, 2011). Zinc intoxication is a consequence of inhalation, ingestion, or manipulation of metal. Free intracellular Zn^{2+}, which is present during intoxication, generates oxidative stress in neurons and astrocytes and modulates neuronal activity.

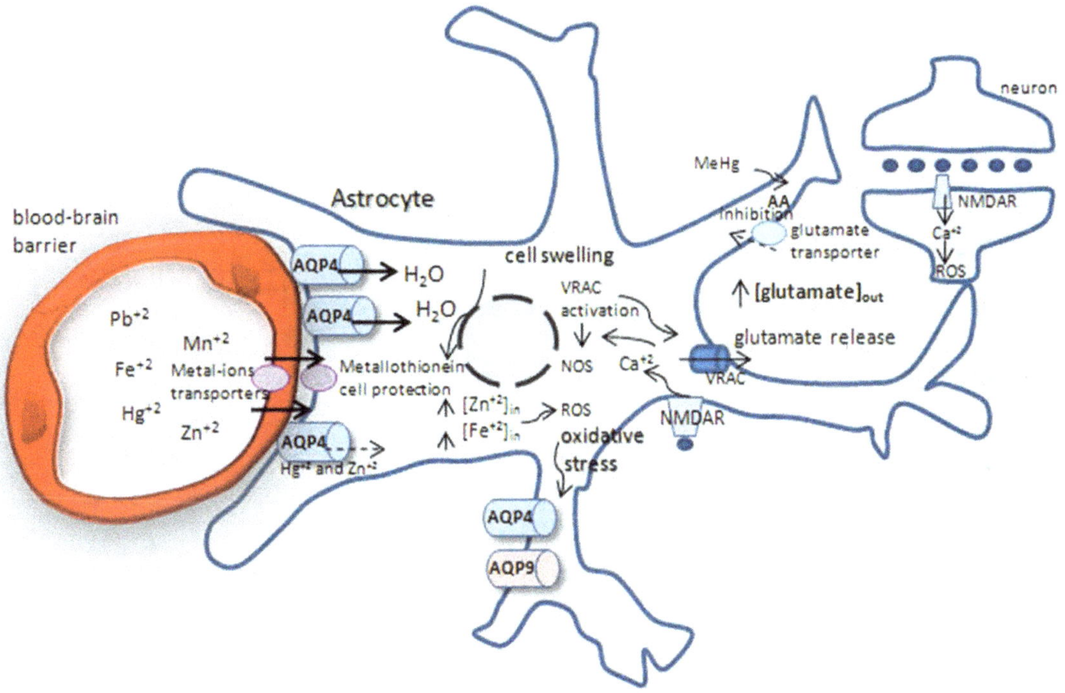

FIGURE 1 | Possible mechanisms involved in brain protection or swelling after metal-ion intoxication. After crossing the blood-brain barrier metal-ions are taken up by astrocytes. Fe^{+2}, Mn^{+2}, Pb^{+2} increase water permeability throughout aquaporin-4 (AQP4), leading to cell swelling and glutamate release from astrocytes by volume-regulated anion channels (VRACs), increasing extracellular glutamate pool. Glutamate acts via NMDA receptor in neurons and astrocytes, increasing $[Ca_i^{+2}]$ and reactive oxygen species (ROS) production, generating oxidative stress. Methylmercury (MeHg) reduces cystein uptake, increasing ROS production. Oxidative stress leads to increase in AQP4 and AQP9 in astrocytes, which leads to cell swelling.

In the brain, Zn^{2+} is mainly distributed in membrane-bound metalloproteins and presynaptic vesicles in glutamatergic neurons. When the amount of free Zn^{2+} increases in the brain, oxidative stress is triggered and activates nitric oxide synthetase (NOS), which in turn releases Zn^{2+} from intracellular stores and activates apoptosis. Increases in free Zn^{2+} promote cellular swelling (Kruczek et al., 2009). Cultured rat astrocytes exposed to a hypo-osmotic milieu (205 mosm/L) increased Zn^{2+} concentrations in the cytoplasm, mitochondria, and nucleus. Hypo-osmotic-dependent zinc increase in astrocytes seems to be trigged by Ca^{2+} and ROS intracellular signaling, as antagonists of the NMDA receptor prevent hypo-osmotic Zn^{2+} increase (Kruczek et al., 2009). Hypo-osmotic effects in astrocytes can be mediated in part by the recently identified AQP4e isoform (Moe et al., 2008). Rat astrocytes transfected with AQP4e and maintained in hypo-osmolar solution (200 mosm/L) showed a transitory increase of AQP4e membrane insertion, concomitant with diminished mobility of the AQPe-carrying vesicles. Depolymerization of vimentin filaments in the cytoskeleton under hypo-osmotic conditions would contribute to the AQPe mobility and membrane insertion (Potokar et al., 2013).

Zinc seems to have an inhibitory effect on water permeability, as demonstrated in AQP4.M23 expressed in proteoliposomes. The Cys178 residue in AQP4 is a potential site for the inhibitory effect of zinc on water permeability, since mutation of this residue resulted in no change in water permeability after zinc exposure (Yukutake et al., 2009).

Iron

Iron is an essential metal in multiple metabolic reactions, including DNA synthesis, enzymatic reactions, and electron transport. Iron accumulation is very deleterious for brain functions due to its wide participation in metabolic reactions (Schipper, 2012; Rouault, 2013). Iron intoxication is not common; however, iron deposition in cells occurs frequently after intracerebral hemorrhage (ICH), a subtype of stroke with high morbidity and mortality in humans.

As early as 24 h after ICH, iron content increases in the perihematomal zone and peaks at day 7. AQP4 expression peaks at day 3 and is maintained until day 7. Brain water content follows the initial increase of AQP4 and then declines slowly until day 14 post ICH onset. AQP4 expression is increased in astrocytes near the perihematomal area. The iron chelator deferoxamine (DFO) reduced iron deposition, brain water content, and AQP4 level in the perihematomal area, demonstrating a correlation between free iron content and brain swelling mediated by AQP4. Additionally, increased iron deposition and brain water permeability are likely to initiate apoptosis in perihematomal areas (Qing et al., 2009).

Cell damage as a result of increased Fe^{2+} is mediated by the NF-κB p65 protein, which activates ROS production and release of proinflammatory cytokines in astrocytes and microglia, respectively, and consequently increases AQP4 and AQP9 in astrocytes (Wang et al., 2015). These studies evidenced increased iron-dependent water permeability in astrocytes mediated by AQP4, showing a role for free iron brain deposition and increased risk of brain damage.

CONCLUSIONS

Metal ions including iron, zinc, and manganese are essential to metabolic functions, protein synthesis, neurotransmission, and antioxidant neuroprotective mechanisms. However, in the CNS, unbalanced essential metal ion amounts, as well as non-essential metal accumulations, are detrimental to brain function.

Toxic amounts of non-essential metals and breakdown of metal ion homeostasis result in changes in brain metabolism and water permeability. These changes are particularly related to increased AQP4 expression in the astrocytes surrounding the BBB, the development of oxidative stress in neurons and astrocytes, and brain swelling, leading to neurodegeneration.

AUTHOR CONTRIBUTIONS

The author confirms being the sole contributor of this work and approved it for publication.

REFERENCES

Agre, P., Bonhivers, M., and Borgnia, M. J. (1998). The aquaporins, blueprints for cellular plumbing systems. *J. Biol. Chem.* 273, 14659–14662. doi: 10.1074/jbc.273.24.14659

Aschner, M. (2000). Manganese: brain transport and emerging research needs. *Environ. Health Perspect.* 108(Suppl. 3), 429–432. doi: 10.1289/ehp.00108s3429

Assentoft, M., Kaptan, S., Fenton, R. A., Hua, S. Z., de Groot, B. L., and MacAulay, N. (2013). Phosphorylation of rat aquaporin-4 at Ser(111) is not required for channel gating. *Glia* 61, 1101–1112. doi: 10.1002/glia.22498

Assentoft, M., Larsen, B. R., Olesen, E. T., Fenton, R. A., and MacAulay, N. (2014). AQP4 plasma membrane trafficking or channel gating is not significantly modulated by phosphorylation at COOH-terminal serine residues. *Am. J. Physiol. Cell Physiol.* 307, C957–C965. doi: 10.1152/ajpcell.00182.2014

Benga, G., Popescu, O., and Pop, V. I. (1985). Water exchange through erythrocyte membranes: p-chloromercuribenzene sulfonate inhibition of water diffusion in ghosts studied by a nuclear magnetic resonance technique. *Biosci. Rep.* 5, 223–228. doi: 10.1007/BF01119591

Erikson, K. M., Dobson, A. W., Dorman, D. C., and Aschner, M. (2004). Manganese exposure and induced oxidative stress in the rat brain. *Sci. Total Environ.* 334–335, 409–416. doi: 10.1016/j.scitotenv.2004.04.044

Gunnarson, E., Axehult, G., Baturina, G., Zelenin, S., Zelenina, M., and Aperia, A. (2005). Lead induces increased water permeability in astrocytes expressing aquaporin 4. *Neuroscience* 136, 105–114. doi: 10.1016/j.neuroscience.2005.07.027

Jung, J. S., Bhat, R. V., Preston, G. M., Guggino, W. B., Baraban, J. M., and Agre, P. (1994). Molecular characterization of an aquaporin cDNA from brain: candidate osmoreceptor and regulator of water balance. *Proc. Natl. Acad. Sci. U.S.A.* 91, 13052–13056. doi: 10.1073/pnas.91.26.13052

Kress, G. J., Dineley, K. E., and Reynolds, I. J. (2002). The relationship between intracellular free iron and cell injury in cultured neurons, astrocytes, and oligodendrocytes. *J. Neurosci.* 22, 5848–5855.

Kruczek, C., Görg, B., Keitel, V., Pirev, E., Kröncke, K. D., Schliess, F., et al. (2009). Hypoosmotic swelling affects zinc homeostasis in cultured rat astrocytes. *Glia* 57, 79–92. doi: 10.1002/glia.20737

Mizuno, D., and Kawahara, M. (2013). The molecular mechanisms of zinc neurotoxicity and the pathogenesis of vascular type senile dementia. *Int. J. Mol. Sci.* 14, 22067–22081. doi: 10.3390/ijms141122067

Moe, S. E., Sorbo J. G., Sogaard, R., Zeuthen, T., Petter Ottersen, O., and Holen, T. (2008). New isoforms of rat aquaporin-4. *Genomics* 91, 367–377. doi: 10.1016/j.ygeno.2007.12.003

Nagelhus, E. A., Horio, Y., Inanobe, A., Fujita, A., Haug, F. M., Nielsen, S., et al. (1999). Immunogold evidence suggests that coupling of K+ siphoning and water transport in rat retinal Müller cells is mediated by a coenrichment of Kir4.1 and AQP4 in specific membrane domains. *Glia* 26, 47–54.

Needleman, H. (2004). Lead Poisoning. *Annu. Rev. Med.* 55, 209–222. doi: 10.1146/annurev.med.55.091902.103653

Ni, M., Li, X., Rocha, J. B., Farina, M., and Aschner, M. (2012). Glia and methylmercury neurotoxicity. *J. Toxicol. Environ. Health A* 75, 1091–1101. doi: 10.1080/15287394.2012.697840

Ni, M., Li, X., Yin, Z., Sidoryk-Węgrzynowicz, M., Jiang, H., Farina, M., et al. (2011). Comparative study on the response of rat primary astrocytes and microglia to methylmercury toxicity. *Glia* 59, 810–820. doi: 10.1002/glia.21153

Nielsen, S., Nagelhus, E. A., Amiry-Moghaddam, M., Bourque, C., Agre, P., and Ottersen, O. P. (1997). Specialized membrane domains for water transport in glial cells: high-resolution immunogold cytochemistry of aquaporin-4 in rat brain. *J. Neurosci.* 17, 171–180.

Nielsen, S., Smith, B. L., Christensen, E. I., and Agre, P. (1993). Distribution of the aquaporin CHIP in secretory and resorptive epithelia and capillary endothelia. *Proc. Natl. Acad. Sci. U.S.A.* 90, 7275–7279. doi: 10.1073/pnas.90.15.7275

Noguchi, Y., Shinozaki, Y., Fujishita, K., Shibata, K., Imura, Y., Morizawa, Y., et al. (2013). Astrocytes protect neurons against methylmercury via ATP/P2Y$_1$ receptor-mediated pathways in astrocytes. *PLoS ONE* 8:e57898. doi: 10.1371/journal.pone.0057898

Paoletti, P., Ascher, P., and Neyton, J. (1997). High-affinity zinc inhibition of NMDA NR1-NR2A receptors. *J. Neurosci.* 17, 5711–5725.

Park, J. D., and Zheng, W. (2012). Human exposure and health effects of inorganic and elemental mercury. *J. Prev. Med. Public Health.* 45, 344–352. doi: 10.3961/jpmph.2012.45.6.344

Potokar, M., Stenovec, M., Jorgačevski, J., Holen, T., Kreft, M., Ottersen, O. P., et al. (2013). Regulation of AQP4 surface expression via vesicle mobility in astrocytes. *Glia* 61, 917–928. doi: 10.1002/glia.22485

Qing, W. G., Dong, Y. Q., Ping, T. Q., Lai, L. G., Fang, L. D., Min, H. W., et al. (2009). Brain edema after intracerebral hemorrhage in rats: the role of iron overload and aquaporin 4. *J. Neurosurg.* 110, 462–468. doi: 10.3171/2008.4.JNS17512

Rao, K. V., Jayakumar, A. R., Reddy, P. V., Tong, X., Curtis, K. M., and Norenberg, M. D. (2010). Aquaporin-4 in manganese-treated cultured astrocytes. *Glia* 58, 1490–1499. doi: 10.1002/glia.21023

Rouault, T. A. (2013). Iron metabolism in the CNS: implications for neurodegenerative diseases. *Nat. Rev. Neurosci.* 14, 551–564. doi: 10.1038/nrn3453

Schipper, H. M. (2012). Neurodegeneration with brain iron accumulation-clinical syndromes and neuroimaging. *Biochim. Biophys. Acta* 1822, 350–360. doi: 10.1016/j.bbadis.2011.06.016

Shi, L. B., and Verkman, A. S. (1996). Selected cysteine point mutations confer mercurial sensitivity to the mercurial-insensitive water channel MIWC/AQP-4. *Biochemistry* 35, 538–544. doi: 10.1021/bi9520038

Tamano, H., and Takeda, A. (2011). Dynamic action of neurometals at the synapse. *Metallomics* 3, 656–661. doi: 10.1039/c1mt00008j

Tchounwou, P. B., Yedjou, C. G., Patlolla, A. K., and Sutton, D. J. (2012). Heavy metal toxicity and the environment. *EXS* 101, 133–164. doi: 10.1007/978-3-7643-8340-4_6

Valko, M., Morris, H., and Cronin, M. T. D. (2005). Metals, toxicity and oxidative stress. *Curr. Med. Chem.* 12, 1161–1208. doi: 10.2174/0929867053764635

Wang, B. F., Cui, Z. W., Zhong, Z. H., Sun, Y. H., Sun, Q. F., Yang, G. Y., et al. (2015). Curcumin attenuates brain edema in mice with intracerebral hemorrhage through inhibition of AQP4 and AQP9 expression. *Acta Pharmacol. Sin.* 36, 939–948. doi: 10.1038/aps.2015.47

Yamamoto, M., Takeya, M., Ikeshima-Kataoka, H., Yasui, M., Kawasaki, Y., Shiraishi, M., et al. (2012). Increased expression of aquaporin-4 with methylmercury exposure in the brain of the common marmoset. *J. Toxicol. Sci.* 37, 749–763. doi: 10.2131/jts.37.749

Yang, B., Brown, D., and Verkman, A. S. (1996). The mercurial insensitive water channel (AQP-4) forms orthogonal arrays in stably transfected Chinese hamster ovary cells. *J. Biol. Chem.* 271, 4577–4580. doi: 10.1074/jbc.271.9.4577

Yasui, M., Hazama, A., Kwon, T. H., Nielsen, S., Guggino, W. B., and Agre, P. (1999). Rapid gating and anion permeability of an intracellular aquaporin. *Nature* 402, 184–187. doi: 10.1038/46045

Ye, B. J., Kim, B. G., Jeon, M. J., Kim, S. Y., Kim, H. C., Jang, T. W., et al. (2016). Evaluation of mercury exposure level, clinical diagnosis and treatment for mercury intoxication. *Ann. Occup. Environ. Med.* 28:5. doi: 10.1186/s40557-015-0086-8

Yukutake, Y., Hirano, Y., Suematsu, M., and Yasui, M. (2009). Rapid and reversible inhibition of aquaporin-4 by zinc. *Biochemistry* 48, 12059–12061. doi: 10.1021/bi901762y

Yukutake, Y., Tsuji, S., Hirano, Y., Adachi, T., Takahashi, T., Fujihara, K., et al. (2008). Mercury chloride decreases the water permeability of aquaporin-4-reconstituted proteoliposomes. *Biol. Cell* 100, 355–363. doi: 10.1042/BC20070132

Yuste, J. E., Tarragon, E., Campuzano, C. M., and Ros-Bernal, F. (2015). Implications of glial nitric oxide in neurodegenerative diseases. *Front. Cell Neurosci.* 9:322. doi: 10.3389/fncel.2015.00322

4

Interhemispheric Resting-State Functional Connectivity Predicts Severity of Idiopathic Normal Pressure Hydrocephalus

Yousuke Ogata[1,2,3*], *Akihiko Ozaki*[4], *Miho Ota*[1,5], *Yurie Oka*[1], *Namiko Nishida*[6], *Hayato Tabu*[6], *Noriko Sato*[7,8] *and Takashi Hanakawa*[1,3*]

[1] Department of Advanced Neuroimaging, Integrative Brain Imaging Center, National Center of Neurology and Psychiatry, Kodaira, Japan, [2] Biointerfaces Unit, Institute of Innovative Research, Tokyo Institute of Technology, Yokohama, Japan, [3] Department of Functional Brain Research, National Institute of Neuroscience, National Center of Neurology and Psychiatry, Kodaira, Japan, [4] Social Welfare Organization Saiseikai Imperial Gift Foundation, Inc., Osaka Saiseikai Nakatsu Hospital, Osaka, Japan, [5] Department of Mental Disorder Research, National Institute of Neuroscience, National Center of Neurology and Psychiatry, Kodaira, Japan, [6] Kitano Hospital, Tazuke Kofukai Medical Research Institute, Osaka, Japan, [7] Department of Radiology, National Center of Neurology and Psychiatry Hospital, Kodaira, Japan, [8] Department of Clinical Neuroimaging, Integrative Brain Imaging Center, National Center of Neurology and Psychiatry, Kodaira, Japan

Edited by:
Manuel Fernando Casanova,
University of Louisville, United States

Reviewed by:
Zsigmond Tamás Kincses,
University of Szeged, Hungary
Zhong Yin,
University of Shanghai for Science and Technology, China

***Correspondence:**
Yousuke Ogata
ogata@cns.pi.titech.ac.jp
Takashi Hanakawa
hanakawa@ncnp.go.jp

Idiopathic normal pressure hydrocephalus (iNPH) is characterized by a clinical triad (gait disturbance, dementia, and urinary incontinence), and by radiological findings of enlarged ventricles reflecting disturbance of central spinal fluid circulation. A diagnosis of iNPH is sometimes challenging, and the pathophysiological mechanisms underlying the clinical symptoms of iNPH remain largely unknown. Here, we used an emerging MRI technique, resting-state functional connectivity MRI (rsfcMRI), to develop a subsidiary diagnostic technique and to explore the underlying pathophysiological mechanisms of iNPH. rsfcMRI data were obtained from 11 patients with iNPH and 11 age-matched healthy volunteers, yielding rsfcMRI-derived functional connectivity (FC) from both groups. A linear support vector machine classifier was trained to distinguish the patterns of FCs of the patients with iNPH from those of the healthy volunteers. After dimensional reduction, the support vector machine successfully classified the two groups with an accuracy of 80%. Moreover, we found that rsfcMRI-derived FC carried information to predict the severity of the triad in iNPH. FCs relevant to the classification of severity were mainly based on interhemispheric connectivity, suggesting that disruption of the corpus callosum fibers due to ventricular enlargement may explain the triad of iNPH. The present results support the usefulness of rsfcMRI as a tool to understand pathophysiology of iNPH, and also to help with its clinical diagnosis.

Keywords: resting-state functional connectivity MRI, idiopathic normal pressure hydrocephalus, functional connectivity, supervised machine learning, support-vector machine, interhemispheric connectivity

INTRODUCTION

Idiopathic normal pressure hydrocephalus (iNPH) is a cryptogenic disorder characterized clinically by a triad (gait disturbance, cognitive impairment and urinary incontinence), and radiologically by enlarged cerebral ventricles because of non-obstructive disturbance of cerebrospinal fluid (CSF) circulation (Ishikawa, 2004). The diagnosis of iNPH is important, because it is one of the few treatable dementias; namely, the clinical symptoms can be often relieved by a shunt operation. Although typical iNPH shows characteristic neuroradiological findings (Kitagaki et al., 1998; Ishikawa et al., 2008; Mori et al., 2012), the diagnosis of iNPH remains challenging in atypical cases, because no functional biomarkers of iNPH have been established (Leinonen et al., 2011; Jingami et al., 2015). The clinical guidelines of iNPH in Japan recommend a "tap test" involving the drainage of a small amount of CSF (30–50 ml) by a lumbar puncture to predict the effectiveness of a shunt operation. However, the tap test has limitations: it is an invasive procedure and carries some risks of adverse events, such as headache. Additionally, although a positive tap test result has a high predictive value for shunt operation outcomes, a negative result has a low predictive value because of a high false negative rate (Sakakibara et al., 2012). Thus, it is important to develop non-invasive and reliable diagnostic methods for iNPH. In particular, a functional neuroimaging method would not only help with a diagnosis of iNPH, but would also provide insight into the pathophysiological mechanisms of iNPH.

Recently, resting-state functional connectivity MRI (rsfcMRI) has drawn attention as a tool to help with a clinical diagnosis and the evaluation of neuropsychiatric disease. For rsfcMRI, participants are not required to perform demanding cognitive tasks, instead they only have to lie quietly in an MRI scanner. This property is advantageous for the application of rsfcMRI to patients with dementia, who might have difficulty in performing cognitive tasks. In fact, rsfcMRI has recently been applied to neuropsychiatric disorders (Greicius et al., 2004; Damoiseaux et al., 2006; Zhang et al., 2010; Khoo et al., 2015; Takamura and Hanakawa, 2017). In particular, Khoo et al. reported that resting-state functional connectivity (RSFC) was reduced in the default mode network (DMN) in iNPH patients, and that the reduction of the RSFC in DMN was positively correlated with symptoms of iNPH (Khoo et al., 2015). This pioneering study indicates that RSFCs may provide a useful biomarker for the assessment of iNPH. However, an alteration of RSFCs other than DMN remains unclear, because the analysis was limited to the DMN. Thus, it is important to test the contribution of multiple large-scale brain networks to the diagnosis of patients with iNPH. In this regard, an emerging method for a multivariate RSFC analysis is the application of machine-learning classification algorithms (Craddock et al., 2009; Arbabshirani et al., 2013). For example, Craddock and colleagues successfully applied support-vector machine (SVM) classification to identifying a pattern of RSFCs representing major depressive disorder (Craddock et al., 2009). A previous study (Arbabshirani et al., 2013) demonstrated that SVM with RSFC features could classify more accurately patients with neuropsychiatric disease than other linear classification methods. In addition, the SVM is particularly suitable to deal with the classification task with limited number of the training instances, and high feature dimensionality. This availability of SVM is suitable to clinical neuroimaging studies where typically just a limited number of dataset is available.

Recently, several researchers used SVM to examine the diagnostic, and prognostic potential of structural MRI, functional MRI, and rsfcMRI in various areas of neurological, and psychiatric disorders, including mild cognitive impairment, probable dementia of Alzheimer type, major depression, bipolar disorder, and schizophrenia (Chen et al., 2011; Costafreda et al., 2011; Orru et al., 2012; Wee et al., 2012; Zeng et al., 2012).

However, to our knowledge, machine-learning classification has not been applied to iNPH. A supervised machine-learning classification algorithm uses multivariate datasets such as whole-brain RSFC, and is able to classify the data into predetermined categories (i.e., iNPH and healthy). Moreover, a multivariate pattern analysis on RSFC has the potential to classify the severity of disease, like the iNPH grading scale (iNPH-GS).

In this study, we applied SVM to rsfcMRI data to test the hypothesis that differences in RSFCs might differentiate between iNPH patients, and healthy volunteers, and might also discriminate across the severity stages of iNPH symptoms.

METHODS

Participants

Eleven patients with iNPH (iNPH group; 5 male, 6 female; average age ± *SD*: 78.2 ± 6.8 years) and 11 age-matched healthy controls (HC group; 4 male, 7 female; average age ± *SD*: 69.8 ± 13.6) participated in the study. The two groups did not significantly differ in terms of age (two-sample *t*-test, $p = 0.07$) or sex (chi-square test, $p = 0.53$). Nine out of 11 patients fulfilled the criteria for probable iNPH (Ishikawa, 2004; Yamashita et al., 2014): (1) age of 60 years or older; (2) presence of at least one of the classic triad (gait disturbance, cognitive impairment, and urinary incontinence); (3) ventricular dilation with Evans' index >.3; (4) normal CSF pressure and content; (5) exclusion of other neurological or non-neurological disorder; and (6) a positive CSF tap test. Two patients were diagnosed as possible iNPH because the result of a CSF tap test was equivocal. The general clinical status of the iNPH patients was assessed with the iNPH grading scale (iNPH-GS) (Kubo et al., 2008). The iNPH-GS grades the severity of three main categories of symptoms (cognitive impairment, gait disturbance, and urinary disturbance) with five levels ranging from 0 (normal) to 4 (severe). Additionally, cognitive impairment was assessed with the Mini-Mental State Examination (MMSE), and the Frontal Assessment Battery (FAB). From the HC group, only the MMSE was available. The score of the MMSE showed significant differences between the iNPH group (22.8 ± 4.3, mean ± *SD*) and the HC group (28.9 ± 1.0) $[T_{(20)} = 3.93, p < 0.001]$. The profiles and clinical information of the iNPH patients are summarized in **Table 1**.

The iNPH patients were enrolled at the Kitano Hospital and the healthy participants were enrolled at the National Center of Neurology and Psychiatry. All participants gave their informed consent prior to their inclusion in the study according to the study protocol approved by the institutional ethics committee.

rsfcMRI Acquisition

For rsfcMRI, the participants were scanned for 7 min with a 3T-MRI system (Achieva 3.0TX, Philips Medical Systems, Best, The Netherlands). The participants were asked to stay relaxed and to close their eyes, but not to fall asleep, in a comfortable position

TABLE 1 | Profiles of the iNPH patients and healthy controls.

	Age group	MMSE	FAB	iNPH-GS gait	iNPH-GS cognition	iNPH-GS urinary	CSF tap test
iNPH1	80–85	17	10	3	3	0	Positive
iNPH2	80–85	25	11	2	1	1	Positive
iNPH3	70–75	22	10	2	2	0	Positive
iNPH4	70–75	16	9	3	3	3	Positive
iNPH5	76–80	19	6	3	2	2	Positive
iNPH6	70–75	28	13	2	2	2	Positive
iNPH7	80–85	25	6	2	2	0	Positive
iNPH8	66–70	29	13	1	2	0	Negative
iNPH9	76–80	25	17	1	1	0	Negative
iNPH10	76–80	25	16	2	2	4	Positive
iNPH11	86–90	20	12	2	3	2	Positive
iNPH (mean ± *SD*)	78.2 ± 6.8	22.8 ± 4.3	11.2 ± 3.5	2.1 ± 0.7	2.1 ± 0.7	1.3 ± 1.4	
Control (mean ± *SD*)	69.8 ± 13.6	28.9 ± 1.0	NA	NA	NA	NA	NA

MMSE, Mini-Mental State Examination; FAB, Frontal Assessment Battery; iNPH-GS, idiopathic normal pressure hydrocephalus grading scale; NA, not available.

within the scanner. They were also instructed not to think about anything in particular, and not to imagine specific figures or scenes. RsfcMRI data were acquired with a T_2*-weighted echo-planer imaging (EPI) sequence using the following parameters: repetition time (TR) = 3,000 ms, echo time (TE) = 30 ms, flip angle (FA) = 90°, 3-mm slice thickness with a 1-mm gap, voxel size = 1.875 × 1.875 × 3 mm, and 34 slices (descending order). In total, 120 volumes were acquired, and the first 4 volumes were discarded to exclude signal changes arising from T1 saturation effects.

Extracting Functional Connectivity

Preprocessing of the rsfcMRI data was conducted with Statistical Parametric Mapping 8 (SPM8, Well-come Department of Imaging Neuroscience, London, UK) implemented on MATLAB (MATHWORKS, Inc., MA, USA). After slice-timing correction was applied to the EPI images, the images were realigned to the first image, using a rigid-body transformation for correcting head motion. Then, the images were spatially normalized to the EPI image template conforming to the Montreal Neurological Institute (MNI) space, using the SPM normalization algorithm. These normalized images were resampled to a 3 × 3 × 3-mm^3 voxel size. The normalized EPI images were then spatially smoothed with an isotropic Gaussian kernel of 6-mm full width at half maximum. In addition, we computed gray matter, white matter and cerebrospinal fluid (CSF) images as binary masks for later use. High-quality three-dimensional anatomical images were available for the healthy controls, but not for the iNPH patients due to the limitation of scanning time. To avoid introducing a bias to the WM/CSF mask images between the groups, we directly segmented the normalized EPI images into GM, WM, and CSF images in both groups, by using a segmentation algorithm implemented in SPM8. The purpose of the segmentation here was to create masks for WM and CSF to compute signals to be regressed out from the data (denoising). This is recommended for the analysis of rsfMRI since signals from CSF and WM produce pseudo-correlations, resulting in non-zero mean and large standard deviations of the functional connectivity data (Whitfield-Gabrieli and Nieto-Castanon, 2012) For the quality check of our de-noising procedure using the EPI-derived WM, and CSF masks, we computed the degree to which false correlation was corrected by removing the signal from WM, and CSF. The QC results showed that the distribution of correlation coefficients was reasonably corrected to nearby zero mean and small standard deviation (before removal; average of mean = 0.18, average of standard deviation = 0.40, after removal; average of mean = 0.09, average of standard deviation = 0.21). Judging from this QC result, we believe that segmentation procedure has provided WM/CSF signals of reasonable quality to reduce the pseudo-correlation.

After these preprocessing steps, the CONN toolbox (Whitfield-Gabrieli and Nieto-Castanon, 2012) was used for conducting a region-of-interest (ROI)-to-ROI analysis to compute RSFC, indexing the degree of correlation between MRI signal time-courses in each pair of ROIs. For defining ROIs, 90 ROIs were defined according to the automated anatomical labeling (AAL) template implemented in the WFU Pickatlas (Tzourio-Mazoyer et al., 2002; Maldjian et al., 2003). First, we used standard AAL ROIs to compute FC. However, in this procedure, some ROIs overlapped the enlarged ventricles only in the iNPH group. To reduce the effects of the ventricle enlargement onto signals from ROIs, we next created modified AAL ROIs, by removing the intersection of the AAL, and the iNPH ventricle template. The iNPH ventricle template represented a map of voxels affected by enlarged ventricle in a group of iNPH patients compared with a group of healthy elderly subjects (Yamashita et al., 2010). We applied the same set of the modified AAL ROIs to the iNPH patients and healthy subjects. Because the results of SVM classification were essentially the same between the standard and modified AAL versions, we only described the results from the modified AAL approach for simplicity. For the removal of signals of no interest, signals correlated with six motion parameters from the realignment procedure and signals derived from the entire WM and CSF mask were regressed out in each participant, by using a general linear model-based multiple regression.

After that, a signal time-series averaged across voxels was extracted from each ROI. Next, all of the confound-removed time course data underwent band-pass filtering of 0.001–0.1 Hz. Then, the correlation coefficient of the BOLD signal time-course was computed between all the pairs of ROIs, and Fisher's z-transform was applied for each coefficient, yielding an FC matrix including all the ROI pairs in each participant.

Classification Analysis Using Support-Vector Machine

We tested whether RSFC information could classify each participant into the iNPH group or the HC group. To do so, we used a linear SVM, a machine-learning algorithm implemented in the e1071 machine-learning package of R version 3.1.3. SVM is a method for classifying data consisting of multi-dimensional features. SVM labels each data input by computing a hyperplane that best classifies the data in the feature space. Under the context of supervised machine learning, SVM identifies the closest data to a hyperplane as sample (or representative) data, and reconfigures the hyperplane to maximize the distance between the sample data with different labels. We used a z-transformed FC between each ROI pair as a feature and computed weights on the FC for successful classification of the iNPH and HC groups. We also tested if RSFC was able to predict the severity of iNPH patients (i.e., iNPH-GS). For the prediction of iNPH-GS, multi-class SVM with a one-against-all classification method was used. Because the iNPH-GS score of iNPH participants in the present cohort varied from 0 to 3 in the gait assessment, from 0 to 3 in the cognitive assessment, from 0 to 4 in the urinary assessment, these scores were set as a label for classification. Because of the limited number of participants, we included data from healthy volunteers for the training of SVM. Because iNPH-GS assessment was not available for the HC group, the label of these data was assumed to be 0 (normal). First, all the FC pairs were fed in to the SVM algorithm in both analyses as feature quantity. All of the features were scaled internally to zero mean and unit variance. The SVM model was constructed with parameters as follows: linear kernel function, C-classification algorithm, and cost factor = 1. Also, to avoid a bias arising from the asymmetry of labels, we defined class the weight vector as 1 divided by number of each labels (Chang and Lin, 2011). Second, we used a feature selection method with a t-test filter to reduce the feature dimension in view of the excess of features against the number of data samples (Craddock et al., 2009). For the t-test filter, we applied a two-sample t-test on the FC comparing between iNPH and HC, and then employed FC with a difference (p-value threshold = 0.05). To validate the SVM model for predicting a new data set, we employed a leave-one-out cross validation (LOOCV) procedure. In the LOOCV analysis, an SVM was trained with FC from a randomly selected 21 out of the 22 participants. After learning, the performance of the SVM classifier was tested to classify the remaining participant. After this procedure was repeated until the FC from every participant had become the test data, we calculated the classification accuracy as the number of correct labels divided by the number of LOOCV tests. To evaluate the specificity of classification accuracy for iNPH patients, we limited the LOOCV test round to the data derived from the iNPH patients in the iNPH-GS classification. A binomial test was used to determine the significance of the classification accuracy.

RESULTS

Classification between iNPH and HC

When the SVM was trained with all 4,005 pairs of the FC (no feature selection), the classifier was able to distinguish iNPH from HC with an accuracy of 63% (**Figure 1**), which was not significantly different from chance level (binominal test, 14 of 22 LOOCV tests, $p = 0.28$). However, when the SVM was trained with 476 features after the feature selection (t-test filtering), classification accuracy was 81% (**Figure 1**), which was significantly above chance level (18 of 22 tests, $p < 0.01$).

To clarify which FC was important for the classification, we assessed SVM weights, representing the degree of contribution of each FC to the classification. We found that relatively high weights were placed onto the FC between the left superior temporal pole and left inferior frontal operculum, the bilateral insula, the left middle temporal pole, and right hippocampus, the right superior medial frontal cortex, and left superior orbitofrontal cortex, and the left paracentral lobule, and left medial frontal cortex. Interhemispheric connectivity accounted for more than half (56%) of the FCs that contributed to the classification after the t-test filtering. **Figure 2**, **Table 2** show the top 20 FC with high-level weights. These 20 weights accounted for 15.6% of the total weights.

Prediction of iNPH-GS

We next tested whether the RSFCs contained information about the severity of iNPH-related symptoms. Specifically, we applied SVM with LOOCV to FCs to predict the level of gait disturbance,

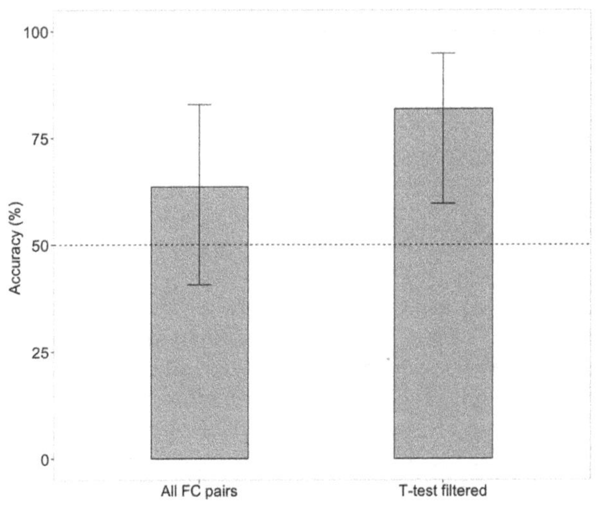

FIGURE 1 | Classification accuracy without **(left)** and with **(right)** future selection. Error bars mean 95% confidence interval from a binomial test.

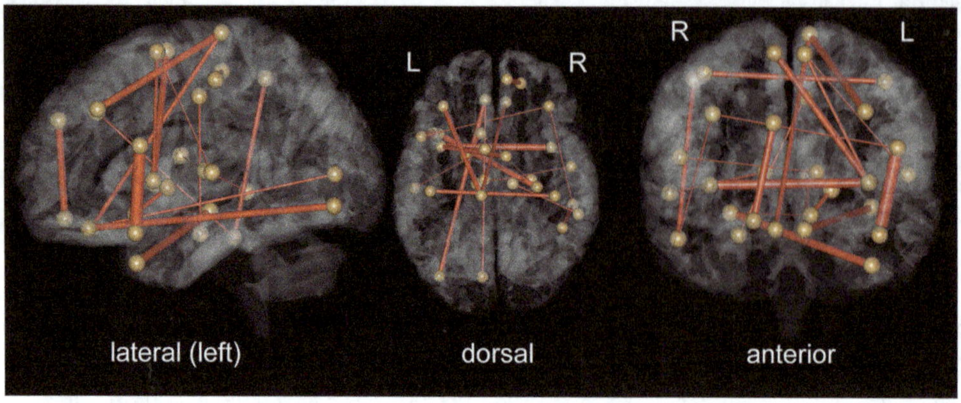

FIGURE 2 | Top 20 functional connectivity pairs contributing to the classification between iNPH and HC groups in the views from the left **(left)**, top **(middle)**, front **(right)**. The spheres represent the barycenter of ROIs, and the lines connecting spheres stand for edges with high SVM weights listed in **Table 2**. The thickness of the lines represents relative SVM weights.

TABLE 2 | SVM weights contributing to the classification of iNPH and HC.

Functional connectivity	Weight of SVM
L superior temporal pole–L inferior frontal operculum	0.0072
R insula–L insula	0.0064
L middle temporal pole–R hippocampus	0.0061
R superior frontal gyrus, medial orbital–L superior frontal gyrus, orbital part	0.0059
L paracentral lobule–L medial frontal cortex	0.0059
L inferior occipital gyrus–L gyrus rectus	0.0058
L insula–R supplementary motor area	0.0058
R postcentral gyrus–L postcentral gyrus	0.0055
R inferior temporal gyrus–R inferior parietal gyrus	0.0054
L paracentral lobule–R gyrus rectus	0.0053
L pallidum–L olfactory cortex	0.0052
L insula–L supplementary motor area	0.0049
L calcarine fissure–L gyrus rectus	0.0048
R parahippocampal gyrus–L median cingulate gyrus	0.0047
R inferior temporal gyrus–R middle frontal gyrus	0.0046
R middle temporal gyrus–R thalamus	0.0046
L superior temporal gyrus–L supplementary motor area	0.0045
L inferior frontal gyrus, opercular part–R middle frontal gyrus	0.0045
L thalamus–R rolandic operculum	0.0044
R hippocampus–L olfactory cortex	0.0043

cognitive impairment and urinary incontinence as indexed by iNPH-GS. This was done after the feature selection by applying t-test filtering comparing the two groups as described above. We found that FC contained significant information concerning the severity of iNPH (**Figure 3**). Classification accuracy was significantly higher than chance when we limited the test round to the data derived from the iNPH patients: 81% for the iNPH-GS cognition (9 out of 11 tests, $p < 0.05$ by a binominal test), 55% for the iNPH-GS gait (6 out of 11 tests, $p < 0.001$), and 72% for the iNPH-GS urinary score (8 tests of 11 tests, $p < 1.0 \times 10^{-7}$).

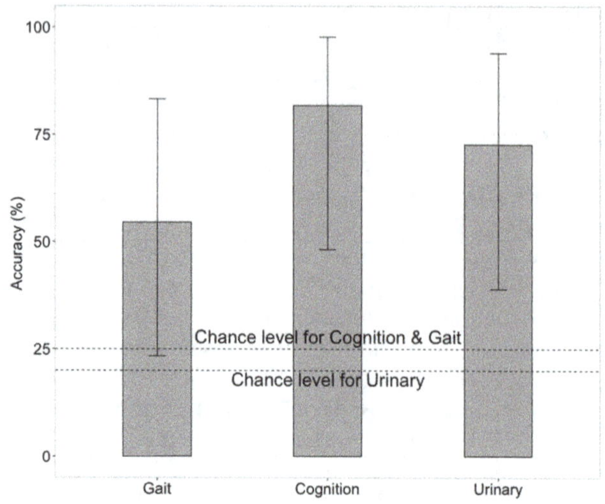

FIGURE 3 | Classification accuracy for severity of iNPH symptoms when we limited the test round to the data derived from the iNPH patients, using functional connectivity as the classification feature. Error bars mean 95% confidence interval of binomial test.

For all the three symptoms, the assessment of SVM weights indicated the importance of inter-hemispheric functional connectivity. The top 30 FCs with high contributions to classification are shown in **Tables 3–5**; **Figure 4**. The sum of these top 30 weights accounts for 16.9% of the total weights for iNPH-GS gait, 16.4% for iNPH-GS cognition, and 15.0% for iNPH-GS urinary incontinence.

To confirm the significance of inter-hemispheric FC for classification, we calculated the sum of weights of inter-hemispheric FC and that of intra-hemispheric FC, all of which contributed to the prediction of iNPH-GS (**Table 6**).

The results showed greater contribution of the inter-hemispheric FC than that of the intra-hemispheric FC significantly for gait ($p = 0.02$, Wilcoxon rank-sum test),

TABLE 3 | SVM weight for classification with iNPH grading scale for gait disturbance.

Functional connectivity	Weight of SVM
iNPH-GS gait	
R postcentral gyrus–L postcentral gyrus	0.048
R paracentral lobule–L paracentral lobule	0.047
R median cingulate gyri–L median cingulate gyri	0.047
R superior frontal gyrus, medial orbital–L superior frontal gyrus, medial orbital	0.046
R cuneus–R calcarine fissure	0.046
R superior frontal gyrus, medial orbital–R superior frontal gyrus, dorsolateral	0.042
R cuneus–L calcarine fissure	0.041
L superior occipital gyrus–L calcarine fissure	0.039
R paracentral lobule–R supplementary motor area	0.038
R inferior frontal gyrus, orbital part–L inferior frontal gyrus, orbital part	0.036
R supplementary motor area–R precentral gyrus	0.036
L paracentral lobule–R supplementary motor area	0.036
L paracentral lobule–R postcentral gyrus	0.036
R angular gyrus–R middle frontal gyrus, orbital part	0.035
L supplementary motor area–L precentral gyrus	0.034
R supplementary motor area–L precentral gyrus	0.033
R inferior temporal gyrus–L inferior temporal gyrus	0.032
R postcentral gyrus–R supplementary motor area	0.032
L paracentral lobule–R precentral gyrus	0.031
L superior frontal gyrus, medial orbital–R superior frontal gyrus, dorsolateral	0.030
R rolandic operculum–L rolandic operculum	0.030
R inferior frontal gyrus, opercular part–R middle frontal gyrus	0.030
R insula–L insula	0.030
R middle temporal gyrus–L superior temporal gyrus	0.030
R precuneus–R superior frontal gyrus, dorsolateral	0.028
R superior frontal gyrus, medial orbital–R middle frontal gyrus	0.028
R hippocampus–L hippocampus	0.028
L middle frontal gyrus, orbital part–L superior frontal gyrus, orbital part	0.028
R inferior frontal gyrus, opercular part–L inferior frontal gyrus, opercular part	0.028
L inferior frontal gyrus, orbital part–L superior frontal gyrus, orbital part	0.028

Bold fonts indicate interhemispheric connectivity.

TABLE 4 | SVM weight for classification with iNPH grading scale for cognitive impairment.

Functional connectivity	Weight of SVM
iNPH-GS cognition	
R superior frontal gyrus, medial orbital–L superior frontal gyrus, medial orbital	0.053
R superior frontal gyrus, medial orbital–R superior frontal gyrus, dorsolateral	0.050
R median cingulate gyri–L median cingulate gyri	0.049
R postcentral gyrus–L postcentral gyrus	0.047
R paracentral lobule–L paracentral lobule	0.046
R cuneus–R calcarine fissure	0.045
R cuneus–L calcarine fissure	0.041
R insular cortex–L insular cortex	0.041
L superior occipital gyrus–L calcarine fissure	0.038
L supplementary motor area–L precentral gyrus	0.038
R supplementary motor area–R precentral gyrus	0.036
R precuneus–R angular gyrus	0.036
R inferior frontal gyrus, orbital part–L inferior frontal gyrus, orbital part	0.036
R angular gyrus–R middle frontal gyrus, orbital part	0.035
L paracentral lobule–R supplementary motor area	0.035
R paracentral lobule–R supplementary motor area	0.034
R angular gyrus–R posterior cingulate gyrus	0.034
R hippocampus–L hippocampus	0.033
L paracentral lobule–R postcentral gyrus	0.033
R rolandic operculum–L rolandic operculum	0.033
R inferior frontal gyrus, opercular part–R middle frontal gyrus	0.033
R superior frontal gyrus, medial orbital–R middle frontal gyrus	0.033
L middle frontal gyrus, orbital part–L superior frontal gyrus, orbital part	0.032
L superior frontal gyrus, medial orbital–R superior frontal gyrus, dorsolateral	0.032
R precuneus–R superior frontal gyrus, dorsolateral	0.032
R postcentral gyrus–R supplementary motor area	0.032
R inferior frontal gyrus, opercular part–L inferior frontal gyrus, opercular part	0.031
R middle temporal gyrus–R precuneus	0.031
R supplementary motor area–L precentral gyrus	0.030
L precuneus–R superior frontal gyrus, dorsolateral	0.029

Bold font indicates interhemispheric connectivity.

cognition ($p = 0.002$), and marginally for urinary symptoms ($p = 0.07$).

DISCUSSION

The SVM classifier, combined with feature selection, was able to learn differences in high-dimensional FCs between the iNPH patients, and the healthy controls, thereby successfully classifying each participant with an accuracy of 80%. Considering the importance, and difficulty of a clinical diagnosis of iNPH, rsfcMRI is promising as a tool for providing a biomarker for the diagnosis of iNPH. Furthermore, the assessment of the spatial distribution of FC contributing to classification has shed light on the pathophysiology of iNPH.

FCs having relevance to the classification of iNPH included the superior temporal pole, middle temporal pole, insula, orbitofrontal cortex, and medial frontal cortex. Almost all of these areas were located near the enlarged cerebral sulci (i.e., increased CSF space) in iNPH patients as shown in a previous voxel-based morphometry study (Yamashita et al., 2010, 2014). In a study by Lenfeldt et al. (2008), the left dorsal premotor cortex and bilateral supplementary motor areas (SMA) showed enhanced activation during hand motor task performance after a three-day continuous CSF drainage in iNPH patients (Lenfeldt et al., 2008). In the present study, FC between insula and SMA, and between bilateral postcentral gyri showed relatively high

TABLE 5 | SVM weight for classification with iNPH grading scale for urinary incontinence.

Functional connectivity	Weight of SVM
iNPH-GS urinary	
R superior frontal gyrus, medial orbital–L superior frontal gyrus, medial orbital	0.047
R median cingulate gyri–L median cingulate gyri	0.043
R superior frontal gyrus, medial orbita–R superior frontal gyrus, dorsolateral	0.042
R postcentral gyrus–L postcentral gyrus	0.036
R paracentral lobule–L paracentral lobule	0.035
R superior frontal gyrus, medial orbital–R middle frontal gyrus	0.034
R cuneus–R calcarine fissure	0.034
R cuneus–L calcarine fissure	0.034
R hippocampus–L hippocampus	0.032
R insular cortex–L insular cortex	0.032
R inferior frontal gyrus, orbital part–L inferior frontal gyrus, orbital part	0.032
R precuneus–R superior frontal gyrus, dorsolateral	0.032
R inferior frontal gyrus, opercular part–R middle frontal gyrus	0.031
L superior frontal gyrus, medial orbital–R superior frontal gyrus, dorsolateral	0.031
L supplementary motor area–L precentral gyrus	0.030
R angular gyrus–R middle frontal gyrus, orbital part	0.030
L precuneus–R superior frontal gyrus, dorsolateral	0.029
R supplementary motor area–R precentral gyrus	0.029
L superior occipital gyrus–L calcarine fissure	0.028
R inferior frontal gyrus, opercular part–L inferior frontal gyrus, opercular part	0.028
L paracentral lobule–R supplementary motor area	0.028
L inferior frontal gyrus, orbital part–L superior frontal gyrus, orbital part	0.028
L inferior frontal gyrus, opercular part–L middle frontal gyrus	0.028
L paracentral lobule–R postcentral gyrus	0.027
R middle temporal gyrus–R superior frontal gyrus, dorsolateral	0.027
R rolandic operculum–L rolandic operculum	0.027
R angular gyrus–R posterior cingulate gyrus	0.027
L paracentral lobule–R precentral gyrus	0.026
R postcentral gyrus–R supplementary motor area	0.026
L postcentral gyrus–R supplementary motor area	0.026

Bold font indicates interhemispheric connectivity.

contribution to the classification of iNPH, and HC as indexed by the SVM weights. Additionally, it is suggested that that the effectiveness of CSF drainage possibly results from the reversal of subcortical chronic ischemia, especially in the periventricular zones (Momjian et al., 2004; Malm and Eklund, 2006; Lenfeldt et al., 2008). Our results suggest that the contribution of periventricular areas to the iNPH-HC classification may indicate the abnormality of these FCs because of the compression of fiber connections by enlarged ventricles.

Moreover, the prediction of iNPH-GS indicated the relevance of inter-hemispheric connectivity to the discrimination of the triad: gait disturbance, cognitive impairment, and urinary incontinence. This finding is consistent with the idea that damage to the inter-hemispheric connections via the corpus callosum may underlie the pathophysiology of iNPH. A majority of previous diffusion tensor imaging studies have observed lower fractional anisotropy (FA) values in the corpus callosum in iNPH patients than in normal controls. For instance, Koyama et al. showed that there was a conspicuous decline in FA values in the corpus callosum in iNPH patients, and that the degree of FA reduction was associated with the severity of gait disturbance, which is the most frequent clinical manifestation of iNPH (Koyama et al., 2012, 2013). Consistent with this result, the reduction of FA in the corpus callosum is correlated with gait disturbance and cognitive decline in patients with age-related white matter changes (Iseki et al., 2015). In this study, the corpus callosum connections are suggested to mediate information relevant to gait planning.

Previous imaging studies suggest that the micturition center is located in the pons, and that SMA is involved in the inhibitory control of the micturition reflex (Fukuyama et al., 1996; Zhang et al., 2005). Because we did not include the pons in the ROI set, the results of the present study would mainly reflect the decline of functional connections to and from the SMA related to the inhibitory control of micturition. The insular cortex and cingulate cortex are thought to be involved in the regulation of the bladder filling sensation and void control (Fowler et al., 2008; de Groat et al., 2015). In our results, the interhemispheric connectivity of cingulate cortex, and insular cortex showed respectively high weights for iNPH-GS urinary classification (see **Table 5**).

To account for cognitive impairment in iNPH, the present finding of inter-hemispheric disconnectivity in iNPH is consistent with the findings that the severity of Alzheimer's disease is correlated with the reduction of volume and FA in the corpus callosum (Chaim et al., 2007; Tomaiuolo et al., 2007). Additionally, Khoo and coworkers have demonstrated that the reduction of RSFC in the DMN was positively correlated with iNPH-GS cognition and urinary incontinence in the iNPH patients (Khoo et al., 2015). Consistent with this result, the present study showed that interhemispheric connectivity in the medial orbital part of the superior frontal gyrus, a part of the DMN, had high weight for all symptoms for iNPH-GS classification. Several researchers reported that white matter alterations in NPH include not only the reduction of FA, but also the alteration of mean diffusivity (MD) and radial diffusivity (RD) (Hattingen et al., 2010; Kanno et al., 2011). In addition, a recent study by Horinek et al. demonstrated reduced FA in the corpus callosum and increased FA, MD, and RD in the cortico-fugal fibers in NPH patients (Horinek et al., 2016). It is possible that the alteration of interhemispheric FC in the iNPH patients shown here is founded on the structural changes of the white matter indexed by those diffusion measures. In sum, the present study suggests the importance of interhemispheric functional connectivity in accounting for the triad of iNPH. For the treatment of iNPH, it is well-recognized that the symptoms are relievable by a shunt operation. The improvement of iNPH triads by CSF drainage can be explained by the idea that a shunt operation releases the compression of the corpus callosum and restores the inter-hemispheric functional connectivity. In a study

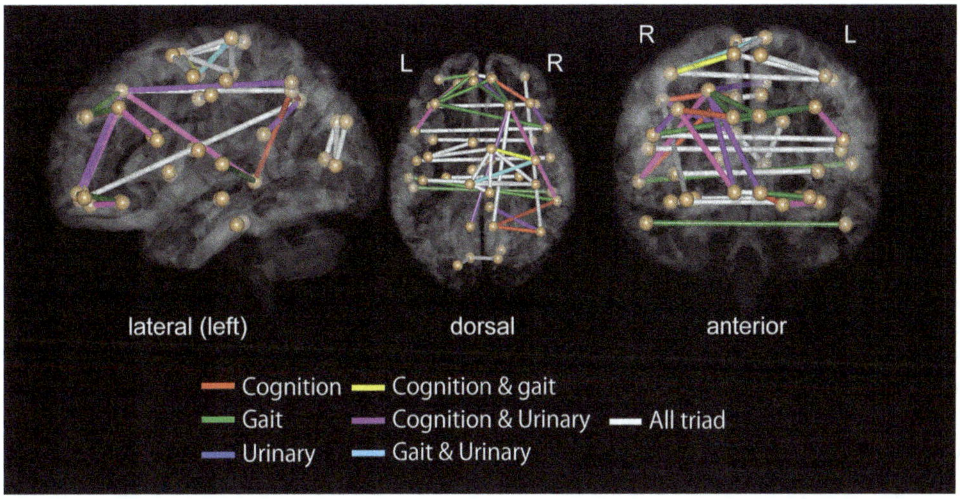

FIGURE 4 | Top 30 functional connectivity with higher SVM weights in classification for iNPH grading scale as viewed from the left **(left)**, top **(middle)**, and front **(right)**. Spheres represent the barycenter of each ROI, and lines between spheres stand for connections that showed higher SVM weights listed in **Tables 3–5**.

TABLE 6 | Sum of SVM weights from inter-hemispheric and intra-hemispheric connectivity contributing to prediction of iNPH-GS.

	iNPH-GS gait	iNPH-GS cognition	iNPH-GS urinary
Inter-hemispheric connectivity	3.361	3.568	4.057
Intra-hemispheric connectivity	2.873	3.190	3.441

by Scheel et al. (2012), abnormality of the corpus callosum FA in iNPH patients showed a trend toward normalization following shunt surgery. It is likely that the enlarged ventricles compressed the corpus callosum, affecting inter-hemispheric functional connectivity. The present findings also suggest that the degree of such compression and the resulting functional disconnectivity are correlated with the severity of iNPH symptoms.

This study has several limitations. First, the present data are derived from a relatively small number of participants. Moreover, we acquired data with the same MRI aperture and EPI sequences, but in different hospital sites. This was for a purely practical reason; scanning of the healthy population was not possible in one hospital, and iNPH patients were not available in the other hospital. It is possible that differences in the sites affected the characteristics of the MRI data, because between-site reliability might be relatively low compared with test-retest reliability (Friedman et al., 2008). However, Turner and collages carried out a multi-site rsfcMRI study on schizophrenia patients, and suggested that critical RSFC information important for disease classification was preserved when the scanner model, and scanning parameters were the same. In the present study, we used the same MRI model, and scanning parameters. Therefore, we believe that the difference in site did not critically impair the RSFC information important for the disease/severity classification.

Second, we were not able to associate the present findings with the information regarding treatment of iNPH, such as responsiveness to a CSF tap test. Aoki et al. (2013, 2015) found that responders to a shunt operation showed higher variance in the power of beta-frequency electroencephalography oscillations in the right fronto-temporo-occipital region than non-responders. Because a CSF tapping test is an invasive procedure and carries some risks of adverse events, we agree that predicting the responsiveness to a CSF tap test beforehand is of clinical benefit. However, we only had two negative responders to a tap test, precluding further analysis between responders, and non-responders. The question of whether rsfcMRI-derived functional connectivity can predict the responsiveness to CSF drainage should be tested in the future.

Finally, it may be possible to enhance classification accuracy by improving the machine learning algorithm. Recently, many methods have been proposed such as linear discrimination analysis, random forest, and sparse logistic regression (Yamashita et al., 2008). We used SVM for the machine-learning classifier, because SVM does not need many samples under the condition that the number of feature dimensions is optimally reduced (Hua et al., 2005). Moreover, classification accuracy may be further improved by optimizing the cost function, kernel type, and classification algorithm. However, considering the computational cost, the exploration of the huge parameter space is beyond the scope of the present study. Future challenges include the improvement of classification accuracy by optimizing the classifiers and feature selection methods. Future challenges include the improvement of classification accuracy by optimizing the classifiers and feature selection methods.

CONCLUSION

In conclusion, a machine-learning algorithm combined with rsfcMRI data was able to discriminate between patients with iNPH and elderly controls. This result indicates that iNPH patients have abnormalities in the RSFC, especially in inter-hemispheric functional connectivity, which contributed to the classification of clinical stages. RsfcMRI may have the potential to discriminate iNPH from other neurological diseases, contributing to a differential diagnosis of iNPH.

AUTHOR CONTRIBUTIONS

YOg designed the study, performed analyses and literature review, and drafted the manuscript. AO, MO, NN, HT, NS recruited healthy volunteers and iNPH patients and performed experiments. YOk developed experimental and analytic programs. TH designed the study and supervised the research and revised the manuscript. All the authors read and approved the final manuscript.

ACKNOWLEDGMENTS

This study was in part supported by the Strategic Research Program for Brain Science of BMI Technologies for Clinical Application carried out under the Strategic Research Program for Brain Sciences and Brain Mapping by Integrated Neurotechnologies for Disease Studies (Brain/MINDS), Health Labor Science Research Grants from Japan Agency for Medical Research and development (AMED) and KAKENHI (26120008 and 16H03306) from MEXT, the Research Grant from Saiseikai, and the Intramural Research Grant for Neurological and Psychiatric Disorders of National Center of Neurology and Psychiatry, Japan, to TH. This study was partially supported by JSPS KAKENHI Grant Number 15K16080 to YOg. This study was also in part supported by JSPS KAKENHI Grant Number 15K10378 to NN.

REFERENCES

Aoki, Y., Kazui, H., Tanaka, T., Ishii, R., Wada, T., Ikeda, S., et al. (2015). Noninvasive prediction of shunt operation outcome in idiopathic normal pressure hydrocephalus. *Sci. Rep.* 5:775. doi: 10.1038/srep07775

Aoki, Y., Kazui, H., Tanaka, T., Ishii, R., Wada, T., Ikeda, S., et al. (2013). EEG and neuronal activity topography analysis can predict effectiveness of shunt operation in idiopathic normal pressure hydrocephalus patients. *NeuroImage* 3, 522–530. doi: 10.1016/j.nicl.2013.10.009

Arbabshirani, M. R., Kiehl, K. A., Pearlson, G. D., and Calhoun, V. D. (2013). Classification of schizophrenia patients based on resting-state functional network connectivity. *Front. Neurosci.* 7:133. doi: 10.3389/fnins.2013.00133

Chaim, T. M., Duran, F. L., Uchida, R. R., Perico, C. A., de Castro, C. C., and Busatto, G. F. (2007). Volumetric reduction of the corpus callosum in Alzheimer's disease *in vivo* as assessed with voxel-based morphometry. *Psychiatry Res.* 154, 59–68. doi: 10.1016/j.pscychresns.2006.04.003

Chang, C. C., and Lin, C. J. (2011). LIBSVM: a library for support vector machines. *Acm Trans. Intell. Syst. Technol.* 2:27. doi: 10.1145/1961189.1961199

Chen, G., Ward, B. D., Xie, C., Li, W., Wu, Z., Jones, J. L., et al. (2011). Classification of Alzheimer disease, mild cognitive impairment, and normal cognitive status with large-scale network analysis based on resting-state functional MR imaging. *Radiology* 259, 213–221. doi: 10.1148/radiol.10100734

Costafreda, S. G., Fu, C. H. Y., Picchioni, M., Toulopoulou, T., McDonald, C., Kravariti, E., et al. (2011). Pattern of neural responses to verbal fluency shows diagnostic specificity for schizophrenia and bipolar disorder. *BMC Psychiatry* 11:18. doi: 10.1186/1471-244X-11-18

Craddock, R. C., Holtzheimer, P. E. III, Hu, X. P., and Mayberg, H. S. (2009). Disease state prediction from resting state functional connectivity. *Magn. Reson. Med.* 62, 1619–1628. doi: 10.1002/mrm.22159

Damoiseaux, J. S., Rombouts, S., Barkhof, F., Scheltens, P., Stam, C. J., Smith, S. M., et al. (2006). Consistent resting-state networks across healthy subjects. *Proc. Natl. Acad. Sci. U.S.A.* 103, 13848–13853. doi: 10.1073/pnas.0601417103

de Groat, W. C., Griffiths, D., and Yoshimura, N. (2015). Neural control of the lower urinary tract. *Compr. Physiol.* 5, 327–396. doi: 10.1002/cphy.c130056

Fowler, C. J., Griffiths, D., and de Groat, W. C. (2008). The neural control of micturition. *Nat. Rev. Neurosci.* 9, 453–466. doi: 10.1038/nrn2401

Friedman, L., Stern, H., Brown, G. G., Mathalon, D. H., Turner, J., Glover, G. H., et al. (2008). Test-retest and between-site reliability in a multicenter fMRI study. *Hum. Brain Mapp.* 29, 958–972. doi: 10.1002/hbm.20440

Fukuyama, H., Matsuzaki, S., Ouchi, Y., Yamauchi, H., Nagahama, Y., Kimura, J., et al. (1996). Neural control of micturition in man examined with single photon emission computed tomography using 99mTc-HMPAO. *Neuroreport* 7, 3009–3012. doi: 10.1097/00001756-199611250-00042

Greicius, M. D., Srivastava, G., Reiss, A. L., and Menon, V. (2004). Default-mode network activity distinguishes Alzheimer's disease from healthy aging: evidence from functional MRI. *Proc. Natl. Acad. Sci. U.S.A.* 101, 4637–4642. doi: 10.1073/pnas.0308627101

Hattingen, E., Jurcoane, A., Melber, J., Blasel, S., Zanella, F. E., Neumann-Haefelin, T., et al. (2010). Diffusion tensor imaging in patients with adult chronic idiopathic hydrocephalus. *Neurosurgery* 66, 917–924. doi: 10.1227/01.NEU.0000367801.35654.EC

Horinek, D., Stepan-Buksakowska, I., Szabo, N., Erickson, B. J., Toth, E., Sulc, V., et al. (2016). Difference in white matter microstructure in differential diagnosis of normal pressure hydrocephalus and Alzheimer's disease. *Clin. Neurol. Neurosurg.* 140, 52–59. doi: 10.1016/j.clineuro.2015.11.010

Hua, J., Xiong, Z., Lowey, J., Suh, E., and Dougherty, E. R. (2005). Optimal number of features as a function of sample size for various classification rules. *Bioinformatics* 21, 1509–1515. doi: 10.1093/bioinformatics/bti171

Iseki, K., Fukuyama, H., Oishi, N., Tomimoto, H., Otsuka, Y., Nankaku, M., et al. (2015). Freezing of gait and white matter changes: a tract-based spatial statistics study. *J. Clin. Mov. Disord.* 2:1. doi: 10.1186/s40734-014-0011-2

Ishikawa, M. (2004). Clinical guidelines for idiopathic normal pressure hydrocephalus. *Neurol. Med. Chir.* 44, 222–223. doi: 10.2176/nmc.44.222

Ishikawa, M., Hashimoto, M., Kuwana, N., Mori, E., Miyake, H., Wachi, A., et al. (2008). Guidelines for management of idiopathic normal pressure hydrocephalus. *Neurol. Med. Chir.* 48, S1–S23. doi: 10.2176/nmc.48.S1

Jingami, N., Asada-Utsugi, M., Uemura, K., Noto, R., Takahashi, M., Ozaki, A., et al. (2015). Idiopathic normal pressure hydrocephalus has a different cerebrospinal fluid biomarker profile from Alzheimer's disease. *J. Alzheimers. Dis.* 45, 109–115. doi: 10.3233/JAD-142622

Kanno, S., Abe, N., Saito, M., Takagi, M., Nishio, Y., Hayashi, A., et al. (2011). White matter involvement in idiopathic normal pressure hydrocephalus: a voxel-based diffusion tensor imaging study. *J. Neurol.* 258, 1949–1957. doi: 10.1007/s00415-011-6038-5

Khoo, H. M., Kishima, H., Tani, N., Oshino, S., Maruo, T., Hosomi, K., et al. (2015). Default mode network connectivity in patients with idiopathic normal pressure hydrocephalus. *J. Neurosurg.* 124, 350–358. doi: 10.3171/2015.1.JNS141633

Kitagaki, H., Mori, E., Ishii, K., Yamaji, S., Hirono, N., and Imamura, T. (1998). CSF spaces in idiopathic normal pressure hydrocephalus: morphology and volumetry. *Am. J. Neuroradiol.* 19, 1277–1284.

Koyama, T., Marumoto, K., Domen, K., and Miyake, H. (2013). White matter characteristics of idiopathic normal pressure hydrocephalus: a diffusion tensor tract-based spatial statistic study. *Neurol. Med. Chir.* 53, 601–608. doi: 10.2176/nmc.oa2012-0307

Koyama, T., Marumoto, K., Domen, K., Ohmura, T., and Miyake, H. (2012). Diffusion tensor imaging of idiopathic normal pressure hydrocephalus: a voxel-based fractional anisotropy study. *Neurol. Med. Chir.* 52, 68–74. doi: 10.2176/nmc.52.68

Kubo, Y., Kazui, H., Yoshida, T., Kito, Y., Kimura, N., Tokunaga, H., et al. (2008). Validation of grading scale for evaluating symptoms of idiopathic normal-pressure hydrocephalus. *Dement. Geriatr. Cogn. Disord.* 25, 37–45. doi: 10.1159/000111149

Leinonen, V., Menon, L. G., Carroll, R. S., Dello Iacono, D., Grevet, J., Jaaskelainen, J. E., et al. (2011). Cerebrospinal fluid biomarkers in idiopathic normal pressure hydrocephalus. *Int. J. Alzheimers. Dis.* 2011:312526. doi: 10.4061/2011/312526

Lenfeldt, N., Larsson, A., Nyberg, L., Andersson, M., Birgander, R., Eklund, A., et al. (2008). Idiopathic normal pressure hydrocephalus: increased supplementary motor activity accounts for improvement after CSF drainage. *Brain* 131, 2904–2912. doi: 10.1093/brain/awn232

Maldjian, J. A., Laurienti, P. J., Kraft, R. A., and Burdette, J. H. (2003). An automated method for neuroanatomic and cytoarchitectonic atlas-based interrogation of fMRI data sets. *Neuroimage* 19, 1233–1239. doi: 10.1016/S1053-8119(03)00169-1

Malm, J., and Eklund, A. (2006). Idiopathic normal pressure hydrocephalus. *Pract. Neurol.* 6, 14–27. doi: 10.1136/jnnp.2006.088351

Momjian, S., Owler, B. K., Czosnyka, Z., Czosnyka, M., Pena, A., and Pickard, J. D. (2004). Pattern of white matter regional cerebral blood flow and autoregulation in normal pressure hydrocephalus. *Brain* 127, 965–972. doi: 10.1093/brain/awh131

Mori, E., Ishikawa, M., Kato, T., Kazui, H., Miyake, H., Miyajima, M., et al. (2012). Guidelines for management of idiopathic normal pressure hydrocephalus: second edition. *Neurol. Med. Chir.* 52, 775–809. doi: 10.2176/nmc.52.775

Orru, G., Pettersson-Yeo, W., Marquand, A. F., Sartori, G., and Mechelli, A. (2012). Using support vector machine to identify imaging biomarkers of neurological and psychiatric disease: a critical review. *Neurosci. Biobehav. Rev.* 36, 1140–1152. doi: 10.1016/j.neubiorev.2012.01.004

Sakakibara, R., Uchida, Y., Ishii, K., Kazui, H., Hashimoto, M., Ishikawa, M., et al. (2012). Correlation of right frontal hypoperfusion and urinary dysfunction in iNPH: A SPECT study. *Neurourol. Urodyn.* 31, 50–55. doi: 10.1002/nau.21222

Scheel, M., Diekhoff, T., Sprung, C., and Hoffmann, K.-T. (2012). Diffusion tensor imaging in hydrocephalus-findings before and after shunt surgery. *Acta Neurochir.* 154, 1699–1706. doi: 10.1007/s00701-012-1377-2

Takamura, T., and Hanakawa, T. (2017). Clinical utility of resting-state functional connectivity magnetic resonance imaging for mood and cognitive disorders. *J. Neural Transm.* 124, 821–839. doi: 10.1007/s00702-017-1710-2

Tomaiuolo, F., Scapin, M., Di Paola, M., Le Nezet, P., Fadda, L., Musicco, M., et al. (2007). Gross anatomy of the corpus callosum in Alzheimer's disease: regions of degeneration and their neuropsychological correlates. *Dement. Geriatr. Cogn. Disord.* 23, 96–103. doi: 10.1159/000097371

Tzourio-Mazoyer, N., Landeau, B., Papathanassiou, D., Crivello, F., Etard, O., Delcroix, N., et al. (2002). Automated anatomical labeling of activations in SPM using a macroscopic anatomical parcellation of the MNI MRI single-subject brain. *Neuroimage* 15, 273–289. doi: 10.1006/nimg.2001.0978

Wee, C. Y., Yap, P. T., Zhang, D. Q., Denny, K., Browndyke, J. N., Potter, G. G., et al. (2012). Identification of MCI individuals using structural and functional connectivity networks. *Neuroimage* 59, 2045–2056. doi: 10.1016/j.neuroimage.2011.10.015

Whitfield-Gabrieli, S., and Nieto-Castanon, A. (2012). Conn: a functional connectivity toolbox for correlated and anticorrelated brain networks. *Brain Connect.* 2, 125–141. doi: 10.1089/brain.2012.0073

Yamashita, F., Sasaki, M., Saito, M., Mori, E., Kawaguchi, A., Kudo, K., et al. (2014). Voxel-based morphometry of disproportionate cerebrospinal fluid space distribution for the differential diagnosis of idiopathic normal pressure hydrocephalus. *J. Neuroimaging* 24, 359–365. doi: 10.1111/jon.12049

Yamashita, F., Sasaki, M., Takahashi, S., Matsuda, H., Kudo, K., Narumi, S., et al. (2010). Detection of changes in cerebrospinal fluid space in idiopathic normal pressure hydrocephalus using voxel-based morphometry. *Neuroradiology* 52, 381–386. doi: 10.1007/s00234-009-0610-z

Yamashita, O., Sato, M., Yoshioka, T., Tong, F., and Kamitani, Y. (2008). Sparse estimation automatically selects voxels relevant for the decoding of fMRI activity patterns. *Neuroimage* 42, 1414–1429. doi: 10.1016/j.neuroimage.2008.05.050

Zeng, L. L., Shen, H., Liu, L., Wang, L. B., Li, B. J., Fang, P., et al. (2012). Identifying major depression using whole-brain functional connectivity: a multivariate pattern analysis. *Brain* 135, 1498–1507. doi: 10.1093/brain/aws059

Zhang, H., Reitz, A., Kollias, S., Summers, P., Curt, A., and Schurch, B. (2005). An fMRI study of the role of suprapontine brain structures in the voluntary voiding control induced by pelvic floor contraction. *Neuroimage* 24, 174–180. doi: 10.1016/j.neuroimage.2004.08.027

Zhang, H.-Y., Wang, S.-J., Liu, B., Ma, Z.-L., Yang, M., Zhang, Z.-J., et al. (2010). Resting brain connectivity: changes during the progress of Alzheimer disease. *Radiology* 256, 598–606. doi: 10.1148/radiol.10091701

5

Cathodal Transcranial Direct Current Stimulation Improves Focal Hand Dystonia in Musicians

Sara Marceglia [1,2†], *Simona Mrakic-Sposta* [1,3†], *Manuela Fumagalli* [1], *Roberta Ferrucci* [1,4], *Francesca Mameli* [1], *Maurizio Vergari* [1], *Sergio Barbieri* [1,4] *and Alberto Priori* [1,4,5*]

[1] Fondazione IRCCS Ca' Granda Ospedale Maggiore Policlinico, Milan, Italy, [2] Dipartimento di Ingegneria e Architettura, Università degli Studi di Trieste, Trieste, Italy, [3] Istituto di Bioimmagini e di Fisiologia Molecolare, Consiglio Nazionale delle Ricerche, Segrate, Italy, [4] "Aldo Ravelli" Center for Neurotechnology and Experimental Brain Therapeutics, University of Milan, Milan, Italy, [5] Department of Health Sciences, University of Milan and ASST Santi Paolo e Carlo, Milan, Italy

Edited by:
Takashi Hanakawa,
National Center of Neurology and Psychiatry, Japan

Reviewed by:
Shinichi Furuya,
Sony Computer Science Laboratories, Japan
Makii Muthalib,
Université de Montpellier, France
Milton Cesar Biagioni,
NYU School of Medicine, United States

***Correspondence:**
Alberto Priori
alberto.priori@unimi.it

† These authors have contributed equally to this work.

Focal hand dystonia (FHD) in musicians is a movement disorder causing abnormal movements and irregularities in playing. Since weak electrical currents applied to the brain induce persistent excitability changes in humans, cathodal tDCS was proposed as a possible non-invasive approach for modulating cortical excitability in patients with FHD. However, the optimal targets and modalities have still to be determined. In this pilot study, we delivered cathodal (2 mA), anodal (2 mA) and sham tDCS over the motor areas bilaterally for 20 min daily for five consecutive days in two musicians with FHD. After cathodal tDCS, both patients reported a sensation of general wellness and improved symptoms of FHD. In conclusion, our pilot results suggest that cathodal tDCS delivered bilaterally over motor-premotor (M-PM) cortex for 5 consecutive days may be effective in improving symptoms in FHD.

Keywords: cathodal transcranial direct current stimulation, neuromodulation, tDCS, focal hand dystonia, musician

INTRODUCTION

Focal hand dystonia (FHD) in musicians is a movement disorder characterized by irregularities in playing due to involuntary muscular activation in both the hand and arms (Cho and Hallett, 2016; Stahl and Frucht, 2017). FHD generally occurs in people who have spent a long period of time performing repetitive skilled motor tasks (Cho and Hallett, 2016). Furthermore, FHD produces excessive co-contraction of agonists and antagonists of hand and forearm muscles resulting in a slow, stiff-appearing movement and causing pain (MacKinnon, 2002; Garraux et al., 2004). Being a network disorder that involves several brain areas, FHD has a complex pathophysiology including several general abnormalities as the loss of inhibition, sensory dysfunction, and abnormal plasticity (Cho and Hallett, 2016). Functional neuroimaging studies showed alterations in the topography and increased activation of somatosensory and motor cortices (Zeuner and Molloy, 2008; Hinkley et al., 2009). Even though the causes of this disabling condition remain unclear, maladaptive plasticity has been proposed as driver for FHD in musicians (Konczak and Abbruzzese, 2013).

Despite several new therapeutic strategies proposed, botulinum toxin injection is the preferred therapy for FHD, even though some results suggest that it does not effectively improve symptoms (Hallett et al., 2009; Lungu and Ahmad, 2016). External shock waves therapy (Trompetto et al., 2009), prolonged immobilization of the affected arm (Priori et al., 2001), thalamic deep brain stimulation (Cho et al., 2009), repetitive Transcranial Magnetic Stimulation (rTMS) (Edwards et al., 2008), and transcranial Direct Current Stimulation (tDCS) (Cho and Hallett, 2016) are among the alternatives explored.

In particular, tDCS is a non-invasive technique that induces prolonged changes in brain excitability and influences motor and cognitive performances (Nitsche and Paulus, 2000; Priori, 2003; Ardolino et al., 2005; Priori et al., 2008; Brunoni et al., 2013; Zhao et al., 2017). In the past 10 years, tDCS has been proposed as adjunctive treatment for several neurological and neuropsychiatric conditions (Fregni et al., 2006; Ferrucci et al., 2008a,b; Monti et al., 2008; Mrakic-Sposta et al., 2008; Cogiamanian et al., 2009; Lefaucheur et al., 2017).

Cathodal tDCS was applied in FHD, but the results were controversial, mainly for the heterogeneity of the stimulation protocols tested (Buttkus et al., 2010, 2011; Benninger et al., 2011; Furuya et al., 2014), in terms of electrode montage, tDCS duration and intensity, as well as the number of treatments administered. Also, tDCS was either performed when the patient was at rest, or while the patient was trained (Cho and Hallett, 2016). Biparietal tDCS (two electrodes with different polarities on the head) applied over days during neurorehabilitation could improve therapy effectiveness in FHD (Furuya and Altenmüller, 2015; Rosset-Llobet et al., 2015) and bilateral tDCS (two electrodes with the same polarity on the head) is thought to improve symptoms in subjects showing bi-manual impairments (Pixa et al., 2017). Evidence of increased excitability or loss of inhibition at multiple levels including premotor and motor cortex, somatosensory cortex and cerebellum (Beck et al., 2008; Brighina et al., 2009; Delnooz et al., 2012) support the hypothesis that cathodal tDCS could improve symptoms by reducing excitability, even though the optimal protocol is still to be determined (Cho and Hallett, 2016).

In this pilot study, we applied bilateral anodal, cathodal, and sham tDCS over the motor—premotor cortices for 5 consecutive days in two musicians with FHD, to (1) test whether cathodal tDCS was superior to anodal and sham tDCS in controlling FHD symptoms in musicians, and (2) preliminarily assess the use of a 5-days protocol in terms of safety and efficacy.

METHODS

Patients

After signing their informed consent, two musicians with FHD were recruited for tDCS treatment application. The study was approved by the local Ethic Committee and it was in agreement with the principles stated in the Declaration of Helsinki. All the assessments were performed by an experienced neurologist and the diagnosis was made according to the recommendations found in the literature (Rosset-Llobet et al., 2009).

Patient 1

The first patient was a right-handed 38 years-old man, in whom FHD symptoms manifested first at the age of 18. He began playing piano when he was 11 years-old. At present, he teaches in a secondary school and plays as concert pianist.

Musician's FHD was diagnosed at the age of 22, but the disease progressively exacerbated. In the past time, the therapeutic intervention with Transcutaneous Electrical Nerve Stimulator (TENS) did not improve symptoms. Anatomic Magnetic Resonance Imaging (MRI) brain scan was normal and electroencephalogram (EEG) did not show any sign of epileptic seizures. At the time, focal dystonia interested the middle finger of the right hand and the left hand.

Presently, despite the drug treatment (anticholinergics: 12 mg/day, carbidopa/levodopa: 500 mg/day), dystonic tremor is present at rest and when the right hand is tired or weak (Lee et al., 2015).

Patient 2

The second patient was a right-handed, 44-years-old man. He began playing the accordion at the age of 11. At present, he teaches in a secondary school and plays saxophone, accordion, and clarinet.

First symptoms (cramps) appeared on the right hand at the age of 30. The patient was treated with botulinum toxin injections in hand and forearm muscles without any improvement.

At present, FHD symptoms were predominantly on the right hand, particularly the fifth finger with a subjective complaint extending to the wrist and the distal forearm. The patient complained initial symptoms to the left hand, too. The patient is not currently taking any pharmacological treatment. Anatomic MRI was normal and EEG did not show any sign of epileptic seizures. Electroneurography (ENG) showed normal motor and sensory conduction parameters; electromyography (EMG) showed a reduced disynaptic and presynaptic inhibition of H reflex in the right flexor carpi radialis (0 ms = 100%; 20 ms = 86%), compatible with a diagnosis of FHD.

Clinical Assessment at Baseline

Musician's FHD was evaluated at baseline (see **Table 1**) using the following rating scales: the *Symptom Severity Scale (SSS)* that consists of 10 questions that evaluate direct and indirect disease manifestations; the *Functional Status Scale (FSS)*, a 12-item disability scale that comprises an assessment of performances

TABLE 1 | Clinical Examination at baseline in both patients.

CLINICAL EXAMINATION T0 (Baseline Evaluation)		
Scale	**Patient 1**	**Patient 2**
FSS	11/36	2/36
TC	3	2
SSS	28/43	24/43
FMS	2	3
MMPI-2	Hy 74 (cut-off ≤ 65; $z = 2.6$)	Normal
CBA	IP-F ($z = -1.73$)	Normal
	IP-1 ($z = -1.9$)	
	MOCQ/R1 ($z = 2.23$)	

FSS, Functional Status Scale; TC, Tubiana and Chamagen Scale; SSS, Symptom Severity Scale; FMS, Fahn Marsden Scale; MMPI-2, Minnesota Multiphasic Personality Inventory Scales; [Hy, Hysteri]; CBA, Cognitive Behavioral Assessment [IP-F=Fear; IP-1=Fear: Calamity; MOCQ/R = Obsessions and compulsing:checking].

of daily activities possibly affected by FHD or hand weakness. The SSS and FSS, which were originally designed for carpal tunnel syndrome, were adapted to FHD in order to investigate its manifestations.

The *Fahn Marsden Scale (FMS)* (Fahn, 1989) was used to quantify generalized or focal dystonia in nine body areas, including eyes, mouth, speech and swallowing, neck, trunk, and right and left arm and leg. The *Tubiana and Chamagne (TC)* (Tubiana and Chamagne, 1983) scale is a classification of severity of focal dystonia in musicians, and it was used to monitor the evolution of the treatment. The scale comprises four stages of severity of dystonia.

Psychological assessment was executed using the *Minnesota Multiphasic Personality Inventory Scales (MMPI-2)* (Butcher et al., 2001) and the *Cognitive Behavioural Assessment 2.0 (CBA-2.0)* (Sanavio and Vidotto, 1996). The MMPI-2 is a well-known and widely used psychological test consisting of 567 true-false items. It traditionally yields scores on four validity scales and 10 clinical scales, although numerous other scales may be scored. For this study, the clinical, select content (Anxiety, Depression, Negative Treatment Indicators) and supplementary (Ego Strength) scales were considered. The CBA 2.0 battery includes a series of questionnaires that investigate broad issues of potential clinical interest and identify areas of dysfunction in the current life of the subjects. Subjective mood, wellness and pain at the hands were evaluated using five 100 mm *Visual Analog Scales (VAS)* (happy/unhappy; wellness/unease; left hand pain/no left hand pain; right hand pain/no right hand pain, tired/no tired).

Performance Assessment

The effects of tDCS on FHD were evaluated through the following tasks administered before and after each tDCS treatment:

Copy of an Archimedes Spiral

Patients were asked to copy a spiral template printed in black on a paper with their dominant arm. The template was 132.31 cm long. The quantitative value was defined through the length of the drawn Archimedean spiral: $L = pi*N*R$ with $N = R/t$; where: $t =$ spiral's step, $N =$ number of rpm, $R =$ max radius of spiral. We compared the spiral template length to the length of the drawn spiral. The presence of tremor was qualitatively evaluated by four independent judges blinded to the stimulation polarity on a 0–3 scale (0 = absence of tremor, 1 = slight tremor, 2 = medium tremor, 3 = important tremor).

Follow with a Pen the Edge of the Spiral

Patients were asked to follow the spiral line with the pen maintaining a constant distance of 2 mm from the printed line. The task was evaluated by four judges blinded to the stimulation polarity on a 0–3 scale about the presence of tremor (0 = absence of tremor; 1 = slight tremor, 2 = medium tremor, 3 = important tremor).

Copy of Sample Pictures

Patients had to copy different figures (cube, pyramid, and more complex figures) and a 10 cm line. Four blind judges evaluated the presence of constructive apraxia on a 0–3 scale (0 = perfect copy; 1 = very similar copy, 2 = incomplete copy, 3 = very incomplete copy) and the presence of tremor (0–3 scale with 0 = absence of tremor, 1 = slight tremor, 2 = medium tremor, 3 = important tremor).

Copy of a List of Words

Eight lists of 33 words were created using the Lists for Writing. Each list was composed by words (verbs, adjectives, concrete and abstract nouns, all of them both regular and irregular) and non-words. Four blind judges evaluated the quality of writing on a 0–1 scale (0 = good writing; 1 = bad writing symptom of a weak and tired hand), and the presence of tremor (0–3 scale with 0 = absence of tremor, 1 = slight tremor, 2 = medium tremor, 3 = important tremor). The % difference from pre-treatment evaluation was considered for the analysis.

Execution of a Musical Scale and Exercises with the Instrument

Patients executed a musical scale and several technical exercises with their instrument. More specifically, for the piano, the patient was asked to play a two-octave C-major scale, right and left hand, 10 sequences; for the clarinet, the patient was asked to play a two-octave C-major scale.

Adverse events were collected throughout the whole session.

Experimental Protocol

This was a double-blind experiment in which both the patients and the judges were blind to the type of stimulation delivered. Both patients underwent three 5-days sessions, one for sham, one for cathodal, and one for anodal tDCS, in random order (**Figure 1**). Three washout weeks elapsed between each session (anodal, cathodal, sham). After a baseline clinical assessment at the beginning of the 5-day session, each day included (1) pre-tDCS performance evaluation; (2) bilateral tDCS at 2 mA intensity per side over the motor/premotor areas (M-PM) of the cerebral cortex (above C3/C4, FC3/FC4 according to the international 10–20 electrode placement system) for 20 min; and (3) post-tDCS performance evaluation. At the end of the 5-days session, FHD symptoms were re-assessed through the SSS, the TC, and the FSS (**Figure 1**).

Follow-up examinations, including both symptom and performance assessments were conducted at 1 (T1) and 10 (T2) days after the end of each 5-days session.

tDCS

tDCS was delivered to the scalp with two "Eldith DC Stimulator" (Neuroconn GmbH, Germany), each connected to a pair of thick (0.3 mm) rounded saline-soaked sponge electrodes, one (active electrode) placed over the scalp and the other (reference electrode) over the right deltoid muscle. Cathodal and anodal tDCS (C-tDCS and A-tDCS) polarity referred to the two electrodes over the scalp. The wide electrode surface (scalp electrodes 48 cm^2; deltoid electrode 64 cm^2) avoided the possible harmful effects of high current density. For sham tDCS (S-tDCS),

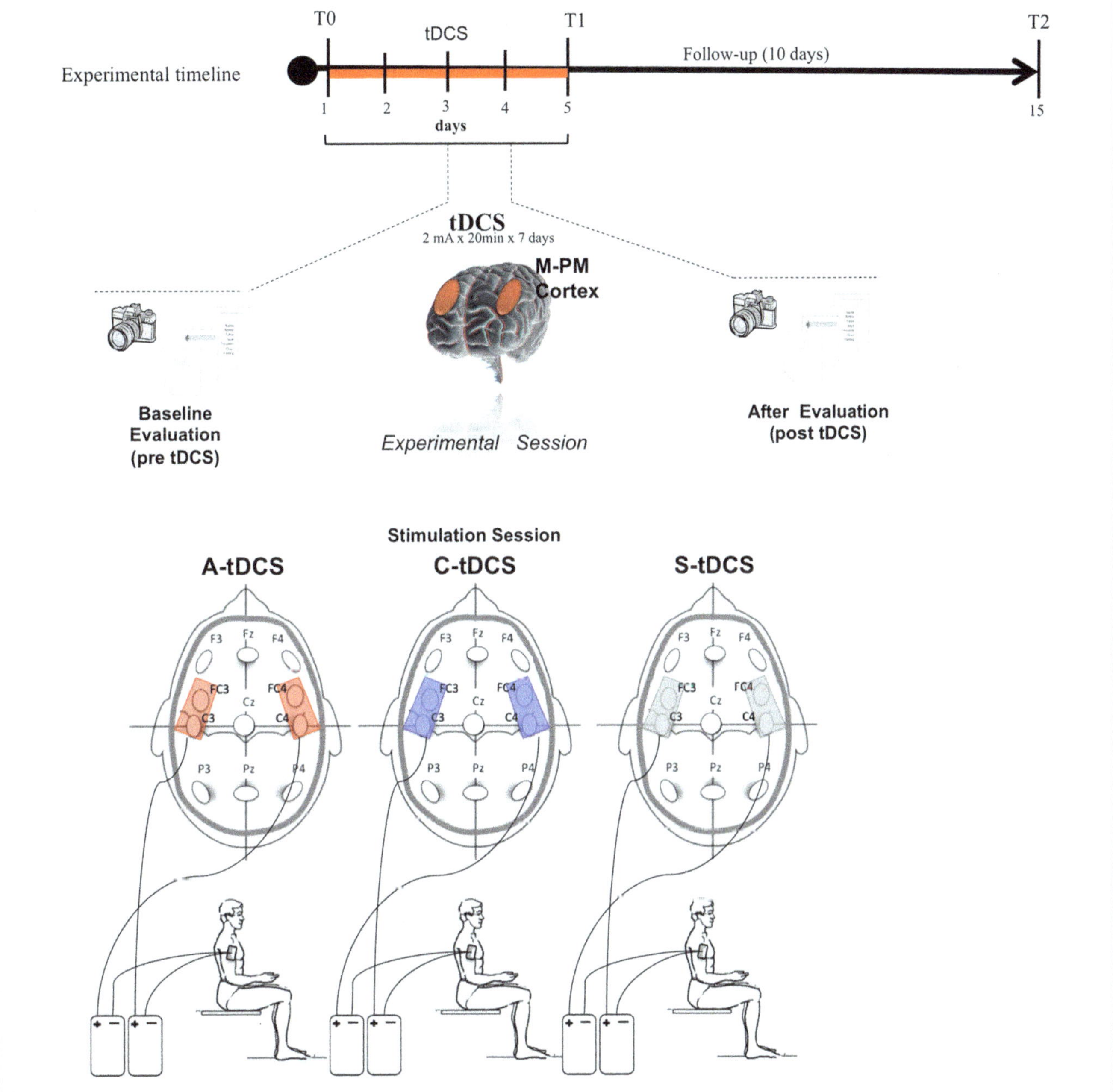

FIGURE 1 | Transcranial Direct Current Stimulation (tDCS) experimental protocol. tDCS was applied bilaterally over the scalp on the motor-premotor cortex (M-PM) for 5 consecutive days. Patients were assessed in the first (T0) and the last day (T1) and after 10 days from ended tDCS (T2).

electrodes were placed as for real stimulation but the stimulator was turned off after 10 s. Hence, the patients felt an initial itching sensation similar to that induced at the beginning of real tDCS but received no stimulation.

To guarantee safety we applied, to each stimulation site, current at a density of 0.0416 mA/cm^2 and delivered a total charge of 0.049 C/cm^2. These intensities are far below the threshold for tissue damage (Nitsche et al., 2003a; Liebetanz et al., 2009; Lefaucheur et al., 2017).

Data Analysis

Considering the low number of subjects reported, we performed only descriptive statistics.

Percentage changes, defined as [(after tDCS-before tDCS)/before tDCS], were used for the analysis to assess tDCS effects. When applicable, the percentage changes of variables evaluated by the independent judges were averaged, to obtain the trend over the entire 5-days session. Data are reported as [mean $\pm$ *SD*].

RESULTS

The patients did not report any adverse effects during stimulation sessions and were not able to distinguish active (anodal or cathodal) and sham stimulation.

Copy of an Archimedes Spiral

Quantitative evaluation showed that whereas S-tDCS and A-tDCS left patients' performance unchanged, after C-tDCS both patients could draw a complete *Copy of an Archimedes spiral* (template length 100%, **Figure 2A**). The time elapsing before each patient could draw a complete spiral differed in the two patients: patient 1 drew a complete spiral 1 day after the entire 5-day C-tDCS session, whereas patient 2 achieved a complete spiral immediately after the first C-tDCS application (day 1) in the post-C-tDCS assessment. Conversely, when sham and anodal sessions ended, both patients could draw a spiral that was 20–30% shorter than the printed one. At T2, the beneficial effect of C-tDCS ended (**Figure 2B**). Qualitative analysis showed that C-tDCS reduced tremor, whereas A-tDCS and S-tDCS did not (**Figures 2C–G**).

Follow with a Pen the Edge of the Spiral and Copy of a Sample Pictures

In the *Follow the edge of a spiral with a pen* task both patients improved at T1 of the C-tDCS session and worsened after A-tDCS (**Figures 3A,B**).

In both patients, tremor decreased (patient 1: −33%; patient 2: −62%) while patients were "*copying sample pictures*" immediately after a single C-tDCS session. At T2, the effect of C-tDCS persisted (% change at T2 C-tDCS, Patient 1: −9%; patient 2: −30%; **Figures 4A,B**).

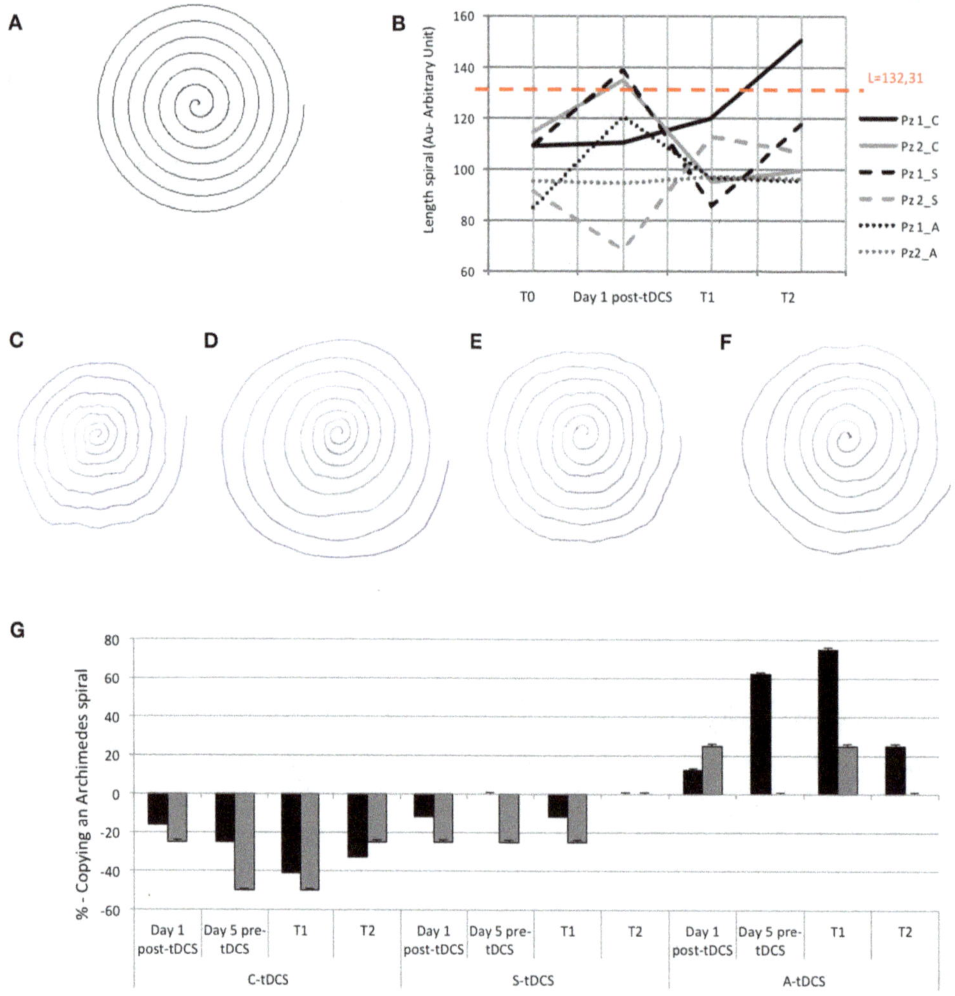

FIGURE 2 | (A) Copy of an Archimedes spiral task: template of Archimedean Spiral; **(B)** The lines show quantitative evaluation in both patients at T0, at day 1 after tDCS, at T1, and at T2. The red dashed line is the length of the sample spiral (132.31 mm), black lines refer to patient 1 and gray lines to patient 2. The full is C-tDCS, the dashed line is A-tDCS and the dotted line s S-tDCS session; **(C)** Copy of Archimedean Spiral the first day after C-tDCS treatment in patient 1; **(D)** Copy of Archimedean Spiral at T1 of the C-tDCS session in patient 1; **(E)** Copy of Archimedean Spiral at the first day after A-tDCS treatment in patient 1; **(F)** Copy of Archimedean Spiral at T1 of the A-tDCS session in patient 1. **(G)** The histogram shows tremor in qualitative analysis in the percentage differences after tDCS in both patients. 0% is baseline (pre-tDCS—T0).

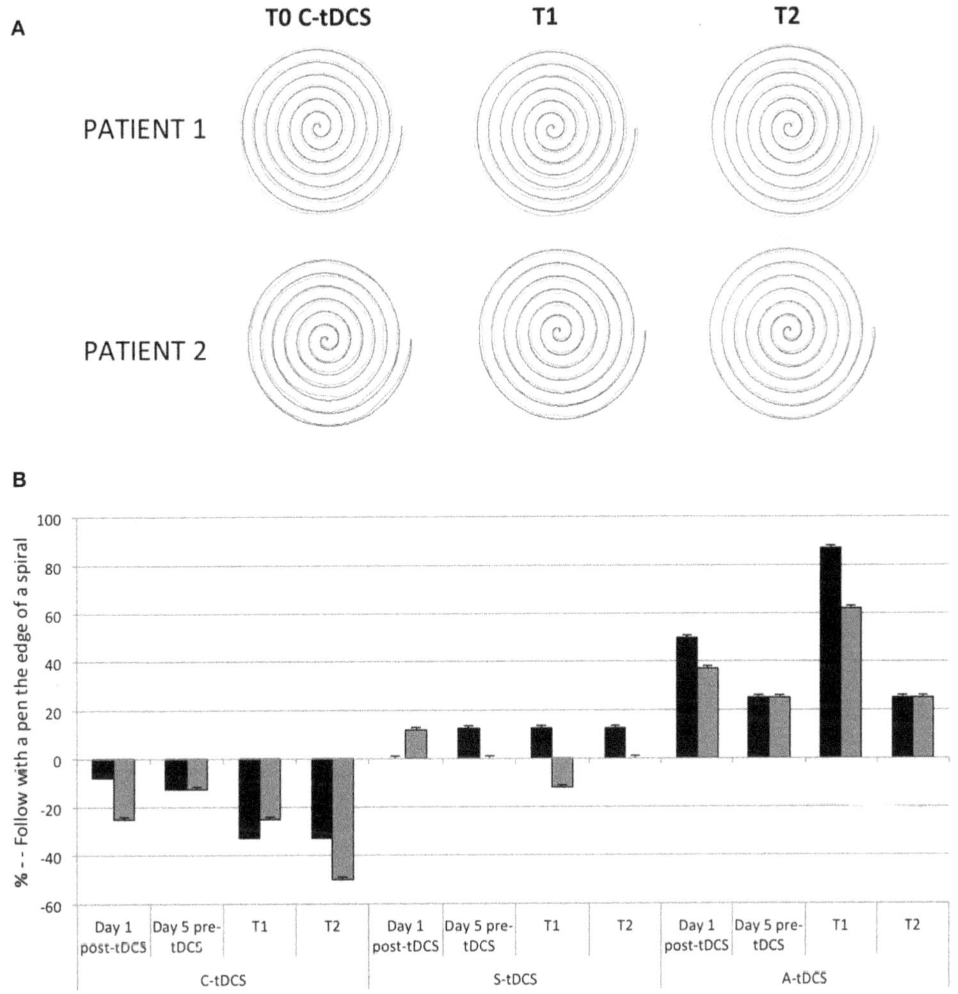

FIGURE 3 | (A) Follow with a pen the edge of the spiral at pre (T0) and post C-tDCS (T1 and T2) in both patients. **(B)** The histogram showed the qualitative analysis in the percentage differences after tDCS in both patients. 0% is baseline (pre-tDCS—T0).

Copy of a List of Words

Either way, before and after tDCS (anodal, cathodal, and sham), the quality of writing was good in both patients, with no presence of bad writing due to a weak or tired hand and tremor.

FHD Symptoms and Playing

FSS, TC, and SSS values improved in both patients after C-tDCS. At T1, FSS decreased by 9% in patient 1 and 100% in patient 2, TC decreased by 33% in patient 1 and 100% in patient 2, SSS decreased by 3% in patient 1 and 46% in patient 2. After A-tDCS, only some values improved: FSS decreased in patient 1 by 35 and 100% in patient 2, TC did not change in patient 1 and 2, SSS decreased by 13% in patient 1 and 5% in patient 2 (**Table 2**).

Patient 1 reported a subjective improvement and decrease of pain at the right hand only after C-tDCS. He also reported subjective improvement of prono-supination movement in the left hand (**Figures 5A,B**).

Patient 2 reported a subjective improvement after cathodal tDCS: the right hand was more toned, he had a better control of the 5th finger, fewer shots, and less hand/art fatigue (**Figures 5C,D**).

VAS

Both patients reported a sensation of general wellness, of happiness, of reduction of hand pain and an improvement of rest particularly after C-tDCS (at T1). In details, for health/wellness: patient 1, 21 vs. 32 vs. 19% (S-C-A-tDCS, respectively); patient 2, 0 vs. 4 vs. 0%; happy/unhappy: patient 1, 20 vs. 55 vs. 43%; patient 2, 0 vs. 8 vs. 2%; pain/no pain right hand patient 1, 13 vs. 37 vs. 0%; patient 2, 0 vs. 0 vs. 0%; pain/no pain left hand patient 1, 2 vs. 68 vs. 3%; patient 2, 0 vs. 0 vs. 0%; tired/not tired patient 1, 18 vs. 42 vs. 24%; patient 2, 0 vs. 5 vs. 7%).

DISCUSSION

Musician's FHD is a difficult disease, with little therapeutic options while bringing to early termination of their professional life. We showed that cathodal tDCS delivered bilaterally for

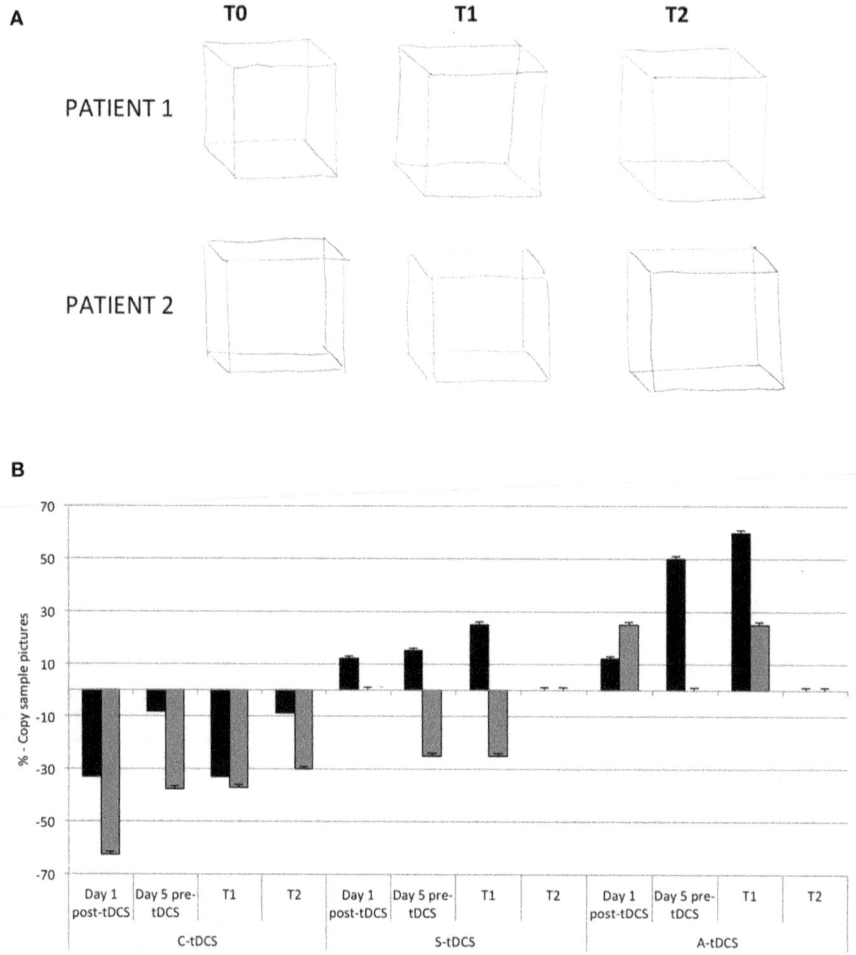

FIGURE 4 | (A) The tremor graft pre (T0), and post (T1 and T2) C-tDCS in both patients. **(B)** The histogram showed qualitative analysis in the percentage differences of tremor after tDCS in both patients. Zero percent is baseline (pre-tDCS—T0).

5 consecutive days is feasible and safe, and that it transiently improves motor performances, subjective perception of pain and fatigue, and subjective perception of playing in two musicians with FHD.

Our findings, while proposing a new stimulation protocol, are in line with the conclusions of the recent review by Cho and Hallet who reported the potential therapeutic use of non-invasive brain stimulation to treat FHD (Cho and Hallett, 2016). Considering the current state-of-the-art, there are few studies investigating the effects of cathodal tDCS in FHD, but none of them applied a 5-days bilateral (two electrodes with the same polarity on the head) M1 tDCS protocol nor it found improvements lasting for 10 days. More specifically, of the seven tDCS studies mentioned in the review (Rosset-Llobet et al., 2009; Buttkus et al., 2010, 2011; Benninger et al., 2011; Furuya et al., 2014; Sadnicka et al., 2014), four have applied electrodes on M1 but only one reported positive effects (Furuya et al., 2014). Unlike the others, the authors combined cathodal tDCS on the affected M1 with anodal tDCS on the unaffected M1 in pianists, finding that rhythmic accuracy of sequential finger movements improved and was retained 4 days after intervention.

Following the Furuya S and colleagues' suggestion of working on the two sides of the head contemporarily, we applied tDCS bilaterally (two electrodes with the same polarity on the two head sides) over the M-PM cortex in two musicians with FHD and bilateral symptoms, sharing the idea of a possible advantage over mono-lateral stimulation. The M-PM cortex was chosen as tDCS target because it is believed to encode the motor programs responsible for skilled finger movement (Karni et al., 1995; Gentner et al., 2010). In addition, bilateral tDCS was shown to improve symptoms occurring on both sides of the body (Pixa et al., 2017), similarly to our two patients, who had both hands affected by symptoms (at least in an initial phase). Then, considering the positive results of applying tDCS for one week (5 days) in other hyperkinetic disorders (Mrakic-Sposta et al., 2008), and considering the boosting effects of tDCS applied over days during neurorehabilitation (Furuya and Altenmüller, 2015; Rosset-Llobet et al., 2015), we chose the 5-days protocol.

After 5 consecutive days of cathodal tDCS, both our patients experienced consistent improvements in tremor, slight improvement of finger postures during playing, and diminished pain in the hands and arms, without experiencing any side

TABLE 2 | Clinical assessment of both patients before and after 5-days tDCS session.

CLINICAL ASSESSMENT												
	T0 (Before tDCS)						T1 (5 days after tDCS)					
Scale	Patient 1			Patient 2			Patient 1			Patient 2		
	C-tDCS	S-tDCS	A-tDCS	C-tDCS	S-tDCS	A-tDCS	C-tDCS	S-tDCS	A-tDCS	C-tDCS	S-tDCS	A-tDCS
FSS	11/36	12/36	17/36	2/36	2/36	2/36	10/36	11/36	11/36	0/36	0/36	0/36
TC	3	3	3	2	2	2	4	3	3	4	2	3
SSS	28/43	28/43	29/43	24/43	17/43	20/43	27/43	29/43	25/43	13/43	18/43	19/43

FSS, Functional Status Scale; TC, Tubiana and Chamagen Scale; SSS, Symptom Severity Scale.

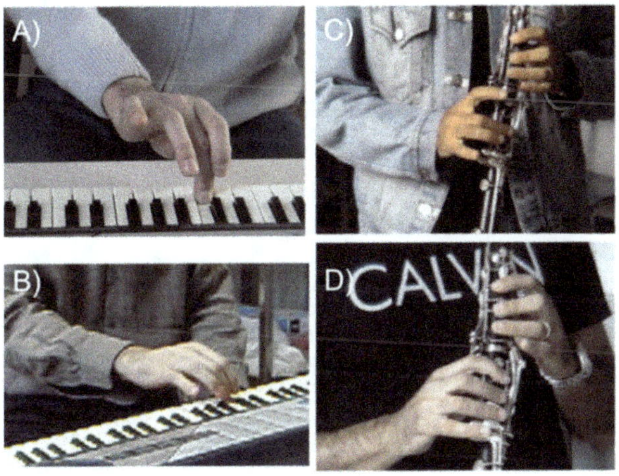

FIGURE 5 | Typical patterns of dystonia posture in a pianist **(A)** and clarinet **(C)** at baseline (T0). In **(B,D)** the patients after 5-days of C-tDCS (T1).

effect. Moreover, our patients, who were blinded to the treatment received, reported a positive subjective impression of how C-tDCS affected their pain, tiredness, mood, and wellness. Conversely, in line with the study by Quartarone et al. (2005), where anodal tDCS was shown to up regulate brain excitability in patients with writer's cramp, A-tDCS worsened the symptoms in our patients. Collectively, our results suggest that cathodal tDCS treatment might help to produce steady, more accurate arm movements, but not to stabilize abnormal fine finger movements. Because cathodal tDCS reduces brain excitability (Nitsche et al., 2003b), bilateral cathodal tDCS delivered over the motor areas could have down regulated excitability in the underlying brain areas by recovering the inadequate motor cortical inhibition responsible for excessive excitation and near synchronous co-contractions of agonists and antagonists (Nitsche et al., 2003b; Ardolino et al., 2005; Byl, 2007). Our application of bi-hemispheric C-tDCS seemed to help recovering patient's bilateral symptoms and overall condition. We can hence hypothesize that, in presence of bilateral symptoms, tDCS should be delivered bilaterally (two electrodes with the same polarity on the two head sides) whereas, in presence of unilateral symptoms (Furuya et al., 2014), tDCS preferable application may be bipolar (two different polarities on the head). Moreover, the 5-days protocol resulted to be effective in providing beneficial effects at least for 2 weeks, confirming that over-days tDCS sessions may be more effective than single-shot tDCS sessions in promoting brain plasticity, especially if combined with neurorehabilitation therapy (Rosset-Llobet et al., 2015).

Finally, our experiment differs from all the others reported in the literature for both the electrode montage (bilateral tDCS) and the stimulation protocol (5 consecutive days). This could partly explain why our results are more consistent than those obtained by other groups (Cho and Hallett, 2016).

However, this was a double-subject studies that allows observing individual responses, but not generalizing its results to the whole population of FHD musicians, as inherent limitation of the experimental design. Although, no definitive conclusions can be derived from 2 subjects, our results should be interpreted in the context of the novel target of stimulation (bilateral M-PM for patients with initial bilateral symptoms) and stimulation protocol (5 consecutive days) that may be considered as new factors in future trials. Also, we haven't assessed any biomarker to better understand the potential pathophysiological mechanisms of tDCS that should be included in further studies.

In conclusion, a 5-days treatment with cathodal tDCS could be a safe and low-cost effective adjuvant in the therapy of involuntary flexion or extension of hand and limbs and in hand pain and the bilateral electrode montage over PM-M areas could favorably impact FHD in musicians with bilateral symptoms.

ETHICS STATEMENT

The study was carried out in accordance with the recommendations of the Ethical Committee of the Fondazione IRCCS Ca'Granda Ospedale Maggiore Policlinico with written informed consent from all subjects. All subjects gave written informed consent in accordance with the Declaration of Helsinki.

AUTHOR CONTRIBUTIONS

SM and SMS designed the study, conducted the experiment, analyzed data, and drafted the manuscript and figures. MF, RF, and FM designed and administered the cognitive tasks and reviewed the manuscript. MV administered tDCS and reviewed the manuscript. SB evaluated the patients, provided clinical advice and scales, and reviewed the manuscript. AP ideated the study, coordinated the research protocol, and finalized the manuscript.

ACKNOWLEDGMENTS

The work was supported by the grant GR-2011-02352807 from the Italian Ministry of Health.

REFERENCES

Ardolino, G., Bossi, B., Barbieri, S., and Priori, A. (2005). Non-synaptic mechanisms underlie the after-effects of cathodal transcutaneous direct current stimulation of the human brain. *J. Physiol.* 568, 653–663. doi: 10.1113/jphysiol.2005.088310

Beck, S., Richardson, S. P., Shamim, E. A., Dang, N., Schubert, M., and Hallett, M. (2008). Short intracortical and surround inhibition are selectively reduced during movement initiation in focal hand dystonia. *J. Neurosci.* 28, 10363–10369. doi: 10.1523/JNEUROSCI.3564-08.2008

Benninger, D. H., Lomarev, M., Lopez, G., Pal, N., Luckenbaugh, D. A., and Hallett, M. (2011). Transcranial direct current stimulation for the treatment of focal hand dystonia. *Mov. Disord.* 26, 1698–1702. doi: 10.1002/mds.23691

Brighina, F., Romano, M., Giglia, G., Saia, V., Puma, A., Giglia, F., et al. (2009). Effects of cerebellar TMS on motor cortex of patients with focal dystonia: a preliminary report. *Exp. Brain Res.* 192, 651–656. doi: 10.1007/s00221-008-1572-9

Brunoni, A. R., Boggio, P. S., Ferrucci, R., Priori, A., and Fregni, F. (2013). Transcranial direct current stimulation: challenges, opportunities, and impact on psychiatry and neurorehabilitation. *Front. Psychiatry* 4:19. doi: 10.3389/fpsyt.2013.00019

Butcher, J., Graham, J., Ben-Porath, Y., Tellegen, A., Dahlstrom, W., and Kaemmer, B. (2001). *MMPI-2: Manual for Administration and Scoring.* Minneapolis, MN: University of Minnesota Press.

Buttkus, F., Baur, V., Jabusch, H.-C., de la Cruz Gomez-Pellin, M., Paulus, W., Nitsche, M. A., et al. (2011). Single-session tDCS-supported retraining does not improve fine motor control in musician's dystonia. *Restor. Neurol. Neurosci.* 29, 85–90. doi: 10.3233/RNN-2011-0582

Buttkus, F., Weidenmüller, M., Schneider, S., Jabusch, H. C., Nitsche, M. A., Paulus, W., et al. (2010). Failure of cathodal direct current stimulation to improve fine motor control in musician's dystonia. *Mov. Disord. Off. J. Mov. Disord. Soc.* 25, 389–394. doi: 10.1002/mds.22938

Byl, N. N. (2007). Learning-based animal models: task-specific focal hand dystonia. *ILAR J.* 48, 411–431. doi: 10.1093/ilar.48.4.411

Cho, C. B., Park, H. K., Lee, K. J., and Rha, H. K. (2009). Thalamic deep brain stimulation for Writer's Cramp. *J. Korean Neurosurg. Soc.* 46:52. doi: 10.3340/jkns.2009.46.1.52

Cho, H. J., and Hallett, M. (2016). Non-invasive brain stimulation for treatment of focal hand dystonia: update and future direction. *J. Mov. Disord.* 9, 55–62. doi: 10.14802/jmd.16014

Cogiamanian, F., Barbieri, S., and Priori, A. (2009). Novel nonpharmacologic perspectives for the treatment of task-specific focal hand dystonia. *J. Hand Ther.* 22, 156–161. doi: 10.1016/j.jht.2008.11.008

Delnooz, C. C. S., Helmich, R. C., Medendorp, W. P., Van de Warrenburg, B. P. C., and Toni, I. (2012). Writer's cramp: increased dorsal premotor activity during intended writing. *Hum. Brain Mapp.* 34, 613–625. doi: 10.1002/hbm.21464

Edwards, M. J., Talelli, P., and Rothwell, J. C. (2008). Clinical applications of transcranial magnetic stimulation in patients with movement disorders. *Lancet Neurol.* 7, 827–840. doi: 10.1016/S1474-4422(08)70190-X

Fahn, S. (1989). "Assessment of the primary dystonias," in *Quantification of Neurologic Deficit*, ed T. Munsat (Oxford: Butterworths), 241–270.

Ferrucci, R., Mameli, F., Guidi, I., Mrakic-Sposta, S., Vergari, M., Marceglia, S., et al. (2008a). Transcranial direct current stimulation improves recognition memory in Alzheimer disease. *Neurology* 71, 493–498. doi: 10.1212/01.wnl.0000317060.43722.a3

Ferrucci, R., Marceglia, S., Vergari, M., Cogiamanian, F., Mrakic-Sposta, S., Mameli, F., et al. (2008b). Cerebellar transcranial direct current stimulation impairs the practice-dependent proficiency increase in working memory. *J. Cogn. Neurosci.* 20, 1687–1697. doi: 10.1162/jocn.2008.20112

Fregni, F., Boggio, P. S., Lima, M. C., Ferreira, M. J. L., Wagner, T., Rigonatti, S. P., et al. (2006). A sham-controlled, phase II trial of transcranial direct current stimulation for the treatment of central pain in traumatic spinal cord injury. *Pain* 122, 197–209. doi: 10.1016/j.pain.2006.02.023

Furuya, S., and Altenmüller, E. (2015). Acquisition and reacquisition of motor coordination in musicians: virtuosity and disorder of musicians. *Ann. N.Y. Acad. Sci.* 1337, 118–124. doi: 10.1111/nyas.12659

Furuya, S., Nitsche, M. A., Paulus, W., and Altenmüller, E. (2014). Surmounting retraining limits in Musicians' dystonia by transcranial stimulation: noninvasive stimulation for FD. *Ann. Neurol.* 75, 700–707. doi: 10.1002/ana.24151

Garraux, G., Bauer, A., Hanakawa, T., Wu, T., Kansaku, K., and Hallett, M. (2004). Changes in brain anatomy in focal hand dystonia. *Ann. Neurol.* 55, 736–739. doi: 10.1002/ana.20113

Gentner, R., Gorges, S., Weise, D., aufm Kampe, K., Buttmann, M., and Classen, J. (2010). Encoding of motor skill in the corticomuscular system of musicians. *Curr. Biol.* 20, 1869–1874. doi: 10.1016/j.cub.2010.09.045

Hallett, M., Benecke, R., Blitzer, A., and Comella, C. L. (2009). Treatment of focal dystonias with botulinum neurotoxin. *Toxicon* 54, 628–633. doi: 10.1016/j.toxicon.2008.12.008

Hinkley, L. B. N., Webster, R. L., Byl, N. N., and Nagarajan, S. S. (2009). Neuroimaging characteristics of patients with focal hand dystonia. *J. Hand Ther.* 22, 125–134. doi: 10.1016/j.jht.2008.11.002

Karni, A., Meyer, G., Jezzard, P., Adams, M. M., Turner, R., and Ungerleider, L. G. (1995). Functional MRI evidence for adult motor cortex plasticity during motor skill learning. *Nature* 377, 155–158. doi: 10.1038/377155a0

Konczak, J., and Abbruzzese, G. (2013). Focal dystonia in musicians: linking motor symptoms to somatosensory dysfunction. *Front. Hum. Neurosci.* 7:297. doi: 10.3389/fnhum.2013.00297

Lee, A., Schoonderwaldt, E., Chadde, M., and Altenmüller, E. (2015). Analysis of dystonic tremor in musicians using empirical mode decomposition. *Clin. Neurophysiol.* 126, 147–153. doi: 10.1016/j.clinph.2014.04.013

Lefaucheur, J.-P., Antal, A., Ayache, S. S., Benninger, D. H., Brunelin, J., Cogiamanian, F., et al. (2017). Evidence-based guidelines on the therapeutic use of transcranial direct current stimulation (tDCS). *Clin. Neurophysiol.* 128, 56–92. doi: 10.1016/j.clinph.2016.10.087

Liebetanz, D., Koch, R., Mayenfels, S., König, F., Paulus, W., and Nitsche, M. A. (2009). Safety limits of cathodal transcranial direct current stimulation in rats. *Clin. Neurophysiol.* 120, 1161–1167. doi: 10.1016/j.clinph.2009.01.022

Lungu, C., and Ahmad, O. (2016). Update on the use of botulinum toxin therapy for focal and task-specific dystonias. *Semin. Neurol.* 36, 41–46. doi: 10.1055/s-0035-1571211

MacKinnon, S. E. (2002). Pathophysiology of nerve compression. *Hand Clin.* 18, 231–241. doi: 10.1016/S0749-0712(01)00012-9

Monti, A., Cogiamanian, F., Marceglia, S., Ferrucci, R., Mameli, F., Mrakic-Sposta, S., et al. (2008). Improved naming after transcranial direct current stimulation in aphasia. *J. Neurol. Neurosurg. Psychiatr.* 79, 451–453. doi: 10.1136/jnnp.2007.135277

Mrakic-Sposta, S., Marceglia, S., Mameli, F., Dilena, R., Tadini, L., and Priori, A. (2008). Transcranial direct current stimulation in two patients with Tourette syndrome. *Mov. Disord.* 23, 2259–2261. doi: 10.1002/mds.22292

Nitsche, M. A., Liebetanz, D., Lang, N., Antal, A., Tergau, F., and Paulus, W. (2003a). Safety criteria for transcranial direct current stimulation (tDCS) in humans. *Clin. Neurophysiol.* 114, 2220–2222. doi: 10.1016/S1388-2457(03)00235-9

Nitsche, M. A., Nitsche, M. S., Klein, C. C., Tergau, F., Rothwell, J. C., and Paulus, W. (2003b). Level of action of cathodal DC polarisation induced inhibition of the human motor cortex. *Clin. Neurophysiol.* 114, 600–604. doi: 10.1016/S1388-2457(02)00412-1

Nitsche, M. A., and Paulus, W. (2000). Excitability changes induced in the human motor cortex by weak transcranial direct current stimulation. *J. Physiol.* 527(Pt 3), 633–639. doi: 10.1111/j.1469-7793.2000.t01-1-00633.x

Pixa, N. H., Steinberg, F., and Doppelmayr, M. (2017). Effects of high-definition anodal transcranial direct current stimulation applied simultaneously to both primary motor cortices on bimanual sensorimotor performance. *Front. Behav. Neurosci.* 11:130. doi: 10.3389/fnbeh.2017.00130

Priori, A. (2003). Brain polarization in humans: a reappraisal of an old tool for prolonged non-invasive modulation of brain excitability. *Clin. Neurophysiol.* 114, 589–595. doi: 10.1016/S1388-2457(02)00437-6

Priori, A., Mameli, F., Cogiamanian, F., Marceglia, S., Tiriticco, M., Mrakic-Sposta, S., et al. (2008). Lie-specific involvement of dorsolateral prefrontal cortex in deception. *Cereb. Cortex* 18, 451–455. doi: 10.1093/cercor/bhm088

Priori, A., Pesenti, A., Cappellari, A., Scarlato, G., and Barbieri, S. (2001). Limb immobilization for the treatment of focal occupational dystonia. *Neurology* 57, 405–409. doi: 10.1212/WNL.57.3.405

Quartarone, A., Rizzo, V., Bagnato, S., Morgante, F., Sant'Angelo, A., Romano, M., et al. (2005). Homeostatic-like plasticity of the primary motor hand area is impaired in focal hand dystonia. *Brain J. Neurol.* 128, 1943–1950. doi: 10.1093/brain/awh527

Rosset-Llobet, J., Candia, V., Fàbregas i Molas, S., Dolors Rosinés i Cubells, D., and Pascual-Leone, A. (2009). The challenge of diagnosing focal hand dystonia in musicians. *Eur. J. Neurol.* 16, 864–869. doi: 10.1111/j.1468-1331.2009.02610.x

Rosset-Llobet, J., Fàbregas-Molas, S., and Pascual Leone, Á. (2015). Effect of transcranial direct current stimulation on neurorehabilitation of task-specific dystonia: a double-blind, randomized clinical trial. *Med. Probl. Perform. Art.* 30, 178–184.

Sadnicka, A., Hamada, M., Bhatia, K. P., Rothwell, J. C., and Edwards, M. J. (2014). Cerebellar stimulation fails to modulate motor cortex plasticity in writing dystonia. *Mov. Disord.* 29, 1304–1307. doi: 10.1002/mds.25881

Sanavio, E., and Vidotto, G. (Eds.). (1996). *CBA-2.0: 10 Anni di Ricerche.* Torino: Upsel.

Stahl, C. M., and Frucht, S. J. (2017). Focal task specific dystonia: a review and update. *J. Neurol.* 264, 1536–1541. doi: 10.1007/s00415-016-8373-z

Trompetto, C., Avanzino, L., Bove, M., Marinelli, L., Molfetta, L., Trentini, R., et al. (2009). External shock waves therapy in dystonia: preliminary results. *Eur. J. Neurol.* 16, 517–521. doi: 10.1111/j.1468-1331.2008.02525.x

Tubiana, R., and Chamagne, P. (1983). Occupational "cramps" of the upper limb. *Ann. Chir. Main* 2, 134–142. doi: 10.1016/S0753-9053(83)80091-X

Zeuner, K. E., and Molloy, F. M. (2008). Abnormal reorganization in focal hand dystonia–sensory and motor training programs to retrain cortical function. *Neurorehabilitation* 23, 43–53.

Zhao, H., Qiao, L., Fan, D., Zhang, S., Turel, O., Li, Y., et al. (2017). Modulation of brain activity with noninvasive transcranial direct current stimulation (tdcs): clinical applications and safety concerns. *Front. Psychol.* 8:685. doi: 10.3389/fpsyg.2017.00685

6

Arsenic Exposure Induces Unscheduled Mitotic S Phase Entry Coupled with Cell Death in Mouse Cortical Astrocytes

Nang T. T. Htike[1], *Fumihiko Maekawa*[2], *Haruka Soutome*[1], *Kazuhiro Sano*[2], *Sho Maejima*[3], *Kyaw H. Aung*[1], *Masaaki Tokuda*[4] *and Shinji Tsukahara*[1,3*]

[1] Area of Regulatory Biology, Division of Life Science, Graduate School of Science and Engineering, Saitama University, Saitama, Japan, [2] Center for Health and Environmental Risk Research, National Institute for Environmental Studies, Tsukuba, Japan, [3] Area of Life-NanoBio, Division of Strategy Research, Graduate School of Science and Engineering, Saitama University, Saitama, Japan, [4] Department of Cell Physiology, Faculty of Medicine/Graduate School of Medicine, Kagawa University, Kagawa, Japan

Edited by:
Eric W. Roubos,
Radboud University Nijmegen,
Netherlands

Reviewed by:
Francisco Capani,
University of Buenos Aires (UBA) and
National Scientific and Technical
Research Council (CONICET),
Argentina
Remco H. S. Westerink,
Utrecht University, Netherlands

***Correspondence:**
Shinji Tsukahara
stsuka@mail.saitama-u.ac.jp

There is serious concern about arsenic in the natural environment, which exhibits neurotoxicity and increases the risk of neurodevelopmental disorders. Adverse effects of arsenic have been demonstrated in neurons, but it is not fully understood how arsenic affects other cell types in the brain. In the current study, we examined whether sodium arsenite ($NaAsO_2$) affects the cell cycle, viability, and apoptosis of *in vitro*-cultured astrocytes isolated from the cerebral cortex of mice. Cultured astrocytes from transgenic mice expressing fluorescent ubiquitination-based cell cycle indicator (Fucci) were subjected to live imaging analysis to assess the effects of $NaAsO_2$ (0, 1, 2, and 4 μM) on the cell cycle and number of cells. Fucci was designed to express monomeric Kusabira Orange2 (mKO2) fused with the ubiquitylation domain of hCdt1, a marker of G1 phase, and monomeric Azami Green (mAG) fused with the ubiquitylation domain of hGem, a marker of S, G2, and M phases. $NaAsO_2$ concentration-dependently decreased the peak levels of the mAG/mKO2 emission ratio when the ratio had reached a peak in astrocytes without $NaAsO_2$ exposure, which was due to attenuating the increase in the mAG-expressing cell number. In contrast, the mAG/mKO2 emission ratio and number of mAG-expressing cells were concentration-dependently increased by $NaAsO_2$ before their peak levels, indicating unscheduled S phase entry. We further examined the fate of cells forced to enter S phase by $NaAsO_2$. We found that most of these cells died up to the end of live imaging. In addition, quantification of the copy number of the glial fibrillary acidic protein gene expressed specifically in astrocytes revealed a concentration-dependent decrease caused by $NaAsO_2$. However, $NaAsO_2$ did not increase the amount of nucleosomes generated from DNA fragmentation and failed to alter the gene expression of molecules relevant to unscheduled S phase entry-coupled apoptosis (p21, p53, E2F1, E2F4, and Gm36566). These findings suggest that $NaAsO_2$ adversely affects the cell cycle and viability of astrocytes by inducing unscheduled S phase entry coupled with cell death that may be caused by mechanisms other than apoptosis.

Keywords: astrocytes, sodium arsenite, cell cycle, cell death, live imaging

INTRODUCTION

Several environmental chemicals are suspected to exert deleterious effects on development of the brain, which may result in an increased risk of neurodevelopmental disorders such as autism, attention-deficit hyperactivity disorder, and cerebral palsy (Grandjean and Landrigan, 2006, 2014). Arsenic is one of these environmental toxicants that disrupt brain development. According to a long-term prospective study of survivors of arsenic poisoning from the Morinaga milk incident in Japan, arsenic poisoning during infancy leads to a risk of mortality from neurological diseases in adulthood (Tanaka et al., 2010). Epidemiological studies suggest that chronic consumption of arsenic-contaminated water causes a reduction in the cognitive performance of school-age children (Calderon et al., 2001; Tsai et al., 2003; Wasserman et al., 2007). Thus, arsenic exposure via drinking water may be a risk factor for neurodevelopmental disorders.

Animal studies support the notion that developmental exposure to arsenic increases the risk of neurodevelopmental disorders. Exposure to sodium arsenite ($NaAsO_2$), an inorganic arsenical compound, via drinking water during gestational and/or postnatal periods causes impairment of spatial learning and memory, neuromotor reflex alteration, and spontaneous locomotor deficits in adult rats (Rodriguez et al., 2002; Xi et al., 2009). Offspring of female mice, which had been chronically exposed to $NaAsO_2$ via drinking water, display depression-like behavior (Martinez et al., 2008), and exhibit deficits in a hippocampus-dependent learning tasks (Martinez-Finley et al., 2009) during adulthood. Thus, $NaAsO_2$ exposure during developmental periods and the associated adverse effects on brain development induce behavioral abnormalities, although the toxic mechanisms of arsenic remain to be elucidated.

In vitro studies of neurons have revealed that $NaAsO_2$ induces apoptotic cell death in primary cultured neurons (Namgung and Xia, 2001; Wong et al., 2005) and neuronal cell lines (Koike-Kuroda et al., 2010; Keim et al., 2012). In addition, $NaAsO_2$ disrupts neuritogenesis in primary cultured neurons (Maekawa et al., 2013) and neuronal cell lines (Frankel et al., 2009; Aung et al., 2013). We previously reported that $NaAsO_2$-induced apoptosis is mediated by activation of caspase-3 (Koike-Kuroda et al., 2010), and that inhibition of neuritogenesis by $NaAsO_2$ is caused by alterations in the expression of cytoskeletal genes tau, tubulin, and neurofilament (Aung et al., 2013), and suppression of glutamate AMPA receptor expression (Maekawa et al., 2013). The toxic mechanisms by which developmental exposure to $NaAsO_2$ impairs the aforementioned brain functions and behaviors remain to be uncovered. However, based on *in vitro* studies of neurons, inorganic arsenic adversely affects the fate and maturation processes of young neurons, which may lead to abnormal formation of the neural circuits responsible for the brain functions and behaviors.

In addition to neurons, there may be other target cells of arsenic in the developing brain. Astrocytes are the largest population of glial cells, which are more abundant in the brain compared with neurons, and contribute to the formation and maintenance of the blood–brain barrier (BBB). The BBB is composed of endothelial cells, which line capillary blood vessels and connect to each other via tight junctions, and astrocytes surrounding blood capillaries via their end feet (Abbott, 2002). The BBB is not considered as a perfect barrier, although it contributes to protection of the brain against circulating xenobiotics that disrupt brain functions. The developing brain is considered to be vulnerable to toxic chemicals compared with the adult brain. One of the reasons is that the immature BBB during early development provides only partial protection against entry of chemicals into the brain (Zheng et al., 2003). Arsenite and arsenate are transferred to offspring through the placenta of pregnant mice that are exposed via drinking water, and arsenic species easily crossing the immature BBB accumulate in the brains of newborn offspring (Jin et al., 2006). Astrocytes are therefore the first brain cells that appear to be targeted by inorganic arsenic when it is transferred from the blood to the brain. Arsenite inhibits glutamate metabolism in astrocytes by reducing the activity and expression of glutamine synthase and glutamate transporters (Zhao et al., 2012). Synapse formation of primary cultured neurons is impaired by culture in conditioned medium from arsenite-exposed astrocytes (Wang et al., 2013). Taken together, the neurotoxicity of inorganic arsenic may be, at least in part, caused by its effects on astrocytes.

During brain development, neuron generation occurs first, followed by the generation of glial cells. In the cerebral cortex of rodents, astrocyte generation begins on embryonic day 18 following neurogenesis during embryonic days 12–18, and the number of astrocytes peaks in the neonatal period (Miller and Gauthier, 2007). It is assumed that neurotoxicant exposure during the developmental period affects not only neurogenesis but also the generation and proliferation of astrocytes, followed by altering the cell numbers. A reduced number of cortical glial cells is related to the pathological changes of schizophrenia and depression, indicating a causal link between glial cell abnormalities and psychiatric disorders (Cotter et al., 2001). In primary cultured rat astrocytes, inorganic arsenic decreases cell viability and increases DNA damage (Catanzaro et al., 2010). Such toxic effects of arsenite are stronger than those of arsenate (Jin et al., 2004). However, the mechanisms by which inorganic arsenic reduces the viability of astrocytes are largely unknown. Fluorescent ubiquitination-based cell cycle indicator (Fucci), which consists of monomeric Kusabira Orange2 (mKO2) fused with the ubiquitylation domain of human Cdt1 to monitor G1 phase and monomeric Azami Green (mAG) fused with the ubiquitylation domain of human Geminin to monitor S/G2/M phases, is useful to visualize the dynamics of cell cycle progression (Niwa et al., 1991; Sakaue-Sawano et al., 2008). In this study, we carried out live imaging analysis of primary cultured astrocytes originating from the cerebral cortex of Fucci transgenic (tg) mice to determine whether $NaAsO_2$ exposure decreases cell viability by affecting the cell cycle. Additionally, we examined the effects of $NaAsO_2$ exposure on the viability, apoptotic cell death, and expression of genes related to the cell cycle and apoptosis in cultured cortical astrocytes.

MATERIALS AND METHODS

Animals

Fucci tg mice were bred and maintained at the National Institute for Environmental Studies (Tsukuba, Japan). Wild-type C57BL/6J mice (Sankyo Labo Service, Tokyo, Japan) were bred at Saitama University (Saitama, Japan). They were housed under a controlled temperature (23 ± 2°C) and photoperiod (12:12, light:dark) with free access of tap water and standard chow. Animal procedures were conducted according to the approval and guidelines of Animal Care and Use Committee at the National Institute of Environmental Studies and Saitama University.

In vitro Culture of Astrocytes

Fucci tg and C57BL/6J mice were sacrificed on postnatal days 1 or 2 (postnatal day 1 = day of birth). After isolation of the cerebral cortex from the brain, the meninges were removed and the cortex tissue were placed in ice-cold Dulbecco's modified Eagle's medium (Sigma-Aldrich, St. Louis, MO, USA) supplemented with 3.7 mg/L sodium bicarbonate (Sigma-Aldrich), 10 mL/L antibiotic antifungal solution (Sigma-Aldrich), which contained 10,000 units penicillin, 10 mg streptomycin, and 25 µg amphotericin B per mL, and 10% fetal bovine serum (FBS; Gibco-Invitrogen, Carlsbad, CA, USA), which is hereafter referred to as culture medium (pH 7.2). Cells were isolated from the cerebral cortex in fresh culture medium by gentle mechanical trituration, seeded on poly-L-ornithine (15 µg/L)-precoated culture dishes or plates, and maintained in culture medium at 37°C in a humidified atmosphere with 5% CO_2. The culture medium was changed at 3 days after seeding, followed by medium changes at intervals of 3–4 days.

Cells obtained from Fucci tg mice were seeded on a four-compartment glass bottom dish (Greiner Bio-One, Kremsmünster, Austria) at 1×10^5 cells per compartment ($1.9\ cm^2$), cultured for more than 1 week, and then applied to fluorescence microscopy (see Section Fluorescence Microscopy of Fucci-Expressing Astrocytes) and live imaging analyses (see Section Time-Lapse Analysis of Fucci-Expressing Astrocytes). Cells obtained from C57BL/6J mice were seeded on a 6-well culture plate (Asahi Glass, Tokyo, Japan) at 3×10^5 cells per well ($9.4\ cm^2$) and cultured until 90–100% confluence. The cells were re-seeded onto new culture plates at 1×10^5 cells per well after trypsinization and then used to analyze the protein expression of glial fibrillary acidic protein (GFAP), a marker of astrocytes (see Section Analysis of GFAP Immunoreactivity), and the GFAP gene copy number (see Section Analysis of GFAP Gene Copy Numbers). For gene expression analysis (see Section Analysis of mRNA Levels), the cells were re-seeded at 4×10^5 cells per well after trypsinization. For apoptosis analysis, the cells were re-seeded on a 96-well culture plate (Asahi glass) at 5×10^3 cells per well (see Section Apoptosis Assay). All culture dishes and plates were precoated with poly-L-ornithine (15 µg/L) before use.

Analysis of GFAP Immunoreactivity

To check the purity of cells in primary culture, we performed immunocytochemistry of GFAP. Cultured cells fixed with 4% paraformaldehyde were reacted with a polyclonal rabbit anti-GFAP antibody (1:500; Dako, Glostrup, Denmark) at 4°C overnight and then Alexa Fluor 647 goat anti-rabbit IgG (1:400; Life Technology, Carlsbad, CA, USA) for 30 min at room temperature. 4,6-Diamidino-2-phenylindole (DAPI) staining was performed to count the total cell number.

Fluorescence Microscopy of Fucci-Expressing Astrocytes

To determine the cell cycle duration of astrocytes, we observed astrocytes from Fucci tg mice under a fluorescence microscope (BioZero 8100; Keyence, Osaka, Japan) equipped with an mKO2 filter (excitation filter: 542AF15; emission filter: 585QM30; dichroic mirror: 560 DRLP; Opto science, Tokyo, Japan) and a mAG filter (excitation filter: 475QM20; emission filter: 518QM32; dichroic mirror: 500DRLP; Opto science). First, the cell cycle of each astrocyte was synchronized by serum starvation. Culturing in medium supplemented with a low concentration of FBS (0.5%) for 72 h is effective to increase the population of cells at G1 phase (Khammanit et al., 2008). Therefore, 30–40% confluent astrocytes were incubated in culture medium supplemented with 0.1% FBS for 3 days. The astrocytes were again incubated in culture medium containing 10% FBS, and fluorescence images of mKO2 and mAG were captured every 6 h for 150 h using an objective lens (Plan Fluor ELWD DM 20 × C, NA 0.45; Nikon, Tokyo, Japan) and a CCD camera in the BioZero 8100 fluorescence microscope. In each culture, digital images were obtained in three regions ($0.58\ mm^2$/region, $1.74\ mm^2$ in total) that were randomly selected in the culture dish. Fluorescence microscopy was performed in four primary cultures derived from different animals.

Image analysis of mKO2 and mAG expression was performed with BZ-II analyzer software (Keyence). The digital images were modified to remove the background signal, and the red-green-blue (RGB) digital images of mKO2 and mAG were converted to monochromatic color images (red, mKO2; green, mAG). The monochromatic color images of mKO2 and mAG were merged at each time point to determine the intensities of mKO2 and mAG expression in the same region, which were obtained by measuring the brightness of the red and green signals, respectively. After measuring the brightness values of red and green signals in the same region of each merged image, the mAG/mKO2 emission ratio was calculated by dividing the brightness value of the green signal by that of the red signal. The mAG/mKO2 emission ratio at each time point was calibrated using the ratio of the same area at 0 h after the end of serum starvation, which was set at 100.

Time-Lapse Analysis of Fucci-Expressing Astrocytes

Exposure to $NaAsO_2$ and Live Imaging

$NaAsO_2$ (Wako Pure Chemical Industries, Osaka, Japan) was dissolved in sterile-filtered water (Sigma-Aldrich) at a concentration of 100 mM. The $NaAsO_2$ solution (100 mM) was further diluted with culture medium to obtain the indicated concentrations. Primary cultured Fucci-expressing astrocytes were subjected to serum starvation (see Section Fluorescence Microscopy of Fucci-Expressing Astrocytes) to synchronize the cell cycle. After synchronization, the cells were exposed to $NaAsO_2$ in culture medium at concentrations of 0, 1, 2, or 4 μM. Immediately after starting $NaAsO_2$ exposure, astrocytes were placed in an incubation chamber (Tokai Hit, Shizuoka, Japan) equipped to the BioZero 8100 fluorescence microscope. In the incubation chamber, the temperature was controlled at 37°C and the CO_2 concentration was maintained at 5%. Time-lapse fluorescence imaging began at 1 h and ended at 73 h after initiation of $NaAsO_2$ exposure. Fluorescence images of mKO2 and mAG expression, and bright field images were captured every 2 h. The digital image data were obtained from three regions (0.58 mm^2/region, 1.74 mm^2 in total) that were randomly selected in each culture dish compartment. Live imaging of Fucci-expressing astrocytes was performed in six primary cultures derived from different animals.

Image Analysis

We analyzed the intensity of mKO2 and mAG signal emissions, the number of cells expressing mKO2 and mAG, and the cell fate after S phase entry using the digital image data from live imaging. Image analyses were performed using the BZ-II analyzer software. The images were modified to remove the background signal and change the RGB colors of mKO2 and mAG to monochromatic colors. The modified images were used for analysis as described below.

The monochromatic color images of mKO2 (red) and mAG (green) were merged at each time point to measure the intensities of mKO2 and mAG in the same region, which were obtained by measuring the brightness of red and green signals, respectively. The mAG/mKO2 emission ratio was then calculated by dividing the brightness value of the green signal by that of the red signal. The mAG/mKO2 emission ratio at each time point was calibrated using the ratio of the same area at 5 h after $NaAsO_2$ exposure, which was set at 100.

To count cells expressing mKO2 and mAG, we used the monochromatic color images for each fluorescent protein, which were obtained every 8 h from 1 h after initiation of $NaAsO_2$ exposure. After counting the number of mKO2- and mAG-expressing cells, the value at each time point was then calibrated using the number of cells in the same area at 1 h after $NaAsO_2$ exposure, which was set at 100.

To analyze cell fate after S phase entry, the digital images of mKO2, mAG, and bright field, which were obtained from astrocytes with or without exposure to 4 μM $NaAsO_2$, were merged at each time point. The merged images at all-time points were then saved as a movie file to observe temporal changes in the expression of mKO2 and mAG, and the morphology of target cells. Target cells were astrocytes that expressed mAG at 41 h in the control group and at 9 h in the $NaAsO_2$-exposed group after initiation of $NaAsO_2$ exposure, because the population of mAG-expressing cells at these time points was the largest during live imaging for each group. These cells were traced until the end of live imaging to determine their viability. Live cells were defined as cells that expressed mAG followed by expression of mKO2 with normal morphology. Dead cells were defined as cells that expressed mAG followed by loss of fluorescent signals with abnormal morphology. A total of 434 cells in the control group and 426 cells in the $NaAsO_2$-exposed group were followed up to determine their cell fate. For each group, the total cell number was defined as 100%, and the percentages of live and dead cell populations were calculated.

Analysis of GFAP Gene Copy Numbers

Exposure to $NaAsO_2$ and DNA Extraction

Astrocytes originating from the cerebral cortex of C57BL/6J mice were incubated in culture medium containing $NaAsO_2$ at concentrations of 0, 1, 2, or 4 μM for 73 h. The astrocytes were then rinsed in Dulbecco's phosphate-buffered saline without calcium and magnesium, and collected in microcentrifuge tubes by scraping the culture plates filled with the buffer. After centrifugation (10,000 rpm, 10 min), the resulting cell pellet was subjected to extraction of total DNA with a DNeasy blood and tissue kit (Qiagen, Hilden, Germany). DNA samples were obtained from eight independent primary cultures derived from different animals.

Real-Time PCR

Real-time PCR was performed using a LightCycler 96 (Roche Diagnostics, Mannheim, Germany). To prepare standard samples for the GFAP gene, a partial fragment of the mouse GFAP gene (430 bp from 13,801 to 14,230 nt) was cloned by insertion of the DNA fragment into the pCR2.1-TOPO vector supplied in a TOPO TA cloning kit (Invitrogen). The plasmid vector containing a copy of the GFAP gene was serially diluted with nuclease-free water at 3.2×10^4, 8.0×10^3, 2.0×10^3, 5.0×10^2, and 1.25×10^2 copies per 2 μl. Two microliters of the standards and unknown samples containing total DNA extracted from the cultured cells were amplified in a 20 μl reaction mixture containing 200 nM of each primer (forward: 5′-TCCTTTCCACCTCCGCTAAC-3′; reverse: 5′-GTTGGGTCTTGCCTGTCTTC-3′) and 10 μl of 2× SYBR Premix Ex Taq (Takara Bio, Otsu, Japan). Real-time PCR conditions were initial activation of Taq polymerase for 30 s at 95°C, followed by 40 cycles of 5 s at 95°C for denaturation, and then 30 s at 60°C for annealing and extension with a temperature transition rate of 20°C/s. After real-time PCR, melting curve analysis was carried out to demonstrate the specificity of the PCR product (estimated amplicon size: 138 bp), resulting in a melting curve with a single peak (data not shown). After measurement of the GFAP gene copy number in each sample, the values were expressed as a percentage of the value obtained from cells without $NaAsO_2$ exposure, whose viability was set at 100%.

Apoptosis Assay

Primary cultured astrocytes originating from the cerebral cortex of C57BL/6J mice were subjected to serum starvation (see Section Fluorescence Microscopy of Fucci-Expressing Astrocytes) to synchronize the cell cycle and then incubated in culture medium containing $NaAsO_2$ at concentrations of 0, 2, or 4 μM for 72 h. The effects of $NaAsO_2$ on DNA fragmentation was examined using a Cell Death Detection ELISA Plus Assay kit (Roche Diagnosis) in accordance with the manufacturer's protocol. This assay was performed using six independent primary cultures derived from different animals. The amount of nucleosomes generated from DNA fragmentation is expressed as relative to that in the controls, which was set at 100% for each culture derived from the same animal.

Analysis of mRNA Levels

Exposure to $NaAsO_2$, RNA Extraction, and Reverse Transcription

Primarily cultured astrocytes were subjected to serum starvation (see Section Fluorescence Microscopy of Fucci-Expressing Astrocytes) to synchronize the cell cycle and then exposed to 0 or 4 μM $NaAsO_2$ in culture medium for 9 and 41 h. After exposure, total RNA was extracted and purified with an RNeasy Mini kit (Qiagen) in accordance with the manufacturer's protocol. For each sample, total RNA (650 ng) was reverse transcribed into cDNA in a final reaction volume of 20 μl using a PrimeScript RT Reagent kit (Takara Bio) in accordance with the manufacturer's protocol.

Real-Time PCR

To measure the gene expression levels of molecules involved in unscheduled S phase entry and apoptosis, p21, p53, E2F1, E2F4, and Gm36566, real-time PCR was performed using a LightCycler 96 (Roche Diagnostics). Equal amounts of cDNA from each sample were combined together and serially diluted with EASY dilution (Takara Bio) to prepare standard samples for each gene. One microliter of standards and diluted unknown samples were amplified in a 10 μl reaction mixture containing 5 μl of 2× SYBR Premix Ex Taq (Takara Bio) and 100 nM of each primer for specific genes (see **Table 1**). The real-time PCR settings were the same as those described in Section Real-Time PCR. The amounts of the mRNAs for target genes in each sample were normalized to the mRNA level of the housekeeping gene cyclophilin B (CPB) in the same sample. The normalized mRNA level of each target gene was expressed relative to that in the controls, which was set at 100%. The percentage values were averaged from five different primary cultures.

Statistical Analysis

Two-way factorial analysis of variance (ANOVA) for repeated measures was used to examine the effects of $NaAsO_2$ and time on the mAG/mKO2 emission ratio. One-way ANOVA was performed to determine the difference among groups with respect to the number of cells expressing mAG and mKO2, the copy number of the GFAP gene, and the amount of nucleosomes generated from DNA fragmentation. When significant overall effects were detected by one-way ANOVA, the Tukey–Kramer test was used for *post-hoc* analysis. Two-way ANOVA was performed to determine the effects of concentrations and exposure time of $NaAsO_2$ on the mRNA levels of target genes. Differences in the populations of live and dead cells between groups with or without exposure to $NaAsO_2$ were analyzed by the nonparametric Mann–Whitney U-test.

TABLE 1 | Primer sequences used for real-time PCR.

	Forward primer sequence (5′–3′)	Reverse primer sequence (5′–3′)	NCBI reference sequence
p21	TAGCTCCTTCCCTGG GATTC	ATAGCAAAGGGGCAG AAAAG	AF035683
p53	GCTTCTCCGAAGACT GGATG	GTCCATGCAGTGAGG TGATG	AB020317
Gm36566	TCCCATTCCCCTATC TGTGT	GCTATTCTCTGCTCC GATCC	XM_011247417
E2F1	ACTGTGACTTTGGGG ACCTG	CAGAGGGTATGGATC GTGCT	L21973
E2F4	CTGGCACTTGTGACT GTGCT	AGCACCACCCTCTCT CTGAA	NM_148952
CPB	AGACTGTTCCAAAAA CAGTGGA	GATGCTCTTTCCTCC TGTGC	M60456

RESULTS

Immunoreactivity of GFAP in Cultured Cells

Microscopy and counting DAPI-stained cells with or without GFAP immunoreactivity showed that most DAPI-stained cells exhibited GFAP-immunoreactive signals (98 ± 0.4% in four primary cultures derived from different animals; **Figure 1**). Thus, cells that were isolated from the mouse brains and cultured *in vitro* were astrocytes expressing GFAP.

Cell Cycle Distribution of Fucci-Expressing Astrocytes

Most primary cultured astrocytes from the cerebral cortex of Fucci tg mice expressed mKO2 after their cell cycles were synchronized by serum starvation (**Figure 2A**). mAG-expressing astrocytes emerged at 12 h after synchronization of the cell cycle. Forty-two hours after synchronization was the first time that expression of mAG reached a peak. mAG expression then decreased and the second peak of mAG expression occurred at 66 h after synchronization. This cycle of mAG expression was repeated during fluorescence microscopic observation.

The emission ratio of mAG to mKO2 in Fucci-expressing astrocytes changed over time (**Figure 2B**). The mAG/mKO2 emission ratio was low until 12–18 h after synchronization of the

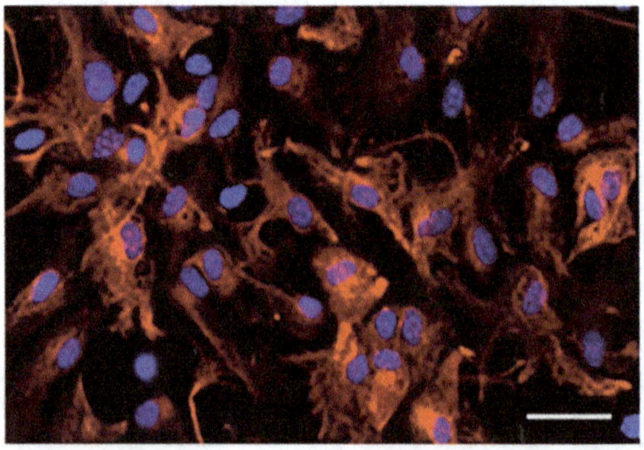

FIGURE 1 | Digital photomicrograph of primary cultured astrocytes. Astrocytes were immunostained for GFAP (red) and counterstained with DAPI (blue). Scale bar: 50 μm.

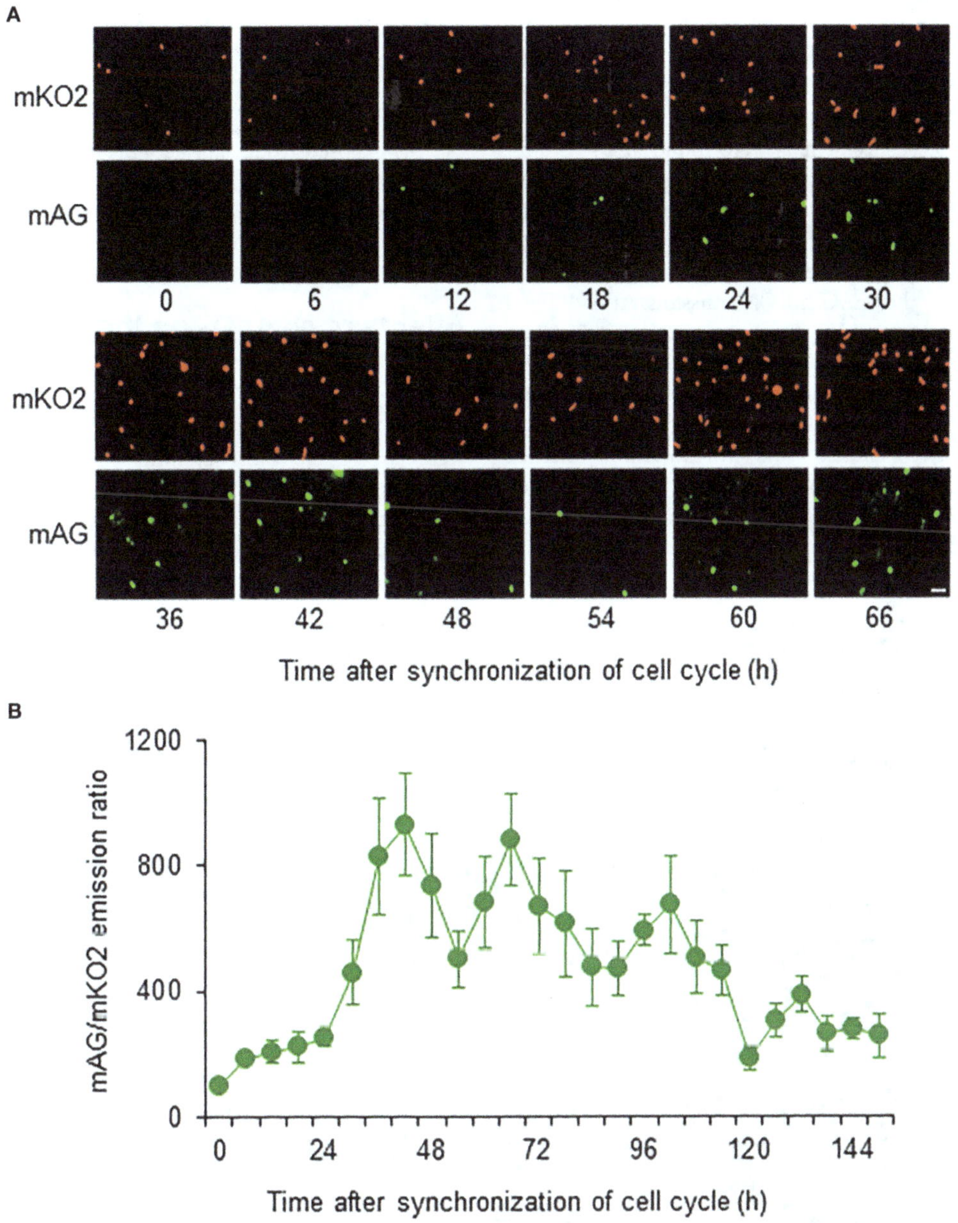

FIGURE 2 | Temporal changes in mAG and mKO2 emission signals of Fucci-expressing astrocytes. After astrocytes were serum starved for 72 h to synchronize the cell cycle, they were cultured in medium containing 10% FBS and applied to cell cycle monitoring. **(A)** Time-lapse images of mAG and mKO2 emission signals after the original fluorescent colors were converted to pseudocolors (mAG, green; mKO2, red). Scale bar: 50 μm. **(B)** Temporal changes in the mAG/mKO2 emission ratio of Fucci-expressing astrocytes. All data points are the means $\pm$ standard error of the mean (SEM) of four primary cultures derived from different animals. The mAG/mKO2 emission ratio at each time point was calibrated using the ratio at 0 h after the cells were cultured in 10% FBS-containing medium, which was set at 100.

cell cycle. The ratio dramatically increased from 24 to 42 h after synchronization of the cell cycle and then decreased until 54 h after synchronization. The ratio increased again and reached a peak at 66 h after synchronization of the cell cycle in four primary cultures derived from different animals. The cyclic changes in the mAG/mKO2 emission ratio were observed four times during the analysis period. The mean interpeak interval of the mAG/mKO2 emission ratio for each culture was 30, 28, 32, and 30 h. When these values were represented as the cell cycle duration in each culture, the mean of four different experiments was 30 $\pm$ 0.82 h, indicating that the cell cycle duration of Fucci-expressing astrocytes is ~30 h.

Effects of $NaAsO_2$ on the Cell Cycle of Astrocytes

Fucci-expressing astrocytes mostly emitted mKO2 fluorescence signals at the beginning of live imaging with or without $NaAsO_2$ exposure, while little emission of mAG signals was observed (**Figure 3**; Supplementary Movies 1–4). In control and $NaAsO_2$ (1 and 2 μM)-exposed groups, astrocytes emitting mAG fluorescence signals were frequently observed between 33 and 49 h after initiation of $NaAsO_2$ exposure, which then decreased over time. On the other hand, in astrocytes exposed to 4 μM $NaAsO_2$, mAG fluorescence signals were found at 5–9 h after $NaAsO_2$ exposure. In some astrocytes exposed to 4 μM $NaAsO_2$, the fluorescent emissions of mAG and mKO2 had disappeared after 31 h of exposure to $NaAsO_2$.

Two-way ANOVA for repeated measures indicated that the temporal changes in the mAG/mKO2 emission ratio differed significantly among groups [$F_{(3, 175)} = 49.3$, $p < 0.05 \times 10^{-26}$], over time [$F_{(34, 175)} = 2.91$, $p < 0.000005$], and by interactions between the main factors [$F_{(102, 525)} = 1.84$, $p < 0.00001$]. In control and $NaAsO_2$ (1 and 2 μM)-exposed groups, the mAG/mKO2 emission ratio was low and maintained a stable level until 23 h after $NaAsO_2$ exposure, which then increased over time and reached a peak at 39–45 h after $NaAsO_2$ exposure, followed by a gradual decrease until the end of live imaging (**Figure 4**). The peak levels of the mAG/mKO2 emission ratio in $NaAsO_2$ (1 and 2 μM)-exposed groups were lower than those in the control group. The temporal change in the mAG/mKO2 emission ratio of the $NaAsO_2$ (4 μM)-exposed group was different from that of other groups. In the $NaAsO_2$ (4 μM)-exposed group, a peak of the mAG/mKO2 emission ratio was found at 7 h after initiation of $NaAsO_2$ exposure, whereas no obvious peak in the ratio was observed when the ratio showed a peak in the control and $NaAsO_2$ (1 and 2 μM)-exposed groups.

Effects of $NaAsO_2$ on the Number of Fucci-Expressing Astrocytes

In control and $NaAsO_2$ (1 μM)-exposed groups, the numbers of mAG-expressing cells at 33 and 41 h after $NaAsO_2$ exposure were larger than those at other time points for each group (**Figure 5A**). Compared with the control group, the number of mAG-expressing cells was significantly ($p < 0.05$) smaller at 41 h after $NaAsO_2$ exposure in the $NaAsO_2$ (2 μM)-exposed group

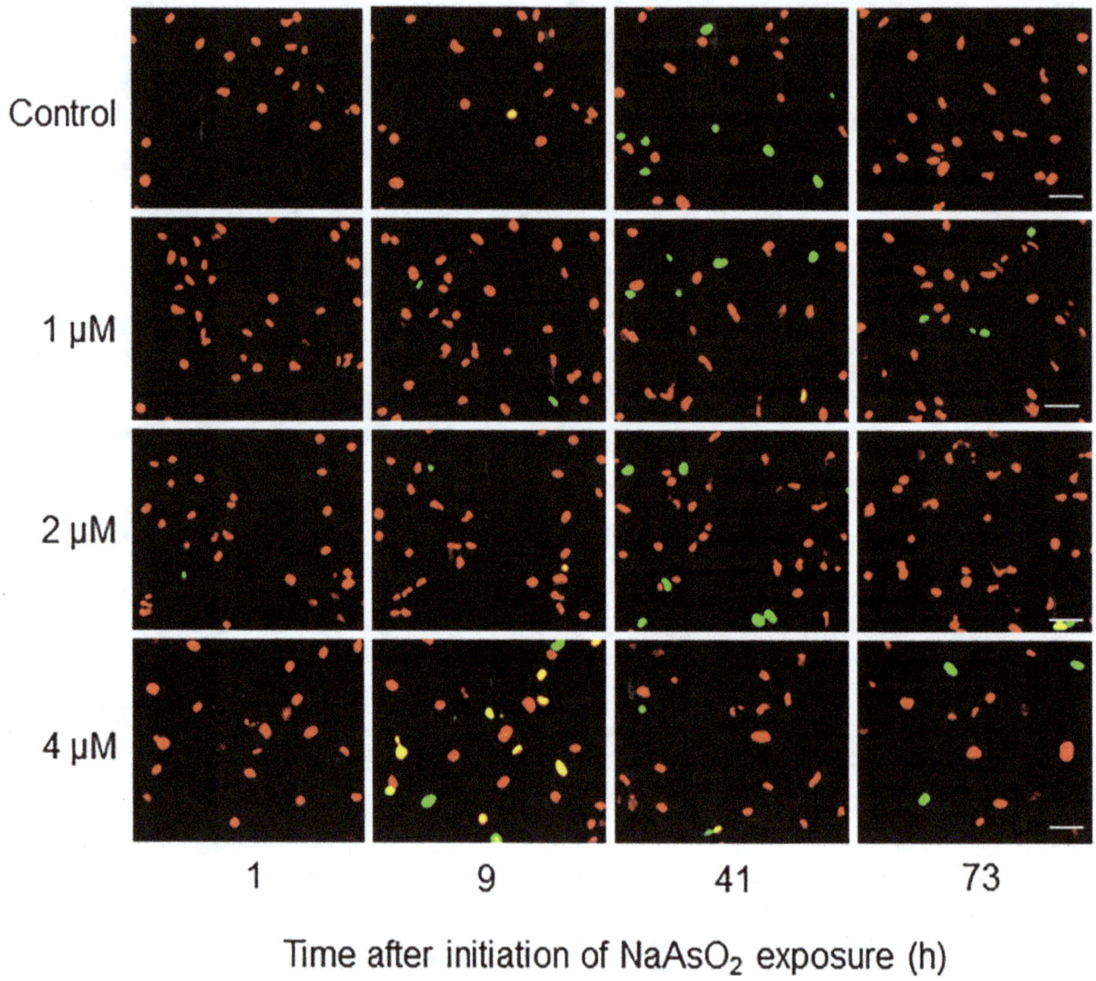

FIGURE 3 | Time-lapse images of Fucci-expressing astrocytes after initiation of $NaAsO_2$ exposure. Images of mAG and mKO2 signals were merged after the original colors were converted to pseudocolors (mAG, green; mKO2, red). Images were obtained from Fucci-expressing astrocytes exposed to $NaAsO_2$ at concentrations of 0 (control), 1, 2, or 4 μM for 1–73 h. Scale bar: 50 μm.

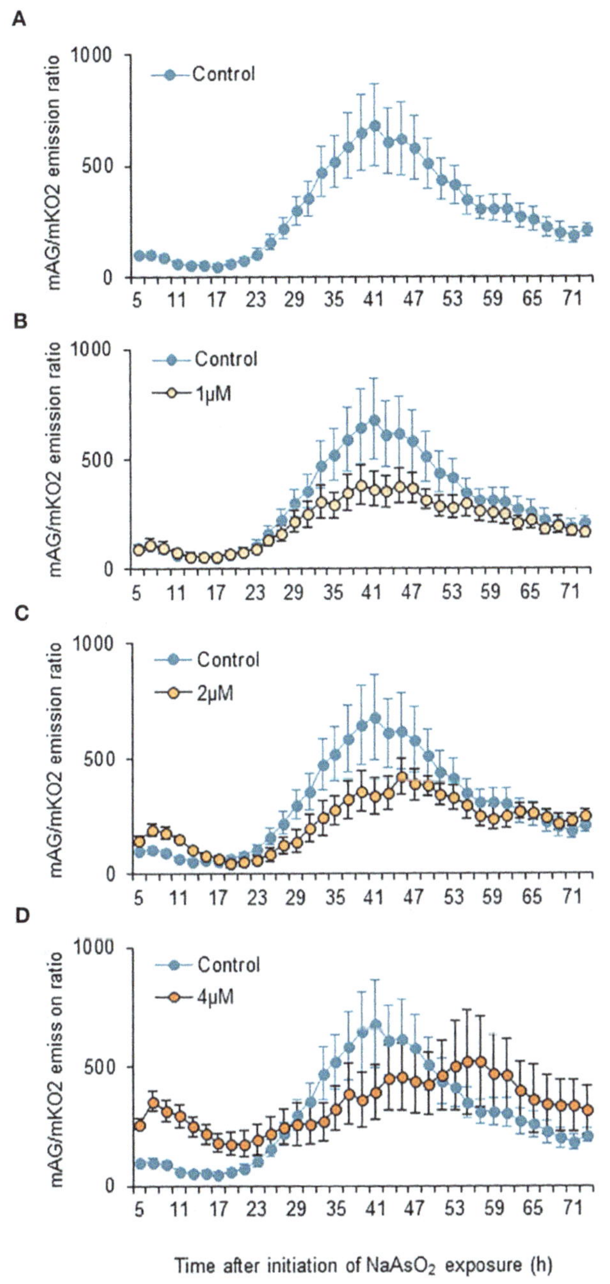

FIGURE 4 | Effects of $NaAsO_2$ exposure on the mAG/mKO2 emission ratio of Fucci-expressing astrocytes. Temporal changes in the mAG/mKO2 emission ratio of the control group **(A)** and groups exposed to $NaAsO_2$ at 1 μM **(B)**, 2 μM **(C)**, or 4 μM **(D)** from 5 to 72 h after initiation of $NaAsO_2$ exposure. Significant effects of the concentration and time of $NaAsO_2$ exposure and the interaction between the concentration and time on the ratio were found in two-way ANOVA for repeated measures. The ratio at each time point was calibrated using the ratio at 5 h after $NaAsO_2$ exposure, which was set at 100. All data are the means ± SEM of six primary cultures derived from different animals.

and at 25, 33, and 41 h after $NaAsO_2$ exposure in the $NaAsO_2$ (4 μM)-exposed group. In the $NaAsO_2$ (4 μM)-exposed group, the number of mAG-expressing cells was highest at 9 h after $NaAsO_2$ exposure, which was significantly ($p < 0.05$) larger than that in the control group.

There was tendency toward an increase in the number of cells expressing mKO2 from the beginning to the end of live imaging in control and $NaAsO_2$ (1 μM)-exposed groups (**Figure 5B**). At 57, 65, and 73 h after $NaAsO_2$ exposure, the total number of mKO2-expressing cells showed a concentration-dependent decrease, although there was no significant difference in the number of mKO2-expressing cells among the groups at each time point.

Effects of $NaAsO_2$ on Cell Death after S Phase Entry

To analyze cell fate after S phase entry, we traced Fucci-expressing astrocytes that emitted mAG fluorescence signals at 41 h in the control group and at 9 h after initiation of $NaAsO_2$ exposure in the $NaAsO_2$ (4 μM)-exposed group. As a result, most cells in the control group were alive at the end of live imaging, because the fluorescent emission signals changed from mAG to mKO2, and the morphology was normal (**Figure 6A**). Conversely, in most astrocytes of the $NaAsO_2$ (4 μM)-exposed group, the emission signal of mAG, which was observed at 9 h after $NaAsO_2$ exposure, had disappeared by the end of live imaging (**Figure 6B**). In addition, the cells did not express mKO2 and exhibited abnormal morphology with a debris-like structure. The population of live cells after S phase entry was significantly ($p < 0.01$) larger in the control group than in the $NaAsO_2$ (4 μM)-exposed group (**Figure 6C**). In contrast, the population of dead cells after S phase entry was significantly ($p < 0.01$) larger in the $NaAsO_2$-exposed group than in the control group.

Effects of $NaAsO_2$ on the Copy Number of the GFAP Gene and DNA Fragmentation

Exposure to $NaAsO_2$ for 73 h significantly [$F_{(3, 28)} = 4.30$, $p < 0.05$] reduced the GFAP gene copy number in a concentration-dependent manner (**Figure 7**). The copy number of the GFAP gene in the $NaAsO_2$ (4 μM)-exposed group was significantly ($p < 0.05$) smaller than that in the control group. We found no significant effect of lower $NaAsO_2$ concentrations.

The amount of nucleosomes generated from DNA fragmentation in astrocytes did not significantly [$F_{(1, 15)} = 2.21$, $p = 0.14$] change after exposure to $NaAsO_2$ (2 and 4 μM) for 72 h (**Figure 8**).

Effect of $NaAsO_2$ on the mRNA Expression of Apoptotic Markers and Cell Cycle Regulators

We did not find any significant effects of $NaAsO_2$ exposure on the mRNA levels of E2F1, E2F4, Gm36566, p21, or p53 in astrocytes (**Figure 9**). The mRNA levels of E2F1, E2F4, and p21, but not Gm36566 and p53, changed over time after synchronization of the cell cycle of astrocytes. The mRNA levels of E2F1 [$F_{(1, 16)} = 300.69$, $p < 0.01 \times 10^{-9}$] and p21 [$F_{(1, 16)} = 37.74$, $p < 0.00005$] were significantly higher at 41 h than 9 h after synchronization of the cell cycle, while the mRNA levels of E2F4 [$F_{(1, 16)} = 16.28$, $p < 0.001$] were higher at 9 h than 41 h after synchronization.

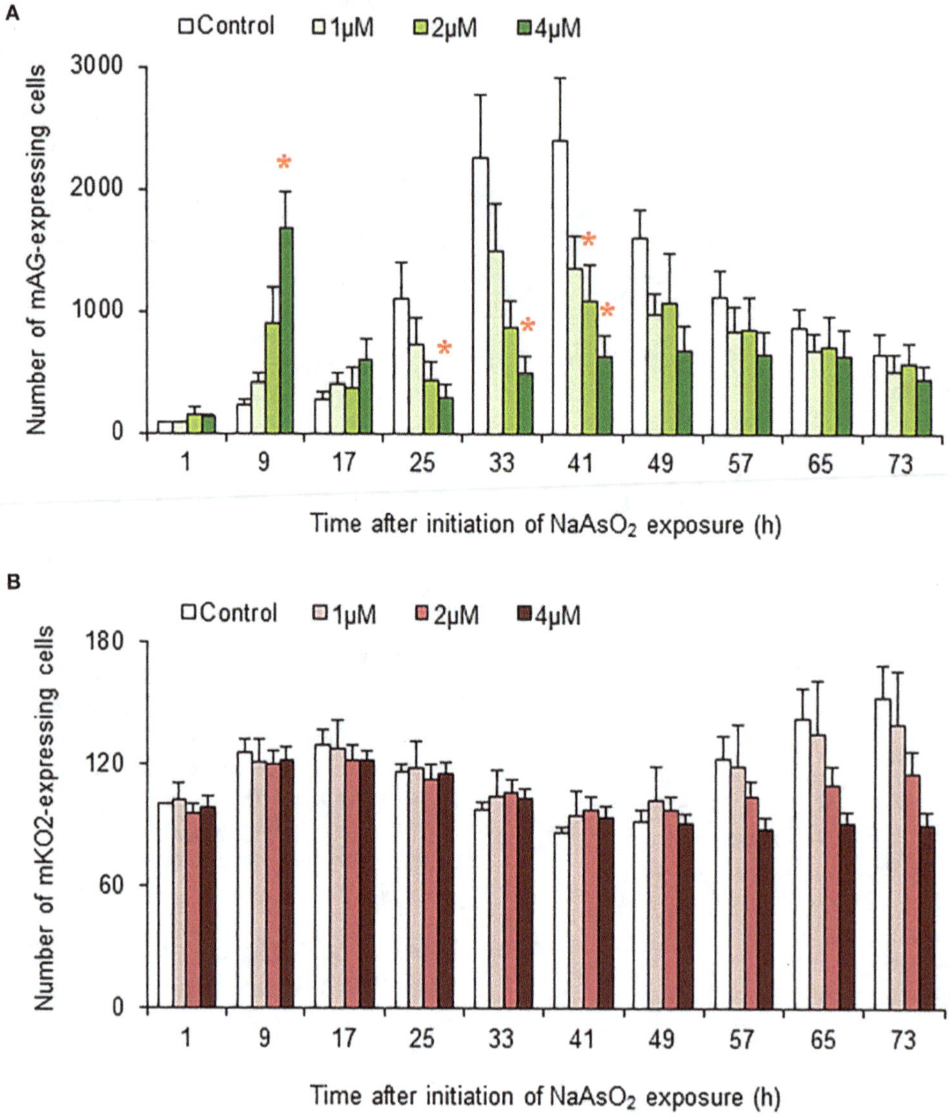

FIGURE 5 | Effects of $NaAsO_2$ exposure on the number of Fucci-expressing astrocytes. The number of cells expressing mAG **(A)** and mKO2 **(B)** at the indicated time point after initiation of $NaAsO_2$ exposure. The value for each time point was calibrated with the number of cells in the control group at 1 h after $NaAsO_2$ exposure, which was set at 100. All data are the means ± SEM of six primary cultures derived from different animals. $^*p < 0.05$ vs. control at the same time point.

DISCUSSION

There is serious concern about contamination of ground water with arsenic, because chronic consumption of arsenic-contaminated water causes an impairment of cognitive functions (Calderon et al., 2001; Tsai et al., 2003; Wasserman et al., 2007). The World Health Organization recommends a limit of 0.01 mg/L (0.01 ppm) arsenic in water (World Health Organization, 2011). However, arsenic contamination in tube well water was found in Bangladesh at a concentration of more than 0.3 mg/L (0.3 ppm; Smith et al., 2000). In a native Andean population living in a part of Argentina, where drinking water contains arsenic at about 0.2 mg/L (0.2 ppm), the concentrations of arsenic were 9 μg/L in cord blood, 11 μg/L in maternal blood, 34 μg/kg in placenta, and 2.3 μg/kg in breast milk (0.009, 0.011, 0.034, and 0.0023 ppm, respectively; Concha et al., 1998a,b). According to a study measuring the accumulated levels of arsenic in newborn mice of mothers that were chronically exposed to $NaAsO_2$ (10–80 ppm) during the gestational period via drinking water, the accumulated level of arsenic in the brain was higher than that in the liver and blood, and ranged from ~100 to 700 ng/g (0.1–0.7 ppm; Markowski et al., 2011). We previously reported that $NaAsO_2$ at 0.5–10 μM induced cell death and suppressed neuritogenesis of cultured neurons (Koike-Kuroda et al., 2010; Aung et al., 2013; Maekawa et al., 2013). In this study, to examine whether $NaAsO_2$ at the micromolar concentrations affect cultured astrocytes, we set the exposure concentrations

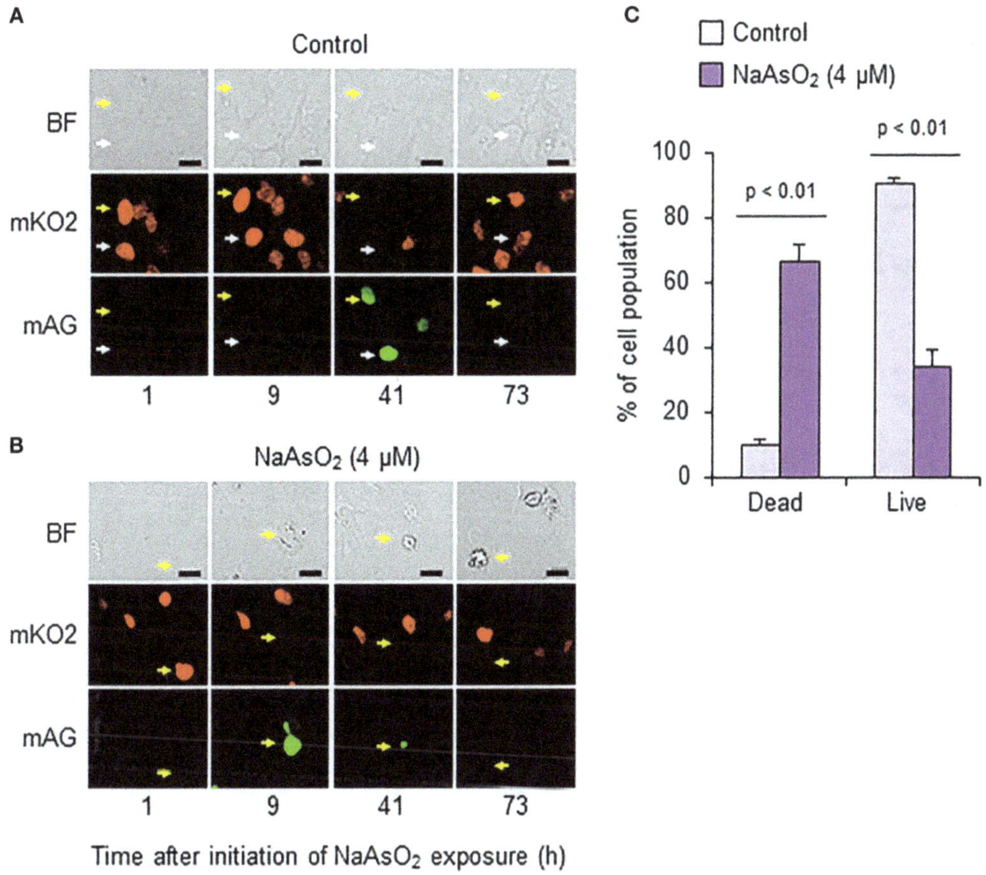

FIGURE 6 | Effects of $NaAsO_2$ exposure on cell fate after S phase entry. Digital photomicrograph of Fucci-expressing astrocytes captured with bright field (BF) and emission of mKO2 and mAG after pseudocolor conversion from the original fluorescent colors (mKO2, red; mAG, green) in control and $NaAsO_2$ (4 μM)-exposed groups **(A,B)**. Yellow and white arrows indicate the same cell or area. Scale bar: 20 μm. Cell population after Fucci-expressing cells entered S phase **(C)**. The percentage values of dead and live cells after S phase entry were calculated with the total number of cells that entered S phase, which was set at 100%. Values are the means ± SEM of six primary cultures derived from different animals.

of $NaAsO_2$ at 1, 2, and 4 μM (equivalent to 0.129, 0.258, and 0.516 ppm, respectively), which were similar to environmental pollution levels and higher than human exposure levels by ~200-times or less.

It is known that cultured cells undergo phototoxic damage induced by frequent illumination with excitation light under a fluorescence microscope (Cervinka et al., 2008). Our previous study revealed that serum supplementation (the combination of 1% horse serum and 0.5% FBS) is vital to protect PC12 cells from phototoxic damage and enables live cell imaging without phototoxic damage (Koike-Kuroda et al., 2010). On the other hand, the doubling time of primary cultured astrocytes from the rat cerebral cortex is 6 days under the culture condition of 2% fetal calf serum (Geisert et al., 1996). This finding indicates that culturing astrocytes with serum supplementation at low concentrations is not beneficial for live imaging to monitor the cell cycle of astrocytes, because it requires a longer time (more than 6 days), which would increase the risk of phototoxic damage. Therefore, to promote cell proliferation and shorten the doubling time of astrocytes, we performed live imaging analysis of primary cultured Fucci-expressing astrocytes under the culture condition of 10% FBS. The duration of the cell cycle in Fucci-expressing astrocytes subjected to live imaging corresponded to that determined by fluorescence microscopy, suggesting that the live imaging technique in our current study could monitor the cell cycle without severe phototoxic damage.

Live imaging analysis of Fucci-expressing astrocytes showed that $NaAsO_2$ exposure significantly altered the cell cycle. The cell population entering S phase, when the cell population had reached to a peak level in the control group without $NaAsO_2$ exposure, was decreased by $NaAsO_2$ in a concentration-dependent manner. In contrast, the cell population entering unscheduled S phase at 9 h after initiation of $NaAsO_2$ exposure was increased by $NaAsO_2$ in a concentration-dependent manner. The findings in our current study suggest that $NaAsO_2$ exposure disrupts the cell cycle and forces astrocytes to enter S phase at an unscheduled timing. In particular, 4 μM $NaAsO_2$ had significant effects to disrupt cell cycle regulation and induce unscheduled S phase entry. Moreover, we traced the morphology

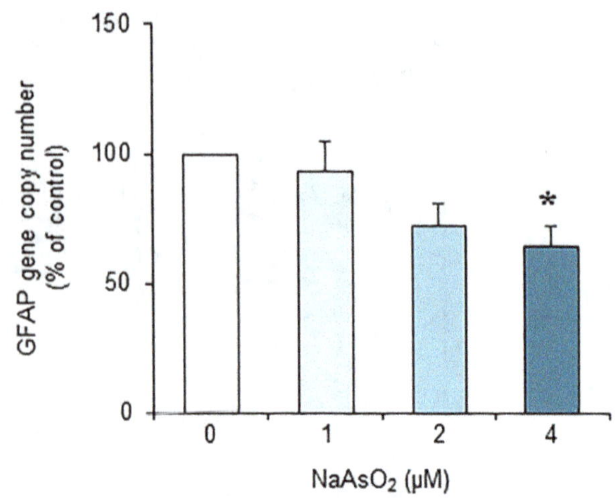

FIGURE 7 | Effects of $NaAsO_2$ exposure on the copy number of the GFAP gene. The GFAP gene copy number is presented as a percentage of the control. Values are the means ± SEM of eight primary cultures derived from different animals. $^*p < 0.05$ vs. control.

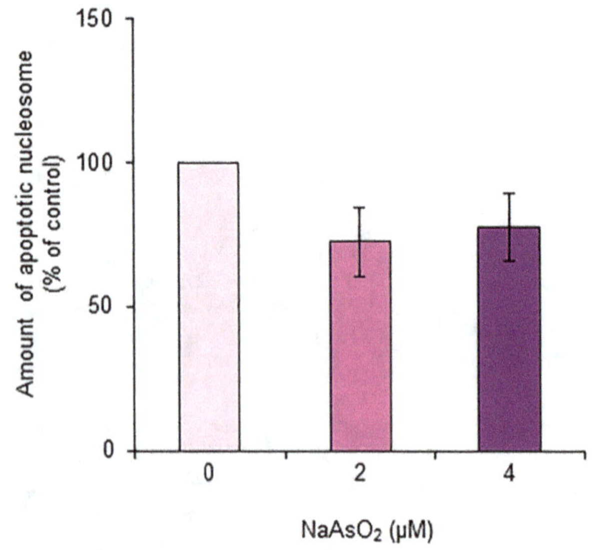

FIGURE 8 | Amount of apoptotic nucleosomes in astrocytes. The amount of apoptotic nucleosomes was assayed in astrocytes exposed to $NaAsO_2$ (0, 2, and 4 μM) and is represented as a percentage of the control. Values are the means ± SEM of six primary cultures derived from different animals.

as well as mKO2 and mAG expression of Fucci-expressing astrocytes to determine the fate of astrocytes that underwent unscheduled S phase entry induced by 4 μM $NaAsO_2$. As a result, more than 60% of astrocytes that entered S phase at 9 h after $NaAsO_2$ exposure had died, with disappearance of fluorescent mKO2 and mAG signals, and transforming debris-like structures until the end of live imaging. We also measured the copy number of the GFAP gene at 73 h after $NaAsO_2$ exposure, and found a significant decrease in the gene copy number induced by 4 μM $NaAsO_2$. Taken together, it appears likely that $NaAsO_2$ exposure at 4 μM decreases the number of astrocytes by inducing unscheduled S phase entry-coupled cell death. There is a report showing a slight increase in the viability of cultured rat cerebellar astrocytes by $NaAsO_2$ exposure at 1 μM for 24 h, but higher concentrations (5–50 μM) decrease the cell viability (An et al., 2016). In contrast, there is a report indicating that the cell viability is unaffected even when cultured rat astrocytes are exposed to 0.3 mM arsenite for 8 h, but it is decreased at 24 h after exposure (Koehler et al., 2014). Although the detailed mechanisms are largely unknown, arsenic may have dual effects to increase or decrease cell viability, which are dependent on the concentration and exposure time. Our current study supports the notion that arsenic decreases the viability of cultured astrocytes, and suggests that decreased cell viability is due to the reduction of cell number induced by unscheduled S phase entry-coupled cell death.

It is well-known that unscheduled S phase entry is linked to apoptotic cell death after DNA damage (Dimova and Dyson, 2005; Cho and Liang, 2011). The live imaging analysis in our current study showed that the mAG/mKO2 emission ratio and the number of mAG-expressing cells increased faster with $NaAsO_2$ exposure, indicating that up-regulation of geminin expression at an unscheduled timing is induced by $NaAsO_2$ exposure. It has been reported that overexpression of geminin induces apoptotic cell death (Shreeram et al., 2002). In this context, we speculated that apoptosis is responsible for the unscheduled S phase entry-coupled cell death induced by $NaAsO_2$ exposure. To test this hypothesis, we examined the effects of $NaAsO_2$ on the amount of nucleosomes generated from DNA fragmentation in astrocytes. However, in contrast to our expectations, we did not find any significant effect of $NaAsO_2$ on the amount of nucleosomes generated from DNA fragmentation. In addition, we examined whether $NaAsO_2$ exposure affected the expression levels of certain molecules involved in unscheduled S phase entry and apoptosis. We measured the mRNA levels of p53, a principal regulator of apoptosis (Fridman and Lowe, 2003; Cho and Liang, 2011), E2F1, an S phase gene transcriptional activator and programed cell death inducer (Hou et al., 2000; Pardee et al., 2004; Dimova and Dyson, 2005; Lazzerini Denchi and Helin, 2005; Cho and Liang, 2011), E2F4, an S phase gene transcriptional suppressor (Dimova and Dyson, 2005), p21, a cyclin dependent kinase inhibitor (Cho and Liang, 2011) and unscheduled S phase inducer (Bedelbaeva et al., 2010), and Gm36566, the mouse ortholog of Killin, which acts as a S-phase-coupled apoptosis regulator (Cho and Liang, 2011). Considering the results of the apoptosis assay with reference to the amount of nucleosomes, the gene expression of these molecules was not significantly affected by $NaAsO_2$ exposure, although the mRNA levels of E2F1, E2F4, and p21 had temporally changed with or without $NaAsO_2$ exposure. Taken together, the unscheduled S phase entry that occurred in astrocytes after $NaAsO_2$ exposure may be induced without alteration of the expression of these molecules. In addition, the subsequent cell death may be

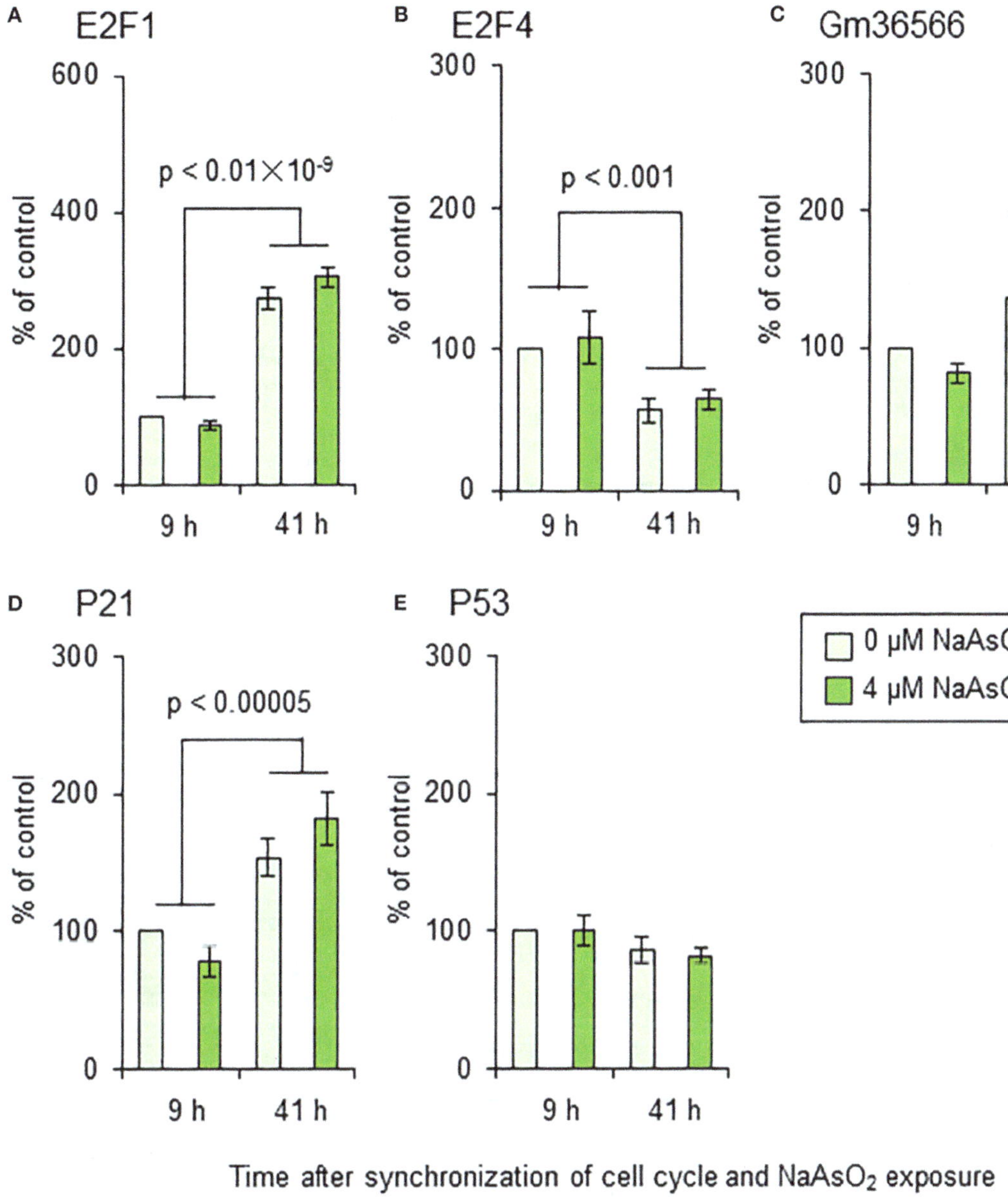

FIGURE 9 | mRNA levels of E2F1 (A), E2F4 (B), Gm36566 (C), p21 (D), and p53 (E) in astrocytes. Astrocytes were exposed to $NaAsO_2$ (0 and 4 μM) for 9 and 41 h. The mRNA level of each gene was normalized to that of CPB and are expressed relative to that of the control (0 μM for 9 h), which was set at 100%. Values are the means ± SEM of five primary cultures derived from different animals.

caused by mechanisms other than apoptosis. However, the mechanisms were not determined in this study. Further studies are needed to clarify the molecular mechanisms of arsenic toxicity, which induce unscheduled S phase entry-coupled cell death in astrocytes.

In summary, we examined the effects of $NaAsO_2$ exposure on the cell cycle, viability, and apoptotic cell death of cultured mouse cerebral astrocytes. The results of these analyses suggest that 4 μM $NaAsO_2$ significantly induces unscheduled S phase entry that is coupled with cell death by mechanisms other than apoptosis.

AUTHOR CONTRIBUTIONS

ST and FM designed the study; NH, HS, KS, and KA performed live imaging analyses; NH, HS, and SM performed molecular analyses; NH and ST wrote the manuscript; FM and MT critically revised the manuscript.

Science and Technology of Japan (23310043 and 15K14556 to ST; 24590307, 15K08223, and 15K14556 to FM), grants from the National Institute for Environmental Studies [1011AF005 and 1416AT001] and a grant from the National Center for Child Health and Development (25-3) to FM.

REFERENCES

Abbott, N. J. (2002). Astrocyte-endothelial interactions and blood-brain barrier permeability. *J. Anat.* 200, 629–638. doi: 10.1046/j.1469-7580.2002.00064.x

An, Y., Liu, T., Liu, X., Zhao, L., and Wang, J. (2016). Rac1 and Cdc42 play important roles in arsenic neurotoxicity in primary cultured rat cerebellar astrocytes. *Biol. Trace Elem. Res.* 170, 173–182. doi: 10.1007/s12011-015-0456-7

Aung, K. H., Kurihara, R., Nakashima, S., Maekawa, F., Nohara, K., Kobayashi, T., et al. (2013). Inhibition of neurite outgrowth and alteration of cytoskeletal gene expression by sodium arsenite. *Neurotoxicology* 34, 226–235. doi: 10.1016/j.neuro.2012.09.008

Bedelbaeva, K., Snyder, A., Gourevitch, D., Clark, L., Zhang, X. M., Leferovich, J., et al. (2010). Lack of p21 expression links cell cycle control and appendage regeneration in mice. *Proc. Natl. Acad. Sci. U.S.A.* 107, 5845–5850. doi: 10.1073/pnas.1000830107

Calderon, J., Navarro, M. E., Jimenez-Capdeville, M. E., Santos-Diaz, M. A., Golden, A., Rodriguez-Leyva, I., et al. (2001). Exposure to arsenic and lead and neuropsychological development in Mexican children. *Environ. Res.* 85, 69–76. doi: 10.1006/enrs.2000.4106

Catanzaro, I., Schiera, G., Sciandrello, G., Barbata, G., Caradonna, F., Proia, P., et al. (2010). Biological effects of inorganic arsenic on primary cultures of rat astrocytes. *Int. J. Mol. Med.* 26, 457–462. doi: 10.3892/ijmm_00000485

Cervinka, M., Cervinkova, Z., and Rudolf, E. (2008). The role of time-lapse fluorescent microscopy in the characterization of toxic effects in cell populations cultivated *in vitro Toxicol. In Vitro* 22, 1382–1386. doi: 10.1016/j.tiv.2008.03.011

Cho, Y. J., and Liang, P. (2011). S-phase-coupled apoptosis in tumor suppression. *Cell Mol. Life Sci.* 68, 1883–1896. doi: 10.1007/s00018-011-0666-x

Concha, G., Vogler, G., Lezcano, D., Nermell, B., and Vahter, M. (1998a). Exposure to inorganic arsenic metabolites during early human development. *Toxicol. Sci.* 44, 185–190. doi: 10.1093/toxsci/44.2.185

Concha, G., Vogler, G., Nermell, B., and Vahter, M. (1998b). Low-level arsenic excretion in breast milk of native Andean women exposed to high levels of arsenic in the drinking water. *Int. Arch. Occup. Environ. Health* 71, 42–46. doi: 10.1007/s004200050248

Cotter, D. R., Pariante, C. M., and Everall, I. P. (2001). Glial cell abnormalities in major psychiatric disorders: the evidence and implications. *Brain Res. Bull.* 55, 585–595. doi: 10.1016/S0361-9230(01)00527-5

Dimova, D. K., and Dyson, N. J. (2005). The E2F transcriptional network: old acquaintances with new faces. *Oncogene* 24, 2810–2826. doi: 10.1038/sj.onc.1208612

Frankel, S., Concannon, J., Brusky, K., Pietrowicz, E., Giorgianni, S., Thompson, W. D., et al. (2009). Arsenic exposure disrupts neurite growth and complexity *in vitro*. *Neurotoxicology* 30, 529–537. doi: 10.1016/j.neuro.2009.02.015

Fridman, J. S., and Lowe, S. W. (2003). Control of apoptosis by p53. *Oncogene* 22, 9030–9040. doi: 10.1038/sj.onc.1207116

Geisert, E. E. Jr., Yang, L., and Irwin, M. H. (1996). Astrocyte growth, reactivity, and the target of the antiproliferative antibody, TAPA. *J. Neurosci.* 16, 5478–5487.

Grandjean, P., and Landrigan, P. J. (2006). Developmental neurotoxicity of industrial chemicals. *Lancet* 368, 2167–2178. doi: 10.1016/S0140-6736(06)69665-7

Grandjean, P., and Landrigan, P. J. (2014). Neurobehavioural effects of developmental toxicity. *Lancet Neurol.* 13, 330–338. doi: 10.1016/S1474-4422(13)70278-3

Hou, S. T., Callaghan, D., Fournier, M. C., Hill, I., Kang, L., Massie, B., et al. (2000). The transcription factor E2F1 modulates apoptosis of neurons. *J. Neurochem.* 75, 91–100. doi: 10.1046/j.1471-4159.2000.0750091.x

Jin, Y., Sun, G., Li, X., Li, G., Lu, C., and Qu, L. (2004). Study on the toxic effects induced by different arsenicals in primary cultured rat astroglia. *Toxicol. Appl. Pharmacol.* 196, 396–403. doi: 10.1016/j.taap.2004.01.015

Jin, Y., Xi, S., Li, X., Lu, C., Li, G., Xu, Y., et al. (2006). Arsenic speciation transported through the placenta from mother mice to their newborn pups. *Environ. Res.* 101, 349–355. doi: 10.1016/j.envres.2005.11.006

Keim, A., Rossler, O. G., Rothhaar, T. L., and Thiel, G. (2012). Arsenite-induced apoptosis of human neuroblastoma cells requires p53 but occurs independently of c-Jun. *Neuroscience* 206, 25–38. doi: 10.1016/j.neuroscience.2012.01.001

Khammanit, R., Chantakru, S., Kitiyanant, Y., and Saikhun, J. (2008). Effect of serum starvation and chemical inhibitors on cell cycle synchronization of canine dermal fibroblasts. *Theriogenology* 70, 27–34. doi: 10.1016/j.theriogenology.2008.02.015

Koehler, Y., Luther, E. M., Meyer, S., Schwerdtle, T., and Dringen, R. (2014). Uptake and toxicity of arsenite and arsenate in cultured brain astrocytes. *J. Trace Elem. Med. Biol.* 28, 328–337. doi: 10.1016/j.jtemb.2014.04.007

Koike-Kuroda, Y., Kakeyama, M., Fujimaki, H., and Tsukahara, S. (2010). Use of live imaging analysis for evaluation of cytotoxic chemicals that induce apoptotic cell death. *Toxicol. In Vitro* 24, 2012–2020. doi: 10.1016/j.tiv.2010.07.022

Lazzerini Denchi, E., and Helin, K. (2005). E2F1 is crucial for E2F-dependent apoptosis. *EMBO Rep.* 6, 661–668. doi: 10.1038/sj.embor.7400452

Maekawa, F., Tsuboi, T., Oya, M., Aung, K. H., Tsukahara, S., Pellerin, L., et al. (2013). Effects of sodium arsenite on neurite outgrowth and glutamate AMPA receptor expression in mouse cortical neurons. *Neurotoxicology* 37, 197–206. doi: 10.1016/j.neuro.2013.05.006

Markowski, V. P., Currie, D., Reeve, E. A., Thompson, D., and Wise, J. P. Sr. (2011). Tissue-specific and dose-related accumulation of arsenic in mouse offspring following maternal consumption of arsenic-contaminated water. *Basic Clin. Pharmacol. Toxicol.* 108, 326–332. doi: 10.1111/j.1742-7843.2010.00660.x

Martinez, E. J., Kolb, B. L., Bell, A., Savage, D. D., and Allan, A. M. (2008). Moderate perinatal arsenic exposure alters neuroendocrine markers associated with depression and increases depressive-like behaviors in adult mouse offspring. *Neurotoxicology* 29, 647–655. doi: 10.1016/j.neuro.2008.05.004

Martinez-Finley, E. J., Ali, A. M., and Allan, A. M. (2009). Learning deficits in C57BL/6J mice following perinatal arsenic exposure: consequence of lower corticosterone receptor levels? *Pharmacol. Biochem. Behav.* 94, 271–277. doi: 10.1016/j.pbb.2009.09.006

Miller, F. D., and Gauthier, A. S. (2007). Timing is everything: making neurons versus glia in the developing cortex. *Neuron* 54, 357–369. doi: 10.1016/j.neuron.2007.04.019

Namgung, U., and Xia, Z. (2001). Arsenic induces apoptosis in rat cerebellar neurons via activation of JNK3 and p38 MAP kinases. *Toxicol. Appl. Pharmacol.* 174, 130–138. doi: 10.1006/taap.2001.9200

Niwa, H., Yamamura, K., and Miyazaki, J. (1991). Efficient selection for high-transfectants with a novel eukaryotic vector. *Gene* 108, 193–199.

Pardee, A. B., Li, C. J., and Reddy, G. P. (2004). Regulation in S phase by E2F. *Cell Cycle* 3, 1091–1094. doi: 10.4161/cc.3.9.1143

Rodriguez, V. M., Carrizales, L., Mendoza, M. S., Fajardo, O. R., and Giordano, M. (2002). Effects of sodium arsenite exposure on development and behavior in the rat. *Neurotoxicol. Teratol.* 24, 743–750. doi: 10.1016/S0892-0362(02)00313-6

Sakaue-Sawano, A., Kurokawa, H., Morimura, T., Hanyu, A., Hama, H., Osawa, H., et al. (2008). Visualizing spatiotemporal dynamics of multicellular cell-cycle progression. *Cell* 132, 487–498. doi: 10.1016/j.cell.2007.12.033

Shreeram, S., Sparks, A., Lane, D. P., and Blow, J. J. (2002). Cell type-specific responses of human cells to inhibition of replication licensing. *Oncogene* 21, 6624–6632. doi: 10.1038/sj.onc.1205910

Smith, A. H., Lingas, E. O., and Rahman, M. (2000). Contamination of drinking-water by arsenic in Bangladesh: a public health emergency. *Bull. World Health Organ.* 78, 1093–1103.

Tanaka, H., Tsukuma, H., and Oshima, A. (2010). Long-term prospective study of 6104 survivors of arsenic poisoning during infancy due to contaminated milk powder in 1955. *J. Epidemiol.* 20, 439–445. doi: 10.2188/jea.JE20090131

Tsai, S. Y., Chou, H. Y., The, H. W., Chen, C. M., and Chen, C. J. (2003). The effects of chronic arsenic exposure from drinking water on the neurobehavioral development in adolescence. *Neurotoxicology* 24, 747–753. doi: 10.1016/S0161-813X(03)00029-9

Wang, Y., Zhao, F., Liao, Y., Jin, Y., and Sun, G. (2013). Effects of arsenite in astrocytes on neuronal signaling transduction. *Toxicology* 303, 43–53. doi: 10.1016/j.tox.2012.10.024

Wasserman, G. A., Liu, X., Parvez, F., Ahsan, H., Factor-Litvak, P., Kline, J., et al. (2007). Water arsenic exposure and intellectual function in 6-year-old children in Araihazar, Bangladesh. *Environ. Health Perspect.* 115, 285–289. doi: 10.1289/ehp.9501

World Health Organization (2011). *Guidelines for Drinking-Water Quality, 4th Edn.* Geneva: WHO press.

Wong, H. K., Fricker, M., Wyttenbach, A., Villunger, A., Michalak, E. M., Strasser, A., et al. (2005). Mutually exclusive subsets of BH3-only proteins are activated by the p53 and c-Jun N-terminal kinase/c-Jun signaling pathways during cortical neuron apoptosis induced by arsenite. *Mol. Cell Biol.* 25, 8732–8747. doi: 10.1128/MCB.25.19.8732-8747.2005

Xi, S., Sun, W., Wang, F., Jin, Y., and Sun, G. (2009). Transplacental and early life exposure to inorganic arsenic affected development and behavior in offspring rats. *Arch. Toxicol.* 83, 549–556. doi: 10.1007/s00204-009-0403-5

Zhao, F., Liao, Y., Jin, Y., Li, G., Lv, X., and Sun, G. (2012). Effects of arsenite on glutamate metabolism in primary cultured astrocytes. *Toxicol. In Vitro* 26, 24–31. doi: 10.1016/j.tiv.2011.10.003

Zheng, W., Aschner, M., and Ghersi-Egea, J. F. (2003). Brain barrier systems: a new frontier in metal neurotoxicological research. *Toxicol. Appl. Pharmacol.* 192, 1–11. doi: 10.1016/S0041-008X(03)00251-5

7

MRI-Guided Regional Personalized Electrical Stimulation in Multisession and Home Treatments

*Andrea Cancelli [1], Carlo Cottone [1], Alessandro Giordani [2], Giampiero Asta [1], Domenico Lupoi [2], Vittorio Pizzella [3,4] and Franca Tecchio [1,5]**

[1] Laboratory of Electrophysiology for Translational Neuroscience, Istituto di scienze e tecnologie della cognizione (ISTC), Consiglio Nazionale Delle Ricerche (CNR), Rome, Italy, [2] AFaR Division, Fatebenefratelli Foundation for Health Research and Education, Rome, Italy, [3] Department of Neuroscience, Imaging and Clinical Sciences, Università degli Studi G. d'Annunzio Chieti e Pescara, Chieti, Italy, [4] Institute for Advanced Biomedical Technologies, Università degli Studi G. d'Annunzio Chieti e Pescara, Chieti, Italy, [5] Institute of Neurology, Catholic University of the Sacred Heart, Rome, Italy

Edited by:
*Takashi Hanakawa,
National Center of Neurology and Psychiatry, Japan*

Reviewed by:
*Satoshi Tanaka,
Hamamatsu University School of Medicine, Japan
Nico Sollmann,
Technische Universität München, Germany*

***Correspondence:**
*Franca Tecchio
franca.tecchio@cnr.it*

The shape and position of the electrodes is a key factor for the efficacy of transcranial electrical stimulations (tES). We have recently introduced the Regional Personalized Electrode (RePE), a tES electrode fitting the personal cortical folding, that has been able to differentiate the stimulation of close by regions, in particular the primary sensory (S1) and motor (M1) cortices, and to personalize tES onto such an extended cortical district. However, neuronavigation on individual brain was compulsory for the correct montage. Here, we aimed at developing and testing a neuronavigation-free procedure for easy and quick positioning RePE, enabling multisession RePE-tES at home. We used off-line individual MRI to shape RePE via an *ad-hoc* computerized procedure, while an *ad-hoc* developed Adjustable Helmet Frame (AHF) was used to properly position it in multisession treatments, even at home. We used neuronavigation to test the RePE shape and position obtained by the new computerized procedure and the re-positioning obtained via the AHF. Using Finite Element Method (FEM) model, we also estimated the intra-cerebral current distribution induced by transcranial direct current stimulation (tDCS) comparing RePE vs. non-RePE with fixed reference. Additionally, we tested, using FEM, various shapes, and positions of the reference electrode taking into account possible small displacements of RePE, to test feasibility of RePE-tES sessions at home. The new RePE neuronavigation-free positioning relies on brain MRI space distances, and produced a mean displacement of 3.5 ± 0.8 mm, and the re-positioning of 4.8 ± 1.1 mm. Higher electric field in S1 than in M1 was best obtained with the occipital reference electrode, a montage that proved to feature low sensitivity to typical RePE millimetric displacements. Additionally, a new tES accessory was developed to enable repositioning the electrodes over the scalp also at home, with a precision which is acceptable according to the modeling-estimated intracerebral currents. Altogether, we provide here a procedure to simplify and make easily applicable RePE-tDCS, which enables efficacious personalized treatments.

Keywords: regional personalized electrode (RePE), transcranial electrical stimulation (tES), computational modeling, primary somatosensory and motor cortex (S1, M1), tDCS home treatments, non-invasive brain stimulation (NIBS)

INTRODUCTION

Advances in analyzing structural and functional brain features using powerful non-invasive neuroimaging methods are nowadays yielding intriguing insights into brain circuits, their variability across individuals, and their relationship to behavior (Van Essen, 2013; Kopell et al., 2014). If properly exploited, this knowledge can enhance the neuromodulation efficacy of transcranial Electrical Stimulation (tES), and transcranial Direct Current Stimulation (tDCS) in particular, by tuning the dimension, position and shape of the electrodes to the brain networks of interest (Murphy et al., 2009; Tecchio et al., 2014; Galletta et al., 2015; Cancelli et al., 2016, 2017; Grimaldi et al., 2016).

Following the need to concentrate the stimulation on the entire bilateral primary somatosensory representation of the whole body (S1), we recently introduced a new MRI-based neuronavigated procedure to customize brain stimulation through the use of the Regional Personalized Electrode (RePE) (Tecchio et al., 2013). The higher efficacy of personalized vs. non-personalized electrode in targeting the whole region was demonstrated experimentally (Cancelli et al., 2015a), and further confirmed by a recent modeling study (Parazzini et al., 2017). RePE targeting S1 (RePE-S1) was employed in two randomized clinical trials (RCT) showing an efficacy of this personalized 5-day tDCS against fatigue in multiple sclerosis (MS), thus we called the treatment Fatigue Relief in Multiple Sclerosis, FaReMuS (Tecchio et al., 2014; Cancelli et al., 2017). In the 2014 group, the mean fatigue reduction was 28% of the baseline after Real stimulation and 8% after Sham, $p = 0.016$. In the 2017 group, the fatigue symptoms reduction were 42% after Real and 20% after Sham, $p = 0.012$. We observed 7 responders, defined as the patients who changed the fatigue level more or equal to 20% of her/his baseline, in the 2014 group, and 9 in the 2017 one. The relevance of the target selection to effectively relieve fatigue can be perceived from the fact that other two tDCS trials, in which every parameter but the electrode shape and position were identical to those of the efficacious FaReMuS neuromodulation (Tecchio et al., 2014; Cancelli et al., 2017), did not produce the desired effects (Ferrucci et al., 2014; Saiote et al., 2014).

RePE-S1 electrode is shaped according to the projection onto the scalp of the individual cortical folding of the Rolandic sulcus. The projection was obtained by a neuronavigated procedure as the minimal distance from the scalp of the central sulcus reconstructed from the individual brain MRI (Tecchio et al., 2013). We conceived that the treatment should target the entire body somatosensory representation, as both limbs are impaired in people with MS and typically both sides. For this reason we decided to target the entire Rolandic sulcus post-central wall (Fischl et al., 2004; Destrieux et al., 2010). For simplicity, we selected from the left to the right Sylvian sulci, including the secondary somatosensory representation. In fact, as discussed above our main aim was to avoid frontal motor areas, while a wider parietal involvement was acceptable consistently with the literature (Pellicano et al., 2010; Engström et al., 2013; Vecchio et al., 2017).

Despite the promising results in relieving fatigue in people with multiple sclerosis (Tecchio et al., 2014; Cancelli et al., 2017), the application of RePE is still difficult because of the burdensome and complicated set up, that requires an experienced operator for the manually neuronavigated shaping of RePE with the patient affected by multiple sclerosis present along the entire shaping procedure, and an accurate neuronavigated positioning at the beginning of every stimulation session.

The tDCS treatments typically require multiple sessions. In fact, the duration of tES treatments, with one stimulation per day, ranges from 2 sessions (against alcohol or smoke craving, Boggio et al., 2008; Fregni et al., 2008) to 30 sessions (to support motor function in stroke patients, Hesse et al., 2011). In clinical contexts, the 5 consecutive day application is common in several diseases, including depression (Fregni et al., 2006b; Nitsche et al., 2009), pain (Zhu et al., 2017), and stroke (Boggio et al., 2007). The possibility of a simple home treatment set-up, easily manageable by the patient without special assistance, would therefore greatly increase the impact of RePE.

By theoretical computational modeling analysis, we tested here the relevance of RePE shape and position in terms of the tDCS differential efficacy on S1 with respect to primary motor cortex (M1) using a personalized vs. a non-personalized electrode. Computational modeling exploits high resolution MRI and accurate brain models based on Finite Element Method (FEM) to predict the electric field induced in each voxel of the brain during tDCS, thus allowing for an optimization of the tDCS montage, i.e., the maximization of the current flowing in the target region with respect to the other brain areas; in other words the maximization of the target region dosage (Antal et al., 2017).

We first aimed here to present and test a new MRI-based procedure to shape a RePE without the need for the neuronavigation technique, therefore bypassing the simultaneous presence of the patient and the experienced operator. Furthermore, we present a positioning technique that takes advantage of the scalp-space distances calculated on the 3D MRI reconstruction of the subject's head.

In the perspective of applying FaReMus at people home, we had here the second aim of introducing a procedure for easy and accurate repositioning of the electrode in a domiciliary environment (Pérez-Borrego et al., 2014; Charvet et al., 2015). We developed an adjustable helmet frame (AHF) to maintain the position of RePE during stimulation, and to allow an easy repositioning of RePE in multisession tDCS treatments even at the patient's home.

METHODS

The whole procedure was tested on 14 healthy volunteers (10 females, 4 males; age range 25–56 years, mean age 33.9 ± 11.0 years), eligible to the study in absence of clinical evidence or history of neurological or vascular diseases and with no pharmacological treatments. All participants provided written informed consent for participation in the study, as approved by the "Lazio 1-San Camillo Forlanini" Ethics Committee.

Each subject underwent a structural brain MRI exam with a 1.5 T scanner (Achieva, Philips Medical Systems, Best, The Netherlands). The acquisition protocol consisted of one 3D high resolution anatomical sequence empirically optimized to increase gray/white matter image contrast (T1-weighted Turbo Field Echo TR/TE/FA = 9.5 ms/4 ms/8°; 2,562 matrix resulting in an in-plane resolution 0.98 × 0.98 mm, slice thickness 1.2 mm, 160 coronal contiguous slice).

Computerized RePE-S1 Shape

As a preliminary step, we manually traced the central sulcus on the standard MNI152_T1_1 mm_brain MR template, thus avoiding the use of neuronavigation in shaping the RePE-S1. A total of 123 points were selected in the middle of the pre- and post-central sulcus (CS) walls, one for each of the 123 sagittal slices passing across the template central sulcus. These points span from the Sylvian sulcus of the left hemisphere to the same sulcus of the right hemisphere (MNI_CS).

The computerized process for shaping the individual RePE-S1 electrode (**Figure 1**) from her/his brain MRI consisted of the following steps:

1. Scalp and brain tissues were segmented from individual original MRIs (iMRI) using the Brain Extraction Tool (BET) of FSL (iBrain and iScalp);
2. iBrain images were spatially normalized with respect to the standard MNI152_T1_1 mm_brain MR template by means of the FMRIB's Linear Image Registration Tool (FLIRT) and the related transformation was saved as a matrix (TM);
3. The 123 MNI_CS points were automatically mapped onto the iMRI of each subject using the inverted spatial normalization matrix [TM^{-1}, convert xfm & img2img] to obtain the 123 points on iMRI (iCS);
4. The iCS was projected onto the external surface of the 3D iScalp using an in-house software (iCSS), applying the minimal distance brain-scalp tissues for each point.
5. The iCSS were then projected to a plan, performing the iCSS on a plan (iCSSp).
6. RePE-S1 was designed using AutoCAD software (Autodesk AutoCAD 2017). The iCCSp coordinates were imported into the software in the native space and replicated at a distance of 2 cm from the original trace. Then, the two 2D iCCS were connected laterally to form a polygon.
7. The shape of RePE was exported in the PDF format and printed to be cut into sponge or conductive silicon electrodes.

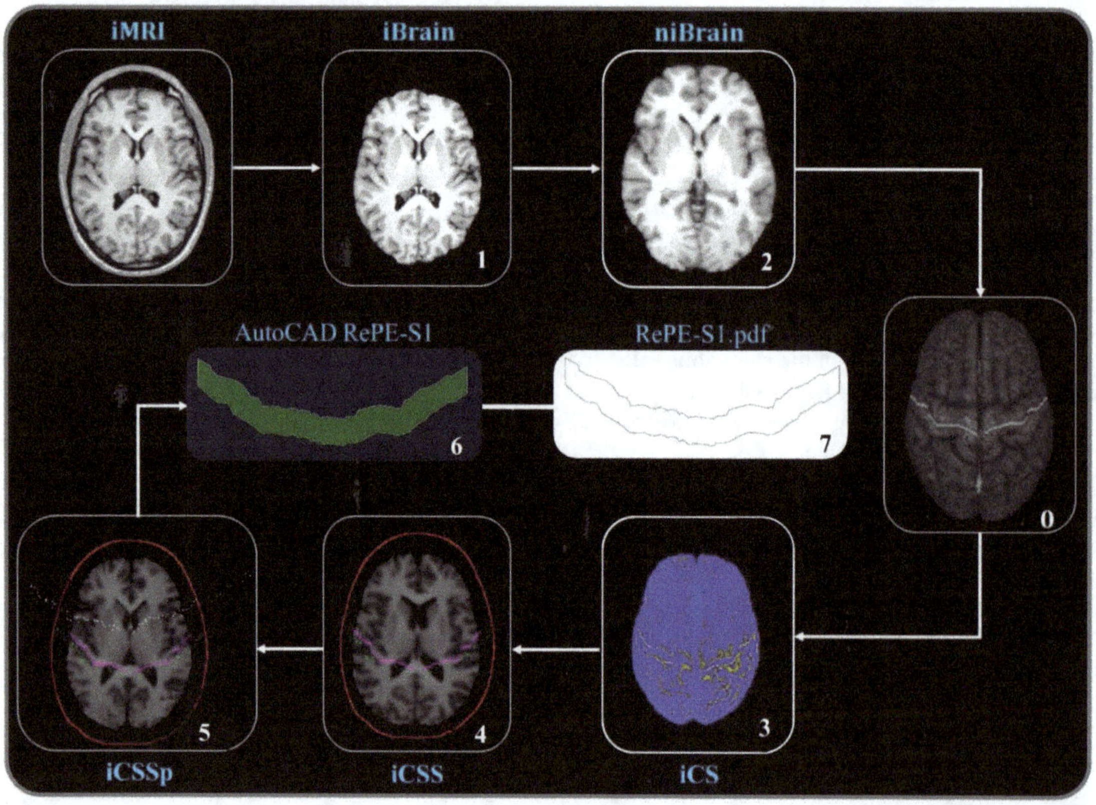

FIGURE 1 | Computerized procedure to shape RePE. As detailed in the Methods, the steps from the individual brain MRI (iMRI), with segmentation of the brain (iBrain, 1), transformed into MNI standard model (niBrain, 2), where the central sulcus identified points are stored (once for every person, thus no number in the process applied in individual subject, 0) and retro projected obtaining the individual central sulcus (iCS, 3), projected on the scalp (iCSS, 4), and further projected on a planar surface (iCSSp, 5) so that by AutoCAD the RePE area is obtained (6) and printed (7).

RePE Positioning Based on the 3D MRI Head Model

To position RePE-S1 over the scalp of each subject in a way that the electrode would overlap her/his iCCS coordinates (minimal distance to the target region), we developed an MRI-based procedure to place each RePE-S1 in relation to the selected external landmarks on the subject's scalp. In particular, we used the following individual head points: Nasion (N, **Figure 2A**); Inion (I, **Figure 2B**); the central and lateral points of RePE-S1 located on the iCSS (RePE-S1_C, RePE-S1_L, RePE-S1_R, **Figure 2C**) with RePE-S1_C positioned on the line connecting Nasion and Inion. Then, over the 3D-rendered head, we measured the distances between N and the above defined three points: N-RePE-S1_C, N-RePE-S1_L, N-RePE-S1_R (**Figures 2D–F**). Given these three values, an operator can position RePE-S1 using the following procedure. She/he should place the zero (0) of a flexible meter on N and extend the meter to I (**Figure 2G**). Then he/she can center RePE-S1_C at distance N-RePE-S1_C from N, along the N-I line. Then he/she can adjust the RePE orientation through the N-RePE-S1_L and RePE-S1_R distances (**Figures 2H,I**).

An Adaptable Helmet Frame [AHF] for the Electrode Repositioning in Multisession tDCS Treatment

We developed an Adaptable Helmet Frame (AHF) using a plastic cyclist helmet (**Figure 3**). The helmet frame was equipped with an adjustable mechanism to comfortably fit the individual head of

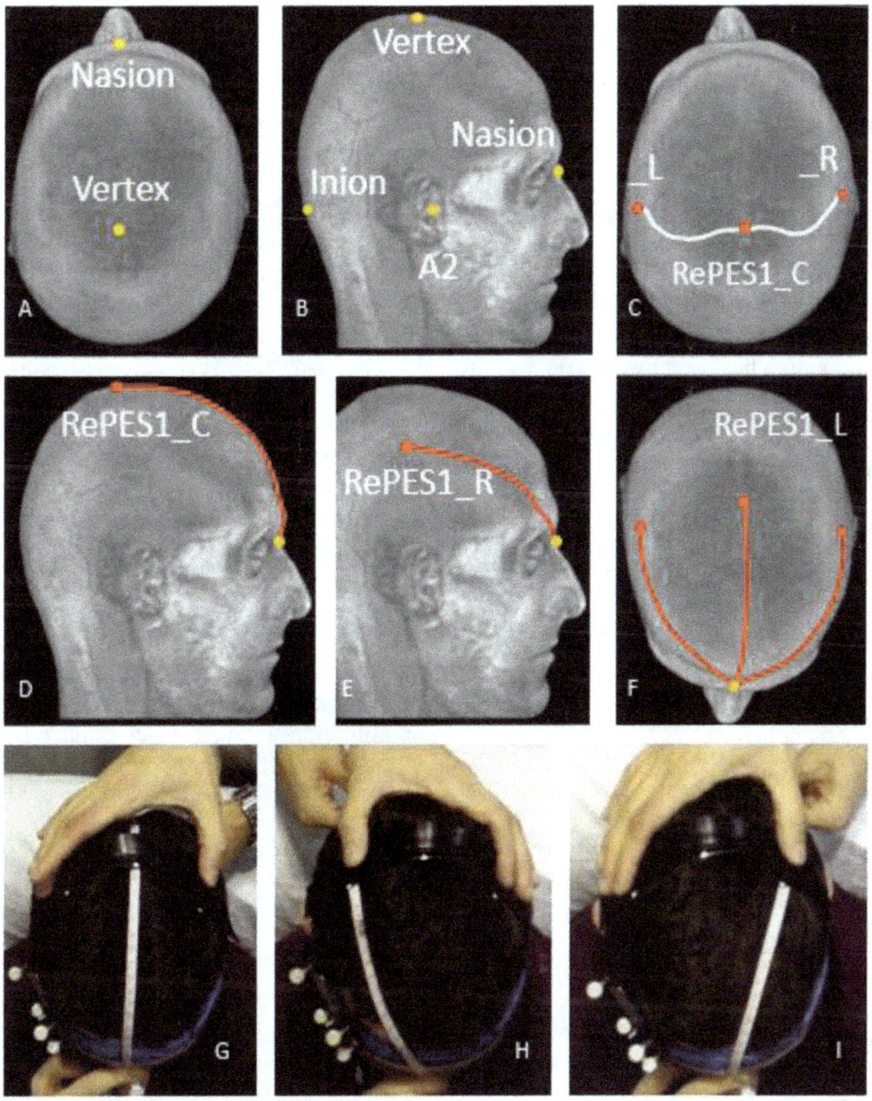

FIGURE 2 | RePE positioning with 3D MRI-derived head space distances. As detailed in the Method section, representation of the curves on the scalp **(A–F)**, whose lengths derived from the individual 3D head model allow positioning RePE **(G–I)**.

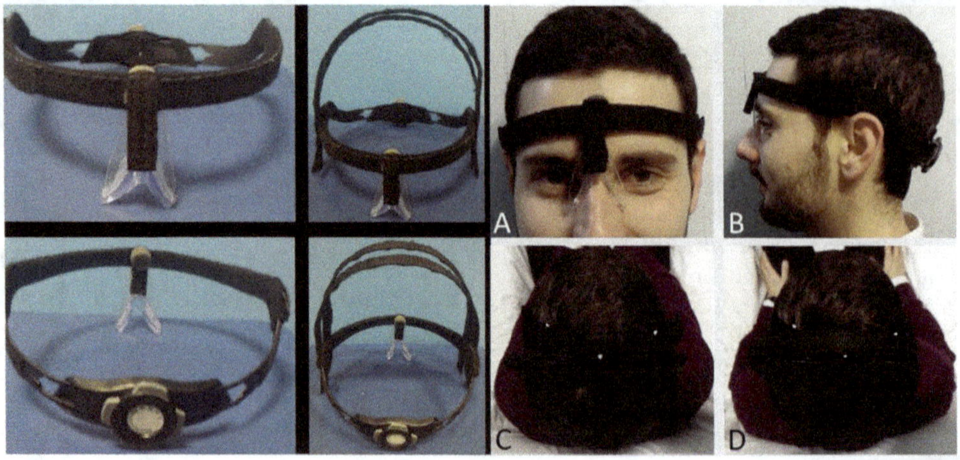

FIGURE 3 | AHF for multisession RePE repositioning. Left: Adaptable Helmet Frame (AHF) without (left) and with (right) the Velcro strips to fix RePE. The occipital cathode electrode is fixed under the adjustable mechanism. Right: As detailed in the Methods, steps **(A,B)** allow positioning and re-positioning the AHF in same position. **(C,D)** fix the RePE position with respect to the AHF. Informed consent was obtained from the participant wearing the AHF to publish the image.

the subject, and it was integrated with a nasal support and Velcro bands to firmly fix the electrodes in the desired position.

Once RePE has been properly positioned, the operator can fix the AHF taking care not to move RePE electrode. In detail, (1) she/he positions the AHF so that the nasal support rests well on the nose (**Figure 3A**) and the inferior border lays over the top of the ears (**Figure 3B**). In this way, the AHF is always set in the same position. Thereafter, she/he (2) adapts the circumference to the individual head using the adjustment mechanism, and (3) fixes the electrode to the AHF stably with the two coronal Velcro strips (**Figures 3C,D**).

Neuronavigated Procedure to Evaluate the RePE Positioning and Re-positioning

We used neuronavigation (SofTaxic Neuronavigation System ver. 2.0, www.softaxic.com, E.M.S., Bologna, Italy) to test the repeatability of the RePE positioning based on the 3D MRI head model (**Figure 4A**), and to test the stability of the RePE AHF repositioning (**Figure 4B**).

We marked 27 points along the entire length of the electrode: the central point, 13 points on the left and 13 on the right of the central point (0.5 cm between points, RePEpoints, **Figure 4C**).

We collected the coordinates of RePEpoints in the individual MRI space, after positioning the electrode along the central sulcus projected on the scalp using the 3D-head space anatomical landmarks system, and repeated the procedure five times. For comparison, we also collected the RePEpoints positions when positioning RePE using the neuronavigated procedure. Finally, we calculated the distances between the corresponding RePEpoints and the points of the central sulcus projected onto the scalp (**Figure 1**).

To test the repeatability of the repositioning tool, we properly fixed the electrode into the AHF, we digitized the RePEpoints coordinates, and then we removed the AHF. We repeated the digitization of the RePE position after wearing AHF over 5 consecutive days.

Statistical Analysis

Evaluation of the Identification of the Computerized Individual Central Sulcus

To evaluate the ability of the computerized procedure to locate the individual central sulcus, we compared the 123 iCSS points with those obtained by manually tracing the central sulcus on individual MRIs projected on the scalp (Manual iCSS).

Two independent researchers (a neuroradiologist—DL and a biomedical engineer with specific training in MRI data analysis—AC) selected every sagittal image where the central sulcus appeared on the individual segmented brain and recorded one point (X, Y, Z) for each slice. Accordingly, the number of points of Manual iCSS varied across subjects between a minimum of 102 and a maximum of 117. We projected the Manual iCS onto the external surface of the 3D iScalp using the same software that was used for the Computerized procedure (Manual iCSS).

We quantified the accuracy of the Computerized iCSS identification as the point-to-point Euclidean distance to the Manual iCSS set (nearest points) and the Intra-Class Correlation (ICC) between Computerized iCSS and Manual iCSS.

RePE Position Accuracy

We evaluated the repeatability of RePE position using the Euclidean distances of the RePEpoints from the corresponding projections on the scalp of the central sulcus points. In order to detect possible systematic positioning errors, we submitted the differences of the 3D coordinates (x, y, z) for the 27 points in successive positions to an analysis of variance (ANOVA) with the Positioning Error (Rep2-1, Rep3-1, Rep4-1, Rep5-1) and Positioning Method (Neuronavigation, 3D MRI-head distances) as within-subject factors. Any systematic displacement will correspond with significant Positioning Error effect. We performed all statistical analysis using SPSS (IBM).

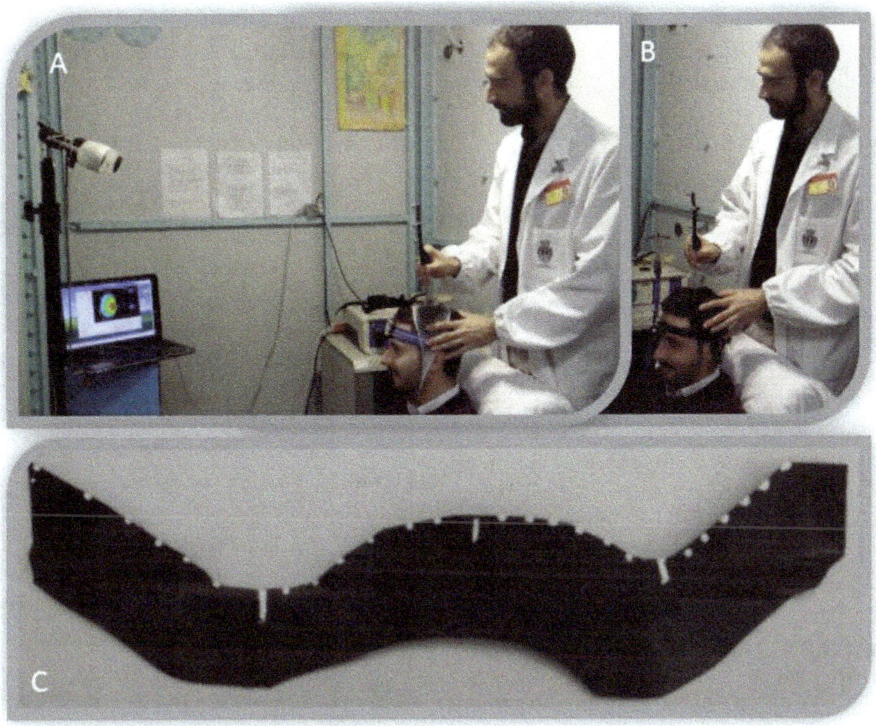

FIGURE 4 | Neuronavigation setup used to estimate RePE positioning systems. Top: As detailed in the Methods, experimental neuronavigated procedure to test the RePE positioning via the MRI-derived 3D-head model measures **(A)** and via the AHF **(B)**. Informed consent was obtained from the participants executing the procedure and wearing RePE to publish the image. **(C)** RePE with the testing point used for the neuronavigated procedure.

Intracerebral Current Induced by RePE: MRI-Derived Finite Element Method

The electric field (EF) distributions induced into the brain by RePE S1 and non-RePE were computed using a FEM forward model. Several configurations were analyzed: different positions of RePE-S1 and different return electrode locations. One MRI scan of a 39 year old adult male head was segmented using an algorithm developed in-house for automated tissue compartment segmentation (Huang et al., 2013). Adaptive volumetric meshing was applied to the tissue segmentation in ScanIP (Simpleware Ltd, Exeter, UK) with a compound coarseness of −15 (maximum edge length 1.85 mm, target minimum 0.775 mm, target Jacobian minimum 0.1). The resulting meshes consisted of $>10^7$ quadratic tetrahedral elements and $>1.5 \cdot 10^6$ degrees of freedom. Further refined meshes were found to have no noticeable effect on simulation results. The mesh was imported into COMSOL Multiphysics 4.3 (Burlington, MA) to simulate quasi-static volume conductor physics, since this approximation is acceptable for tES (Smith, 1992; Nathan et al., 1993; Eshel et al., 1995). The overall volume was divided in seven compartments with different electrical conductivity (Datta et al., 2011; Parazzini et al., 2011; Wagner et al., 2014; Galletta et al., 2015; Cancelli et al., 2016) representing: gray matter ($\sigma = 0.276$ S·m^{-1}), white matter ($\sigma = 0.126$ S·m^{-1}), cerebral spinal fluid (CSF, $\sigma = 1.65$ S·m^{-1}), skull ($\sigma = 10^{-2}$ S·m^{-1}), air ($\sigma = 10^{-4}$ S·m^{-1}), fat $\sigma = 0.025$ S·m^{-1}), and skin ($\sigma = 0.465$ S·m^{-1}). Two additional masks including the Post and Anterior Central Gyruses were created and intersected with gray matter to segment the Primary Somatosensory and Motor Area, respectively, for a quantitative evaluation of the electric field generated at the target. The electrodes were imported into ScanCAD (Simpleware Ltd, Exeter, UK) for manual positioning over the scalp of the 3D model. During transcranial electrical stimulation (tES), a conductive gel ($\sigma = 0.3$ S·m^{-1}) is interposed between the silicon electrode and the scalp. The adopted model was modified accordingly.

Within COMSOL, the Laplace equation $\nabla(\sigma\nabla V) = 0$, with σ being the electric conductivity and V the electric potential, was solved considering the Neumann boundary conditions. COMSOL implemented a linear system solver of conjugate gradients with a relative tolerance of 10^{-6} mA of current stimulation which was applied for all the montages, so a boundary condition of orthogonal current density was implemented to the anode and the cathode. For each electrode, the current value was divided by the skin-electrode contact area and was applied as a current density boundary condition and assigned to the mesh nodes as current loads representing the right-hand-side of the linear system of equations.

RePE-S1 vs. Non-RePE-S1 Bilateral Stimulation

Two different electrodes of 35 cm^2, RePE over S1 and a non-personalized electrode (semi-curved pad 17.5 × 2 cm, Cancelli et al., 2015a; Parazzini et al., 2017) placed in three different locations were examined as anodes (**Figure 5**). A standard electrode with twice the area of the anodes [70 cm^2, in order to decrease the current density under the return electrode (Tecchio et al., 2014, 2015; Cancelli et al., 2015a,b, 2017)] was used as a cathode centered over Oz.

We examined four montages:

- Montage RePE A: RePE-S1 designed and positioned over S1 as detailed in sections Computerized RePE-S1 shape and RePE Positioning Based on the 3D MRI Head Model;
- Montage Non-RePE A: non-RePE over hand/mouth S1;
- Montage Non-RePE B: non-RePE centered on Cz of the 10–10 International System (IS);
- Montage Non-RePE C: non-RePE centered on CPz of the IS.

Reference Electrode Evaluation

Following the results of the montages described in section Reference Evaluation in RePE tDCS, no more computations involving either the non-RePE anode or positions behind the Central Sulcus of RePE-S1 were run. Sixteen montages with RePE-S1 were evaluated with the aim of optimizing the RePE stimulation: four different reference electrodes (pad over Oz, Neck, Shoulders and a strip around the head, **Figure 6**), each with four different positions of RePE-S1, with the anterior border of RePE-S1 overlapping the CS scalp projection (RePE A), 0.5 cm ahead of the CS scalp projection (RePE B), or 1 and 1.5 cm ahead (RePE C and RePE D).

RESULTS

Computerized RePE Design

Computerized Individual Central Sulcus on the Scalp

The mean average distance across points and subjects of iCSS and manual iCSS sets was 2.9 ± 3.2 mm, and the mean intra-class correlation was 0.999 ± 0.0013 (ICC).

RePE Positioning and Re-positioning

RePE Position Based on Head Fiducials

The coordinates of the RePE position did not differ between neuronavigated positioning and new computerized positioning based on the distances derived from the 3D-head model, as indicated by the *Positioning Method* factor [$F_{(3, 3)} = 0.263$, $p = 0.849$]. The mean repetition error in terms of the Euclidean distance was 3.0 mm for neuronavigation and 3.5 mm for anatomical landmark-system across all repetitions (**Table 1**). When compared with paired-sample *t*-test, no differences were found [$t_{(9)} = -1.110$, $p = 0.296$]. No systematic displacement occurred in any direction, as indicated by the *Positioning Error* factor [$F_{(9, 45)} = 0.768, p = 0.646$].

Adaptable Helmet Frame [AHF] for the Electrode Repositioning in Multisession tDCS Treatment

The mean repositioning error in terms of the Euclidean distance was 4.8 ± 1.1 mm across all repetitions and subjects. The ANOVA design analyzing the coordinate differences displayed that no systematic displacement occurred in any direction (**Table 2**). In fact, *Positioning Error* factor was [$F_{(3, 24)} = 0.086, p = 0.967$].

Electric Field Distribution Analysis

RePE-S1 vs. Non-RePE-S1 Bilateral Stimulation

The different shape and position of the electrode used as anode and cathode (**Figure 5**) played a key role in determining the boundaries of the cortical area that was stimulated. Specifically, RePE A generated a cortical EF diffused uniformly from the central sulcus to the occipital area, position of the return electrode. Therefore, the stimulation affected the entire S1 with an average EF (EF_{AVE}) of 0.152 V/m for the 1.5 mA/35 cm^2 current density, while the EF was minimized in M1 ($EF_{AVE} = 0.134$ V/m). In the montage non-RePE A the non-personalized electrode was placed ahead of the Central Sulcus and the stimulation involved both the entire S1 ($EF_{AVE} = 0.153$ V/m) and M1 ($EF_{AVE} = 0.140$ V/m). The montage non-RePE B generated a similar EF magnitude to that of RePE A in the central section of S1, but decreasing toward the Sylvian Fissure (**Figure 5**). This is conceivably because the non-personalized electrode didn't follow the convolutions of the entire Post Central Gyrus. Thus, the resulting average EF in S1 was lower than RePE A, $EF_{AVE} = 0.114$ V/m. The montage non-RePE C was placed posteriorly to S1 so the stimulation barely affected both S1 ($EF_{AVE} = 0.083$ V/m) and M1 ($EF_{AVE} = 0.078$ V/m).

The maximum ratio between the EF induced in S1 and M1, was obtained by montage RePE A ($EF_{AVE}{}^{S1} > 13\%\ EF_{AVE}{}^{M1}$).

Reference Evaluation in RePE tDCS

The computational analysis using various positions of the RePE anode with different cathodes revealed that the highest efficacy is obtained using a standard reference electrode on Oz, placed oppositely to the area in which the induced EF is required to be low (in this case, M1). The average EF obtained with all the RePE positions with Oz reference (**Figure 6** bottom, **Table 3**) is the highest (0.91 V/m) in the Left, Central and Right part of S1, even if the effect in the central part is similar in M1. Indeed, the other reference choices cannot discriminate between the EF in M1 and S1 at all. In particular the Neck and Shoulder reference induced maximal EF only in the lateral parts (L and R, 0.09 V/m) of the target region. The strip reference causes a low EF from Left to Right both in S1 and M1 (0.58 V/m).

Comparing the positions of the RePE anode over the scalp, best efficacy is obtained by the RePE A position ($EF_{S1}/EF_{M1} = 1.13$). RePE B, with a slip of 5 mm from Position A toward the projection of M1, generated similar EF at the target ($EF_{S1}/EF_{M1} = 1.12$), while RePE C and RePE D (1 and 1.5 cm form Position A) significantly decreased performances.

DISCUSSION

The main achievement of this study is the double development of an easy and effective tool to shape and position a tES electrode personalized for stimulating a specific cortical district, and for repositioning it for a multi-sessions protocol, specifically designed to be used by the patient at home.

When the stimulation target is a limited cortical area, modeling suggests that a ring configuration of HD electrodes is the most appropriate montage for focusing current into such area

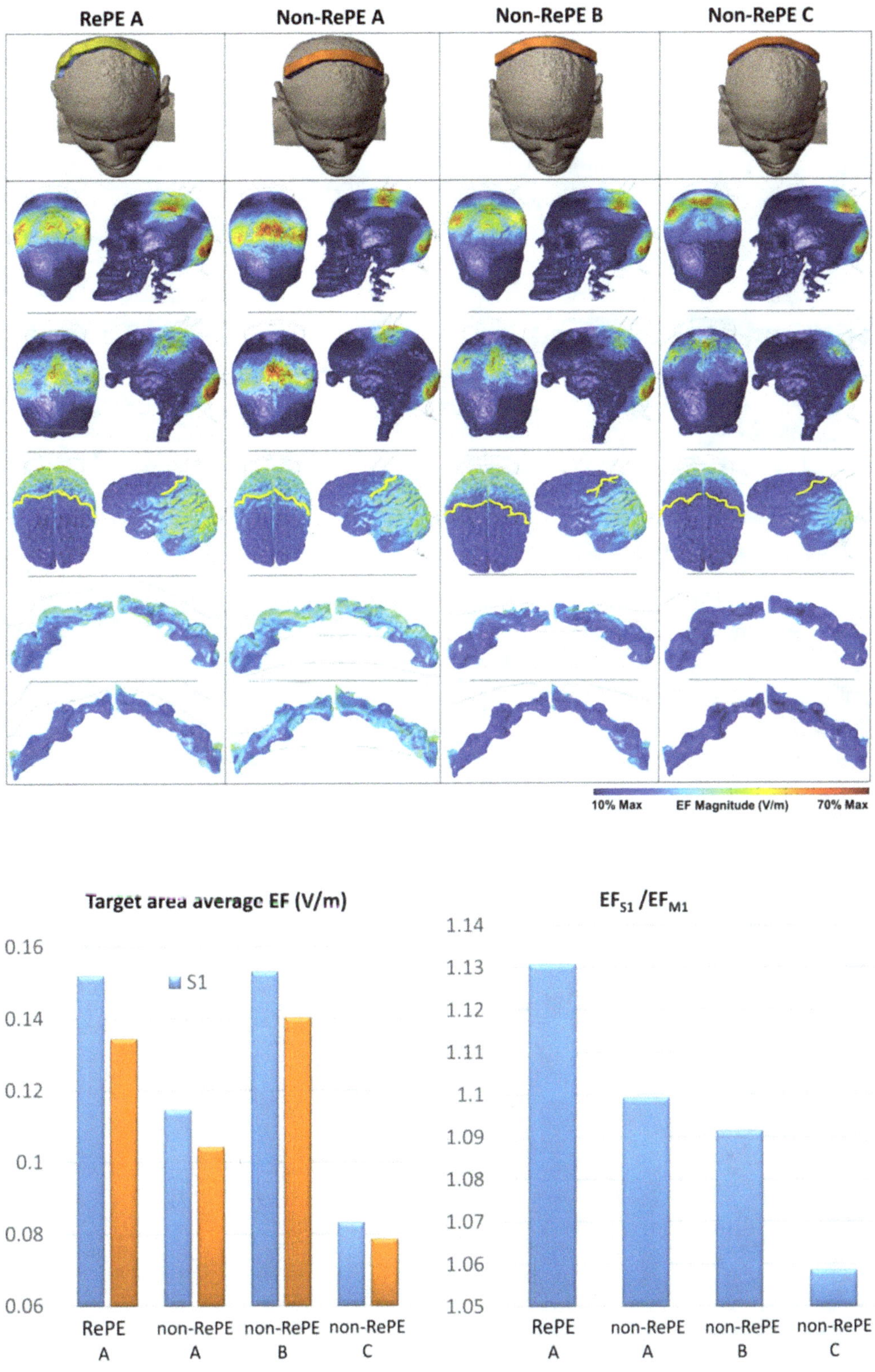

FIGURE 5 | Modeling: RePE-S1 vs. non-RePE-S1 comparison. Top: First row: The four anodal electrodes tested against the same reference with twice the RePE's area positioned on Oz: personalized S1 electrode positioned 0.5 cm frontal to the scalp projection of the central sulcus (RePE A), the non-personalized strip shaped to overlay Cz and from C3 to C4 (Non-RePE) with a part on hand/mouth S1 (A), on Cz (B), or on CPz (C). From the second row: electric field amplitude (EF) on the scalp (second row), dura mater (third row), cortical surface (fourth row), and S1 post-central (fifth row) and M1 pre-central gyri (sixth row). Bottom: Average EF (V/m) in the whole body S1 (light blue) and M1 (orange) for the four montages (Left) and the ratio in S1 with respetct to M1 (Right).

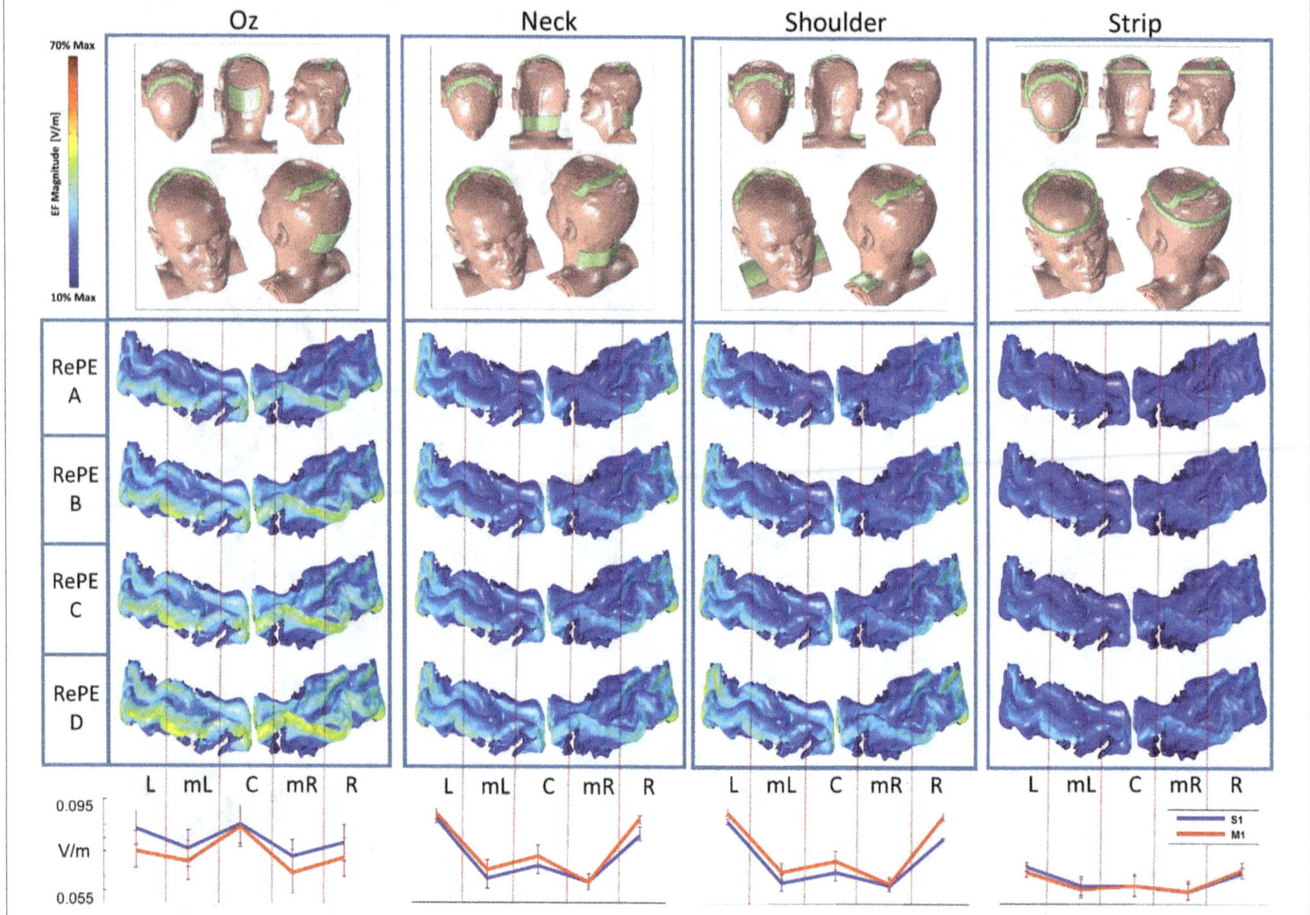

FIGURE 6 | Modeling: Reference evaluation in RePE tDCS. **(Top)** For each of the reference electrode position (Oz, neck, shoulders, and a ring centered on RePE) the electric field amplitude (EF) on the cortical strip including the S1 and M1 cortical gyri for the four RePE positions: with the anterior border fitting the CS scalp projection (RePE A), 0.5 cm (RePE B), or 1 cm (RePE C) and 1.5 cm ahead (RePE D). **(Bottom)** Average EF (V/m) in the five sections (Left L, medio-Left mL, central C, medio-Right mR, and Right R) of S1 (blue) and M1 (red), averaged across the RePE positions, for the four reference electrodes.

TABLE 1 | RePE positioning via 3D head MRI distances vs. Neuronavigation.

Session	Neuronavigation (mm)				3D head model MRI distances (mm)			
	Distance	*X*	*Y*	*Z*	Distance	*X*	*Y*	*Z*
1	3.1 ± 1.4	1.1 ± 2.9	0.5 ± 2.8	−0.8 ± 2.7	3.7 ± 0.6	1.9 ± 2.7	−3.1 ± 4.1	2.0 ± 3.9
2	2.6 ± 1.5	0.4 ± 3.0	−0.6 ± 3.1	−0.4 ± 2.2	2.5 ± 0.5	1.5 ± 2.7	−2.3 ± 4.3	2.8 ± 4.9
3	2.7 ± 1.3	0.9 ± 2.1	−1.9 ± 1.6	0.7 ± 2.3	3.7 ± 0.5	−2.0 ± 3.7	2.3 ± 4.4	0.9 ± 3.7
4	3.4 ± 1.1	1.4 ± 3.3	0.0 ± 2.2	0.5 ± 2.4	4.2 ± 0.7	2.0 ± 3.0	2.0 ± 2.7	−3.9 ± 2.6
5	3.0 ± 0.6	1.3 ± 2.7	−1.4 ± 4.2	1.2 ± 3.6	3.8 ± 1.2	0.8 ± 3.5	−0.2 ± 4.6	2.5 ± 5.0
Overall	3.0 ± 1.2	1.0 ± 2.8	−0.7 ± 2.8	0.2 ± 2.6	3.5 ± 0.8	0.8 ± 3.3	−2.8 ± 4.3	0.3 ± 2.1

Mean displacements between each of the 27 RePEpoints in each electrode and the corresponding point of the scalp projection of the central sulcus, both as Euclidean distance (Distance) and the differences of each of the three Cartesian coordinates (x, y, z), when the personalized electrode was positioned either using the neuronavigated procedure or the distances derived from the 3D-head model from individual MRI.

(Datta et al., 2009; Cancelli et al., 2016). On the contrary, the idea of the RePE-tDCS came out from the necessity to uniformly stimulate an extended cortical region (S1) and to minimize the degree to which EF was induced in the adjacent region (M1). The present procedure makes this personalized stimulation more easy and affordable.

The results obtained through computational modeling support the idea that RePE-tDCS is a valid montage for

TABLE 2 | RePE position by adaptable helmet frame [AHF].

Day	Distance	*X*	*Y*	*Z*
1	4.8 ± 1.4	−2.0 ± 1.9	0.9 ± 1.4	0.8 ± 1.2
2	4.9 ± 1.1	−0.7 ± 3.6	3.0 ± 3.1	−1.0 ± 2.4
3	4.7 ± 1.0	0.8 ± 1.2	2.8 ± 0.4	0.7 ± 2.3
4	4.9 ± 1.1	−2.1 ± 2.8	0.6 ± 3.8	1.1 ± 2.4
5	4.6 ± 0.7	−2.0 ± 3.9	0.8 ± 4.2	0.5 ± 2.8
Overall	4.8 ± 1.1	−0.7 ± 2.7	1.6 ± 2.6	0.4 ± 2.4

Mean displacements between each of the 27 RePEpoints in each electrode positioning with the AHF and the corresponding point of the scalp projection of the central sulcus, both as Euclidean distance (Distance) and the differences of each of the three Cartesian coordinates (x, y, z).

differentiating the tDCS dose between two contiguous areas. A non-RePE electrode cannot reach the same efficiency in terms of local specificity of the induced EF, regardless of its position on the scalp. On the other hand, it is clear that in any standard tDCS montage, i.e., with 2 electrodes, the position of the second electrode is crucial in managing the direction of the current flow. Because of the high conductivity of the CSF, the EF generated by tDCS is diffused between the two electrodes. Therefore, the electrode shape is not the unique parameter which should be considered in a RePE-montage optimization. To realize a correct RePE-tDCS, the shape and position of the reference electrode are essential (**Figure 6**). In both extra cephalic standard electrode references—neck and shoulders—and a strip around the head, the current flow did not affect the cortex as much as utilizing an occipital electrode. The four positions used to test RePE suggest that the tDCS dose is more differentiated between the two areas when the edge of the electrode, opposite to the reference, is close to the boundary delimiting the two areas (RePE A). On the other hand, a similar EF magnitude is obtained using a position of the anode that is 0.5 cm away (RePE B). This suggests that a position displacement of <5 mm does not affect the stimulation.

The computerized procedure we developed to design RePE identifies the edge of the target area on the MNI model and retro-transforms it onto the individual MRI coordinates. We evaluated the accuracy of this step through a control test, and we observed errors to the order of 2–3 mm with respect to the visual inspection of manual tracing, as tested by two independent MRI analysis experts.

The computerized procedure, processing the individual MRI using standard well-tested software, offers multiple advantages relative to manual protocols including:

(1) a significant time reduction in the electrode preparation; (2) no need to have the patient in the laboratory for the RePE preparation; (3) no need for a neuronavigation system; (4) the reduction of the variability in the RePE shape, depending on the experience of the researcher or technician who prepares the electrode.

In the present investigation, we used a 3D T1 sequence (MPRAGE) on a 1.5 T MRI scanner to obtain anatomical scans. In some experiments we tested lower resolution images in order to consider the minimal requirement of the quality of scans necessary to apply the proposed computerized procedure. The

TABLE 3 | Reference evaluation in RePE tDCS.

Montage	Oz					Neck					Shoulders					Strip				
	L	mL	C	mR	R	L	mL	C	mR	R	L	mL	C	mR	R	L	mL	C	mR	R
RePE A	1.135	1.090	1.029	1.144	1.101	0.993	0.945	0.960	0.991	0.967	0.974	0.942	0.946	0.992	0.923	1.071	1.038	1.008	1.003	1.006
RePE B	1.139	1.091	1.026	1.124	1.093	0.994	0.964	0.960	1.026	0.932	0.977	0.948	0.950	1.006	0.916	1.065	1.056	1.016	1.026	0.983
RePE C	1.126	1.076	1.022	1.103	1.094	0.991	0.967	0.961	1.024	0.929	0.974	0.952	0.952	1.008	0.912	1.057	1.056	1.011	1.022	0.980
RePE D	1.106	1.062	1.011	1.061	1.073	0.981	0.962	0.960	1.006	0.919	0.966	0.950	0.952	0.996	0.902	1.036	1.040	1.000	0.991	0.964

Electric field in S1 and M1 ratio delivered by the 16 montages in the five different portions of the target regions.

scans do not require high-resolution 3D sequences, but the sulcus can be well identified using almost any acquisition sequence (i.e., T1, T2, Flair) in any direction axial, sagittal and coronal, with a voxel resolution around 1 mm^2 and maximum 3 mm of slice thickness.

The present paper provides a simple and low-cost procedure for the tES electrode positioning and re-positioning (AHF), using easily recognizable anatomical scalp landmarks in any tES multisession treatments. Being a non-invasive brain stimulation, tDCS painlessly delivers electrical current of low intensity through the skull to selected areas of the brain (Nitsche et al., 2000; Antal et al., 2017), and offers a very high safety profile. Several double-blind studies proved multisession tDCS treatments to have negligible side effects offering an analgesic effect against chronic pain (Soler et al., 2010; Brietzke et al., 2016), to relieve symptoms in attention deficits and depression (Gögler et al., 2016; Cachoeira et al., 2017), in addition to relieving fatigue in multiple sclerosis. The suitability and repeatability consistent with those obtained via neuronavigation further simplify tES procedures, making them largely suitable for multisession home treatments and clinical protocols (Pérez-Borrego et al., 2014; Amatya et al., 2015; Charvet et al., 2015).

The test of the whole procedure is performed only for the single post-central gyrus RePE shape and position. This is a limitation of the present study. However, it is conceivable that the presented procedure can be easily exported to other extended cortical targets, like (almost) all bilateral associative cortices. While in the case of the central sulcus we proved that our procedure was appropriate, for different sulci that show greater variability between individuals other brain normalization procedures that take into account all cortical folding (Destrieux et al., 2010) might be evaluated. In the present work, we developed an automatized procedure to shape and position an electrode to focus the neuromodulation effect on a cortical area, limiting as much as possible the direct effects on contiguous cortical areas. We developed this procedure, based on individual brain MRI, since we documented that the personalization of the electrode is necessary to modify the excitability of the entire area of the postcentral gyrus from the left to the right Silvian sulcus (Cancelli et al., 2015a).

Future perspectives in the field of transportation research will consider to build and strengthen easy to use methods for other personalized tES. The relevance of the homologous areas balance in different neurological and psychiatric disorders (Fregni et al., 2006a; Ferrucci et al., 2009; Nitsche et al., 2009), and the indication that equal bilateral stimulation impinge positively counteracting pathological imbalances (Pahor and Jaušovec, 2018; Tseng et al., 2018), suggests that developing electrodes to target such bilateral representations will be more frequent in future. Conceivably, to build electrodes that take into account the specific individual cortical folding is an advantage in focusing the stimulation of high-definition tES (Edwards et al., 2013; Moreno-Duarte et al., 2014; Malavera et al., 2015; De Ridder et al., 2017). In fact, we devoted this work to develop an easy applicable tool to stimulate a specific cortical region in individual patients, without the need of neuronavigation, and we underlined that other RePE to target other cortical folding can be shaped and positioned via the procedure offered in the present work. Nevertheless, specific cases require proper modeling analyses in selecting the proper montage, specifically defining the reference in use.

CONCLUSIONS

We provide a model-based investigation of the RePE tDCS accompanied by a simple, low-cost procedure to easily apply it. We tested the technique for the stimulation of the primary somatosensory area, but the procedure, if supported by a correct application of the return electrode, can potentially be applied to any cortical region to differentiate the EF induced at the target region. Furthermore, as a complete and computerized design, positioning and re-positioning of the electrodes establishes a relevant advancement for any home tES treatment.

AUTHOR CONTRIBUTIONS

FT and AC: contributed to conception and design of the study; AC, GA, CC, AG, and DL: acquired and analyzed the data; AC, FT, and VP: drafted and finally revised the manuscript and the figures.

ACKNOWLEDGMENTS

The authors are sincerely grateful to all involved for the time and cooperation required to participate in the study and thank Massimiliano Marconi and Daniele Spizzichino for the support in collecting MRI and Prof. Filippo Carducci and Eng. Giulia Santi for important steps in the computerized procedure of the RePE shaping. This work was supported by:

1) FISM—Fondazione Italiana Sclerosi Multipla—Cod. 2014/R/22 [FaReMuS CuNeH], and
2) PNR-CNR Aging Program 2012–2018.

REFERENCES

Amatya, B., Galea, M. P., Kesselring, J., and Khan, F. (2015). Telerehabilitation for persons with multiple sclerosis. *Cochrane Database Syst. Rev.* 4:CD010508. doi: 10.1002/14651858.CD010508.pub2

Antal, A., Alekseichuk, I., Bikson, M., Brockmöller, J., Brunoni, A. R., Chen, R., et al. (2017). Low intensity transcranial electric stimulation: safety, ethical, legal regulatory and application guidelines. *Clin. Neurophysiol.* 128, 1774–1809. doi: 10.1016/j.clinph.2017.06.001

Boggio, P. S., Nunes, A., Rigonatti, S. P., Nitsche, M. A., Pascual-Leone, A., and Fregni, F. (2007). Repeated sessions of noninvasive brain DC stimulation is associated with motor function improvement in stroke patients. *Restor. Neurol. Neurosci.* 25, 123–129.

Boggio, P. S., Sultani, N., Fecteau, S., Merabet, L., Mecca, T., Pascual-Leone, A., et al. (2008). Prefrontal cortex modulation using transcranial DC stimulation reduces alcohol craving: a double-blind, sham-controlled study. *Drug Alcohol Depend.* 92, 55–60. doi: 10.1016/j.drugalcdep.2007.06.011

Brietzke, A. P., Rozisky, J. R., Dussan-Sarria, J. A., Deitos, A., Laste, G., Hoppe, P. F., et al. (2016). Neuroplastic effects of transcranial direct current stimulation on painful symptoms reduction in chronic hepatitis C: a phase II randomized, double blind, sham controlled trial. *Front. Neurosci.* 9:498. doi: 10.3389/fnins.2015.00498

Cachoeira, C. T., Leffa, D. T., Mittelstadt, S. D., Mendes, L. S. T., Brunoni, A. R., Pinto, J. V., et al. (2017). Positive effects of transcranial direct current stimulation in adult patients with attention-deficit/hyperactivity disorder – A pilot randomized controlled study. *Psychiatry Res.* 247, 28–32. doi: 10.1016/j.psychres.2016.11.009

Cancelli, A., Cottone, C., Di Giorgio, M., Carducci, F., and Tecchio, F. (2015a). Personalizing the electrode to neuromodulate an extended cortical region. *Brain Stimul.* 8, 555–560. doi: 10.1016/j.brs.2015.01.398

Cancelli, A., Cottone, C., Giordani, A., Migliore, S., Lupoi, D., Porcaro, C., et al. (2017). Personalized bilateral whole body somatosensory cortex stimulation to relieve fatigue in multiple sclerosis. *Mult. Scler.* doi: 10.1177/1352458517720528. [Epub ahead of print].

Cancelli, A., Cottone, C., Tecchio, F., Truong, D. Q., Dmochowski, J., and Bikson, M. (2016). A simple method for EEG guided transcranial electrical stimulation without models. *J. Neural Eng.* 13:36022. doi: 10.1088/1741-2560/13/3/036022

Cancelli, A., Cottone, C., Zito, G., Di Giorgio, M., Pasqualetti, P., and Tecchio, F. (2015b). Cortical inhibition and excitation by bilateral transcranial alternating current stimulation. *Restor. Neurol. Neurosci.* 33, 105–114. doi: 10.3233/RNN-140411

Charvet, L. E., Kasschau, M., Datta, A., Knotkova, H., Stevens, M. C., Alonzo, A., et al. (2015). Remotely-supervised transcranial direct current stimulation (tDCS) for clinical trials: guidelines for technology and protocols. *Front. Syst. Neurosci.* 9:26. doi: 10.3389/fnsys.2015.00026

Datta, A., Baker, J. M., Bikson, M., and Fridriksson, J. (2011). Individualized model predicts brain current flow during transcranial direct-current stimulation treatment in responsive stroke patient. *Brain Stimul.* 4, 169–174. doi: 10.1016/j.brs.2010.11.001

Datta, A., Bansal, V., Diaz, J., Patel, J., Reato, D., and Bikson, M. (2009). Gyri-precise head model of transcranial direct current stimulation: improved spatial focality using a ring electrode versus conventional rectangular pad. *Brain Stimul.* 2, 201–207. doi: 10.1016/j.brs.2009.03.005

De Ridder, D., Perera, S., and Vanneste, S. (2017). State of the art: novel applications for cortical stimulation. *Neuromodulation* 20, 206–214. doi: 10.1111/ner.12593

Destrieux, C., Fischl, B., Dale, A., and Halgren, E. (2010). Automatic parcellation of human cortical gyri and sulci using standard anatomical nomenclature. *Neuroimage* 53, 1–15. doi: 10.1016/j.neuroimage.2010.06.010

Edwards, D., Cortes, M., Datta, A., Minhas, P., Wassermann, E. M., and Bikson, M. (2013). Physiological and modeling evidence for focal transcranial electrical brain stimulation in humans: a basis for high-definition tDCS. *Neuroimage* 74, 266–275. doi: 10.1016/j.neuroimage.2013.01.042

Engström, M., Flensner, G., Landtblom, A. M., Ek, A. C., and Karlsson, T. (2013). Thalamo-striato-cortical determinants to fatigue in multiple sclerosis. *Brain Behav.* 3, 715–728. doi: 10.1002/brb3.181

Eshel, Y., Witman, S., Rosenfeld, M., and Abboud, S. (1995). Correlation between skull thickness asymmetry and scalp potential estimated by a numerical model of the head. *IEEE Trans. Biomed. Eng.* 42, 242–249. doi: 10.1109/10.364510

Ferrucci, R., Bortolomasi, M., Vergari, M., Tadini, L., Salvoro, B., Giacopuzzi, M., et al. (2009). Transcranial direct current stimulation in severe, drug-resistant major depression. *J. Affect. Disord.* 118, 215–219. doi: 10.1016/j.jad.2009.02.015

Ferrucci, R., Vergari, M., Cogiamanian, F., Bocci, T., Ciocca, M., Tomasini, E., et al. (2014). Transcranial direct current stimulation (tDCS) for fatigue in multiple sclerosis. *Neuro Rehabilitation* 34, 121–127. doi: 10.3233/NRE-131019

Fischl, B., van der Kouwe, A., Destrieux, C., Halgren, E., Ségonne, F., Salat, D. H., et al. (2004). Automatically parcellating the human cerebral cortex. *Cereb. Cortex* 14, 11–22. doi: 10.1093/cercor/bhg087

Fregni, F., Boggio, P. S., Nitsche, M. A., Marcolin, M. A., Rigonatti, S. P., and Pascual-Leone, A. (2006a). Treatment of major depression with transcranial direct current stimulation. *Bipolar Disord.* 8, 203–204. doi: 10.1111/j.1399-5618.2006.00291.x

Fregni, F., Gimenes, R., Valle, A. C., Ferreira, M. J., Rocha, R. R., Natalle, L., et al. (2006b). A randomized, sham-controlled, proof of principle study of transcranial direct current stimulation for the treatment of pain in fibromyalgia. *Arthritis Rheum.* 54, 3988–3998. doi: 10.1002/art.22195

Fregni, F., Liguori, P., Fecteau, S., Nitsche, M. A., Pascual-Leone, A., and Boggio, P. S. (2008). Cortical stimulation of the prefrontal cortex with transcranial direct current stimulation reduces cue-provoked smoking craving: a randomized, sham-controlled study. *J. Clin. Psychiatry* 69, 32–40. doi: 10.4088/JCP.v69n0105

Galletta, E. E., Cancelli, A., Cottone, C., Simonelli, I., Tecchio, F., Bikson, M., et al. (2015). Use of computational modeling to inform tDCS electrode montages for the promotion of language recovery in post-stroke aphasia. *Brain Stimul.* 8, 1108–1115. doi: 10.1016/j.brs.2015.06.018

Gögler, N., Willacker, L., Funk, J., Strube, W., Langgartner, S., Napiórkowski, N., et al. (2016). Single-session transcranial direct current stimulation induces enduring enhancement of visual processing speed in patients with major depression. *Eur. Arch. Psychiatry Clin. Neurosci.* 267, 671–686. doi: 10.1007/s00406-016-0761-y

Grimaldi, G., Argyropoulos, G. P., Bastian, A., Cortes, M., Davis, N. J., Edwards, D. J., et al. (2016). Cerebellar Transcranial Direct Current Stimulation (ctDCS): a novel approach to understanding cerebellar function in health and disease. *Neuroscientist* 22, 83–97. doi: 10.1177/1073858414559409

Hesse, S., Waldner, A., Mehrholz, J., Tomelleri, C., Pohl, M., and Werner, C. (2011). Combined transcranial direct current stimulation and robot-assisted arm training in subacute stroke patients: an exploratory, randomized multicenter trial. *Neurorehabil. Neural Repair* 25, 838–846. doi: 10.1177/15459683114 13906

Huang, Y., Dmochowski, J. P., Su, Y., Datta, A., Rorden, C., and Parra, L. C. (2013). Automated MRI segmentation for individualized modeling of current flow in the human head. *J. Neural Eng.* 10:066004. doi: 10.1088/1741-2560/10/6/066004

Kopell, N. J., Gritton, H. J., Whittington, M. A., and Kramer, M. A. (2014). Beyond the connectome: the dynome. *Neuron* 83, 1319–1328. doi: 10.1016/j.neuron.2014.08.016

Malavera, A., Vasquez, A., and Fregni, F. (2015). Novel methods to optimize the effects of transcranial direct current stimulation: a systematic review of transcranial direct current stimulation patents. *Expert Rev. Med. Devices* 12, 679–688. doi: 10.1586/17434440.2015.1090308

Moreno-Duarte, I., Morse, L. R., Alam, M., Bikson, M., Zafonte, R., and Fregni, F. (2014). Targeted therapies using electrical and magnetic neural stimulation for the treatment of chronic pain in spinal cord injury. *Neuroimage* 85, 1003–1013. doi: 10.1016/j.neuroimage.2013.05.097

Murphy, D. N., Boggio, P., and Fregni, F. (2009). Transcranial direct current stimulation as a therapeutic tool for the treatment of major depression: insights from past and recent clinical studies. *Curr. Opin. Psychiatry* 22, 306–311. doi: 10.1097/YCO.0b013e32832a133f

Nathan, S. S., Sinha, S. R., Gordon, B., Lesser, R. P., and Thakor, N. V (1993). Determination of current density distributions generated by electrical stimulation of the human cerebral cortex. *Electroencephalogr. Clin. Neurophysiol.* 86, 183–192. doi: 10.1016/0013-4694(93)90006-H

Nitsche, M. A., Boggio, P. S., Fregni, F., and Pascual-Leone, A. (2009). Treatment of depression with transcranial direct current stimulation (tDCS): a review. *Exp. Neurol.* 219, 14–19. doi: 10.1016/j.expneurol.2009.03.038

Nitsche, M. A., Nitsche, M. A., Paulus, W., and Paulus, W. (2000). Excitability changes induced in the human motor cortex by weak transcranial direct current stimulation. *J. Physiol.* 527(Pt 3), 633–639. doi: 10.1111/j.1469-7793.2000.t01-1-00633.x

Pahor, A., and Jaušovec, N. (2018). The effects of theta and gamma tACS on working memory and electrophysiology. *Front. Hum. Neurosci.* 11:651. doi: 10.3389/fnhum.2017.00651

Parazzini, M., Fiocchi, S., Cancelli, A., Cottone, C., Liorni, I., Ravazzani, P., et al. (2017). A computational model of the electric field distribution due to regional personalized or nonpersonalized electrodes to select transcranial electric stimulation target. *IEEE Trans. Biomed. Eng.* 64, 184–195. doi: 10.1109/TBME.2016.2553177

Parazzini, M., Fiocchi, S., Rossi, E., Paglialonga, A., and Ravazzani, P. (2011). Transcranial direct current stimulation: estimation of the electric field and of the current density in an anatomical human head model. *IEEE Trans. Biomed. Eng.* 58, 1773–1780. doi: 10.1109/TBME.2011.2116019

Pellicano, C., Gallo, A., Li, X., Ikonomidou, V. N., Evangelou, I. E., Ohayon, J. M., et al. (2010). Relationship of cortical atrophy to fatigue in patients with multiple sclerosis. *Arch. Neurol.* 67, 447–453. doi: 10.1001/archneurol.2010.48

Pérez-Borrego, Y. A., Campolo, M., Soto-León, V., Rodriguez-Matas, M. J., Ortega, E., and Oliviero, A. (2014). Pain treatment using tDCS in a single patient: telemedicine approach in non-invasive brain simulation. *Brain Stimul.* 7, 334–335. doi: 10.1016/j.brs.2013.11.008

Saiote, C., Goldschmidt, T., Timäus, C., Steenwijk, M. D., Opitz, A., Antal, A., et al. (2014). Impact of transcranial direct current stimulation on fatigue in multiple sclerosis. *Restor. Neurol. Neurosci.* 32, 423–436. doi: 10.3233/RNN-130372

Smith, W. E. (1992). Estimation of the spatio-temporal correlations of biological electrical sources from their magnetic fields. *IEEE Trans. Biomed. Eng.* 39, 997–1004. doi: 10.1109/10.161331

Soler, M. D., Kumru, H., Pelayo, R., Vidal, J., Tormos, J. M., Fregni, F., et al. (2010). Effectiveness of transcranial direct current stimulation and visual illusion on neuropathic pain in spinal cord injury. *Brain* 133, 2565–2577. doi: 10.1093/brain/awq184

Tecchio, F., Cancelli, A., Cottone, C., Ferrucci, R., Vergari, M., Zito, G., et al. (2015). Brain plasticity effects of neuromodulation against multiple sclerosis fatigue. *Front. Neurol.* 6:141. doi: 10.3389/fneur.2015.00141

Tecchio, F., Cancelli, A., Cottone, C., Tomasevic, L., Devigus, B., Zito, G., et al. (2013). Regional personalized electrodes to select transcranial current stimulation target. *Front. Hum. Neurosci.* 7:131. doi: 10.3389/fnhum.2013.00131

Tecchio, F., Cancelli, A., Cottone, C., Zito, G., Pasqualetti, P., Ghazaryan, A., et al. (2014). Multiple sclerosis fatigue relief by bilateral somatosensory cortex neuromodulation. *J. Neurol.* 261, 1552–1558. doi: 10.1007/s00415-014-7377-9

Tseng, P., Iu, K. C., and Juan, C. H. (2018). The critical role of phase difference in theta oscillation between bilateral parietal cortices for visuospatial working memory. *Sci. Rep.* 8:349. doi: 10.1038/s41598-017-18449-w

Van Essen, D. C. (2013). Cartography and connectomes. *Neuron* 80, 775–790. doi: 10.1016/j.neuron.2013.10.027

Vecchio, F., Miraglia, F., Porcaro, C., Cottone, C., Cancelli, A., Rossini, P. M., et al. (2017). Electroencephalography-derived sensory and motor network topology in multiple sclerosis fatigue. *Neurorehabil. Neural Repair* 31, 56–64. doi: 10.1177/1545968316656055

Wagner, S., Rampersad, S. M., Aydin, Ü., Vorwerk, J., Oostendorp, T. F., Neuling, T., et al. (2014). Investigation of tDCS volume conduction effects in a highly realistic head model. *J. Neural Eng.* 11:016002. doi: 10.1088/1741-2560/11/1/016002

Zhu, C. E., Yu, B., Zhang, W., Chen, W., Qi, Q., and Miao, Y. (2017). Effiectiveness and safety of transcranial direct current stimulation in fibromyalgia: a systematic review and meta-analysis. *J. Rehabil. Med.* 49, 2–9. doi: 10.2340/16501977-2179

8

An Emerging Role of micro-RNA in the Effect of the Endocrine Disruptors

Adel Derghal[1], Mehdi Djelloul[1,2], Jérôme Trouslard[1] and Lourdes Mounien[1]*

[1] Aix Marseille University, PPSN, Marseille, France, [2] Department of Cell and Molecular Biology, Karolinska Institute, Stockholm, Sweden

Edited by:
Fumihiko Maekawa,
National Institute for Environmental Studies, Japan

Reviewed by:
Guillaume Gourcerol,
Rouen University Hospital, France
Mohamed Najimi,
Sultan Moulay Slimane University, Morocco
Wataru Yoshioka,
The Jikei University School of Medicine, Japan

***Correspondence:**
Lourdes Mounien
lourdes.mounien@univ-amu.fr

Endocrine-disrupting chemicals (EDCs) are diverse natural and synthetic chemicals that may alter various mechanisms of the endocrine system and produce adverse developmental, reproductive, metabolic, and neurological effects in both humans and wildlife. Research on EDCs has revealed that they use a variety of both nuclear receptor-mediated and non-receptor-mediated mechanisms to modulate different components of the endocrine system. The molecular mechanisms underlying the effects of EDCs are still under investigation. Interestingly, some of the effects of EDCs have been observed to pass on to subsequent unexposed generations, which can be explained by the gametic transmission of deregulated epigenetic marks. Epigenetics is the study of heritable changes in gene expression that occur without a change in the DNA sequence. Epigenetic mechanisms, including histone modifications, DNA methylation, and specific micro-RNAs (miRNAs) expression, have been proposed to mediate transgenerational transmission and can be triggered by environmental factors. MiRNAs are short non-coding RNA molecules that post-transcriptionally repress the expression of genes by binding to 3′-untranslated regions of the target mRNAs. Given that there is mounting evidence that miRNAs are regulated by hormones, then clearly it is important to investigate the potential for environmental EDCs to deregulate miRNA expression and action.

Keywords: micro-RNA, endocrine disruptors, environment

INTRODUCTION

Endocrine-disrupting chemicals (EDCs) are diverse natural and synthetic chemicals that may alter various mechanisms of the endocrine system and produce adverse developmental, reproductive, metabolic, and neurological effects in both humans and wildlife (Henley and Korach, 2006). To date, close to 800 chemicals are known or suspected to be capable of interfering with hormone receptors and/or hormone synthesis and then play a larger role in the causation of many endocrine diseases and disorders (WHO | State of the science of endocrine disrupting chemicals, 2012). Excretion of EDCs is dependent on the nature of the chemical substances. If the substance is non-persistent it is usually predicted that they are metabolized by the liver then finally eliminated from the body through feces and urine. Persistent endocrine disruptors are accumulated especially in adipose tissue and they can be released slowly. One way of excretion of these persistent endocrine disruptors is thought to be from mother to child through breast feeding. It is observed in many studies that the daily intake of breast milk containing organic pollutants may exceed the tolerable limit. It has been established that some EDCs can act directly on hormone receptors as hormone mimics or antagonists. Others can act directly on proteins that control the delivery of a hormone to its target cell or tissue. In addition, EDCs may act synergistically and produce additive effects. Most studies on EDCs have focused on chemicals that affect the reproductive and thyroid axis. However, several studies have suggested that environmental chemicals could affect several physiological systems that lead to metabolic disorders or central nervous system dysfunctions (Casals-Casas and Desvergne, 2011). For instance, neurobehavioral disorders have been associated with hypothalamic-pituitary-adrenal (HPA) axis disruption induced by hydroxyl-polychlorinated biphenyl (PCB; Kimura-Kuroda et al., 2007).

It is particularly difficult to highlight only one mechanism of action shared by the set of EDCs. In fact, the main problem is that there are many and diverse EDCs including industrial chemicals, pesticides, pollutants, and plastic industry compounds. Nevertheless, research on EDCs has revealed that they use a variety of both nuclear receptor- and non-receptor-mediated mechanisms to modulate different components of the endocrine system. For instance Vinclozolin (VCZ), a widely used fungicide with antiandrogenic effects in mammals, is a competitive antagonist of androgen receptor (AR) ligand binding (Kelce et al., 1997). Several studies showed that exposure to VCZ induce masculinized females and feminized males in rodents (Buckley et al., 2006). Interestingly, some of the effects of VCZ have been observed to pass on to subsequent unexposed generations, which can be explained by the gametic transmission of deregulated epigenetic marks (Anway et al., 2005; Stouder and Paoloni-Giacobino, 2010; Guerrero-Bosagna et al., 2012; Skinner et al., 2013). Epigenetic mechanisms, including histone modifications, DNA methylation, and specific micro-RNAs (miRNAs) expression, have been proposed to mediate such transgenerational transmission (Reik et al., 2001; Del-Mazo et al., 2013).

This review provides an insight into the toxicological effects of EDCs and particularly new molecular mechanisms, i.e., miRNAs, involved in the EDCs induced endocrine disruption.

THE DIFFERENT TYPES OF EDCS

The term endocrine disruptors were first introduced by the group of Soto in 1993 that showed that EDCs induced developmental abnormalities (Colborn et al., 1993). The International Program on Chemical Safety (IPCS) in 2002 and World Health Organization in 2013 defined EDCs as "*...an exogenous substance or mixture that alters function(s) of the endocrine system and consequently causes adverse health effects in an intact organism, or its progeny, or (sub) populations. A potential endocrine disruptor is an exogenous substance or mixture that possesses properties that might be expected to lead to endocrine disruption in an intact organism, or its progeny, or (sub) populations.*" To date, EDCs include a large variety of chemical classes such as pesticides [methoxychlor, chlopyrifos, and dichlorodiphenyltrichloroethane (DDT)], pharmaceutical agents [diethylstrilbestrol (DES)], plastic packaging compounds [Bisphenol A (BPA), phthalates], and other industrial products that are used in daily life as fungicides VCZ or solvents/lubricants (dioxins). Some of them but not all are exposed in this paragraph.

A large number of chemicals are used as pesticides. The most important pesticides are organochlorines pesticides (OCPs), organophosphates, or triazines. The most emblematic of the banned OCPs is DDT and the exposure to it persists. The pesticides are involved in a large number of diseases including cancer, diabetes but also neurodegenerative disease as Parkinson or Alzheimer (Mostafalou et al., 2012; Mostafalou and Abdollahi, 2013).

The dioxins are a general name for a family of organochlorines including the polychlorinated dibenzodioxins (PCDDs), the polychlorinated dibenzofurans (PCDFs), and the polychlorinated biphenyls (PCBs). Dioxins are produced by various industrial processes and are commonly regarded as highly toxic compounds that are environmental pollutants and persistent organic pollutants. Among the PCDDs, the 2,3,7,8-Tetrachlorodibenzo-*p*-dioxin (TCDD) is the most potent and toxic compound and became known as a contaminant in Agent Orange, a herbicide used as a weapon in the Vietnam War (Schecter et al., 2006). TCDD was also released into the environment during the Seveso disaster (Sweeney and Mocarelli, 2000). The TCDD and the other toxins have been shown to be involved in different diseases including cancers, thyroid dysfunction, and nervous system degeneration but also type 2 diabetes (Pelclová et al., 2006; Schecter et al., 2006; Mostafalou et al., 2012; Mostafalou and Abdollahi, 2013).

An important number of EDCs are found in plastic products. World plastic production exceeded 300 million tons in 2010 (Halden, 2010). Most abundant of these plastics are phthalates and BPA. These are two most common EDCs and are associated with parental and social behavioral disturbances but also endocrine disease. Phthalates are mainly used as plasticizers in a wide range of common products, and are released into the environment. Phthalate exposure may be through direct use or by indirect means through leaching and general environmental contamination (Aurela et al., 1999). Food products are believed to be the main source of di-(2-ethylhexyl) phthalate (DEHP) and other phthalates in the general population. Fatty foods such as milk, butter, and meats are a major source. In several studies in human and rodents, high and even low doses of phthalates have been shown to change hormone levels as T3, T4, and thyroid-stimulating hormone and cause birth defects (Gayathri et al., 2004; Heudorf et al., 2007; Meeker et al., 2009). BPA is one of the other emblematic plastics used in polycarbonate plastic and polystyrene resins. Interestingly, it has been shown that BPA is detected in 95% of urine sample from a reference population of 394 adults in the United States (Calafat et al., 2005). This higher level of BPA in urine is associated with cardiovascular disease, sterility, and other reproductive diseases but also diabetes and liver abnormalities (Takeuchi et al., 2004; Sugiura-Ogasawara et al., 2005; Lang et al., 2008).

THE TOXICOLOGICAL EFFECTS OF EDCs ON ENDOCRINE AXIS

Reproductive Axis

In the last few years, it has been noticed that the incidence of certain diseases of the reproductive axis has increased (WHO | State of the science of endocrine disrupting chemicals, 2012). It is well-established that estrogen and androgen are involved in sexual differentiation. In this context, EDCs may act as estrogen and or androgen antagonists and induce different sexual disorders in males and females (Diamanti-Kandarakis et al., 2009; Sweeney et al., 2015; Toppari et al., 2016). For instance, DES and phthalates exposure to rats are associated with cryptorchidism or micropenis (Fisher et al., 2003; Li et al., 2003). In human, it has been shown that breast milk dioxin concentration correlated positively with the risk of cryptorchidism in Denmark (Main et al., 2007). It has also been shown that perinatal exposure to low doses of dioxin can permanently reduce sperm quality (Mocarelli et al., 2011). In humans, exposure to PCBs caused a defect in the development of the reproductive system (Staessen et al., 2001). Recently, epidemiological, study suggested that prenatal exposure to PCBs may be also associated with increased risk for cryptorchidism (Koskenniemi et al., 2015).

EDCs are associated with some types of female reproductive axis disorder including polycystic ovarian syndrome (PCOS). PCOS is a problem in which a woman's hormones are out of balance. It can disrupt the menstrual cycle and makes it difficult to become pregnant. If it isn't treated, over time it can lead to serious health problems, such as diabetes and heart disease. Most women with PCOS grow many small cysts on their ovaries. Interestingly, women with PCOS have higher levels of BPA and increased testosterone in these women is consistent with decreased clearance of BPA (Takeuchi et al., 2004, 2006). The cause of PCOS is not fully understood, but the EDCs as well as BPA could play a role in the onset of PCOS. Female rats exhibited sexual precocity as a consequence of exposure to DTT (Rasier et al., 2007).

It has also been shown in the hypothalamic GT1-7 cell line that organochlorine pesticides such as methoxychlor and chlopyrifos altered gonadotropin-releasing hormone (GnRH) gene expression and biosynthesis (Gore, 2002) suggesting that EDCs could affect the different levels or reproductive axis. Interestingly, it has been revealed that the BPA-mediated inhibition of GnRH neuronal activity occurred independent of estrogen receptors via a non-canonical unknown pathway (Klenke et al., 2016).

Thyreotropic Axis

Thyroid hormones (T3 and T4) are important for brain development, for the modulation of metabolism and are associated with many aspects of normal adult physiology. For these reasons, thyreotropic axis disruption induced a large scale of perturbation in adult physiology, development, and metabolism. It has been reported that numerous EDCs can directly affect the normal functioning of the thyroid gland. In numerous studies, it has been shown that different EDCs such as PCBs, BPA, or DTT have thyroid-disrupting effects in animals and humans (Patrick, 2009; Molehin et al., 2016).

The EDCs can affect the thyroid system at different levels such as the transport and/or biosynthesis of the thyroid hormones. It has been shown that PCBs have a high affinity with thyroxin specific binding protein which can affect the thyroid hormone transport (Rickenbacher et al., 1986; McKinney et al., 1987; Darnerud et al., 1996). More precisely, treatment of mice during gestation with PCB as 3,3′, 4,4′-tetrachlorobiphenyl (CB-77) leads to a decrease of free and total T4 in fetal plasma (Darnerud et al., 1996). More recently, the group of Seegal examined the effects of a mixture of PCBs and polybrominated diphenyl ethers (PBDEs) coexposure from gestational day 6 through postnatal day 21, alone and in combination, on T4 levels in rat offspring (Miller et al., 2012, 201). They observed that PCBs and PBDEs induces similar reductions in T4 levels and that coexposure to a mixture of PCBs and PBDEs has additive effects on T4 level in male and female offspring (Miller et al., 2012). In the study of Schmutzler et al., rats (female, ovariectomized) were treated for 12 weeks with different EDCs and an alteration in thyrotropin (TSH) and thyroid hormones (T4, T3) serum levels were observed (Schmutzler et al., 2004). In another set of studies, exposure to phthalates induced thyroid function alterations (Mitchell et al., 1985; Hinton et al., 1986; Price et al., 1988). Interestingly, the treatment of rats for periods of 3 months with di-(2-ethylhexyl) phthalate increased the number and size of lysosomes, hypertrophy of the Golgi apparatus, and dilation of the rough endoplasmic reticulum in thyroid cells and these changes are consistent with persistent hyperactivity in the gland (Price et al., 1988). It has also been shown that EDCs can alter deiodinase activity which is the peroxidase enzyme that is involved in the activation or deactivation of thyroid hormones (Meerts et al., 2002; Viluksela et al., 2004; Noyes et al., 2013).

In human, there is now growing evidence that PCBs but also BPA and phthalates have thyroid-disrupting effects (Boas et al., 2012; Campos and Freire, 2016). For instance, the group of Yoshinaga showed that exposure to hydroxylated-PCBs at environmental levels during the first trimester of pregnancy can affect neonatal thyroid hormone status (Hisada et al., 2014). It has also been shown that early exposure to certain environmental chemicals with endocrine-disruption activity as pesticides may interfere with neonatal thyroid hormone status (Freire et al., 2011).

Central Nervous System

There is strong evidence that there is a correlation between the increasing prevalence of neurodevelopmental disorders and the increase in exposure to pollutants over the past several decades (Weiss and Landrigan, 2000; Landrigan and Goldman, 2011a,b). For instance, since the 1970s, there have been dramatic increases in previously rare neurodevelopmental disorders such as autism which is characterized by some degree of impaired social behavior, communication and language, and a narrow range of interests and activities that are both unique to the individual and carried out repetitively. In the 1970s, autism's prevalence was estimated to be between 4 and 5 in 10,000 children (Wing et al., 1976) but today this value is estimated to be 1 in 110 children (Rice et al., 2007). In a review of the literature performed by de Cock et al., a positive association was found for autism in relation to exposure to different chemicals investigated, which included hazardous air pollutants, pesticides, and BPA (de Cock et al., 2012). In the same study, a relationship between attention deficit hyperactivity disorders and different EDCs including BCPs and pesticides such as chlorpyrifos has been done (de Cock et al., 2012).

The function of central nervous system (CNS) can be affected by EDCs and these effects can be induced by different mechanisms. The most important is the effects of EDCs on different endocrine axis important for CNS functions and development. Evidence that prenatal estrogen exposure is important in neuronal correct development emerged from reports of psychosis in patients prenatally exposed to the synthetic estrogen DES (Katz et al., 1987; Brown, 2009; Inadera, 2015; Negri-Cesi, 2015). Interestingly, several researches indicate that BPA is an estrogenic EDC that alters or interferes with normal endocrine development in various vertebrate and invertebrate species (vom Saal et al., 2007) suggesting a role of BPA in CNS disease. For instance, prenatal exposure to low dose of BPA disturbed neocortical histogenesis in mice (Nakamura et al., 2006, 2007).

As exposed above, BPA is a well-known xenoestrogen (Kuiper et al., 1998; Delfosse et al., 2014; Inadera, 2015). BPA has complex action in the CNS but primarily BPA was exhibited to bind both estrogen receptors α and β (ERα and ERβ) and has also been shown to act as an anti-androgen (Kuiper et al., 1998; Wolstenholme et al., 2011). Interestingly, it has been described endocrine and neuroendocrine abnormalities in schizophrenia (Marx and Lieberman, 1998; Stevens, 2002). In fact, estrogen has been associated with a neuroprotective effect but lower plasma levels of estrogens induced schizophrenia-like syndrome in males and females (Huber et al., 2001; Kaneda and Ohmori, 2005; Segal et al., 2007). Furthermore, neuronal disorders have also been associated with an impairment of HPA axis. For instance, the increase of glucocorticoid concentrations induced hippocampal nerve damage and schizophrenia (Cotter and Pariante, 2002). In rat, corticosterone exposures also lead to degeneration of the prefrontal cortex causing impairments in executive functions such as behavioral flexibility and working memory (Cerqueira et al., 2005). It has been established in baboons that HPA is potentially affected by estrogen (Pepe and Albrecht, 1998; Albrecht et al., 2005). In addition, it has been recently shown that perinatal exposure to low-dose of BPA caused HPA axis dysfunctions (Panagiotidou et al., 2014; Chen et al., 2015; Zhou et al., 2015). Particularly, the administration of low doses of BPA (2 μg/kg.day) to female breeders from gestation day 10 to lactation day 7 induced obvious anxiety/depression-like behaviors in the offspring (Chen et al., 2015). Notably, significant increase in serum corticosterone and adrenocorticotropin, and corticotropin-releasing hormone mRNA were detected in BPA-exposed rats before or after the mild stressor (Chen et al., 2015). Altogether these different observations strongly suggest that BPA and other EDCs could be associated to schizophrenia pathogenesis (Brown, 2009).

Metabolic Disorders

In addition to the reproductive and neuronal developmental effects, there is also evidence that metabolic disorders may be linked to EDCs (Casals-Casas et al., 2008; Newbold et al., 2008). Obesity, diabetes and metabolic syndrome are due to disruption of the energy storage balance endocrine system and thus are potentially sensitive to EDCs. This hypothesis is supported by different epidemiological and animal studies that have shown that a variety of EDCs can influence adipogenesis and obesity (Baillie-Hamilton, 2002; Casals-Casas et al., 2008; Elobeid and Allison, 2008; Newbold et al., 2008; Chen et al., 2009). For instance, the administration of DES to neonatal mice induced overweight associated with an increase of abdominal body fats and inflammatory biomarkers (Newbold et al., 2007). In rats, perinatal exposure to low doses of BPA increased adipogenesis and body weight in adult females (Somm et al., 2009). EDCs are also involved in glucose homeostasis defects. In accordance with this fact, epidemiological studies report that exposure to EDCs may affect the risk of type 2 diabetes (Remillard and Bunce, 2002; Huang et al., 2015; Song et al., 2016). Very low doses of BPA induced hyperinsulenemia and type 2 diabetes (Alonso-Magdalena et al., 2010). In the same way, low doses of BPA and dioxins altered α-cell function and glucagon release which lead to glucose homeostasis defect (Alonso-Magdalena et al., 2005). Interestingly, it has been established that EDCs such as BPA or dioxins are accumulated by adipose tissue and that they are released slowly and have induced glucose homeostasis impairment (Alonso-Magdalena et al., 2011). When administrated to mother mice, BPA induces metabolic disorders in adult male offspring such as an age-related change in food intake, an increase in body weight and liver weight, abdominal adipocyte mass, number and volume, and in serum leptin and insulin, but a decrease in serum adiponectin and in glucose tolerance (Angle et al., 2013). Furthermore, mother mice treated with BPA during gestation, at environmentally relevant doses, exhibit profound glucose intolerance and altered insulin sensitivity as well as increased body weight (Alonso-Magdalena et al., 2015).

MICRO-RNAs AND EDCs

EDCs often act via more than one mechanism. The target cells of the hormones bear receptors specific to a given hormone and will be activated by either a lipid-soluble (permeable to plasma membrane) or water-soluble hormone (binds cell-surface receptor; Casals-Casas and Desvergne, 2011; Wolstenholme et al., 2011; Maqbool et al., 2016). Lipid-soluble hormones (steroid hormones and hormones of the thyroid gland) diffuse through the plasma membrane to enter the target cell and bind to a nuclear receptor (NR) protein that will in turn activates expression of specific genes that influence specific physiological cell activities. Water-soluble hormones (such as insulin) bind to a receptor protein on the plasma membrane of the cell which leads to specific cellular transduction pathways (Casals-Casas and Desvergne, 2011; Maqbool et al., 2016; Wolstenholme et al.,

2011). Because many EDCs are small lipophilic compounds, they can directly interact with a given NR, which presumably perturbs or modulates downstream gene expression.

In parallel with these classical pathways, it appears that EDCs not only involve genetics but also epigenetic mechanisms. Epigenetics is broadly defined as those heritable changes in the genome not dependent upon changes in genetic sequences (e.g., DNA methylation or histone modification). These epigenetic processes control tissue development by controlling gene expression. Thus, a major route by which hormones act during development is by changing the epigenome. These different epigenetic mechanisms also include miRNAs which are short non-coding RNA molecules that post-transcriptionally repress the expression of genes by binding to 3′-untranslated regions (3′UTR) of the target mRNAs. Recently, it appears that miRNAs can be involved in the action of EDCs (Cameron et al., 2016; Klinge, 2015). This part of the review focuses on the regulation of miRNAs by the EDCs which appear as a new molecular mechanism involved in endocrine disruption.

Biogenesis and Action of miRNAs

The miRNAs are short non-coding RNA with a size of 21–26 nucleotides that suppress target gene expression through the inhibition of gene translation and the increase of the degradation of target mRNAs (Bartel, 2004). These small regulatory molecules are involved in a large range of biological processes such as development, cell proliferation, apoptosis, synaptic plasticity, and energy metabolism (Bartel, 2004). The gene regulation and processing as well as the mode of action of miRNAs are conserved over the evolution of a species (Stricklin et al., 2005; Landgraf et al., 2007; Ruby et al., 2007b). In recent decades, research on miRNAs has deepened our understanding of their mechanisms of action and their biological functions. These regulatory RNAs are predicted to modulate the expression of ~30% of protein-coding genes (Lewis et al., 2005). The miRNA can affect translation and mRNA stability by means of RNA-RNA interactions. A number of algorithms allow the identification of the potentially targeted mRNA by miRNA and conversely miRNA modulator of mRNA. Although the regulation of genes by miRNAs is an active area of research, few targets of miRNAs have been experimentally validated in a physiological context.

In parallel with the discovery of new miRNA, the identification of the components of the miRNA maturation and processing machinery is an active area of research (**Figure 1**). The miRNA genes are located throughout the genome, within introns of protein-coding genes and rarely in exons (Rodriguez et al., 2004). Despite the small number of cases studied, it seems that the promoters of miRNAs have the same characteristics as those genes encoding proteins. The genes encode primary RNA (pri-miRNAs) conformation stem-loop, with one or two sequences which produce mature miRNAs (Hutvágner et al., 2001; Lagos-Quintana et al., 2001; Lau et al., 2001). The transcription machinery involves a RNA polymerase II (Lee et al., 2004; Bortolin-Cavaillé et al., 2009). The pri-miRNA is cleaved and polyadenylated at 3′ and 5′ capped in the same manner as the mRNAs (**Figure 1**; Cai et al., 2004). The steps of the pri-miRNA maturation require two endonucleases before they become functional miRNAs (Lee et al., 2003). The first step involves an RNA binding protein, the DiGeorge Syndrome Critical Region 8 (DGCR8) also called Partner of Drosha (PASHA) associated with Drosha (Denli et al., 2004; Gregory et al., 2004; Han et al., 2004). Drosha cleaves sequences on either side of the stem-loop of the pri-miRNA and gives the precursor miRNA (pre-miRNA). Pre-miRNA is exported from the nucleus to the cytoplasm by a karyopherin known as Exportin 5 (Yi et al., 2003; Bohnsack et al., 2004; Lund et al., 2004). In the second step, endonuclease DICER cleaves the pre-miRNA loop region in the cytoplasm, thereby releasing a double-stranded RNA of about 20 nucleotide pairs containing the mature miRNA (Bernstein et al., 2001; Grishok et al., 2001; Hutvágner et al., 2001; Ketting et al., 2001). Like Drosha, DICER is associated with an RNA binding-protein, the human immunodeficiency virus Transactivating Response RNA-Binding Protein (TRBP; Chendrimada et al., 2005; Gregory et al., 2005; Haase et al., 2005). One of the two strands is recognized by a protein of the family of the Argonautes (AGO), most commonly AGO2, which in turn recruits other elements of the RNA-induced silencing complex (RISC; Sontheimer, 2005). The other strand called "star strand" is degraded. An asterisk is associated with the name of the miRNA that is not incorporated into the RISC complex (e.g., miR-488*). However, for some miRNAs, both strands may be incorporated into the RISC complex. In this case, the end of the strand 5′ of the stem-loop is called "5p" and that of strand 3′ is called "3p" (e.g., miR-384-5p and miR-384-3p). In fact, new data indicates that a small fraction of the star strand is incorporated into the RISC complex for most miRNA families (Yang et al., 2011). For these reasons, the nomenclature scheme "–5p/–3p" is increasingly used instead of the terminology "mature/star." The RISC complex/mature miRNA (miRISC) recognizes the target mRNA and induces degradation and/or inactivation of the latter (**Figure 2**).

However, various studies reveal that some families of miRNAs undergo non-canonical pathway maturation. Importantly, some studies described miRNAs called mirtrons which are located in the short sequence of introns. The mirtrons undergo a first processing step, independent of Drosha, by the splicing machinery to give miRNA with a lariat structure. The introns are then processed by the lariat-debranching enzyme to give the pre-miRNAs which carry-on its maturation by the canonical pathway (Okamura et al., 2007; Ruby et al., 2007a). It has also been reported in one case (miR-451) that the cleavage step by DICER is substituted with AGO2 (Cheloufi et al., 2010; Cifuentes et al., 2010).

The miRNA-mRNA Interactions

The action of miRNAs depends on their specific interaction with their targets. In plants, miRNAs bind to their targets with perfect complementarity of bases, which induces a rapid cleavage of the transcript by the ribonuclease activity of AGO (Baumberger and Baulcombe, 2005). In metazoans, the majority of miRNAs partially bind to their targets primarily through a region of so-called seed sequence, located at positions 2–7 from the miRNA 5′-end (Doench and Sharp, 2004; Brennecke et al., 2005). This region binds perfectly on the 3′UTR via complementary

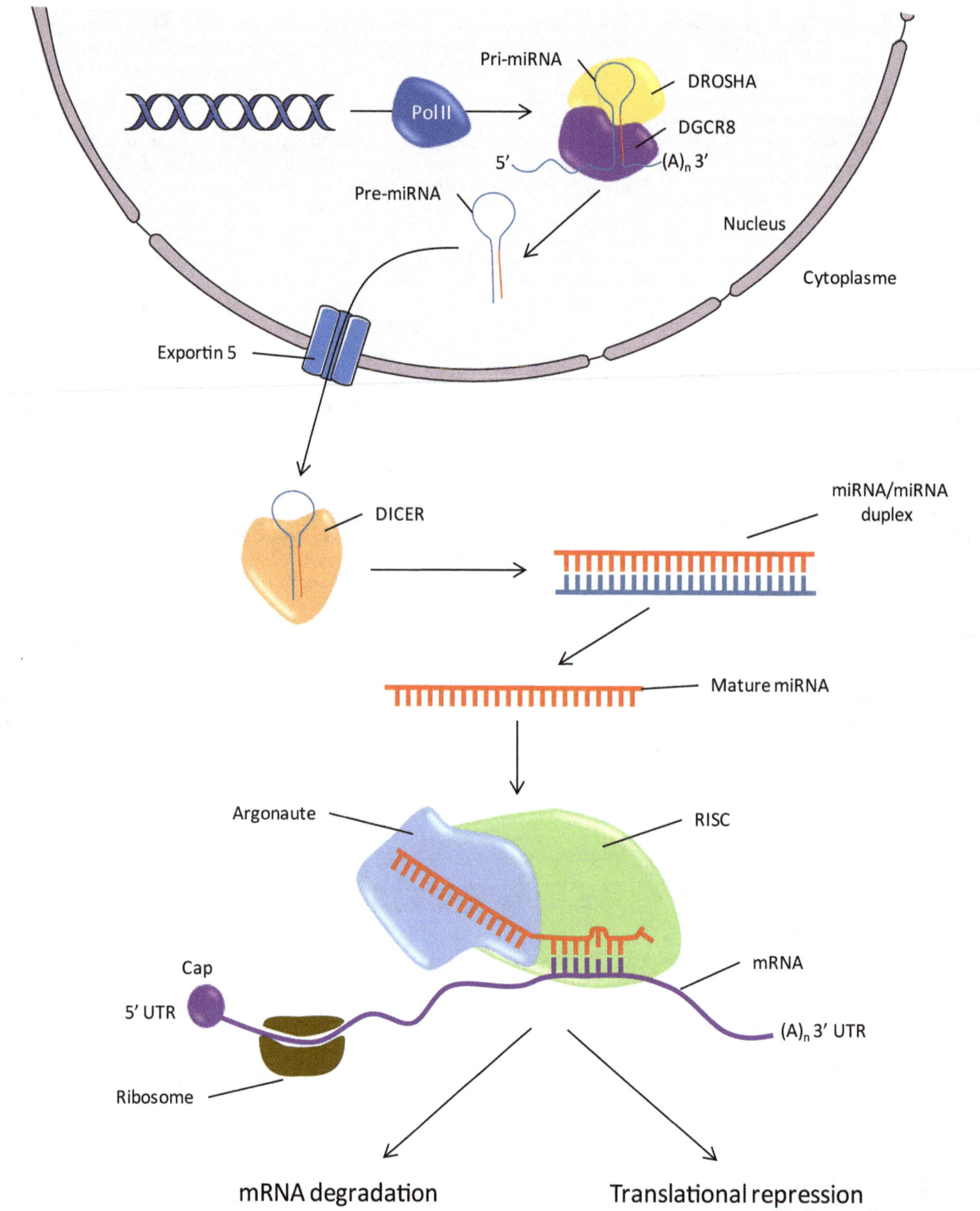

FIGURE 1 | Biogenesis of miRNAs. Pol II, RNA Polymerase II; pri-miR, primary miRNA; pre-miR, precursor miRNA; RISC, RNA-Induced Silencing Complex; 5′ or 3′UTR, 5′ or 3′ untranslated region; DGCR8, DiGeorge Syndrome Critical Region 8; $(A)_n$, Polyadenylation.

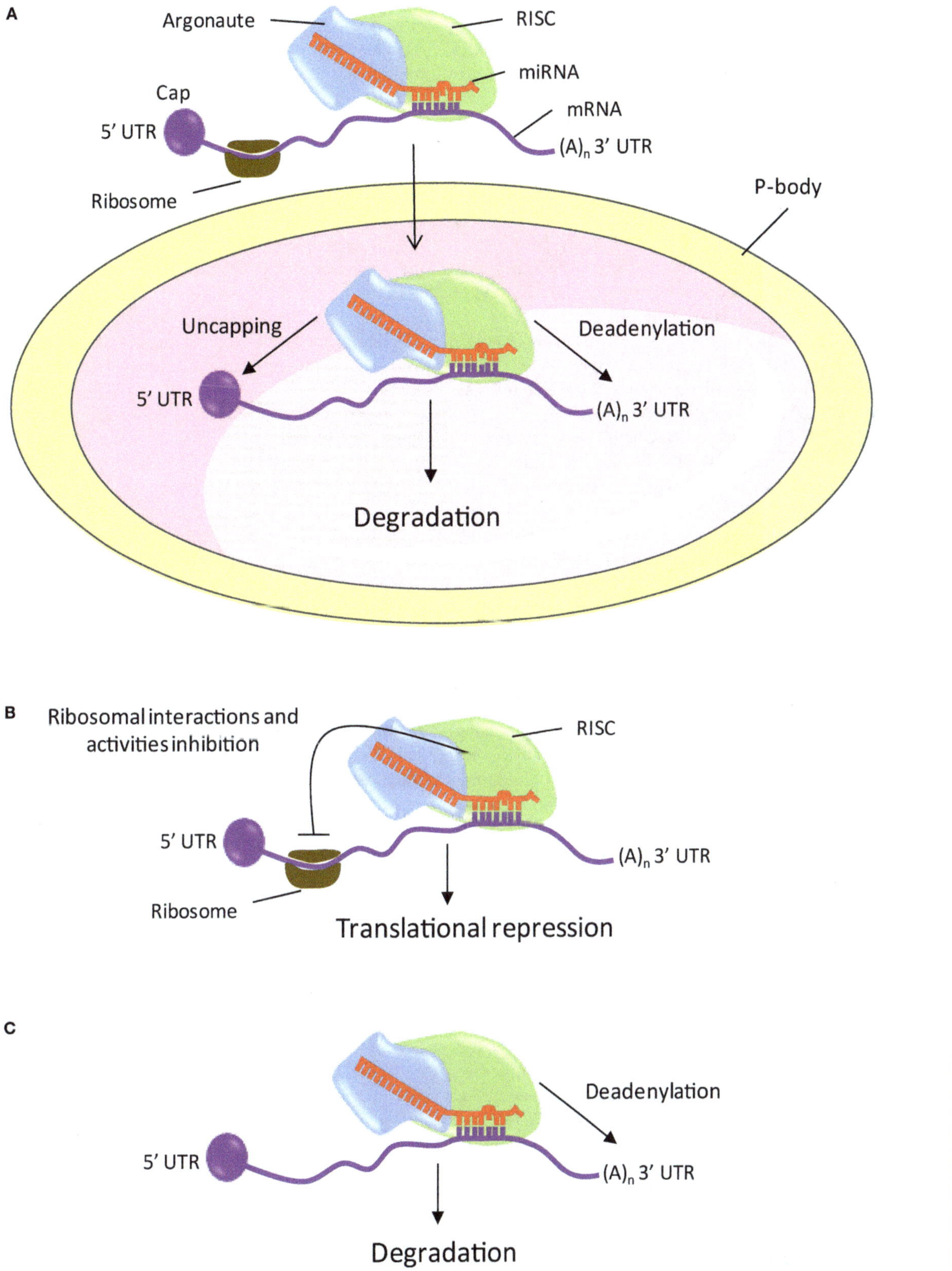

FIGURE 2 | The different mechanisms of mRNA repression or degradation by miRNA. (A) The processing bodies. **(B)** Action on the initiation of translation and repression in post-initiation steps. **(C)** Deadenylation. miRNA, microRNA; P-bodies, processing bodies; RISC, *RNA-Induced Silencing Complex;* 5′ or 3′UTR, 5′ or 3′ untranslated region; $(A)_n$, Polyadenylation.

base interactions. These interactions induce inhibition of the expression of the target mRNA through a blocking of the translation or a degradation of the transcript. The different mechanisms of mRNA repression or degradation by miRNA are briefly described below.

Processing bodies (P-bodies) are cytoplasmic foci containing mRNA degradation enzymes and trinucleotide repeat-containing gene 6A protein (TNRC6A or GW182 for Drosophila). These are involved in the catabolism and/or storage of untranslated mRNA (**Figure 2A**; Eystathioy et al., 2002, 2003; Ingelfinger et al., 2002; van Dijk et al., 2002; Sheth and Parker, 2003). The GW182 proteins are also found in the miRISC complex where they play a key role in the repression induced by miRNAs (Jakymiw et al., 2005; Liu et al., 2005; Eulalio et al., 2008). In addition, the AGO and GW182 proteins, miRNAs and targeted mRNAs are found in the P-bodies (Ding et al., 2005; Liu et al., 2005; Pillai et al., 2005; Sen and Blau, 2005). These studies suggest that targeted mRNAs are repressed or degraded in the P-bodies.

The mechanism by which miRISC inhibits translation is controversial. Several studies indicate a blocking of the initiation of translation, while other studies suggest a repression in post-initiation steps (**Figure 2B**). Indeed, it has been shown that the miRNA targeted mRNAs are associated with fewer ribosomes during elongation than in mRNAs controls (Humphreys et al., 2005; Pillai et al., 2005; Bhattacharyya et al., 2006; Huang et al., 2007; Ding and Grosshans, 2009). The initiation is stopped by the blocking by miRISC of the interaction of the translation ribosomal subunit 60S with mRNA (Chendrimada et al., 2007; Wang et al., 2008). In addition, GW182 recognizes the 5′ cap of the mRNA and prevents the initiation of translation (Eulalio et al., 2008). In the other studies, two mechanisms inducing translation repression after initiation have been described. It has been shown that miRISC promotes the release of ribosomes during elongation, thus blocking translation (Petersen et al., 2006). Another study suggests that the elongation process is maintained without peptide production when mRNA is targeted by a miRNA (Nottrott et al., 2006). The authors suggest that the complex-related proteases miRISC could degrade the native peptides.

Studies showed that repression of many miRNA targets is associated with a deadenylation and degradation (**Figure 2C**; Lim et al., 2005; Giraldez et al., 2006; Wu et al., 2006; Wakiyama et al., 2007; Eulalio et al., 2009). Comparative analysis of large scale proteomic and transcriptomic changes, following overexpression or inhibition of a miRNA in mammalian cells show that the vast majority of targets repressed by a miRNA have decreased their level of mRNA reflecting a lower presence of protein (Baek et al., 2008; Selbach et al., 2008; Hendrickson et al., 2009; Guo et al., 2010). These studies show that repression induced by miRNAs predominantly results in mRNA degradation.

Modulation of miRNA Expression by Hormones

Numerous studies clearly indicated that different hormones modulate miRNA expression in different organs (Hu et al., 2013; Cameron et al., 2016; Derghal et al., 2015; Klinge, 2015). For instance, the treatment with thyroid hormones of hepatocytes cells AML 12 over-expressing miR-206 resulted in decreased miR-206 expression, and a significant increase in two predicted target genes (i.e., Mup1 and Gpd2; Dong et al., 2010).

It has also been shown that estradiol actively controls miRNA production in various tissues such as mammary and ovarian cells (Gupta et al., 2012). More precisely, estrogens modulate miRNA transcription by inactivating RNA polymerase II and precursor miRNA biogenesis by blocking Drosha-mediated processing (Gupta et al., 2012). It also been shown that estrogen regulates miRNA expression in brain and particularly in the hippocampus, the amygdala and paraventricular nucleus (Rao et al., 2013). Recently, it has been established that miR-27a/b and miR-494 regulate tissue factor pathway inhibitor α (TFPIα) expression suggesting a possible role of these miRNAs in the estrogen mediated downregulation of TFPIα involved in breast cancer (Ali et al., 2016).

Several studies indicate that gonadotropins as estrogen can affect miRNA expression (Cohen et al., 2016). In accordance with this, it has been observed variability in miRNA expression profiles in estrogen receptor-positive and -negative breast cancer phenotypes (Iorio et al., 2005; Mattie et al., 2006). As described recently miR-136-3p expression levels were increased after the administration of human chorionic gonadotropin to ovarian cells (Kitahara et al., 2013). Direct action of estrogen on miRNAs expression has been demonstrated in different studies. For instance, an aberrant miRNA expression has been characterized in estrogen-induced rat breast carcinogenesis (Kovalchuk et al., 2007). Using the microarray approach, it has been shown that estrogen can modulate the profile of miRNAs expression in zebrafish model and in human MCF-7 and ZR-75 breast cancer cells (Cohen et al., 2008; Bhat-Nakshatri et al., 2009; Maillot et al., 2009; Ferraro et al., 2012).

Altogether, these different observations suggest that the link between hormones, miRNAs and mRNA targets will lead to an improved understanding of how EDCs affect the different endocrine axis.

Modulation of miRNA Expression by EDCs

A few recent studies report the effect of several EDCs on the expression of miRNAs in fish, animals, or cell lines (Collotta et al., 2013; Vrijens et al., 2015). These disturbances of miRNAs expression profile by EDCs are associated with diseases of the CNS and reproductive axis as well as metabolic disorders (Vrijens et al., 2015).

In humans, it has been shown that several EDCs as DTT or BPA decreased the expression of miR-21 which has a key role in cancer especially in breast cancer development (Tilghman et al., 2012; Sicard et al., 2013). In addition, decreased expression of let-7f is also associated with breast cancer (Sakurai et al., 2012). In the work led by Tilghman et al., DTT (10 μM) or BPA (10 μM) activate ERα in MCF-7 breast cancer cells which down-regulated the expression of miR-21, let-7a-f, miR-15b, and miR-28b and increased the expression miR-638, miR-663, and miR-1915 (Tilghman et al., 2012). In addition, it has been exhibited an important role of miR-19 in BPA-mediated MCF-7 cell proliferation (Li et al., 2014). The xenoestrogens DES also showed a decrease of miR-34b expression in MCF-7 cells (Lee et al., 2011). In rats, the neonatal exposure to the estrogenic analog (i.e., estradiol benzoate) increased the expression of miR-29 in testicular tissue (Meunier et al., 2012). Increased miR-29 expression resulted in a decrease in DNA methyltransferases (DNMT1, 3a and 3b) and antiapoptotic myeloid cell leukemia sequence 1 (Mcl-1) protein levels. Together, the increased miR-29 combined with a subsequent reduction of DNMT and Mcl-1 protein levels may represent a basis of explanation for the adult expression of the germ cell apoptosis phenotype. Interestingly, BPA given to rats at moderate doses is associated with erectile dysfunction, cavernosal lipofibrosis and alterations of global gene transcription including a set of miRNAs expressed in the penile shaft (Kovanecz et al., 2014). In female, prenatal BPA treatment in sheep results in hypergonadotropism and ovarian cycle disruptions (Veiga-Lopez et al., 2013). Interestingly, in this study it has been shown that fetal ovarian miRNAs expression was altered by prenatal BPA with 45 down-regulated (>1.5-fold) at day 65 and 11 down-regulated at day 90 of gestation (Veiga-Lopez et al., 2013). In chicks, several miRNAs (miR-1623, miR-1552-3p, miR-1573, miR-124a, and miR-1764) were down-regulated in the DES-treated chick oviduct compared with control oviduct (Lim and Song, 2015). Interestingly, these miRNAs regulate the expression of vitelline membrane outer layer protein 1, a basic protein present in the outer layer of the vitelline membrane of eggs, plays essential roles in separating the yolk from the egg white (Lim and Song, 2015). There is a growing concern about the potential health effects of exposure to various EDCs during pregnancy and infancy. The placenta is expected to be an effective barrier protecting the developing embryo against some EDCs circulating in maternal blood. However, it has been shown recently that miR-146a was significant overexpressed and correlated significantly with BPA accumulation in the placenta from pregnant women living in a polluted area and undergoing therapeutic abortion due to fetal malformations (De Felice et al., 2015). This observation has been also established in HTR-8 and 3A human placental cells (Avissar-Whiting et al., 2010). These different studies highlight the fact that the EDCs induce miRNA-expression alterations in the reproductive axis.

In the context of CNS disease, Jiang et al. established by *in silico* approach that miR-146a is involved in Alzheimer's disease (Jiang et al., 2013). Interestingly, BPA exposure of human placental cell lines has been shown to alter miRNA expression levels, and specifically, miR-146a was strongly induced by BPA treatment (Avissar-Whiting et al., 2010). Then, miR-146a could be used as a biomarker for Alzheimer's disease after EDCs exposure.

Recently, it has been established that the expression of hepatic miRNA (miR-22b, miR-140, miR-210a, mir-301, miR-457b, and let-7d) is increased in fluoxetine (the active ingredient in Prozac®) exposed female zebrafish (Craig et al., 2014). Interestingly, the miRNAs that were up-regulated were predicted to be responsible for down-regulating pathways such as insulin signaling, cholesterol synthesis, and triglyceride synthesis (Craig et al., 2014). Recently, it was shown that miR-21, 221, 222, and 429 expression levels decreased in the liver of DDT-treated female Wistar rats, whereas increases were observed in cytochrome 1A1 and 2B1 mRNA (Chanyshev et al., 2014; Gulyaeva et al., 2016). By an original approach using DNA-Au bio bar code (DNA-Au) and G-quadruplex-based DNA enzyme, Meng et al. demonstrated that miR-21 expression is increased in BPA-treated human hepatocarcinoma BEL-7402 cells (Meng et al., 2013). In primary mouse hepatocyte, TCCD modulated the expression of miR-503-5p that targeting cyclin D2 which was involved in the discriminative process of p53 signaling and metabolism (Rieswijk et al., 2015). In addition, it also been shown that TCDD regulates the expression of miR-101a and miR-122 and that cyclooxygenase-2, a target gene of miR-101a, plays a significant role in liver damage in mice exposed to TCDD (Yoshioka et al., 2011). Altogether, these observations suggest that the EDCs can induce metabolic disorders through the disturbance of specific miRNAs in the liver.

Altogether, these different studies indicated that miRNAs profile changed in tissue exposed to different EDCs. Potentially, miRNAs can be considered as new biomarkers for EDCs exposure (Vrijens et al., 2015).

CONCLUSION

Despite the high number of studies generated in the past few years on the mechanism of how EDCs act on the different endocrine axis, much still needs to be learnt. To date, very few ecotoxicology studies have considered miRNA in the context of endocrine disruption. In this review, we have seen that exposure to EDCs may lead to modification of miRNAs expression associated with endocrine disruption. However, many questions remain open, for instance (i) what is the impact on the miRNAs expression in different tissues which have suffered chronic low level EDCs exposure, (ii) what are the effects of the exposure either to a single EDC or to a complex mixture of different chemicals. Further, studies are warranted to evaluate if miRNAs may act as a causal link between EDCs exposure and their effect on health or if they can be used as a diagnostic or prognostic tools.

AUTHOR CONTRIBUTIONS

LM and AD wrote the manuscript. MD and JT helped with manuscript preparation.

ACKNOWLEDGMENTS

This research was supported by funding obtained from Aix-Marseille University, the "Région Provence-Alpes-Côte d'Azur," the "Conseil Général des Bouches-du-Rhône" (PACA, CG13) and Benjamin Delessert foundation. AD is the recipient of a doctoral fellowship from the Ministry of Education. The authors are grateful to O. Knowles for critical reading of the manuscript.

REFERENCES

Albrecht, E. D., Aberdeen, G. W., and Pepe, G. J. (2005). Estrogen elicits cortical zone-specific effects on development of the primate fetal adrenal gland. *Endocrinology* 146, 1737–1744. doi: 10.1210/en.2004-1124

Ali, H. O., Arroyo, A. B., González-Conejero, R., Stavik, B., Iversen, N., Sandset, P. M., et al. (2016). The role of microRNA -27a/b and microRNA-494 in oestrogen mediated downregulation of tissue factor pathway inhibitor α. *J. Thromb. Haemost.* 14, 1226–1237. doi: 10.1111/jth.13321

Alonso-Magdalena, P., García-Arévalo, M., Quesada, I., and Nadal, Á. (2015). Bisphenol-A treatment during pregnancy in mice: a new window of susceptibility for the development of diabetes in mothers later in life. *Endocrinology* 156, 1659–1670. doi: 10.1210/en.2014-1952

Alonso-Magdalena, P., Laribi, O., Ropero, A. B., Fuentes, E., Ripoll, C., Soria, B., et al. (2005). Low doses of bisphenol A and diethylstilbestrol impair Ca2+ signals in pancreatic alpha-cells through a nonclassical membrane estrogen receptor within intact islets of Langerhans. *Environ. Health Perspect.* 113, 969–977. doi: 10.1289/ehp.8002

Alonso-Magdalena, P., Quesada, I., and Nadal, A. (2011). Endocrine disruptors in the etiology of type 2 diabetes mellitus. *Nat. Rev. Endocrinol.* 7, 346–353. doi: 10.1038/nrendo.2011.56

Alonso-Magdalena, P., Vieira, E., Soriano, S., Menes, L., Burks, D., Quesada, I., et al. (2010). Bisphenol A exposure during pregnancy disrupts glucose homeostasis in mothers and adult male offspring. *Environ. Health Perspect.* 118, 1243–1250. doi: 10.1289/ehp.1001993

Angle, B. M., Do, R. P., Ponzi, D., Stahlhut, R. W., Drury, B. E., Nagel, S. C., et al. (2013). Metabolic disruption in male mice due to fetal exposure to low but not high doses of bisphenol A (BPA): evidence for effects on body weight, food intake, adipocytes, leptin, adiponectin, insulin and glucose regulation. *Reprod. Toxicol.* 42, 256–268. doi: 10.1016/j.reprotox.2013.07.017

Anway, M. D., Cupp, A. S., Uzumcu, M., and Skinner, M. K. (2005). Epigenetic transgenerational actions of endocrine disruptors and male fertility. *Science* 308, 1466–1469. doi: 10.1126/science.1108190

Aurela, B., Kulmala, H., and Söderhjelm, L. (1999). Phthalates in paper and board packaging and their migration into Tenax and sugar. *Food Addit. Contam.* 16, 571–577. doi: 10.1080/026520399283713

Avissar-Whiting, M., Veiga, K. R., Uhl, K. M., Maccani, M. A., Gagne, L. A., Moen, E. L., et al. (2010). Bisphenol A exposure leads to specific microRNA alterations in placental cells. *Reprod. Toxicol.* 29, 401–406. doi: 10.1016/j.reprotox.2010.04.004

Baek, D., Villén, J., Shin, C., Camargo, F. D., Gygi, S. P., and Bartel, D. P. (2008). The impact of microRNAs on protein output. *Nature* 455, 64–71. doi: 10.1038/nature07242

Baillie-Hamilton, P. F. (2002). Chemical toxins: a hypothesis to explain the global obesity epidemic. *J. Altern. Complement. Med.* 8, 185–192. doi: 10.1089/107555302317371479

Bartel, D. P. (2004). MicroRNAs: genomics, biogenesis, mechanism, and function. *Cell* 116, 281–297. doi: 10.1016/S0092-8674(04)00045-5

Baumberger, N., and Baulcombe, D. C. (2005). Arabidopsis ARGONAUTE1 is an RNA Slicer that selectively recruits microRNAs and short interfering RNAs. *Proc. Natl. Acad. Sci. U.S.A.* 102, 11928–11933. doi: 10.1073/pnas.0505461102

Bernstein, E., Caudy, A. A., Hammond, S. M., and Hannon, G. J. (2001). Role for a bidentate ribonuclease in the initiation step of RNA interference. *Nature* 409, 363–366. doi: 10.1038/35053110

Bhat-Nakshatri, P., Wang, G., Collins, N. R., Thomson, M. J., Geistlinger, T. R., Carroll, J. S., et al. (2009). Estradiol-regulated microRNAs control estradiol response in breast cancer cells. *Nucleic Acids Res.* 37, 4850–4861. doi: 10.1093/nar/gkp500

Bhattacharyya, S. N., Habermacher, R., Martine, U., Closs, E. I., and Filipowicz, W. (2006). Relief of microRNA-mediated translational repression in human cells subjected to stress. *Cell* 125, 1111–1124. doi: 10.1016/j.cell.2006.04.031

Boas, M., Feldt-Rasmussen, U., and Main, K. M. (2012). Thyroid effects of endocrine disrupting chemicals. *Mol. Cell. Endocrinol.* 355, 240–248. doi: 10.1016/j.mce.2011.09.005

Bohnsack, M. T., Czaplinski, K., and Görlich, D. (2004). Exportin 5 is a RanGTP-dependent dsRNA-binding protein that mediates nuclear export of pre-miRNAs. *RNA* 10, 185–191. doi: 10.1261/rna.5167604

Bortolin-Cavaillé, M.-L., Dance, M., Weber, M., and Cavaillé, J. (2009). C19MC microRNAs are processed from introns of large Pol-II, non-protein-coding transcripts. *Nucleic Acids Res.* 37, 3464–3473. doi: 10.1093/nar/gkp205

Brennecke, J., Stark, A., Russell, R. B., and Cohen, S. M. (2005). Principles of microRNA-target recognition. *PLoS Biol.* 3:e85. doi: 10.1371/journal.pbio.0030085

Brown, J. S. (2009). Effects of bisphenol-A and other endocrine disruptors compared with abnormalities of schizophrenia: an endocrine-disruption theory of schizophrenia. *Schizophr. Bull.* 35, 256–278. doi: 10.1093/schbul/sbm147

Buckley, J., Willingham, E., Agras, K., and Baskin, L. S. (2006). Embryonic exposure to the fungicide vinclozolin causes virilization of females and alteration of progesterone receptor expression *in vivo*: an experimental study in mice. *Environ. Health Glob. Access Sci. Source* 5:4. doi: 10.1186/1476-069X-5-4

Cai, X., Hagedorn, C. H., and Cullen, B. R. (2004). Human microRNAs are processed from capped, polyadenylated transcripts that can also function as mRNAs. *RNA* 10, 1957–1966. doi: 10.1261/rna.7135204

Calafat, A. M., Kuklenyik, Z., Reidy, J. A., Caudill, S. P., Ekong, J., and Needham, L. L. (2005). Urinary concentrations of bisphenol A and 4-nonylphenol in a human reference population. *Environ. Health Perspect.* 113, 391–395. doi: 10.1289/ehp.7534

Cameron, B. E., Craig, P. M., and Trudeau, V. L. (2016). Implication of microRNA deregulation in the response of vertebrates to endocrine disrupting chemicals. *Environ. Toxicol. Chem. SETAC*, 35, 788–793. doi: 10.1002/etc.3063

Campos, É., and Freire, C. (2016). Exposure to non-persistent pesticides and thyroid function: a systematic review of epidemiological evidence. *Int. J. Hyg. Environ. Health.* doi: 10.1016/j.ijheh.2016.05.006. [Epub ahead of print].

Casals-Casas, C., and Desvergne, B. (2011). Endocrine disruptors: from endocrine to metabolic disruption. *Annu. Rev. Physiol.* 73, 135–162. doi: 10.1146/annurev-physiol-012110-142200

Casals-Casas, C., Feige, J. N., and Desvergne, B. (2008). Interference of pollutants with PPARs: endocrine disruption meets metabolism. *Int. J. Obes. 2005*(32 Suppl. 6), S53–S61. doi: 10.1038/ijo.2008.207

Cerqueira, J. J., Pêgo, J. M., Taipa, R., Bessa, J. M., Almeida, O. F. X., and Sousa, N. (2005). Morphological correlates of corticosteroid-induced changes in prefrontal cortex-dependent behaviors. *J. Neurosci. Off. J. Soc. Neurosci.* 25, 7792–7800. doi: 10.1523/JNEUROSCI.1598-05.2005

Chanyshev, M. D., Kosorotikov, N. I., Titov, S. E., Kolesnikov, N. N., and Gulyaeva, L. F. (2014). Expression of microRNAs, CYP1A1 and CYP2B1 in the livers and ovaries of female rats treated with DDT and PAHs. *Life Sci.* 103, 95–100. doi: 10.1016/j.lfs.2014.03.031

Cheloufi, S., Dos Santos, C. O., Chong, M. M. W., and Hannon, G. J. (2010). A dicer-independent miRNA biogenesis pathway that requires Ago catalysis. *Nature* 465, 584–589. doi: 10.1038/nature09092

Chen, F., Zhou, L., Bai, Y., Zhou, R., and Chen, L. (2015). Hypothalamic-pituitary-adrenal axis hyperactivity accounts for anxiety- and depression-like behaviors in rats perinatally exposed to bisphenol A. *J. Biomed. Res.* 29, 250–258. doi: 10.7555/JBR.29.20140058

Chen, J.-Q., Brown, T. R., and Russo, J. (2009). Regulation of energy metabolism pathways by estrogens and estrogenic chemicals and potential implications in obesity associated with increased exposure to endocrine disruptors. *Biochim. Biophys. Acta* 1793, 1128–1143. doi: 10.1016/j.bbamcr.2009.03.009

Chendrimada, T. P., Finn, K. J., Ji, X., Baillat, D., Gregory, R. I., Liebhaber, S. A., et al. (2007). MicroRNA silencing through RISC recruitment of eIF6. *Nature* 447, 823–828. doi: 10.1038/nature05841

Chendrimada, T. P., Gregory, R. I., Kumaraswamy, E., Norman, J., Cooch, N., Nishikura, K., et al. (2005). TRBP recruits the Dicer complex to Ago2 for microRNA processing and gene silencing. *Nature* 436, 740–744. doi: 10.1038/nature03868

Cifuentes, D., Xue, H., Taylor, D. W., Patnode, H., Mishima, Y., Cheloufi, S., et al. (2010). A novel miRNA processing pathway independent of Dicer requires Argonaute2 catalytic activity. *Science* 328, 1694–1698. doi: 10.1126/science.1190809

Cohen, A., Burgos-Aceves, M. A., and Smith, Y. (2016). Estrogen repression of microRNA as a potential cause of cancer. *Biomed. Pharmacother. Biomèd. Pharmacothérapie* 78, 234–238. doi: 10.1016/j.biopha.2016.01.023

Cohen, A., Shmoish, M., Levi, L., Cheruti, U., Levavi-Sivan, B., and Lubzens, E. (2008). Alterations in micro-ribonucleic acid expression profiles reveal a novel pathway for estrogen regulation. *Endocrinology* 149, 1687–1696. doi: 10.1210/en.2007-0969

Colborn, T., vom Saal, F. S., and Soto, A. M. (1993). Developmental effects of endocrine-disrupting chemicals in wildlife and humans. *Environ. Health Perspect.* 101, 378–384. doi: 10.1289/ehp.93101378

Collotta, M., Bertazzi, P. A., and Bollati, V. (2013). Epigenetics and pesticides. *Toxicology* 307, 35–41. doi: 10.1016/j.tox.2013.01.017

Cotter, D., and Pariante, C. M. (2002). Stress and the progression of the developmental hypothesis of schizophrenia. *Br. J. Psychiatry J. Ment. Sci.* 181, 363–365. doi: 10.1192/bjp.181.5.363

Craig, P. M., Trudeau, V. L., and Moon, T. W. (2014). Profiling hepatic microRNAs in zebrafish: fluoxetine exposure mimics a fasting response that targets AMP-activated protein kinase (AMPK). *PLoS ONE* 9:e95351. doi: 10.1371/journal.pone.0095351

Darnerud, P. O., Morse, D., Klasson-Wehler, E., and Brouwer, A. (1996). Binding of a 3,3′, 4,4′-tetrachlorobiphenyl (CB-77) metabolite to fetal transthyretin and effects on fetal thyroid hormone levels in mice. *Toxicology* 106, 105–114. doi: 10.1016/0300-483X(95)03169-G

de Cock, M., Maas, Y. G. H., and van de Bor, M. (2012). Does perinatal exposure to endocrine disruptors induce autism spectrum and attention deficit hyperactivity disorders? *Acta Paediatr.* 101, 811–818. doi: 10.1111/j.1651-2227.2012.02693.x

De Felice, B., Manfellotto, F., Palumbo, A., Troisi, J., Zullo, F., Di Carlo, C., et al. (2015). Genome-wide microRNA expression profiling in placentas from pregnant women exposed to BPA. *BMC Med. Genomics* 8:56. doi: 10.1186/s12920-015-0131-z

Delfosse, V., Grimaldi, M., le Maire, A., Bourguet, W., and Balaguer, P. (2014). Nuclear receptor profiling of bisphenol-A and its halogenated analogues. *Vitam. Horm.* 94, 229–251. doi: 10.1016/B978-0-12-800095-3.00009-2

Del-Mazo, J., Brieño-Enríquez, M. A., García-López, J., López-Fernández, L. A., and De-Felici, M. (2013). Endocrine disruptors, gene deregulation and male germ cell tumors. *Int. J. Dev. Biol.* 57, 225–239. doi: 10.1387/ijdb.130042jd

Denli, A. M., Tops, B. B. J., Plasterk, R. H. A., Ketting, R. F., and Hannon, G. J. (2004). Processing of primary microRNAs by the Microprocessor complex. *Nature* 432, 231–235. doi: 10.1038/nature03049

Derghal, A., Djelloul, M., Airault, C., Pierre, C., Dallaporta, M., Troadec, J.-D., et al. (2015). Leptin is required for hypothalamic regulation of miRNAs targeting POMC 3′UTR. *Front. Cell. Neurosci.* 9:172. doi: 10.3389/fncel.2015.00172

Diamanti-Kandarakis, E., Bourguignon, J.-P., Giudice, L. C., Hauser, R., Prins, G. S., Soto, A. M., et al. (2009). Endocrine-disrupting chemicals: an Endocrine Society scientific statement. *Endocr. Rev.* 30, 293–342. doi: 10.1210/er.2009-0002

Ding, L., Spencer, A., Morita, K., and Han, M. (2005). The developmental timing regulator AIN-1 interacts with miRISCs and may target the argonaute protein ALG-1 to cytoplasmic P bodies in C. *elegans. Mol. Cell* 19, 437–447. doi: 10.1016/j.molcel.2005.07.013

Ding, X. C., and Grosshans, H. (2009). Repression of C. elegans microRNA targets at the initiation level of translation requires GW182 proteins. *EMBO J.* 28, 213–222. doi: 10.1038/emboj.2008.275

Doench, J. G., and Sharp, P. A. (2004). Specificity of microRNA target selection in translational repression. *Genes Dev.* 18, 504–511. doi: 10.1101/gad.1184404

Dong, H., Paquette, M., Williams, A., Zoeller, R. T., Wade, M., and Yauk, C. (2010). Thyroid hormone may regulate mRNA abundance in liver by acting on microRNAs. *PLoS ONE* 5:e12136. doi: 10.1371/journal.pone.0012136

Elobeid, M. A., and Allison, D. B. (2008). Putative environmental-endocrine disruptors and obesity: a review. *Curr. Opin. Endocrinol. Diabetes Obes.* 15, 403–408. doi: 10.1097/MED.0b013e32830ce95c

Eulalio, A., Huntzinger, E., and Izaurralde, E. (2008). GW182 interaction with Argonaute is essential for miRNA-mediated translational repression and mRNA decay. *Nat. Struct. Mol. Biol.* 15, 346–353. doi: 10.1038/nsmb.1405

Eulalio, A., Huntzinger, E., Nishihara, T., Rehwinkel, J., Fauser, M., and Izaurralde, E. (2009). Deadenylation is a widespread effect of miRNA regulation. *RNA* 15, 21–32. doi: 10.1261/rna.1399509

Eystathioy, T., Chan, E. K. L., Tenenbaum, S. A., Keene, J. D., Griffith, K., and Fritzler, M. J. (2002). A phosphorylated cytoplasmic autoantigen, GW182, associates with a unique population of human mRNAs within novel cytoplasmic speckles. *Mol. Biol. Cell* 13, 1338–1351. doi: 10.1091/mbc.01-11-0544

Eystathioy, T., Jakymiw, A., Chan, E. K. L., Séraphin, B., Cougot, N., and Fritzler, M. J. (2003). The GW182 protein colocalizes with mRNA degradation associated proteins hDcp1 and hLSm4 in cytoplasmic GW bodies. *RNA* 9, 1171–1173. doi: 10.1261/rna.5810203

Ferraro, L., Ravo, M., Nassa, G., Tarallo, R., De Filippo, M. R., Giurato, G., et al. (2012). Effects of oestrogen on microRNA expression in hormone-responsive breast cancer cells. *Horm. Cancer* 3, 65–78. doi: 10.1007/s12672-012-0102-1

Fisher, J. S., Macpherson, S., Marchetti, N., and Sharpe, R. M. (2003). Human "testicular dysgenesis syndrome": a possible model using in-utero exposure of the rat to dibutyl phthalate. *Hum. Reprod. Oxf. Engl.* 18, 1383–1394. doi: 10.1093/humrep/deg273

Freire, C., Lopez-Espinosa, M.-J., Fernández, M., Molina-Molina, J.-M., Prada, R., and Olea, N. (2011). Prenatal exposure to organochlorine pesticides and TSH status in newborns from Southern Spain. *Sci. Total Environ.* 409, 3281–3287. doi: 10.1016/j.scitotenv.2011.05.037

Gayathri, N. S., Dhanya, C. R., Indu, A. R., and Kurup, P. A. (2004). Changes in some hormones by low doses of di (2-ethyl hexyl) phthalate (DEHP), a commonly used plasticizer in PVC blood storage bags & medical tubing. *Indian J. Med. Res.* 119, 139–144.

Giraldez, A. J., Mishima, Y., Rihel, J., Grocock, R. J., Van Dongen, S., Inoue, K., et al. (2006). Zebrafish MiR-430 promotes deadenylation and clearance of maternal mRNAs. *Science* 312, 75–79. doi: 10.1126/science.1122689

Gore, A. C. (2002). Organochlorine pesticides directly regulate gonadotropin-releasing hormone gene expression and biosynthesis in the GT1-7 hypothalamic cell line. *Mol. Cell. Endocrinol.* 192, 157–170. doi: 10.1016/S0303-7207(02)00010-2

Gregory, R. I., Chendrimada, T. P., Cooch, N., and Shiekhattar, R. (2005). Human RISC Couples MicroRNA Biogenesis and Posttranscriptional Gene Silencing. *Cell* 123, 631–640. doi: 10.1016/j.cell.2005.10.022

Gregory, R. I., Yan, K.-P., Amuthan, G., Chendrimada, T., Doratotaj, B., Cooch, N., et al. (2004). The Microprocessor complex mediates the genesis of microRNAs. *Nature* 432, 235–240. doi: 10.1038/nature03120

Grishok, A., Pasquinelli, A. E., Conte, D., Li, N., Parrish, S., Ha, I., et al. (2001). Genes and mechanisms related to RNA interference regulate expression of the small temporal RNAs that control C. *elegans developmental timing. Cell* 106, 23–34. doi: 10.1016/S0092-8674(01)00431-7

Guerrero-Bosagna, C., Covert, T. R., Haque, M. M., Settles, M., Nilsson, E. E., Anway, M. D., et al. (2012). Epigenetic transgenerational inheritance of vinclozolin induced mouse adult onset disease and associated sperm epigenome biomarkers. *Reprod. Toxicol.* 34, 694–707. doi: 10.1016/j.reprotox.2012.09.005

Gulyaeva, L. F., Chanyshev, M. D., Kolmykov, S. K., Ushakov, D. S., and Nechkin, S. S. (2016). Effect of xenobiotics on microrna expression in rat liver. *Biomed. Khim.* 62, 154–159. doi: 10.18097/pbmc20166202154

Guo, H., Ingolia, N. T., Weissman, J. S., and Bartel, D. P. (2010). Mammalian microRNAs predominantly act to decrease target mRNA levels. *Nature* 466, 835–840. doi: 10.1038/nature09267

Gupta, A., Caffrey, E., Callagy, G., and Gupta, S. (2012). Oestrogen-dependent regulation of miRNA biogenesis: many ways to skin the cat. *Biochem. Soc. Trans.* 40, 752–758. doi: 10.1042/BST20110763

Haase, A. D., Jaskiewicz, L., Zhang, H., Lainé, S., Sack, R., Gatignol, A., et al. (2005). TRBP, a regulator of cellular PKR and HIV-1 virus expression, interacts with Dicer and functions in RNA silencing. *EMBO Rep.* 6, 961–967. doi: 10.1038/sj.embor.7400509

Halden, R. U. (2010). Plastics and health risks. *Annu. Rev. Public Health* 31, 179–194. doi: 10.1146/annurev.publhealth.012809.103714

Han, J., Lee, Y., Yeom, K.-H., Kim, Y.-K., Jin, H., and Kim, V. N. (2004). The Drosha-DGCR8 complex in primary microRNA processing. *Genes Dev.* 18, 3016–3027. doi: 10.1101/gad.1262504

Hendrickson, D. G., Hogan, D. J., McCullough, H. L., Myers, J. W., Herschlag, D., Ferrell, J. E., et al. (2009). Concordant regulation of translation and mRNA abundance for hundreds of targets of a human microRNA. *PLoS Biol.* 7:e1000238. doi: 10.1371/journal.pbio.1000238

Henley, D. V., and Korach, K. S. (2006). Endocrine-disrupting chemicals use distinct mechanisms of action to modulate endocrine system function. *Endocrinology* 147, S25–S32. doi: 10.1210/en.2005-1117

Heudorf, U., Mersch-Sundermann, V., and Angerer, J. (2007). Phthalates: toxicology and exposure. *Int. J. Hyg. Environ. Health* 210, 623–634. doi: 10.1016/j.ijheh.2007.07.011

Hinton, R. H., Mitchell, F. E., Mann, A., Chescoe, D., Price, S. C., Nunn, A., et al. (1986). Effects of phthalic acid esters on the liver and thyroid. *Environ. Health Perspect.* 70, 195–210. doi: 10.1289/ehp.8670195

Hisada, A., Shimodaira, K., Okai, T., Watanabe, K., Takemori, H., Takasuga, T., et al. (2014). Associations between levels of hydroxylated PCBs and PCBs in serum of pregnant women and blood thyroid hormone levels and body size of neonates. *Int. J. Hyg. Environ. Health* 217, 546–553. doi: 10.1016/j.ijheh.2013.10.004

Hu, Z., Shen, W.-J., Cortez, Y., Tang, X., Liu, L.-F., Kraemer, F. B., et al. (2013). Hormonal regulation of microRNA expression in steroid producing cells of the ovary, testis and adrenal gland. *PLoS ONE* 8:e78040. doi: 10.1371/journal.pone.0078040

Huang, C.-Y., Wu, C.-L., Yang, Y.-C., Chang, J.-W., Kuo, Y.-C., Cheng, Y.-Y., et al. (2015). Association between Dioxin and diabetes mellitus in an endemic area of exposure in Taiwan: a population-based study. *Medicine (Baltimore).* 94:e1730. doi: 10.1097/md.0000000000001730

Huang, J., Liang, Z., Yang, B., Tian, H., Ma, J., and Zhang, H. (2007). Derepression of microRNA-mediated protein translation inhibition by apolipoprotein B mRNA-editing enzyme catalytic polypeptide-like 3G (APOBEC3G) and its family members. *J. Biol. Chem.* 282, 33632–33640. doi: 10.1074/jbc.M705116200

Huber, T. J., Rollnik, J., Wilhelms, J., von zur Mühlen, A., Emrich, H. M., and Schneider, U. (2001). Estradiol levels in psychotic disorders. *Psychoneuroendocrinology* 26, 27–35. doi: 10.1016/S0306-4530(00)00034-2

Humphreys, D. T., Westman, B. J., Martin, D. I. K., and Preiss, T. (2005). MicroRNAs control translation initiation by inhibiting eukaryotic initiation factor 4E/cap and poly(A) tail function. *Proc. Natl. Acad. Sci. U.S.A.* 102, 16961–16966. doi: 10.1073/pnas.0506482102

Hutvágner, G., McLachlan, J., Pasquinelli, A. E., Bálint, E., Tuschl, T., and Zamore, P. D. (2001). A cellular function for the RNA-interference enzyme Dicer in the maturation of the let-7 small temporal RNA. *Science* 293, 834–838. doi: 10.1126/science.1062961

Inadera, H. (2015). Neurological effects of bisphenol A and its analogues. *Int. J. Med. Sci.* 12, 926–936. doi: 10.7150/ijms.13267

Ingelfinger, D., Arndt-Jovin, D. J., Lührmann, R., and Achsel, T. (2002). The human LSm1-7 proteins colocalize with the mRNA-degrading enzymes Dcp1/2 and Xrnl in distinct cytoplasmic foci. *RNA* 8, 1489–1501. doi: 10.1017/S1355838202021726

Iorio, M. V., Ferracin, M., Liu, C.-G., Veronese, A., Spizzo, R., Sabbioni, S., et al. (2005). MicroRNA gene expression deregulation in human breast cancer. *Cancer Res.* 65, 7065–7070. doi: 10.1158/0008-5472.CAN-05-1783

Jakymiw, A., Lian, S., Eystathioy, T., Li, S., Satoh, M., Hamel, J. C., et al. (2005). Disruption of GW bodies impairs mammalian RNA interference. *Nat. Cell Biol.* 7, 1267–1274. doi: 10.1038/ncb1334

Jiang, W., Zhang, Y., Meng, F., Lian, B., Chen, X., Yu, X., et al. (2013). Identification of active transcription factor and miRNA regulatory pathways in Alzheimer's disease. *Bioinforma. Oxf. Engl.* 29, 2596–2602. doi: 10.1093/bioinformatics/btt423

Kaneda, Y., and Ohmori, T. (2005). Relation between estradiol and negative symptoms in men with schizophrenia. *J. Neuropsychiatry Clin. Neurosci.* 17, 239–242. doi: 10.1176/jnp.17.2.239

Katz, D. L., Frankenburg, F. R., Benowitz, L. I., and Gilbert, J. M. (1987). Psychosis and prenatal exposure to diethylstilbestrol. *J. Nerv. Ment. Dis.* 175, 306–308. doi: 10.1097/00005053-198705000-00011

Kelce, W. R., Lambright, C. R., Gray, L. E., and Roberts, K. P. (1997). Vinclozolin and p,p'-DDE alter androgen-dependent gene expression: *in vivo* confirmation of an androgen receptor-mediated mechanism. *Toxicol. Appl. Pharmacol.* 142, 192–200. doi: 10.1006/taap.1996.7966

Ketting, R. F., Fischer, S. E. J., Bernstein, E., Sijen, T., Hannon, G. J., and Plasterk, R. H. A. (2001). Dicer functions in RNA interference and in synthesis of small RNA involved in developmental timing in C. *elegans. Genes Dev.* 15, 2654–2659. doi: 10.1101/gad.927801

Kimura-Kuroda, J., Nagata, I., and Kuroda, Y. (2007). Disrupting effects of hydroxy-polychlorinated biphenyl (PCB) congeners on neuronal development of cerebellar Purkinje cells: a possible causal factor for developmental brain disorders? *Chemosphere* 67, S412–S420. doi: 10.1016/j.chemosphere.2006.05.137

Kitahara, Y., Nakamura, K., Kogure, K., and Minegishi, T. (2013). Role of microRNA-136-3p on the expression of luteinizing hormone-human chorionic gonadotropin receptor mRNA in rat ovaries. *Biol. Reprod.* 89, 114. doi: 10.1095/biolreprod.113.109207

Klenke, U., Constantin, S., and Wray, S. (2016). BPA directly decreases GnRH neuronal activity via noncanonical pathway. *Endocrinology* 157, 1980–1990. doi: 10.1210/en.2015-1924

Klinge, C. M. (2015). miRNAs regulated by estrogens, tamoxifen, and endocrine disruptors and their downstream gene targets. *Mol. Cell. Endocrinol.* 418(Pt 3), 273–297. doi: 10.1016/j.mce.2015.01.035

Koskenniemi, J. J., Virtanen, H. E., Kiviranta, H., Damgaard, I. N., Matomäki, J., Thorup, J. M., et al. (2015). Association between levels of persistent organic pollutants in adipose tissue and cryptorchidism in early childhood: a case-control study. *Environ. Health Glob. Access Sci. Source* 14, 78. doi: 10.1186/s12940-015-0065-0

Kovalchuk, O., Tryndyak, V. P., Montgomery, B., Boyko, A., Kutanzi, K., Zemp, F., et al. (2007). Estrogen-induced rat breast carcinogenesis is characterized by alterations in DNA methylation, histone modifications and aberrant microRNA expression. *Cell Cycle Georget. Tex* 6, 2010–2018. doi: 10.4161/cc.6.16.4549

Kovanecz, I., Gelfand, R., Masouminia, M., Gharib, S., Segura, D., Vernet, D., et al. (2014). Oral Bisphenol A (BPA) given to rats at moderate doses is associated with erectile dysfunction, cavernosal lipofibrosis and alterations of global gene transcription. *Int. J. Impot. Res.* 26, 67–75. doi: 10.1038/ijir.2013.37

Kuiper, G. G., Lemmen, J. G., Carlsson, B., Corton, J. C., Safe, S. H., van der Saag, P. T., et al. (1998). Interaction of estrogenic chemicals and phytoestrogens with estrogen receptor beta. *Endocrinology* 139, 4252–4263.

Lagos-Quintana, M., Rauhut, R., Lendeckel, W., and Tuschl, T. (2001). Identification of novel genes coding for small expressed RNAs. *Science* 294, 853–858. doi: 10.1126/science.1064921

Landgraf, P., Rusu, M., Sheridan, R., Sewer, A., Iovino, N., Aravin, A., et al. (2007). A mammalian microRNA expression atlas based on small RNA library sequencing. *Cell* 129, 1401–1414. doi: 10.1016/j.cell.2007.04.040

Landrigan, P. J., and Goldman, L. R. (2011a). Children's vulnerability to toxic chemicals: a challenge and opportunity to strengthen health and environmental policy. *Health Aff. (Millwood)* 30, 842–850. doi: 10.1377/hlthaff.2011.0151

Landrigan, P. J., and Goldman, L. R. (2011b). Protecting children from pesticides and other toxic chemicals. *J. Expo. Sci. Environ. Epidemiol.* 21, 119–120. doi: 10.1038/jes.2011.1

Lang, I. A., Galloway, T. S., Scarlett, A., Henley, W. E., Depledge, M., Wallace, R. B., et al. (2008). Association of urinary bisphenol A concentration with medical disorders and laboratory abnormalities in adults. *JAMA* 300, 1303–1310. doi: 10.1001/jama.300.11.1303

Lau, N. C., Lim, L. P., Weinstein, E. G., and Bartel, D. P. (2001). An abundant class of tiny RNAs with probable regulatory roles in Caenorhabditis elegans. *Science* 294, 858–862. doi: 10.1126/science.1065062

Lee, Y., Ahn, C., Han, J., Choi, H., Kim, J., Yim, J., et al. (2003). The nuclear RNase III Drosha initiates microRNA processing. *Nature* 425, 415–419. doi: 10.1038/nature01957

Lee, Y., Kim, M., Han, J., Yeom, K.-H., Lee, S., Baek, S. H., et al. (2004). MicroRNA genes are transcribed by RNA polymerase II. *EMBO J.* 23, 4051–4060. doi: 10.1038/sj.emboj.7600385

Lee, Y.-M., Lee, J.-Y., Ho, C.-C., Hong, Q.-S., Yu, S.-L., Tzeng, C.-R., et al. (2011). miRNA-34b as a tumor suppressor in estrogen-dependent growth of breast cancer cells. *Breast Cancer Res.* 13, R116. doi: 10.1186/bcr3059

Lewis, B. P., Burge, C. B., and Bartel, D. P. (2005). Conserved seed pairing, often flanked by adenosines, indicates that thousands of human genes are microRNA targets. *Cell* 120, 15–20. doi: 10.1016/j.cell.2004.12.035

Li, S., Hursting, S. D., Davis, B. J., McLachlan, J. A., and Barrett, J. C. (2003). Environmental exposure, DNA methylation, and gene regulation: lessons from diethylstilbesterol-induced cancers. *Ann. N.Y. Acad. Sci.* 983, 161–169. doi: 10.1111/j.1749-6632.2003.tb05971.x

Li, X., Xie, W., Xie, C., Huang, C., Zhu, J., Liang, Z., et al. (2014). Curcumin modulates miR-19/PTEN/AKT/p53 axis to suppress bisphenol A-induced MCF-7 breast cancer cell proliferation. *Phytother. Res.* 28, 1553–1560. doi: 10.1002/ptr.5167

Lim, L. P., Lau, N. C., Garrett-Engele, P., Grimson, A., Schelter, J. M., Castle, J., et al. (2005). Microarray analysis shows that some microRNAs downregulate large numbers of target mRNAs. *Nature* 433, 769–773. doi: 10.1038/nature03315

Lim, W., and Song, G. (2015). Differential expression of vitelline membrane outer layer protein 1: hormonal regulation of expression in the oviduct and in ovarian carcinomas from laying hens. *Mol. Cell. Endocrinol.* 399, 250–258. doi: 10.1016/j.mce.2014.10.015

Liu, J., Rivas, F. V., Wohlschlegel, J., Yates, J. R., Parker, R., and Hannon, G. J. (2005). A role for the P-body component GW182 in microRNA function. *Nat. Cell Biol.* 7, 1261–1266. doi: 10.1038/ncb1333

Lund, E., Güttinger, S., Calado, A., Dahlberg, J. E., and Kutay, U. (2004). Nuclear export of microRNA precursors. *Science* 303, 95–98. doi: 10.1126/science.1090599

Maillot, G., Lacroix-Triki, M., Pierredon, S., Gratadou, L., Schmidt, S., Bénès, V., et al. (2009). Widespread estrogen-dependent repression of micrornas involved in breast tumor cell growth. *Cancer Res.* 69, 8332–8340. doi: 10.1158/0008-5472.CAN-09-2206

Main, K. M., Kiviranta, H., Virtanen, H. E., Sundqvist, E., Tuomisto, J. T., Tuomisto, J., et al. (2007). Flame retardants in placenta and breast milk and cryptorchidism in newborn boys. *Environ. Health Perspect.* 115, 1519–1526. doi: 10.1289/ehp.9924

Maqbool, F., Mostafalou, S., Bahadar, H., and Abdollahi, M. (2016). Review of endocrine disorders associated with environmental toxicants and possible involved mechanisms. *Life Sci.* 145, 265–273. doi: 10.1016/j.lfs.2015.10.022

Marx, C. E., and Lieberman, J. A. (1998). Psychoneuroendocrinology of schizophrenia. *Psychiatr. Clin. North Am.* 21, 413–434. doi: 10.1016/S0193-953X(05)70013-7

Mattie, M. D., Benz, C. C., Bowers, J., Sensinger, K., Wong, L., Scott, G. K., et al. (2006). Optimized high-throughput microRNA expression profiling provides novel biomarker assessment of clinical prostate and breast cancer biopsies. *Mol. Cancer* 5:24. doi: 10.1186/1476-4598-5-24

McKinney, J., Fannin, R., Jordan, S., Chae, K., Rickenbacher, U., and Pedersen, L. (1987). Polychlorinated biphenyls and related compound interactions with specific binding sites for thyroxine in rat liver nuclear extracts. *J. Med. Chem.* 30, 79–86. doi: 10.1021/jm00384a014

Meeker, J. D., Sathyanarayana, S., and Swan, S. H. (2009). Phthalates and other additives in plastics: human exposure and associated health outcomes. *Philos. Trans. R. Soc. Lond. B Biol. Sci.* 364, 2097–2113. doi: 10.1098/rstb.2008.0268

Meerts, I. A. T. M., Assink, Y., Cenijn, P. H., Van Den Berg, J. H. J., Weijers, B. M., Bergman, A., et al. (2002). Placental transfer of a hydroxylated polychlorinated biphenyl and effects on fetal and maternal thyroid hormone homeostasis in the rat. *Toxicol. Sci. Off. J. Soc. Toxicol.* 68, 361–371. doi: 10.1093/toxsci/68.2.361

Meng, X., Zhou, Y., Liang, Q., Qu, X., Yang, Q., Yin, H., et al. (2013). Electrochemical determination of microRNA-21 based on bio bar code and hemin/G-quadruplet DNAenzyme. *Analyst* 138, 3409–3415. doi: 10.1039/c3an36788f

Meunier, L., Siddeek, B., Vega, A., Lakhdari, N., Inoubli, L., Bellon, R. P., et al. (2012). Perinatal programming of adult rat germ cell death after exposure to xenoestrogens: role of microRNA miR-29 family in the down-regulation of DNA methyltransferases and Mcl-1. *Endocrinology* 153, 1936–1947. doi: 10.1210/en.2011-1109

Miller, V. M., Sanchez-Morrissey, S., Brosch, K. O., and Seegal, R. F. (2012). Developmental coexposure to polychlorinated biphenyls and polybrominated diphenyl ethers has additive effects on circulating thyroxine levels in rats. *Toxicol. Sci. Off. J. Soc. Toxicol.* 127, 76–83. doi: 10.1093/toxsci/kfs089

Mitchell, F. E., Price, S. C., Hinton, R. H., Grasso, P., and Bridges, J. W. (1985). Time and dose-response study of the effects on rats of the plasticizer di(2-ethylhexyl) phthalate. *Toxicol. Appl. Pharmacol.* 81, 371–392. doi: 10.1016/0041-008X(85)90409-0

Mocarelli, P., Gerthoux, P. M., Needham, L. L., Patterson, D. G., Limonta, G., Falbo, R., et al. (2011). Perinatal exposure to low doses of dioxin can permanently impair human semen quality. *Environ. Health Perspect.* 119, 713–718. doi: 10.1289/ehp.1002134

Molehin, D., Dekker Nitert, M., and Richard, K. (2016). Prenatal exposures to multiple thyroid hormone disruptors: effects on glucose and lipid metabolism. *J. Thyroid Res.* 2016:8765049. doi: 10.1155/2016/8765049

Mostafalou, S., and Abdollahi, M. (2013). Pesticides and human chronic diseases: evidences, mechanisms, and perspectives. *Toxicol. Appl. Pharmacol.* 268, 157–177. doi: 10.1016/j.taap.2013.01.025

Mostafalou, S., Eghbal, M. A., Nili-Ahmadabadi, A., Baeeri, M., and Abdollahi, M. (2012). Biochemical evidence on the potential role of organophosphates in hepatic glucose metabolism toward insulin resistance through inflammatory signaling and free radical pathways. *Toxicol. Ind. Health* 28, 840–851. doi: 10.1177/0748233711425073

Nakamura, K., Itoh, K., Sugimoto, T., and Fushiki, S. (2007). Prenatal exposure to bisphenol A affects adult murine neocortical structure. *Neurosci. Lett.* 420, 100–105. doi: 10.1016/j.neulet.2007.02.093

Nakamura, K., Itoh, K., Yaoi, T., Fujiwara, Y., Sugimoto, T., and Fushiki, S. (2006). Murine neocortical histogenesis is perturbed by prenatal exposure to low doses of Bisphenol A. *J. Neurosci. Res.* 84, 1197–1205. doi: 10.1002/jnr.21020

Negri-Cesi, P. (2015). Bisphenol A interaction with brain development and functions. *Dose Response* 13:1559325815590394. doi: 10.1177/1559325815590394

Newbold, R. R., Padilla-Banks, E., Jefferson, W. N., and Heindel, J. J. (2008). Effects of endocrine disruptors on obesity. *Int. J. Androl.* 31, 201–208. doi: 10.1111/j.1365-2605.2007.00858.x

Newbold, R. R., Padilla-Banks, E., Snyder, R. J., and Jefferson, W. N. (2007). Perinatal exposure to environmental estrogens and the development of obesity. *Mol. Nutr. Food Res.* 51, 912–917. doi: 10.1002/mnfr.200600259

Nottrott, S., Simard, M. J., and Richter, J. D. (2006). Human let-7a miRNA blocks protein production on actively translating polyribosomes. *Nat. Struct. Mol. Biol.* 13, 1108–1114. doi: 10.1038/nsmb1173

Noyes, P. D., Lema, S. C., Macaulay, L. J., Douglas, N. K., and Stapleton, H. M. (2013). Low level exposure to the flame retardant BDE-209 reduces thyroid hormone levels and disrupts thyroid signaling in fathead minnows. *Environ. Sci. Technol.* 47, 10012–10021. doi: 10.1021/es402650x

Okamura, K., Hagen, J. W., Duan, H., Tyler, D. M., and Lai, E. C. (2007). The mirtron pathway generates microRNA-class regulatory RNAs in Drosophila. *Cell* 130, 89–100. doi: 10.1016/j.cell.2007.06.028

Panagiotidou, E., Zerva, S., Mitsiou, D. J., Alexis, M. N., and Kitraki, E. (2014). Perinatal exposure to low-dose bisphenol A affects the neuroendocrine stress response in rats. *J. Endocrinol.* 220, 207–218. doi: 10.1530/JOE-13-0416

Patrick, L. (2009). Thyroid disruption: mechanism and clinical implications in human health. *Altern. Med. Rev.* 14, 326–346.

Pelclová, D., Urban, P., Preiss, J., Lukás, E., Fenclová, Z., Navrátil, T., et al. (2006). Adverse health effects in humans exposed to 2,3,7,8-tetrachlorodibenzo-p-dioxin (TCDD). *Rev. Environ. Health* 21, 119–138. doi: 10.1515/REVEH.2006.21.2.119

Pepe, G. J., and Albrecht, E. D. (1998). Central integrative role of oestrogen in the regulation of placental steroidogenic maturation and the development of the fetal pituitary-adrenocortical axis in the baboon. *Hum. Reprod. Update* 4, 406–419. doi: 10.1093/humupd/4.4.406

Petersen, C. P., Bordeleau, M.-E., Pelletier, J., and Sharp, P. A. (2006). Short RNAs repress translation after initiation in mammalian cells. *Mol. Cell* 21, 533–542. doi: 10.1016/j.molcel.2006.01.031

Pillai, R. S., Bhattacharyya, S. N., Artus, C. G., Zoller, T., Cougot, N., Basyuk, E., et al. (2005). Inhibition of translational initiation by Let-7 MicroRNA in human cells. *Science* 309, 1573–1576. doi: 10.1126/science.1115079

Price, S. C., Chescoe, D., Grasso, P., Wright, M., and Hinton, R. H. (1988). Alterations in the thyroids of rats treated for long periods with di-(2-ethylhexyl) phthalate or with hypolipidaemic agents. *Toxicol. Lett.* 40, 37–46. doi: 10.1016/0378-4274(88)90181-6

Rao, Y. S., Mott, N. N., Wang, Y., Chung, W. C. J., and Pak, T. R. (2013). MicroRNAs in the aging female brain: a putative mechanism for age-specific estrogen effects. *Endocrinology* 154, 2795–2806. doi: 10.1210/en.2013-1230

Rasier, G., Parent, A.-S., Gérard, A., Lebrethon, M.-C., and Bourguignon, J.-P. (2007). Early maturation of gonadotropin-releasing hormone secretion and sexual precocity after exposure of infant female rats to estradiol or dichlorodiphenyltrichloroethane. *Biol. Reprod.* 77, 734–742. doi: 10.1095/biolreprod.106.059303

Reik, W., Dean, W., and Walter, J. (2001). Epigenetic reprogramming in mammalian development. *Science* 293, 1089–1093. doi: 10.1126/science.1063443

Remillard, R. B. J., and Bunce, N. J. (2002). Linking dioxins to diabetes: epidemiology and biologic plausibility. *Environ. Health Perspect.* 110, 853–858. doi: 10.1289/ehp.02110853

Rice, C. E., Baio, J., Van Naarden Braun, K., Doernberg, N., Meaney, F. J., Kirby, R. S., et al. (2007). A public health collaboration for the surveillance of autism spectrum disorders. *Paediatr. Perinat. Epidemiol.* 21, 179–190. doi: 10.1111/j.1365-3016.2007.00801.x

Rickenbacher, U., McKinney, J. D., Oatley, S. J., and Blake, C. C. (1986). Structurally specific binding of halogenated biphenyls to thyroxine transport protein. *J. Med. Chem.* 29, 641–648. doi: 10.1021/jm00155a010

Rieswijk, L., Brauers, K. J. J., Coonen, M. L. J., van Breda, S. G. J., Jennen, D. G. J., and Kleinjans, J. C. S. (2015). Evaluating microRNA profiles reveals discriminative responses following genotoxic or non-genotoxic carcinogen exposure in primary mouse hepatocytes. *Mutagenesis* 30, 771–784. doi: 10.1093/mutage/gev036

Rodriguez, A., Griffiths-Jones, S., Ashurst, J. L., and Bradley, A. (2004). Identification of mammalian microRNA host genes and transcription units. *Genome Res.* 14, 1902–1910. doi: 10.1101/gr.2722704

Ruby, J. G., Jan, C. H., and Bartel, D. P. (2007a). Intronic microRNA precursors that bypass Drosha processing. *Nature* 448, 83–86. doi: 10.1038/nature05983

Ruby, J. G., Stark, A., Johnston, W. K., Kellis, M., Bartel, D. P., and Lai, E. C. (2007b). Evolution, biogenesis, expression, and target predictions of a substantially expanded set of Drosophila microRNAs. *Genome Res.* 17, 1850–1864. doi: 10.1101/gr.6597907

vom Saal, F. S., Akingbemi, B. T., Belcher, S. M., Birnbaum, L. S., Crain, D. A., Eriksen, M., et al. (2007). Chapel Hill bisphenol A expert panel consensus statement: integration of mechanisms, effects in animals and potential to impact human health at current levels of exposure. *Reprod. Toxicol.* 24, 131–138. doi: 10.1016/j.reprotox.2007.07.005

Sakurai, M., Miki, Y., Masuda, M., Hata, S., Shibahara, Y., Hirakawa, H., et al. (2012). LIN28: a regulator of tumor-suppressing activity of let-7 microRNA in human breast cancer. *J. Steroid Biochem. Mol. Biol.* 131, 101–106. doi: 10.1016/j.jsbmb.2011.10.007

Schecter, A., Birnbaum, L., Ryan, J. J., and Constable, J. D. (2006). Dioxins: an overview. *Environ. Res.* 101, 419–428. doi: 10.1016/j.envres.2005.12.003

Schmutzler, C., Hamann, I., Hofmann, P. J., Kovacs, G., Stemmler, L., Mentrup, B., et al. (2004). Endocrine active compounds affect thyrotropin and thyroid hormone levels in serum as well as endpoints of thyroid hormone action in liver, heart and kidney. *Toxicology* 205, 95–102. doi: 10.1016/j.tox.2004.06.041

Segal, M., Avital, A., Berstein, S., Derevenski, A., Sandbank, S., and Weizman, A. (2007). Prolactin and estradiol serum levels in unmedicated male paranoid schizophrenia patients. *Prog. Neuropsychopharmacol. Biol. Psychiatry* 31, 378–382. doi: 10.1016/j.pnpbp.2006.09.016

Selbach, M., Schwanhäusser, B., Thierfelder, N., Fang, Z., Khanin, R., and Rajewsky, N. (2008). Widespread changes in protein synthesis induced by microRNAs. *Nature* 455, 58–63. doi: 10.1038/nature07228

Sen, G. L., and Blau, H. M. (2005). Argonaute 2/RISC resides in sites of mammalian mRNA decay known as cytoplasmic bodies. *Nat. Cell Biol.* 7, 633–636. doi: 10.1038/ncb1265

Sheth, U., and Parker, R. (2003). Decapping and decay of messenger RNA occur in cytoplasmic processing bodies. *Science* 300, 805–808. doi: 10.1126/science.1082320

Sicard, F., Gayral, M., Lulka, H., Buscail, L., and Cordelier, P. (2013). Targeting miR-21 for the therapy of pancreatic cancer. *Mol. Ther. J. Am. Soc. Gene Ther.* 21, 986–994. doi: 10.1038/mt.2013.35

Skinner, M. K., Guerrero-Bosagna, C., Haque, M., Nilsson, E., Bhandari, R., and McCarrey, J. R. (2013). Environmentally induced transgenerational epigenetic reprogramming of primordial germ cells and the subsequent germ line. *PLoS ONE* 8:e66318. doi: 10.1371/journal.pone.0066318

Somm, E., Schwitzgebel, V. M., Toulotte, A., Cederroth, C. R., Combescure, C., Nef, S., et al. (2009). Perinatal exposure to bisphenol a alters early adipogenesis in the rat. *Environ. Health Perspect.* 117, 1549–1555. doi: 10.1289/ehp.11342

Song, Y., Chou, E. L., Baecker, A., You, N.-C. Y., Song, Y., Sun, Q., et al. (2016). Endocrine-disrupting chemicals, risk of type 2 diabetes, and diabetes-related metabolic traits: a systematic review and meta-analysis. *J. Diabetes.* 8, 516–532. doi: 10.1111/1753-0407.12325

Sontheimer, E. J. (2005). Assembly and function of RNA silencing complexes. *Nat. Rev. Mol. Cell Biol.* 6, 127–138. doi: 10.1038/nrm1568

Staessen, J. A., Nawrot, T., Hond, E. D., Thijs, L., Fagard, R., Hoppenbrouwers, K., et al. (2001). Renal function, cytogenetic measurements, and sexual development in adolescents in relation to environmental pollutants: a feasibility study of biomarkers. *Lancet Lond. Engl.* 357, 1660–1669. doi: 10.1016/S0140-6736(00)04822-4

Stevens, J. R. (2002). Schizophrenia: reproductive hormones and the brain. *Am. J. Psychiatry* 159, 713–719. doi: 10.1176/appi.ajp.159.5.713

Stouder, C., and Paoloni-Giacobino, A. (2010). Transgenerational effects of the endocrine disruptor vinclozolin on the methylation pattern of imprinted genes in the mouse sperm. *Reprod. Camb. Engl.* 139, 373–379. doi: 10.1530/rep-09-0340

Stricklin, S. L., Griffiths-Jones, S., and Eddy, S. R. (2005). *C. elegans* noncoding RNA genes. *WormBook Online Rev. C Elegans Biol,* 1–7. doi: 10.1895/wormbook.1.1.1

Sugiura-Ogasawara, M., Ozaki, Y., Sonta, S., Makino, T., and Suzumori, K. (2005). Exposure to bisphenol A is associated with recurrent miscarriage. *Hum. Reprod. Oxf. Engl.* 20, 2325–2329. doi: 10.1093/humrep/deh888

Sweeney, M. F., Hasan, N., Soto, A. M., and Sonnenschein, C. (2015). Environmental endocrine disruptors: effects on the human male reproductive system. *Rev. Endocr. Metab. Disord.* 16, 341–357. doi: 10.1007/s11154-016-9337-4

Sweeney, M. H., and Mocarelli, P. (2000). Human health effects after exposure to 2,3,7,8-TCDD. *Food Addit. Contam.* 17, 303–316. doi: 10.1080/026520300283379

Takeuchi, T., Tsutsumi, O., Ikezuki, Y., Kamei, Y., Osuga, Y., Fujiwara, T., et al. (2006). Elevated serum bisphenol A levels under hyperandrogenic conditions may be caused by decreased UDP-glucuronosyltransferase activity. *Endocr. J.* 53, 485–491. doi: 10.1507/endocrj.K06-032

Takeuchi, T., Tsutsumi, O., Ikezuki, Y., Takai, Y., and Taketani, Y. (2004). Positive relationship between androgen and the endocrine disruptor, bisphenol A, in normal women and women with ovarian dysfunction. *Endocr. J.* 51, 165–169. doi: 10.1507/endocrj.51.165

Tilghman, S. L., Bratton, M. R., Segar, H. C., Martin, E. C., Rhodes, L. V., Li, M., et al. (2012). Endocrine disruptor regulation of microRNA expression in breast carcinoma cells. *PLoS ONE* 7:e32754. doi: 10.1371/journal.pone.0032754

Toppari, J., Rodprasert, W., and Koskenniemi, J. J. (2016). Exposure variation and endocrine disruption of the male reproductive system. *Horm. Res. Paediatr.* 85. doi: 10.1159/000446436. [Epub ahead of print].

van Dijk, E., Cougot, N., Meyer, S., Babajko, S., Wahle, E., and Séraphin, B. (2002). Human Dcp2: a catalytically active mRNA decapping enzyme located in specific cytoplasmic structures. *EMBO J.* 21, 6915–6924. doi: 10.1093/emboj/cdf678

Veiga-Lopez, A., Luense, L. J., Christenson, L. K., and Padmanabhan, V. (2013). Developmental programming: gestational bisphenol-A treatment alters trajectory of fetal ovarian gene expression. *Endocrinology* 154, 1873–1884. doi: 10.1210/en.2012-2129

Viluksela, M., Raasmaja, A., Lebofsky, M., Stahl, B. U., and Rozman, K. K. (2004). Tissue-specific effects of 2,3,7,8-tetrachlorodibenzo-p-dioxin (TCDD) on the activity of 5′-deiodinases I and II in rats. *Toxicol. Lett.* 147, 133–142. doi: 10.1016/j.toxlet.2003.10.025

Vrijens, K., Bollati, V., and Nawrot, T. S. (2015). MicroRNAs as potential signatures of environmental exposure or effect: a systematic review. *Environ. Health Perspect.* 123, 399–411. doi: 10.1289/ehp.1408459

Wakiyama, M., Takimoto, K., Ohara, O., and Yokoyama, S. (2007). Let-7 microRNA-mediated mRNA deadenylation and translational repression in a mammalian cell-free system. *Genes Dev.* 21, 1857–1862. doi: 10.1101/gad.1566707

Wang, B., Yanez, A., and Novina, C. D. (2008). MicroRNA-repressed mRNAs contain 40S but not 60S components. *Proc. Natl. Acad. Sci. U.S.A.* 105, 5343–5348. doi: 10.1073/pnas.0801102105

Weiss, B., and Landrigan, P. J. (2000). The developing brain and the environment: an introduction. *Environ. Health Perspect.* 108(Suppl. 3), 373–374. doi: 10.1289/ehp.00108s3373

WHO | State of the science of endocrine disrupting chemicals (2012). WHO. Available online at: http://www.who.int/ceh/publications/endocrine/en/ (Accessed February 28, 2016).

Wing, L., Yeates, S. R., Brierley, L. M., and Gould, J. (1976). The prevalence of early childhood autism: comparison of administrative and epidemiological studies. *Psychol. Med.* 6, 89–100. doi: 10.1017/S0033291700007522

Wolstenholme, J. T., Rissman, E. F., and Connelly, J. J. (2011). The role of Bisphenol A in shaping the brain, epigenome and behavior. *Horm. Behav.* 59, 296–305. doi: 10.1016/j.yhbeh.2010.10.001

Wu, L., Fan, J., and Belasco, J. G. (2006). MicroRNAs direct rapid deadenylation of mRNA. *Proc. Natl. Acad. Sci. U.S.A.* 103, 4034–4039. doi: 10.1073/pnas.0510928103

Yang, J.-S., Phillips, M. D., Betel, D., Mu, P., Ventura, A., Siepel, A. C., et al. (2011). Widespread regulatory activity of vertebrate microRNA* species. *RNA* 17, 312–326. doi: 10.1261/rna.2537911

Yi, R., Qin, Y., Macara, I. G., and Cullen, B. R. (2003). Exportin-5 mediates the nuclear export of pre-microRNAs and short hairpin RNAs. *Genes Dev.* 17, 3011–3016. doi: 10.1101/gad.1158803

Yoshioka, W., Higashiyama, W., and Tohyama, C. (2011). Involvement of microRNAs in dioxin-induced liver damage in the mouse. *Toxicol. Sci. Off. J. Soc. Toxicol.* 122, 457–465. doi: 10.1093/toxsci/kfr130

Zhou, R., Chen, F., Feng, X., Zhou, L., Li, Y., and Chen, L. (2015). Perinatal exposure to low-dose of bisphenol A causes anxiety-like alteration in adrenal axis regulation and behaviors of rat offspring: a potential role for metabotropic glutamate 2/3 receptors. *J. Psychiatr. Res.* 64, 121–129. doi: 10.1016/j.jpsychires.2015.02.018

9

Chemicals, Nutrition, and Autism Spectrum Disorder

Takeo Fujiwara [1,2]*, *Naho Morisaki* [1], *Yukiko Honda* [1,3], *Makiko Sampei* [1] *and Yukako Tani* [1,2,4]

[1] *Department of Social Medicine, National Research Institute for Child Health and Development, Okura, Setagaya-ku, Tokyo, Japan,* [2] *Department of Global Health Promotion, Tokyo Medical and Dental University, Tokyo, Japan,* [3] *Global Cooperation Institute for Sustainable Cities, Yokohama City University, Yokohama, Japan,* [4] *Department of Health Education and Health Sociology, School of Public Health, The University of Tokyo, Tokyo, Japan*

Edited by:
Shoji F. Nakayama,
National Institute for Environmental Studies, Japan

Reviewed by:
Anne-Simone Parent,
Giga Neurosciences, Belgium
Francisco Gaytán,
University of Cordoba, Spain

***Correspondence:**
Takeo Fujiwara
fujiwara.hlth@tmd.ac.jp

The rapid increase of the prevalence of autism spectrum disorder (ASD) suggests that exposure to chemicals may impact the development of ASD. Therefore, we reviewed literature on the following chemicals, nutrient to investigate their association with ASD: (1) smoke/tobacco, (2) alcohol, (3) air pollution, (4) pesticides, (5) endocrine-disrupting chemicals, (6) heavy metals, (7) micronutrients, (8) fatty acid, and (9) parental obesity as a proxy of accumulation of specific chemicals or nutritional status. Several chemical exposures such as air pollution (e.g., particular matter 2.5), pesticides, bisphenol A, phthalates, mercury, and nutrition deficiency such as folic acid, vitamin D, or fatty acid may possibly be associated with an increased risk of ASD, whereas other traditional risk factors such as smoking/tobacco, alcohol, or polychlorinated biphenyls are less likely to be associated with ASD. Further research is needed to accumulate evidence on the association between chemical exposure and nutrient deficiencies and ASD in various doses and populations.

Keywords: autism spectrum disorder, air pollution, chemicals, pesticide, fatty acid, micronutrients, heavy metal, environment

INTRODUCTION

Autism spectrum disorder (ASD) is a developmental disorder typified by impaired communication and social skills (Grabrucker, 2012). A recent increase in cases of ASD from 4–5 of 10,000 persons in 1966 to 100 cases of 10,000 persons currently (Fombonne, 2009) may not solely be explained by genetic factors (Abrahams and Geschwind, 2010). Thus, it needs to be determined whether environmental factors play a role in the onset of ASD (Grabrucker, 2012), and a recent study using twin samples reported that around 50% of cases of ASD can be explained by environmental factors (Hallmayer et al., 2011).

In the present mini-review, we report several relatively new studies that have evaluated the association between ASD and environmental factors by focusing on chemical or nutritional exposures because these are modifiable factors. These exposures included smoking/tobacco, alcohol, air pollution, pesticides, endocrine-disrupting chemicals, heavy metals, micronutrients, and fatty acid. Parental obesity was also included as an exposure because maternal obesity can be an indicator of exposure to chemicals or nutrition.

SMOKE OR TOBACCO

Although not consistent, most recent population-based studies have suggested that maternal smoking during pregnancy is not directly associated with ASD after adjusting for socioeconomic status (Burstyn et al., 2010; Kalkbrenner et al., 2012; Lee et al., 2012; Tran et al., 2013). For example,

Lee et al. (2012) performed a population-based nested case-control study of 3958 cases of ASD and 38,983 controls in a longitudinal register-based study consisting of individuals aged 4–17 years, and found that maternal smoking during 8–12 weeks of gestation was significantly associated with an increased odds of high-functioning autism in an unadjusted model (odds ratio [OR] = 1.22, 95% confidence interval [CI]: 1.09, 1.36); however, this finding was no longer statistically significant after adjusting for parental socioeconomic status. Additionally, Tran et al. (2013) conducted a population-based nested case-control study comprising 16,185 samples, including 4020 cases of ASD, based on the Finnish National Birth Cohort. Maternal smoking during all pregnancies was not associated with the offsprings' ASD status after adjusting for confounding factors.

Considering that these studies were conducted mostly among Caucasians, the impact of smoking on the development of ASD may differ by race. Zhang et al. (2010) conducted a case-control study using 190 Han children aged 3–21 years with and without autism in China, and found that maternal second-hand smoke exposure during pregnancy, was significantly associated with autism (OR = 3.53, 95% CI: 1.30, 9.56), suggesting that maternal smoking may be associated with ASD among Asians.

ALCOHOL

Few studies have evaluated the impact of maternal alcohol use on the onset of ASD among offspring. Two population-based nested control studies in North European countries reported that maternal alcohol intake during pregnancy was not associated with ASD (Daniels et al., 2008; Eliasen et al., 2010).

AIR POLLUTION

In the last decade, literature on the effect of air pollution exposure during pregnancy on the risk of ASD has grown immensely. Although a large study using direct person-based air sampling is needed, the analytical models used to calculate residence-based effects have become increasingly complex to correctly estimate exposure during a specific time. Regardless of this change in measuring the effect of exposures, most studies have shown a positive association between air pollution exposure and ASD (Suades-Gonzalez et al., 2015). Recent findings support that exposure to particulate matter (PM) $<2.5\ \mu m$ in diameter ($PM_{2.5}$) during the third trimester causes the most detrimental effect on the development of ASD (Kalkbrenner et al., 2015; Raz et al., 2015; Talbott et al., 2015; Weisskopf et al., 2015).

One of the earlier studies that measured air pollution during pregnancy was conducted in 2011 using the distance of one's residence to major roadways as its proxy. Comparing 304 cases of ASD and 259 controls, Volk et al. (2011) reported that mothers of children with ASD were more likely to have lived near a freeway during their third trimester (OR 2.22, CI: 1.16, 4.42) or at the time of delivery (OR 1.86, CI: 1.04, 4.42). This study raised another research question: which type of air pollution has the most effect on the onset of ASD? Evidence of the effect of ozone or nitro-oxides on ASD has been inconclusive (Becerra et al., 2013; Gong T. et al., 2014; Guxens et al., 2016), but maternal exposure to small particles such as diesel PM (Windham et al., 2006; Roberts et al., 2013), PM 2.5 (Becerra et al., 2013; Volk et al., 2013; Raz et al., 2015; Talbott et al., 2015), and PM $<10\ \mu m$ in diameter (PM_{10}) (Volk et al., 2013; Kalkbrenner et al., 2015) has been most consistently reported with an increased risk of ASD. Several case-control studies have investigated the effect of individual hazardous air pollutants (HAP) such as metals and volatile organics on ASD (Windham et al., 2006; Kalkbrenner et al., 2010; Roberts et al., 2013; von Ehrenstein et al., 2014) with all studies conducted in the United States showing that cases of ASD have an elevated exposure of HAP by 1.3–2.0 times. However, two reports from European countries (Guxens et al., 2016) and a separate twin study in Sweden (Gong T. et al., 2014) showed no association of maternal exposure to air pollution and ASD.

Most studies about the effect of air pollution on ASD have been prone to residual confounders such as a low socioeconomic status, which is related to both worse living environments and an increased risk of ASD (Bell and Ebisu, 2012; Shmool et al., 2014).

PESTICIDES

Evidence from previous studies has suggested a strong relationship between pesticide exposure and ASD. Despite the quick turnover in commercial product names, organophosphates (OP) and organochlorines (OC) are still in use despite their neurotoxicity (Kalkbrenner et al., 2014). The association between ASD and pesticides has been observed across studies that measured exposures from residential exposure to agricultural drift (Roberts et al., 2007; Roberts and English, 2013), administered questionnaires on the use of insecticides (Keil et al., 2014), and assessed bio-specimens to detect metabolites (Rauh et al., 2006; Eskenazi et al., 2007; Cheslack-Postava et al., 2013) and numerous pesticides, including but not limited to OC (Roberts et al., 2007; Cheslack-Postava et al., 2013; Roberts and English, 2013; Braun et al., 2014) and OP (Rauh et al., 2006; Eskenazi et al., 2007; Shelton et al., 2014) pesticides.

Shelton et al. (2014) compared 486 cases of ASD and 316 controls, and found an association with OP exposure and ASD, which strengthened later in pregnancy for mothers living within 1.75 km from the agricultural use of OP during their third trimester. They also found increased exposure to pyrethroids in patients with ASD. Eskenazi et al. (2007) and Rauh et al. (2006) reported that cases of ASD had higher OP metabolites during early- to mid-pregnancy. Other case-control studies reported that exposure to imidacloprid through the consistent use of flea/tick pet treatment throughout pregnancy period was associated with ASD (Kalkbrenner et al., 2014; Keil et al., 2014).

ENDOCRINE-DISRUPTING CHEMICALS

Although, polychlorinated biphenyl (PCB) and several dioxins such as tetrachlorodibenzodioxin were banned by the Stockholm Convention in 2001, they are still detected in humans due to their long half-life in the environment, as well as the consumption of predatory fish in which such chemicals tend to accumulate. Other chemicals are still used, such as bisphenol A (BPA), in many canned foods, receipts, toys, and medical equipment, and some chemicals such as polybrominated diphenyl ethers and phthalates may have even increased body burden (Zota et al., 2008, 2014). Studies on these chemicals are sparse with mixed findings.

Associations between ASD and PCB are inconsistent (Kim et al., 2010; Cheslack-Postava et al., 2013; Braun et al., 2014), and the seemingly elevated risks in a pilot study (Cheslack-Postava et al., 2013) have been criticized for possible bias due to lack of adjustment for birth order (Kalkbrenner et al., 2014). Kardas et al. reported higher serum BPA concentrations in a case-control study of 48 cases of ASD and 41 controls, but no measurement of prenatal exposure was reported (Kardas et al., 2016). Braun et al. (2014) and Miodovnik et al. (2011) failed to find any association with the score of Social Responsiveness Scale (SRS), measurement of ASD traits, and maternal BPA serum or urine concentration and in their cohort studies; however, Braun et al. (2009) found that mid-pregnancy BPA concentrations were associated with an increase in externalizing problem behaviors in early childhood.

However, studies on phthalates mostly suggest an association between ASD and phthalates. Miodovnik et al. (2011) studied 137 children and found that higher phthalate metabolites in maternal urine in the third trimester were associated with a lower score on several of the SRS subscales at 7–9 years old (Miodovnik et al., 2011). Larsson et al. (2009) followed 4779 children and reported that those at 1–6 years old living in homes with polyvinyl chloride flooring (a significant source of phthalates) were 2.4 times more likely to be diagnosed with ASD (Larsson et al., 2009). Kardas et al. (2016) also reported higher serum phthalates concentrations in cases of ASD (Kardas et al., 2016). Braun et al. (2014) failed to detect an association between phthalates in maternal urine and ASD, and Phillipat et al. (Philippat et al., 2015) also failed to detect an association between house dust levels of phthalates and ASD; however, Phillipat et al. explained that the lack of association may be due to fact that the measured exposure may have only poorly reflected the actual exposure of phthalates.

HEAVY METALS

There is sufficient evidence that maternal exposure to heavy metals such as lead, mercury, cadmium, and arsenic cause an increase in neurodevelopmental disorders, and restrict fetal and infant growth even at low-level exposures (De Palma et al., 2012; Ornoy et al., 2015). However, less research has been conducted on heavy metals in relation to ASD. Recently, Rossignol et al. (2014) systematically reviewed literature on environmental toxicants and summarized 40 case-control studies that compared a variety of heavy metal concentrations (i.e., lead, mercury, arsenic, cadmium, aluminum, fluoride, manganese, chromium, nickel, uranium, and tin) in blood, hair, brain, teeth, or urine in children with ASD compared to controls, as well as seven similar studies on urinary porphyrin, which is considered to have a heavy metal burden (Rossignol et al., 2014). The most studied metals were mercury (29 studies) and lead (25 studies). Although the urinary porphyrin studies collectively suggest a higher heavy metal burden among children with ASD, a recent study by Dickerson et al. (2015) found that among 2489 children the prevalence of ASD was higher when mothers were living closer to industrial facilities that released arsenic, lead, or mercury.

A meta-analysis of seven studies on the mean hair level of mercury in a total of 343 cases of ASD and 317 controls did not show any significant association between mercury and ASD (De Palma et al., 2012) and neither did a recent cohort study by van Wijngaarden et al. (2013) on 1784 children and young adults. Some studies that assessed blood have found an association between mercury and ASD (Ip et al., 2004; Desoto and Hitlan, 2007; Geier et al., 2010), whereas others have not (Hertz-Picciotto et al., 2010; Stamova et al., 2011; Albizzati et al., 2012; Adams et al., 2013; Rahbar et al., 2013). However, the lack of adjusting for strong protective factors such as fish oil that are ingested concomitantly in many of the studies (Karagas et al., 2012) and the possible conflict of interest with industries (Kern et al., 2015) may be masking existing associations, as studies on air-borne mercury consistently report an association between mercury exposure and ASD (Windham et al., 2006; Roberts et al., 2013).

MICRONUTRIENTS

Micronutrients are essential for neurogenesis and the development of the neuro-network (Curtis and Patel, 2008). Lower levels of magnesium (Strambi et al., 2006), zinc (Adams and Vogelaar, 2005), selenium (Adams and Vogelaar, 2005), vitamin A (Adams and Vogelaar, 2005), vitamin B complex (Adams and Vogelaar, 2005; Pineles et al., 2010), vitamin D (Adams and Vogelaar, 2005; Gong Z. L. et al., 2014; Kocovska et al., 2014), vitamin E (Adams and Vogelaar, 2005), and carnitine (Filipek et al., 2004) in blood, hair, or other tissue among children with ASD have been reported. Further, the association between a deficiency of micronutrients during pregnancy, such as folic acid (Schmidt et al., 2011, 2012; Suren et al., 2013) and vitamin D (Cannell, 2008; Grant and Soles, 2009), have been reported as a risk for offspring developing ASD.

These previous studies advanced to intervention studies to confirm the causality or possibility of using nutrients to treat ASD. Several studies have reported that nutritional intervention showed a trend toward improvement in patients with ASD. For example, a double-blind study on 20 children (age 3–8 years) with ASD who took a broad-based multi-vitamin and mineral supplement suggested the possible benefit of improving general behavior and receptive language, although this finding was not significant (Adams and Holloway, 2004). Another double-blind study reported that supplementing L-carnosine to children (age 3–12 years) with ASD showed statistically significant improvements in the symptoms on ASD (Chez et al., 2002). In another study, it was also reported that oral magnesium and vitamin B6 supplements led to improvements in social interactions, communication, stereotyped restricted behavior, and abnormal/delayed functioning among children (age 1–10 years) with ASD (Mousain-Bosc et al., 2006).

Several studies have reported the association between gender and ASD in the relationship with micronutrients. For example, a study conducted in the Faroe Islands (Kocovska et al., 2014) noted the trend for ASD males having lower levels of vitamin

D and 25(OH)D3. Similarly, another study suggested that the differenteial effects of estrogen and testosterone on vitamin D metabolism might explain the gender difference of ASD (Cannell, 2008).

FATTY ACIDS

As neural development requires essential fatty acids, particularly long-chain omega-3 fatty acids during critical growth periods, and inflammation may be associated with ASD (Ornoy et al., 2015), the fatty acid level may play an important role in the development of ASD. Several studies have shown that both red blood cell and plasma fatty acid composition among cases of ASD differ from those of non-ASD people. Specifically, the levels of omega-3 fatty acids (Vancassel et al., 2001; Bell et al., 2004; Brigandi et al., 2015), docosahexaenoic acid (DHA) (Meguid et al., 2008; Wiest et al., 2009; El-Ansary et al., 2011; Al-Farsi et al., 2013; Brigandi et al., 2015), and arachidonic acid (AA) (Meguid et al., 2008; El-Ansary et al., 2011; Brigandi et al., 2015; Yui et al., 2016) were significantly lower in the red blood cell or plasma of cases of ASD compared to controls, although some studies did not support these claims (Bu et al., 2006; Bell et al., 2010). To date, only one study has examined maternal fatty acid intake during pregnancy is association with ASD (Lyall et al., 2013). Women with higher intake of polyunsaturated fatty acids (PUFA) before and during pregnancy had a reduced risk of having a child with ASD than those with lower PUFA intake. Analysis on specific PUFAs showed that women in the highest quartile of intake of omega-6 fatty acids had a 34% reduction in the risk of having a child with ASD compared with those in the lowest quartile, with similar results for linoleic acid intake. In concern with omega-3 fatty acids, women with very low intakes (i.e., the lowest 5% of the distribution) of had a significantly increased risk of having a child with ASD compared with those in the middle 90% of the distribution.

Reports on the benefits of fatty acid supplementation in children with ASD are inconclusive. Recently, Mankad et al. (2015) conducted a randomized controlled 6-month trial of 1.5 g/day of omega-3 fatty acids or a placebo in 38 children aged 2–5 years with ASD, and found no evidence for the efficacy of omega-3 fatty acids on improving core symptoms (Mankad et al., 2015). However, Ooi et al. (2015) conducted a 12-week open-label study of 1 g/day of omega-3 fatty acids in 41 children aged 7–18 years with ASD, and found significant improvements in the core symptoms and attention problems (Ooi et al., 2015). Yui et al. (2012) conducted a randomized controlled 16-week trial of AA and DHA supplementation or a placebo in 13 individuals aged 6–28 years with autism, and found significant improvements in social withdrawal and communication (Yui et al., 2012). These studies were relatively small, thus the findings may be by coincidental so a further larger randomized controlled trial is needed.

PARENTAL OBESITY

Maternal obesity can be associated with having offspring with ASD due to the accumulation of the aforementioned chemicals, or it can serve as a proxy of poor nutrition (Dodds et al., 2011; Kawicka and Regulska-Ilow, 2013; Ornoy et al., 2015). According to a Swedish cohort study of 333,057 participants, which included 6420 individuals with ASD, maternal overweight or obesity evaluated at the first antenatal visit was associated with having an offspring with ASD (Gardner et al., 2015). However, the association between an elevated maternal body mass index and the risk of ASD was not clear in matched sibling analyses.

In a population-based prospective cohort study of 92,909 children (age 4–13 years), Suren et al. (2014) investigated the association between ASD and paternal obesity recorded in the questionnaires answered by the fathers. They found that paternal obesity was associated with an increasing risk of ASD (adjusted OR: 1.73, 95% CI: 1.07, 2.82), whereas maternal obesity showed only a weak association with ASD (Suren et al., 2014).

SUMMARY AND FUTURE DIRECTIONS

In summary, several chemical exposures such as air pollution (e.g., PM 2.5), pesticides, BPA, phthalates, mercury or lead, and nutrition deficiencies such as folic acid, vitamin D, or fatty acid are possibly associated with the onset of ASD, whereas other traditional risk factors such as smoke/tobacco, alcohol, or PCB are less likely to be associated with ASD. Apparently, no single environmental factor can explain the development of ASD, suggesting that upstream environmental factors such as socioeconomic status need to be considered as risk factors for ASD, which have not been as rigorously investigated (Fujiwara, 2014). Further, few studies have investigated the accumulative or synergistic effect of the different chemical exposures and nutrition deficiencies simultaneously. The impact of multiple exposures to chemicals and nutrient deficiencies, which are suggestive of association with ASD, need to be studied together to assess whether effect is additive or multiplicative. Moreover, not all children exposed to these chemicals or nutrients may have risk of developing ASD, suggesting that some genetic polymorphism related to ASD, such as *CD38* (Higashida et al., 2012), may have an interaction effect with these environmental exposures during the onset of ASD, as studied in the exposure of heavy mental and genetic polymorphism related to metabolism (Rossignol et al., 2014). Moreover, few chemical or nutritional exposures were investigated to elucidate the mechanism of gender difference of ASD prevalence. These uncovered topics need to be investigated in future research.

AUTHOR CONTRIBUTIONS

TF conceived the review focus, conducted literature review, summarized, and finalized the manuscript. NM, YH, MS, and YT reviewed literature, wrote first draft, and finalized the manuscript. All authors approved final version of manuscript.

REFERENCES

Abrahams, B. S., and Geschwind, D. H. (2010). Connecting genes to brain in the autism spectrum disorders. *Arch. Neurol.* 67, 395–399. doi: 10.1001/archneurol.2010.47

Adams, J. B., and Vogelaar, A. T. (2005). "Nutritional abnormalities in autism and effects of nutritional supplementation," in *ASA's 36th National Conference on Autism Spectrum Disorders* (Nashville, TN).

Adams, J. B., Audhya, T., Mcdonough-Means, S., Rubin, R. A., Quig, D., Geis, E., et al. (2013). Toxicological status of children with autism vs. neurotypical children and the association with autism severity. *Biol. Trace Elem. Res.* 151, 171–180. doi: 10.1007/s12011-012-9551-1

Adams, J. B., and Holloway, C. (2004). Pilot study of a moderate dose multivitamin/mineral supplement for children with autistic spectrum disorder. *J. Altern. Complement Med.* 10, 1033–1039. doi: 10.1089/acm.2004.10.1033

Albizzati, A., More, L., Di Candia, D., Saccani, M., and Lenti, C. (2012). Normal concentrations of heavy metals in autistic spectrum disorders. *Minerva Pediatr.* 64, 27–31.

Al-Farsi, Y. M., Waly, M. I., Deth, R. C., Al-Sharbati, M. M., Al-Shafaee, M., Al-Farsi, O., et al. (2013). Impact of nutrition on serum levels of docosahexaenoic acid among Omani children with autism. *Nutrition* 29, 1142–1146. doi: 10.1016/j.nut.2013.03.009

Becerra, T. A., Wilhelm, M., Olsen, J., Cockburn, M., and Ritz, B. (2013). Ambient air pollution and autism in Los Angeles county, California. *Environ. Health Perspect.* 121, 380–386. doi: 10.1289/ehp.1205827

Bell, J. G., Mackinlay, E. E., Dick, J. R., Macdonald, D. J., Boyle, R. M., and Glen, A. C. (2004). Essential fatty acids and phospholipase A2 in autistic spectrum disorders. *Prostaglandins Leukot. Essent. Fatty Acids* 71, 201–204. doi: 10.1016/j.plefa.2004.03.008

Bell, J. G., Miller, D., Macdonald, D. J., Mackinlay, E. E., Dick, J. R., Cheseldine, S., et al. (2010). The fatty acid compositions of erythrocyte and plasma polar lipids in children with autism, developmental delay or typically developing controls and the effect of fish oil intake. *Br. J. Nutr.* 103, 1160–1167. doi: 10.1017/S0007114509992881

Bell, M. L., and Ebisu, K. (2012). Environmental inequality in exposures to airborne particulate matter components in the United States. *Environ. Health Perspect.* 120, 1699–1704. doi: 10.1289/ehp.1205201

Braun, J. M., Kalkbrenner, A. E., Just, A. C., Yolton, K., Calafat, A. M., Sjodin, A., et al. (2014). Gestational exposure to endocrine-disrupting chemicals and reciprocal social, repetitive, and stereotypic behaviors in 4- and 5-year-old children: the HOME study. *Environ. Health Perspect.* 122, 513–520. doi: 10.1289/ehp.1307261

Braun, J. M., Yolton, K., Dietrich, K. N., Hornung, R., Ye, X., Calafat, A. M., et al. (2009). Prenatal bisphenol A exposure and early childhood behavior. *Environ. Health Perspect.* 117, 1945–1952. doi: 10.1289/ehp.0900979

Brigandi, S. A., Shao, H., Qian, S. Y., Shen, Y., Wu, B. L., and Kang, J. X. (2015). Autistic children exhibit decreased levels of essential Fatty acids in red blood cells. *Int. J. Mol. Sci.* 16, 10061–10076. doi: 10.3390/ijms160510061

Bu, B., Ashwood, P., Harvey, D., King, I. B., Water, J. V., and Jin, L. W. (2006). Fatty acid compositions of red blood cell phospholipids in children with autism. *Prostaglandins Leukot. Essent. Fatty Acids* 74, 215–221. doi: 10.1016/j.plefa.2006.02.001

Burstyn, I., Sithole, F., and Zwaigenbaum, L. (2010). Autism spectrum disorders, maternal characteristics and obstetric complications among singletons born in Alberta, Canada. *Chronic Dis. Can.* 30, 125–134.

Cannell, J. J. (2008). Autism and vitamin D. *Med. Hypotheses* 70, 750–759. doi: 10.1016/j.mehy.2007.08.016

Cheslack-Postava, K., Rantakokko, P. V., Hinkka-Yli-Salomaki, S., Surcel, H. M., Mckeague, I. W., Kiviranta, H. A., et al. (2013). Maternal serum persistent organic pollutants in the Finnish Prenatal Study of Autism: a pilot study. *Neurotoxicol. Teratol.* 38, 1–5. doi: 10.1016/j.ntt.2013.04.001

Chez, M. G., Buchanan, C. P., Aimonovitch, M. C., Becker, M., Schaefer, K., Black, C., et al. (2002). Double-blind, placebo-controlled study of L-carnosine supplementation in children with autistic spectrum disorders. *J. Child Neurol.* 17, 833–837. doi: 10.1177/08830738020170111501

Curtis, L. T., and Patel, K. (2008). Nutritional and environmental approaches to preventing and treating autism and attention deficit hyperactivity disorder (ADHD): a review. *J. Altern. Complement. Med.* 14, 79–85. doi: 10.1089/acm.2007.0610

Daniels, J. L., Forssen, U., Hultman, C. M., Cnattingius, S., Savitz, D. A., Feychting, M., et al. (2008). Parental psychiatric disorders associated with autism spectrum disorders in the offspring. *Pediatrics* 121, e1357–e1362. doi: 10.1542/peds.2007-2296

De Palma, G., Catalani, S., Franco, A., Brighenti, M., and Apostoli, P. (2012). Lack of correlation between metallic elements analyzed in hair by ICP-MS and autism. *J. Autism Dev. Disord.* 42, 342–353. doi: 10.1007/s10803-011-1245-6

Desoto, M. C., and Hitlan, R. T. (2007). Blood levels of mercury are related to diagnosis of autism: a reanalysis of an important data set. *J. Child Neurol.* 22, 1308–1311. doi: 10.1177/0883073807307111

Dickerson, A. S., Rahbar, M. H., Han, I., Bakian, A. V., Bilder, D. A., Harrington, R. A., et al. (2015). Autism spectrum disorder prevalence and proximity to industrial facilities releasing arsenic, lead or mercury. *Sci. Total Environ.* 536, 245–251. doi: 10.1016/j.scitotenv.2015.07.024

Dodds, L., Fell, D. B., Shea, S., Armson, B. A., Allen, A. C., and Bryson, S. (2011). The role of prenatal, obstetric and neonatal factors in the development of autism. *J. Autism Dev. Disord.* 41, 891–902. doi: 10.1007/s10803-010-1114-8

El-Ansary, A. K., Bacha, A. G., and Al-Ayahdi, L. Y. (2011). Plasma fatty acids as diagnostic markers in autistic patients from Saudi Arabia. *Lipids Health Dis.* 10:62. doi: 10.1186/1476-511x-10-62

Eliasen, M., Tolstrup, J. S., Nybo Andersen, A. M., Gronbaek, M., Olsen, J., and Strandberg-Larsen, K. (2010). Prenatal alcohol exposure and autistic spectrum disorders–a population-based prospective study of 80,552 children and their mothers. *Int. J. Epidemiol.* 39, 1074–1081. doi: 10.1093/ije/dyq056

Eskenazi, B., Marks, A. R., Bradman, A., Harley, K., Barr, D. B., Johnson, C., et al. (2007). Organophosphate pesticide exposure and neurodevelopment in young Mexican-American children. *Environ. Health Perspect.* 115, 792–798. doi: 10.1289/ehp.9828

Filipek, P. A., Juranek, J., Nguyen, M. T., Cummings, C., and Gargus, J. J. (2004). Relative carnitine deficiency in autism. *J. Autism Dev. Disord.* 34, 615–623. doi: 10.1007/s10803-004-5283-1

Fombonne, E. (2009). Epidemiology of pervasive developmental disorders. *Pediatr. Res.* 65, 591–598. doi: 10.1203/PDR.0b013e31819e7203

Fujiwara, T. (2014). Socioeconomic status and the risk of suspected autism spectrum disorders among 18-month-old toddlers in Japan: a population-based study. *J. Autism Dev. Disord.* 44, 1323–1331. doi: 10.1007/s10803-013-1988-3

Gardner, R. M., Lee, B. K., Magnusson, C., Rai, D., Frisell, T., Karlsson, H., et al. (2015). Maternal body mass index during early pregnancy, gestational weight gain, and risk of autism spectrum disorders: results from a Swedish total population and discordant sibling study. *Int. J. Epidemiol.* 44, 870–883. doi: 10.1093/ije/dyv081

Geier, D. A., Audhya, T., Kern, J. K., and Geier, M. R. (2010). Blood mercury levels in autism spectrum disorder: is there a threshold level? *Acta Neurobiol. Exp. (Wars).* 70, 177–186.

Gong, T., Almqvist, C., Bolte, S., Lichtenstein, P., Anckarsater, H., Lind, T., et al. (2014). Exposure to air pollution from traffic and neurodevelopmental disorders in Swedish twins. *Twin Res. Hum. Genet.* 17, 553–562. doi: 10.1017/thg.2014.58

Gong, Z. L., Luo, C. M., Wang, L., Shen, L., Wei, F., Tong, R. J., et al. (2014). Serum 25-hydroxyvitamin D levels in Chinese children with autism spectrum disorders. *Neuroreport* 25, 23–27. doi: 10.1097/WNR.0000000000000034

Grabrucker, A. M. (2012). Environmental factors in autism. *Front. Psychiatry* 3:118. doi: 10.3389/fpsyt.2012.00118

Grant, W. B., and Soles, C. M. (2009). Epidemiologic evidence supporting the role of maternal vitamin D deficiency as a risk factor for the development of infantile autism. *Dermatoendocrinology* 1, 223–228. doi: 10.4161/derm.1.4.9500

Guxens, M., Ghassabian, A., Gong, T., Garcia-Esteban, R., Porta, D., Giorgis-Allemand, L., et al. (2016). Air pollution exposure during pregnancy and childhood autistic traits in four European population-based cohort studies: the ESCAPE Project. *Environ. Health Perspect.* 124, 133–140. doi: 10.1289/ehp.1408483

Hallmayer, J., Cleveland, S., Torres, A., Phillips, J., Cohen, B., Torigoe, T., et al. (2011). Genetic heritability and shared environmental factors among twin pairs with autism. *Arch. Gen. Psychiatry* 68, 1095–1102. doi: 10.1001/archgenpsychiatry.2011.76

Hertz-Picciotto, I., Green, P. G., Delwiche, L., Hansen, R., Walker, C., and Pessah, I. N. (2010). Blood mercury concentrations in CHARGE Study children with and without autism. *Environ. Health Perspect.* 118, 161–166. doi: 10.1289/ehp.0900736

Higashida, H., Yokoyama, S., Kikuchi, M., and Munesue, T. (2012). CD38 and its role in oxytocin secretion and social behavior. *Horm. Behav.* 61, 351–358. doi: 10.1016/j.yhbeh.2011.12.011

Ip, P., Wong, V., Ho, M., Lee, J., and Wong, W. (2004). Mercury exposure in children with autistic spectrum disorder: case-control study. *J. Child Neurol.* 19, 431–434.

Kalkbrenner, A. E., Braun, J. M., Durkin, M. S., Maenner, M. J., Cunniff, C., Lee, L. C., et al. (2012). Maternal smoking during pregnancy and the prevalence of autism spectrum disorders, using data from the autism and developmental disabilities monitoring network. *Environ. Health Perspect.* 120, 1042–1048. doi: 10.1289/ehp.1104556

Kalkbrenner, A. E., Daniels, J. L., Chen, J. C., Poole, C., Emch, M., and Morrissey, J. (2010). Perinatal exposure to hazardous air pollutants and autism spectrum disorders at age 8. *Epidemiology* 21, 631–641. doi: 10.1097/EDE.0b013e3181e65d76

Kalkbrenner, A. E., Schmidt, R. J., and Penlesky, A. C. (2014). Environmental chemical exposures and autism spectrum disorders: a review of the epidemiological evidence. *Curr. Probl. Pediatr. Adolesc. Health Care* 44, 277–318. doi: 10.1016/j.cppeds.2014.06.001

Kalkbrenner, A. E., Windham, G. C., Serre, M. L., Akita, Y., Wang, X., Hoffman, K., et al. (2015). Particulate matter exposure, prenatal and postnatal windows of susceptibility, and autism spectrum disorders. *Epidemiology* 26, 30–42. doi: 10.1097/EDE.0000000000000173

Karagas, M. R., Choi, A. L., Oken, E., Horvat, M., Schoeny, R., Kamai, E., et al. (2012). Evidence on the human health effects of low-level methylmercury exposure. *Environ. Health Perspect.* 120, 799–806. doi: 10.1289/ehp.1104494

Kardas, F., Bayram, A. K., Demirci, E., Akin, L., Ozmen, S., Kendirci, M., et al. (2016). Increased serum phthalates (MEHP, DEHP) and Bisphenol a concentrations in children with autism spectrum disorder: the role of endocrine disruptors in autism etiopathogenesis. *J. Child Neurol.* 31, 629–635. doi: 10.1177/0883073815609150

Kawicka, A., and Regulska-Ilow, B. (2013). How nutritional status, diet and dietary supplements can affect autism. A review. *Rocz. Panstw. Zakl. Hig.* 64, 1–12.

Keil, A. P., Daniels, J. L., and Hertz-Picciotto, I. (2014). Autism spectrum disorder, flea and tick medication, and adjustments for exposure misclassification: the CHARGE (CHildhood Autism risks from genetics and environment) case-control study. *Environ. Health* 13:3. doi: 10.1186/1476-069X-13-3

Kern, J. K., Geier, D. A., Deth, R. C., Sykes, L. K., Hooker, B. S., Love, J. M., et al. (2015). Systematic assessment of research on autism spectrum disorder and mercury reveals conflicts of interest and the need for transparency in autism research. *Sci. Eng. Ethics.* doi: 10.1007/s11948-015-9713-6. [Epub ahead of print].

Kim, S. M., Han, D. H., Lyoo, H. S., Min, K. J., Kim, K. H., and Renshaw, P. (2010). Exposure to environmental toxins in mothers of children with autism spectrum disorder. *Psychiatry Investig.* 7, 122–127. doi: 10.4306/pi.2010.7.2.122

Kocovska, E., Andorsdottir, G., Weihe, P., Halling, J., Fernell, E., Stora, T., et al. (2014). Vitamin d in the general population of young adults with autism in the faroe islands. *J. Autism Dev. Disord.* 44, 2996–3005. doi: 10.1007/s10803-014-2155-1

Larsson, M., Weiss, B., Janson, S., Sundell, J., and Bornehag, C. G. (2009). Associations between indoor environmental factors and parental-reported autistic spectrum disorders in children 6-8 years of age. *Neurotoxicology* 30, 822–831. doi: 10.1016/j.neuro.2009.01.011

Lee, B. K., Gardner, R. M., Dal, H., Svensson, A., Galanti, M. R., Rai, D., et al. (2012). Brief report: maternal smoking during pregnancy and autism spectrum disorders. *J. Autism Dev. Disord.* 42, 2000–2005. doi: 10.1007/s10803-011-1425-4

Lyall, K., Munger, K. L., O'reilly, É. J., Santangelo, S. L., and Ascherio, A. (2013). Maternal dietary fat intake in association with autism spectrum disorders. *Am. J. Epidemiol.* 178, 209–220. doi: 10.1093/aje/kws433

Mankad, D., Dupuis, A., Smile, S., Roberts, W., Brian, J., Lui, T., et al. (2015). A randomized, placebo controlled trial of omega-3 fatty acids in the treatment of young children with autism. *Mol. Autism* 6, 18. doi: 10.1186/s13229-015-0010-7

Meguid, N. A., Atta, H. M., Gouda, A. S., and Khalil, R. O. (2008). Role of polyunsaturated fatty acids in the management of Egyptian children with autism. *Clin. Biochem.* 41, 1044–1048. doi: 10.1016/j.clinbiochem.2008.05.013

Miodovnik, A., Engel, S. M., Zhu, C., Ye, X., Soorya, L. V., Silva, M. J., et al. (2011). Endocrine disruptors and childhood social impairment. *Neurotoxicology* 32, 261–267. doi: 10.1016/j.neuro.2010.12.009

Mousain-Bosc, M., Roche, M., Polge, A., Pradal-Prat, D., Rapin, J., and Bali, J. P. (2006). Improvement of neurobehavioral disorders in children supplemented with magnesium-vitamin B6. II. Pervasive developmental disorder-autism. *Magnes. Res.* 19, 53–62.

Ooi, Y. P., Weng, S. J., Jang, L. Y., Low, L., Seah, J., Teo, S., et al. (2015). Omega-3 fatty acids in the management of autism spectrum disorders: findings from an open-label pilot study in Singapore. *Eur. J. Clin. Nutr.* 69, 969–971. doi: 10.1038/ejcn.2015.28

Ornoy, A., Weinstein-Fudim, L., and Ergaz, Z. (2015). Prenatal factors associated with autism spectrum disorder (ASD). *Reprod. Toxicol.* 56, 155–169. doi: 10.1016/j.reprotox.2015.05.007

Philippat, C., Bennett, D. H., Krakowiak, P., Rose, M., Hwang, H. M., and Hertz-Picciotto, I. (2015). Phthalate concentrations in house dust in relation to autism spectrum disorder and developmental delay in the CHildhood Autism Risks from Genetics and the Environment (CHARGE) study. *Environ. Health* 14, 56. doi: 10.1186/s12940-015-0024-9

Pineles, S. L., Avery, R. A., and Liu, G. T. (2010). Vitamin B12 optic neuropathy in autism. *Pediatrics* 126, e967–e970. doi: 10.1542/peds.2009-2975

Rahbar, M. H., Samms-Vaughan, M., Loveland, K. A., Ardjomand-Hessabi, M., Chen, Z., Bressler, J., et al. (2013). Seafood consumption and blood mercury concentrations in Jamaican children with and without autism spectrum disorders. *Neurotox. Res.* 23, 22–38. doi: 10.1007/s12640-012-9321-z

Rauh, V. A., Garfinkel, R., Perera, F. P., Andrews, H. F., Hoepner, L., Barr, D. B., et al. (2006). Impact of prenatal chlorpyrifos exposure on neurodevelopment in the first 3 years of life among inner-city children. *Pediatrics* 118, e1845–e1859. doi: 10.1097/00001648-200611001-00247

Raz, R., Roberts, A. L., Lyall, K., Hart, J. E., Just, A. C., Laden, F., et al. (2015). Autism spectrum disorder and particulate matter air pollution before, during, and after pregnancy: a nested case-control analysis within the Nurses' Health Study II Cohort. *Environ. Health Perspect.* 123, 264–270. doi: 10.1289/ehp.1408133

Roberts, A. L., Lyall, K., Hart, J. E., Laden, F., Just, A. C., Bobb, J. F., et al. (2013). Perinatal air pollutant exposures and autism spectrum disorder in the children of Nurses' Health Study II participants. *Environ. Health Perspect.* 121, 978–984. doi: 10.1289/ehp.1206187

Roberts, E. M., and English, P. B. (2013). Bayesian modeling of time-dependent vulnerability to environmental hazards: an example using autism and pesticide data. *Stat. Med.* 32, 2308–2319. doi: 10.1002/sim.5600

Roberts, E. M., English, P. B., Grether, J. K., Windham, G. C., Somberg, L., and Wolff, C. (2007). Maternal residence near agricultural pesticide applications and autism spectrum disorders among children in the California Central Valley. *Environ. Health Perspect.* 115, 1482–1489. doi: 10.1289/ehp.10168

Rossignol, D. A., Genuis, S. J., and Frye, R. E. (2014). Environmental toxicants and autism spectrum disorders: a systematic review. *Transl. Psychiatry* 4, e360. doi: 10.1038/tp.2014.4

Schmidt, R. J., Hansen, R. L., Hartiala, J., Allayee, H., Schmidt, L. C., Tancredi, D. J., et al. (2011). Prenatal vitamins, one-carbon metabolism gene variants, and risk for autism. *Epidemiology* 22, 476–485. doi: 10.1097/EDE.0b013e31821d0e30

Schmidt, R. J., Tancredi, D. J., Ozonoff, S., Hansen, R. L., Hartiala, J., Allayee, H., et al. (2012). Maternal periconceptional folic acid intake and risk of autism spectrum disorders and developmental delay in the CHARGE (CHildhood Autism Risks from Genetics and Environment) case-control study. *Am. J. Clin. Nutr.* 96, 80–89. doi: 10.3945/ajcn.110.004416

Shelton, J. F., Geraghty, E. M., Tancredi, D. J., Delwiche, L. D., Schmidt, R. J., Ritz, B., et al. (2014). Neurodevelopmental disorders and prenatal residential proximity to agricultural pesticides: the CHARGE study. *Environ. Health Perspect.* 122, 1103–1109. doi: 10.1289/ehp.1307044

Shmool, J. L., Kubzansky, L. D., Newman, O. D., Spengler, J., Shepard, P., and Clougherty, J. E. (2014). Social stressors and air pollution across New York City communities: a spatial approach for assessing correlations among multiple exposures. *Environ. Health* 13:91. doi: 10.1186/1476-069X-13-91

Stamova, B., Green, P. G., Tian, Y., Hertz-Picciotto, I., Pessah, I. N., Hansen, R., et al. (2011). Correlations between gene expression and mercury levels in blood of boys with and without autism. *Neurotox. Res.* 19, 31–48. doi: 10.1007/s12640-009-9137-7

Strambi, M., Longini, M., Hayek, J., Berni, S., Macucci, F., Scalacci, E., et al. (2006). Magnesium profile in autism. *Biol. Trace Elem. Res.* 109, 97–104. doi: 10.1385/BTER:109:2:097

Suades-Gonzalez, E., Gascon, M., Guxens, M., and Sunyer, J. (2015). Air pollution and neuropsychological development: a review of the latest evidence. *Endocrinology* 156, 3473–3482. doi: 10.1210/en.2015-1403

Suren, P., Gunnes, N., Roth, C., Bresnahan, M., Hornig, M., Hirtz, D., et al. (2014). Parental obesity and risk of autism spectrum disorder. *Pediatrics* 133, e1128–e1138. doi: 10.1542/peds.2013-3664

Suren, P., Roth, C., Bresnahan, M., Haugen, M., Hornig, M., Hirtz, D., et al. (2013). Association between maternal use of folic acid supplements and risk of autism spectrum disorders in children. *JAMA* 309, 570–577. doi: 10.1001/jama.2012.155925

Talbott, E. O., Arena, V. C., Rager, J. R., Clougherty, J. E., Michanowicz, D. R., Sharma, R. K., et al. (2015). Fine particulate matter and the risk of autism spectrum disorder. *Environ. Res.* 140, 414–420. doi: 10.1016/j.envres.2015.04.021

Tran, P. L., Lehti, V., Lampi, K. M., Helenius, H., Suominen, A., Gissler, M., et al. (2013). Smoking during pregnancy and risk of autism spectrum disorder in a finnish national birth cohort. *Paediatr. Perinat. Epidemiol.* 27, 266–274. doi: 10.1111/ppe.12043

van Wijngaarden, E., Davidson, P. W., Smith, T. H., Evans, K., Yost, K., Love, T., et al. (2013). Autism spectrum disorder phenotypes and prenatal exposure to methylmercury. *Epidemiology* 24, 651–659. doi: 10.1097/EDE.0b013e31829d2651

Vancassel, S., Durand, G., Barthelemy, C., Lejeune, B., Martineau, J., Guilloteau, D., et al. (2001). Plasma fatty acid levels in autistic children. *Prostaglandins Leukot. Essent. Fatty Acids* 65, 1–7. doi: 10.1054/plef.2001.0281

Volk, H. E., Hertz-Picciotto, I., Delwiche, L., Lurmann, F., and Mcconnell, R. (2011). Residential proximity to freeways and autism in the CHARGE study. *Environ. Health Perspect.* 119, 873–877. doi: 10.1289/ehp.1002835

Volk, H. E., Lurmann, F., Penfold, B., Hertz-Picciotto, I., and Mcconnell, R. (2013). Traffic-related air pollution, particulate matter, and autism. *JAMA Psychiatry* 70, 71–77. doi: 10.1001/jamapsychiatry.2013.266

von Ehrenstein, O. S., Aralis, H., Cockburn, M., and Ritz, B. (2014). In utero exposure to toxic air pollutants and risk of childhood autism. *Epidemiology* 25, 851–858. doi: 10.1097/EDE.0000000000000150

Weisskopf, M. G., Kioumourtzoglou, M. A., and Roberts, A. L. (2015). Air pollution and autism spectrum disorders: causal or confounded? *Curr. Environ. Health Rep.* 2, 430–439. doi: 10.1007/s40572-015-0073-9

Wiest, M. M., German, J. B., Harvey, D. J., Watkins, S. M., and Hertz-Picciotto, I. (2009). Plasma fatty acid profiles in autism: a case-control study. *Prostaglandins Leukot. Essent. Fatty Acids* 80, 221–227. doi: 10.1016/j.plefa.2009.01.007

Windham, G. C., Zhang, L., Gunier, R., Croen, L. A., and Grether, J. K. (2006). Autism spectrum disorders in relation to distribution of hazardous air pollutants in the san francisco bay area. *Environ. Health Perspect.* 114, 1438–1444. doi: 10.1289/ehp.9120

Yui, K., Imataka, G., Kawasaki, Y., and Yamada, H. (2016). Down-regulation of a signaling mediator in association with lowered plasma arachidonic acid levels in individuals with autism spectrum disorders. *Neurosci. Lett.* 610, 223–228. doi: 10.1016/j.neulet.2015.11.006

Yui, K., Koshiba, M., Nakamura, S., and Kobayashi, Y. (2012). Effects of large doses of arachidonic acid added to docosahexaenoic acid on social impairment in individuals with autism spectrum disorders: a double-blind, placebo-controlled, randomized trial. *J. Clin. Psychopharmacol.* 32, 200–206. doi: 10.1097/JCP.0b013e3182485791

Zhang, X., Lv, C. C., Tian, J., Miao, R. J., Xi, W., Hertz-Picciotto, I., et al. (2010). Prenatal and perinatal risk factors for autism in china. *J. Autism Dev. Disord.* 40, 1311–1321. doi: 10.1007/s10803-010-0992-0

Zota, A. R., Calafat, A. M., and Woodruff, T. J. (2014). Temporal trends in phthalate exposures: findings from the National Health and Nutrition Examination Survey, 2001-2010. *Environ. Health Perspect.* 122, 235–241. doi: 10.1289/ehp.1306681

Zota, A. R., Rudel, R. A., Morello-Frosch, R. A., and Brody, J. G. (2008). Elevated house dust and serum concentrations of PBDEs in California: unintended consequences of furniture flammability standards? *Environ. Sci. Technol.* 42, 8158–8164. doi: 10.1021/es801792z

10

Remodeling Functional Connectivity in Multiple Sclerosis: A Challenging Therapeutic Approach

Mario Stampanoni Bassi[1,2], *Luana Gilio*[1,2], *Fabio Buttari*[1,2], *Pierpaolo Maffei*[1], *Girolama A. Marfia*[2], *Domenico A. Restivo*[3], *Diego Centonze*[1,2*] *and Ennio Iezzi*[1]

[1] *Unit of Neurology & Unit of Neurorehabilitation, IRCCS Istituto Neurologico Mediterraneo Neuromed, Pozzilli, Italy,* [2] *Multiple Sclerosis Research Unit, Department of Systems Medicine, Tor Vergata University, Rome, Italy,* [3] *Department of Neurology, Nuovo Garibaldi Hospital, Catania, Italy*

Edited by:
Takashi Hanakawa, National Center of Neurology and Psychiatry, Japan

Reviewed by:
Kazumasa Uehara, Arizona State University, United States
Katsuya Ogata, Kyushu University, Japan

***Correspondence:**
Diego Centonze
centonze@uniroma2.it

Neurons in the central nervous system are organized in functional units interconnected to form complex networks. Acute and chronic brain damage disrupts brain connectivity producing neurological signs and/or symptoms. In several neurological diseases, particularly in Multiple Sclerosis (MS), structural imaging studies cannot always demonstrate a clear association between lesion site and clinical disability, originating the "clinico-radiological paradox." The discrepancy between structural damage and disability can be explained by a complex network perspective. Both brain networks architecture and synaptic plasticity may play important roles in modulating brain networks efficiency after brain damage. In particular, long-term potentiation (LTP) may occur in surviving neurons to compensate network disconnection. In MS, inflammatory cytokines dramatically interfere with synaptic transmission and plasticity. Importantly, in addition to acute and chronic structural damage, inflammation could contribute to reduce brain networks efficiency in MS leading to worse clinical recovery after a relapse and worse disease progression. These evidence suggest that removing inflammation should represent the main therapeutic target in MS; moreover, as synaptic plasticity is particularly altered by inflammation, specific strategies aimed at promoting LTP mechanisms could be effective for enhancing clinical recovery. Modulation of plasticity with different non-invasive brain stimulation (NIBS) techniques has been used to promote recovery of MS symptoms. Better knowledge of features inducing brain disconnection in MS is crucial to design specific strategies to promote recovery and use NIBS with an increasingly tailored approach.

Keywords: multiple sclerosis, inflammation, brain networks, functional connectivity, synaptic plasticity, non-invasive brain stimulation

INTRODUCTION

Multiple Sclerosis (MS) is an autoimmune inflammatory disease of the central nervous system (CNS) characterized by white matter demyelinating lesions and gray matter atrophy. MS represents one of the most frequent neurological condition associated with clinical disability in young adults. Symptoms include a huge range of manifestations such as motor/sensory deficits, fatigue, spasticity, cognitive dysfunction, and pain, related to the different neural systems involved. In several neurological disorders, and particularly in MS, structural imaging studies hardly demonstrate clear associations between lesion site and clinical disability. The peculiar discordance between radiological and clinical features is usually referred to as the "clinico-radiological paradox" (Barkhof, 2002). The remote effects of a brain lesion on functionally connected regions and the ongoing rearrangement produced by synaptic plasticity in response to brain damage can concur in determining the discrepancy between structural damage and clinical symptoms.

The concept of diaschisis (von Monakow, 1914; Feeney and Baron, 1986) refers to focal changes in metabolism or neuronal activity in anatomically intact brain regions located away from the lesion (Carrera and Tononi, 2014). Recently, the concept of diaschisis has been applied to complex networks analysis. The connectome is defined as an overall map of neural connections in the brain (Sporns et al., 2005) represented by a set of nodes (i.e., graphs) joined by lines depicted between them (Bullmore and Bassett, 2011). It is possible to explore how network activity is changed by a lesion relying upon its topography within the network architecture (Honey and Sporns, 2008; Alstott et al., 2009; Joyce et al., 2013). Accordingly, the term "connectomal diaschisis" refers to changes in the structural and functional connectome, including disconnections between and reorganization of subgraphs, involving areas located away from the lesion (Carrera and Tononi, 2014). A better definition of diaschisis could contribute to clarify the clinico-radiological paradox in neurological disorders. Understanding how lesions alter brain networks could help to select the appropriate treatment based on the underlying process. However, it is challenging to ascertain whether remote connectivity changes occur following diaschisis or rely on other recovery mechanisms, such as plasticity (either positive or maladaptive) and vicariation (Carrera and Tononi, 2014).

Clinical improvement after brain lesions mainly depends on structural and functional connectivity restoring. Synaptic plasticity is the main mechanism involved, both promoting spontaneous recovery and mediating the beneficial effects of rehabilitation. Non-invasive brain stimulation (NIBS) techniques such as repetitive transcranial magnetic stimulation (rTMS) and transcranial direct current stimulation (tDCS) perturbing local neural activity can subsequently affect the function of distributed brain regions located away from the stimulated area. Therefore, NIBS can be successfully used for testing and modulating brain networks dynamics in physiological and in a number of neuropsychiatric conditions (Shafi et al., 2012).

A number of studies suggest that inflammatory molecules released during MS relapses alter neuronal functioning acting both on synaptic transmission and plasticity (Stampanoni Bassi et al., 2017b). It is therefore reasonable to assume that inflammation in MS could disrupt brain connectivity, even regardless of demyelinating white matter lesions and gray matter atrophy. In addition, as inflammation could restrain brain network reorganization inducing synaptic plasticity alterations, promoting beneficial synaptic plasticity through NIBS could represent a promising therapeutic approach in MS.

In this paper, the main studies exploring brain connectivity in MS with different techniques will be overviewed. We performed a literature search in PubMed in August 2017 using the terms "connectivity" and "multiple sclerosis." We looked for original case-control studies, case series, or cohort studies. We also examined many of the references of the articles found. We excluded studies not available in English language, studies conducted in animals, studies published more than 10 years before, and studies including patients with age <18 years. We will also overview the alterations of synaptic transmission and plasticity described in a MS experimental model (i.e., experimental autoimmune encephalomyelitis, EAE) and in human MS using TMS. The findings supporting the role of inflammation in inducing connectivity dysfunction and the possible role of NIBS in promoting beneficial connectivity for recovery will be discussed.

CONNECTIVITY IN MS

In MS, alterations of brain connectivity have been studied with different techniques. TMS has been used to test cortico-cortical connectivity, checking how a stimulus delivered on a given brain region can influence the excitability of a different region and providing information on effective connectivity (Gerstein and Aertsen, 1985; Friston et al., 1993). Inhibitory connectivity between homologous regions of both primary motor cortices (M1) has been assessed using either a single coil or a double-coil (d-c) approach (**Figure 1**). With a single suprathreshold magnetic pulse given over M1, it is possible to induce inhibitory influences in the contralateral M1 measurable as a suppression of the tonic muscle voluntary activity ipsilateral to the stimulated cortex (ipsilateral silent period, iSP; Wassermann et al., 1991). Interhemispheric inhibition (IHI) can be also studied with d-c TMS when a suprathreshold stimulus delivered over one M1 is able to suppress the test response elicited by a suprathreshold stimulus given over the contralateral M1 at short (10 ms) or longer (40 ms) interstimulus intervals (Ferbert et al., 1992; Murase et al., 2004; Uehara et al., 2013). The two subtypes of IHI are likely mediated by different physiological mechanisms, both depending on GABAB transmission (Kukaswadia et al., 2005; Radhu et al., 2012). IHI40 could depend on an overlapping population of inhibitory neurons activated by the excitatory input from the contralateral M1 (Kukaswadia et al., 2005) whereas IHI10 may be mediated by transcallosal fibers passing through the posterior body and the isthmus of the corpus callosum (CC, Ni et al., 2009). In MS, owing to high prevalence of lesions within the CC, most TMS approaches mainly focused on interhemispheric connectivity (Boroojerdi et al., 1998; Schmierer et al., 2000; Codecà et al., 2010; Wahl et al., 2011). In MS, altered iSP correlated with clinical disability (Schmierer et al., 2000, 2002; Llufriu et al., 2012; Neva et al., 2016) and with central motor conduction time prolongation (Jung et al., 2006). Whereas, some studies showed a correlation between CC lesions and iSP alterations (Lenzi et al., 2007; Llufriu et al., 2012), other studies found that reduced iSP did not correlate with magnetic resonance imaging (MRI) alterations of the CC (Jung et al., 2006). One study reported reduced IHI in early RR-MS even without detectable CC lesions at conventional MRI, making IHI

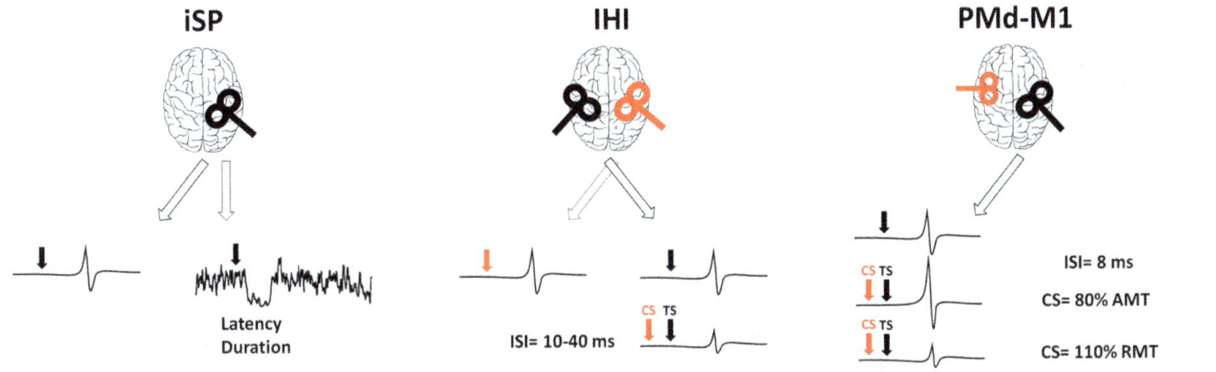

- Slower transcallosal conduction in MS patients ***(Boroojerdi et al., 1998)***
- Abnormalities of iSP in 80% of MS patients ***(Schmirer et al., 2000)***
- Abnormal iSP and CMCT correlated with EDSS. In PP-MS patients only altered iSP correlated with EDSS ***(Schmirer et al., 2002)***
- iSP duration correlated with CMCT and did not correlate with MRI alterations of the CC ***(Jung et al., 2006)***
- iSP duration was negatively correlated with activation in the iM1 on fMRI. iM1 activation correlated with T1-LL and CC alterations ***(Lenzi et al., 2007).***
- iSP latency correlated with EDSS and SDMT. iSP latency correlated with CC area and volume ***(Llufriu et a., 2012).***

- IHI_{10} was reduced in early RR-MS compared with HC. The correlation between CC microstructure and IHI_{10} observed in HC was lacking in MS. These alterations were observed in the absence of macroscopic CC lesions, motor hand/arm dysfunction in the nine-hole-peg test and prolonged CMCT ***(Wahl et al., 2011)***

- MS patients had reduced facilitation compared with HS. Only disabled MS patients showed less inhibition. PMd–M1 interactions did not differ between patients with or without lesions in the CC ***(Codecà et al., 2010)***

FIGURE 1 | Results of the main studies investigating interhemispheric connections in MS. Red coils and arrows represent CS, black coils and arrows depict TS. AMT, active motor threshold; CC, corpus callosum; CMCT, central motor conduction time; CS, conditioning stimulus; EDSS, expanded disability status scale; fMRI, functional magnetic resonance imaging; HC, healthy controls; IHI, interhemispheric inhibition; iM1, ipsilateral primary motor cortex; ISI, interstimulus interval; iSP, ipsilateral silent period; M1, primary motor cortex; PMd, dorsal premotor cortex; PP-MS, primary progressive multiple sclerosis; RMT, resting motor threshold; RR-MS, relapsing-remitting multiple sclerosis; SDMT, symbol digit modality test; T1-LL, T1 lesion load; TS, test stimulus.

failure a possible marker of callosal disconnection also at earlier disease stages (Wahl et al., 2011). Finally, altered connectivity between dorsal premotor cortex and contralateral M1 suggests that also excitatory transcallosal connectivity may be impaired independently of lesion load and site, and even in the absence of clinical disability (Codecà et al., 2010).

Recently, functional MRI (fMRI) gave the opportunity to study the activity of a large number of brain regions. FMRI is a tool able to reveal dynamic changes in brain tissue occurring whilst the subject is awake and fully relaxed (i.e., resting state fMRI, rs-fMRI), or in response to specific behavioral tasks (i.e., task-based fMRI). In MS, task-based fMRI showed increased and widespread brain activations compared to healthy controls, particularly at disease onset (Rocca et al., 2005). Increased activation is generally interpreted as adaptive plastic changes aimed at preventing the clinical manifestations (Pantano et al., 2006; Filippi and Rocca, 2013). Nevertheless, overactivation does not consequently denote adaptive plasticity, as it may be associated to high disability. For instance, diffuse microstructural damage—as shown by combined diffusion tensor imaging (DTI) and fMRI- correlated with increased sensorimotor network activation (Rocca et al., 2002; Lenzi et al., 2007). Intriguingly, increased activation of ipsilateral M1 during hand movements correlated with CC damage and loss of transcallosal inhibition (Lenzi et al., 2007) suggesting that ipsilateral M1 hyperactivation could likely represent a simple epiphenomenon of disease.

The development of methods testing brain connectivity at rest helped to avoid behavioral confounding related to task. In particular, the temporal correlation between neural or hemodynamic spontaneous activity arising from distinct brain regions, namely functional connectivity (FC), describes the intrinsic property of a given area or the influences of a particular area over another region, independently of external stimuli (Biswal et al., 1995; Fox and Raichle, 2007; van den Heuvel and Hulshoff Pol, 2010). In brain networks analysis different types of connectivity can be explored. Structural connectivity is usually referred to the anatomical connections and is evaluated by fiber tractography from DTI to obtain a reliable map of anatomical connection between brain areas. The relationship between structural and functional brain networks has not been yet completely elucidated (Rubinov et al., 2009; Honey et al., 2010; Ponten et al., 2010). Whereas, areas anatomically connected show a greater FC (Honey et al., 2007, 2009; Rubinov et al., 2009; Hermundstad et al., 2013), functional interactions are not limited to directly connected areas (Honey et al., 2007, 2009). A better definition of the complex relationship between structural and functional brain networks could predict how structural damage alters network dynamics (Honey and Sporns, 2008; Kaiser, 2013; van Dellen et al., 2013).

In MS, several studies have described rs-fMRI alterations involving different networks. Increased or decreased FC have been related to disease phenotype, clinical characteristics and neuroradiological findings (**Table 1**). Overall, findings apparently contrast likely due to different methodological approaches, and different clinical phenotypes. In addition, whether FC changes could be compensatory or maladaptive is not yet clear. Longitudinal studies or combining different experimental techniques could contribute to clarify the clinical implications of connectivity changes in MS. In addition, standardized measures should be properly identified to predict the effect of damage, evaluate symptoms evolution and compare the effect of different treatment protocols. Recently, graph based rs-fMRI studies showed that analyzing properties of large-scale brain networks could help to identify reliable measures of brain network functioning. Parameters such as clustering coefficient, path length, network centrality, and modularity, show that brain networks magnify cost efficiency of parallel information processing (Achard and Bullmore, 2007). Moreover, these properties contribute to protect networks from damage (Achard et al., 2006; Achard and Bullmore, 2007). Accordingly, clinical symptoms may occur in MS when structural damage raises to a critical level reducing overall network efficiency (Schoonheim et al., 2015).

INFLAMMATION ALTERS SYNAPTIC TRANSMISSION AND BRAIN CONNECTIVITY

In MS, brain connectivity disruption could rely on the acute and chronic structural damage and also on inflammation. In MS experimental models, inflammatory cytokines induce alterations of synaptic transmission of both glutamatergic and GABAergic transmission, causing synaptic hyperexcitability (Rossi et al., 2011; Mandolesi et al., 2013; Stampanoni Bassi et al., 2017a). Interleukin (IL)-1β represents one of the main inflammatory cytokines involved (Mandolesi et al., 2013).

Synaptic transmission can be explored in humans with TMS and specific protocols are related to different features of synaptic transmission (Ziemann et al., 2008; Rossini et al., 2015). Studies in MS showed that the same inflammatory cytokines induce synaptic alterations similar to those seen in EAE (Rossi et al., 2012a); moreover, the magnitude of these alterations correlated with CNS levels of IL-1β. Furthermore, cerebrospinal fluid from MS patients in active phase of the disease reproduced *in vitro* both the glutamatergic and GABAergic alterations and the neuronal degeneration observed in EAE (Rossi et al., 2012a,b). In addition, different phases and disease phenotypes are associated to specific patterns of alterations. In particular, the relapsing phase of MS is characterized by cortical disinhibition as indexed by reduced contralateral silent period duration and reduced short-interval intracortical inhibition (Caramia et al., 2004).

As inflammatory cytokines alter synaptic functioning, a direct role of neuroinflammation in connectivity dysfunction occurring in MS may be hypothesized. To support this view, few studies showed that in patients with clinically isolated syndrome (CIS) significant FC alterations develop even without white matter lesions or brain atrophy. One study showed significant rs-fMRI changes in a group of patients with CIS manifesting as acute optic neuritis, involving both left and right primary visual cortices and extravisual regions (Wu et al., 2015). Another study explored FC alterations in a group of RR-MS patients and in a group of patients with CIS without brain lesions (Liu et al., 2016), including patients with optic neuritis or spinal cord syndromes. CIS patients showed significantly decreased FC in the visual areas and increased FC in the temporal lobes. It should be highlighted that in both studies altered FC developed also in networks other than the visual system, likely suggesting that acute inflammation may induce diffuse connectivity changes.

It is important to mention another study exploring FC in CIS and RR-MS patients considering graph-based network analysis (Liu et al., 2017). As expected, in RR-MS patients decreased whole brain network efficiency, reduced nodal efficiency, and impaired FC were found. In addition, patients with CIS displayed a similar pattern of alterations. In particular, impaired FC involved the occipital, temporal, and frontal cortices and the insula. Finally, changes in RR-MS did not correlate with white matter lesion load and site, and with gray matter atrophy.

A number of studies showed that also systemic inflammation could affect brain FC. For instance, in healthy individuals, experimental inflammation influences brain activity in the insula and in the cingulate cortex (Hannestad et al., 2012) and alters resting connectivity between the left thalamus and the right posterior cingulate cortex (Labrenz et al., 2016). Furthermore, a study using graph analysis showed that in patients with Hepatitis C the administration of IFN α reduced whole brain network connectivity and efficiency (Dipasquale et al., 2016). Recently, a study showed that IL-6 blood levels covaried with connectivity in the default mode network (Marsland et al., 2017). These studies are in line with previous reports showing that peripheral cytokines may modulate central synaptic transmission altering task-based fMRI (Capuron et al., 2005; Harrison et al., 2009).

Overall, these data suggest that inflammation in MS, altering synaptic transmission, may represent an additional key feature contributing to network dysfunction. It may be hypothesized that, in addition to structural damage, network efficiency can be dramatically disrupted by inflammatory cytokines.

INFLAMMATION, SYNAPTIC PLASTICITY, AND CLINICAL RECOVERY

Recovery after brain injury mainly depends on the ability of surviving neurons to undergo long-term functional changes (Floel and Cohen, 2006). Long-term potentiation (LTP), the most studied form of synaptic plasticity, consists of enduring enhancement of synaptic strength followed by structural rearrangements (Bliss and Gardner-Medwin, 1973). LTP can be virtually induced in all brain areas and may reduce the clinical

TABLE 1 | Main results of studies investigating rs-FC in MS.

Authors	Study population	Main findings
Roosendaal et al., 2010	14 CIS, 31 RR-MS, 41 HCs	Increased rs-FC in several RSNs, including the DMN and sensorimotor network, in CIS compared to HCs and RR-MS. In RR-MS GM atrophy and abnormal WM diffusivity compared to HCs. No changes in CIS. rs-FC and structural MRI or clinical disability did not correlate in CIS and RR-MS.
Rocca et al., 2010	33 SP-MS (18 CI), 24 PP-MS (12 CI), 24 HCs	In SP-MS reduced activity in the DMN, in the medial prefrontal cortex and precentral gyrus, compared with HCs. In PP-MS reduced activity in the precentral gyrus and the ACC compared with HCs. In SP-MS increased ACC activity compared with PP-MS. RS activity in the ACC was reduced particularly in CI. DMN abnormalities correlated with cognitive test and DTI changes in the CC and the cingulum.
Bonavita et al., 2011	36 RR-MS (18 CI and 18 CP), 18 HCs	In RR-MS reduced DMN connectivity in the ACC, reduced in the core and increased at the periphery of the PCC. No correlations between FC changes and global atrophy or T2-LL, but association with regional GM loss. The findings were more marked in CP than CI.
Faivre et al., 2012	13 early RR-MS, 14 HCs	Increased rs-FC in several RSNs in early RR-MS compared with HCs. No correlations between RSNs connectivity and T2-LL or disease duration. Increased rs-FC in cognitive and sensorimotor networks negatively correlated with different cognitive and motor tasks and MSFC scores.
Rocca et al., 2012	85 RR-MS, 40 HCs	In RR-MS decreased rs-FC in different RSNs (salience, executive control, working memory, default mode, sensorimotor, and visual) and increased rs-FC in regions of the executive control and auditory RSNs. Decreased rs-FC was correlated with disability and T2 lesion volumes.
Tona et al., 2014	48 RR-MS, 24 HCs	In RR-MS both increased and decreased connectivity within the thalamic RSN. No significant correlation between thalamic FC and radiologic variables. Increased thalamocortical FC correlated with decreased cognitive performance.
Cruz-Gómez et al., 2014	60 RR-MS (30 CI and 30 CP), 18 HCs	Decreased rs-FC in the DMN in CI compared with CP and HCs. Decreased rs-FC in the LFPN in both CI and CP compared with HCs. Decreased rs-FC in the RFPN and salience network in CI compared with CP. BPF correlated with rs-FC in the DMN, LFPN and RFPN. T1-LL negatively correlated with rs-FC in all explored RSNs.
Louapre et al., 2014	35 RR MS (15 CI and 20 CP), 20 HCs	In CI decreased rs-FC in DMN and ATT compared with CP. In CI decreased rs-FC particularly between the medial prefrontal cortex and the PCC, predicted by PCC atrophy. In CI higher WM LL and more severe GM atrophy in cognitive networks compared with CP. In CP increased rs-FC in ATT compared with HCs.
Zhou et al., 2014	24 RR-MS and 24 HC	The connections of paired DMN subregions showed decreased SC and increased FC in RR-MS patients. SC alterations correlated with EDSS. Decreased SC was correlated to atrophy.
Rocca et al., 2015	69 CP MS, 42 HCs	In CP MS decreased rs-FC between the hippocampi and several cortical–subcortical regions within the DMN. Reduced hippocampal rs-FC correlated with T2-LL, disease duration, depression and disability.
Sbardella et al., 2015	30 RR-MS and 24 HCs	In RR-MS decreased rs-FC in several networks (cerebellar, executive-control, medial-visual, basal ganglia and sensorimotor) and changes in inter-network correlations. CC microstructural damage correlated with FC in cerebellar and auditory networks. No correlations between rs-FC in all explored RSNs and T2-LL.
Liu et al., 2015	35 RR-MS, 35 HC	Compared to HC, the MS group showed significantly decreased FC between thalamus and several brain regions including right middle frontal and parahippocampal gyri, and the left inferior parietal lobule. Increased intra and inter-thalamic FC was observed in MS compared to HC. FC alterations were not correlated with T2-LL, thalamic volume or the presence of thalamic lesions.
Baltruschat et al., 2015	17 RR-MS, 15 HCs	In RR-MS increased FC between left posterior cingulate gyrus/precuneus, and left middle temporal gyrus and left cerebellum. In RR-MS GM bilateral atrophy in posterior cingulate gyrus/precuneus. BPF negatively correlated with FC between left posterior cingulate gyrus/precuneus and left cerebellum.
Rocca et al., 2016	214 MS patients (RR-MS and SP-MS), 55 HC	Global network properties (network degree, global efficiency, hierarchy, path length and assortativity) were abnormal in MS compared with HC and contributed to distinguish CI MS patients from HC, but not the main MS phenotypes. In MS, global and regional network properties were not correlated with T2-LL and normalized brain volume.
d'Ambrosio et al., 2017	187 MS patients (136 RR-MS, 42 SP-MS and 9 PP- MS), (122 CP and 65 CI); 94 HCs	In patients lower GM, WM and thalamic volumes compared with HCs. In patients decreased rs-FC between thalamic subregions and the caudate, cingulate cortex and cerebellum correlated with worse motor performance. Increased rs-FC with the insula correlated with better motor performance. In CI increased rs-FC between thalamic subregions and temporal areas compared with CP. No correlations between thalamic rs-FC and T2-LL.

ACC, anterior cingulate cortex; ATT, attentional network; CC, corpus callosum; CI, cognitive-impaired patients; CIS, clinically isolated syndrome; CP, cognitive-preserved patients; DMN, Default Mode Network; DTI, Diffusion Tensor Imaging; FC, functional connectivity; GM, gray matter; HCs, healthy controls; LFPN, left fronto-parietal network; LL, lesion load; MRI, Magnetic Resonance Imaging; MS, Multiple Sclerosis; MSFC, Multiple Sclerosis Functional Composite Score; PCC, posterior cingulate cortex; PP-MS, primary-progressive MS patients; RFPN, right fronto-parietal network; RR-MS, relapsing-remitting MS patients; rs-FC, resting-state Functional Connectivity; RSN, resting state network; SC, structural connectivity; SP-MS, secondary-progressive MS patients; WM, white matter.

expression of neuronal damage likely restoring the excitability of neurons deprived of their synaptic inputs. Promoting LTP could therefore contribute to maximize network efficiency restoring, delaying the clinical expression of brain damage. The link between LTP and clinical recovery after acute brain lesion first came from animal studies. In rats, neurological deficit after experimental ischemia partly improved 7 days after the infarction and correlated with increased glutamatergic excitatory transmission in surviving neurons, suggesting that recovery was driven by increased excitatory synaptic activity surrounding the damaged area (Centonze et al., 2007c). In humans, the evidence that LTP could be crucial for clinical recovery was first showed in acute stroke patients, comparing the amount of TMS-induced LTP-like plasticity with the degree of recovery 6 months later. Patients with higher TMS-induced LTP displayed a better recovery (Di Lazzaro et al., 2010a). Accordingly, the term LTP reserve has been proposed to indicate the amount of LTP induced by different TMS protocols as significant predictor of clinical recovery.

Physical rehabilitation represents the main treatment option to enhance spontaneous recovery of neurological deficits Albeit early rehabilitation after acute brain lesions can facilitate recovery, the optimal treatment type is still poorly defined (Morreale et al., 2016). It is likely that the beneficial effect of rehabilitation could be mediated by LTP, as shown in animals and also in human studies by the findings that learning a motor skill engages LTP mechanisms triggered by motor practice (Rioult-Pedotti et al., 2000; Muellbacher et al., 2001; Ziemann et al., 2004).

Different studies reported alterations of synaptic plasticity in EAE and MS (Mori et al., 2011, 2012; Di Filippo et al., 2013; Nisticò et al., 2013). An early finding was that MS relapses are associated with impaired LTP-like plasticity as assessed with intermittent theta-burst stimulation (iTBS) (Mori et al., 2011). In a further study, iTBS-induced LTP-like plasticity was explored in RR-MS patients either in acute or stable disease phase, confirming that LTP-like plasticity is reduced in relapsing patients compared to remitting patients (Mori et al., 2012) Remarkably, in the same study, 6-months treatment with interferon (IFN) beta 1-a improved LTP-like plasticity in relapsing patients (Mori et al., 2012).

The association between LTP reserve and clinical recovery has been explored in RR-MS patients using the paired associative stimulation protocol (Mori et al., 2014). In this study, LTP reserve tested at the time of a clinical relapse correlated with clinical recovery 3 months later. Patients with greater LTP reserve showed a better recovery whereas patients with absent or poor LTP reserve displayed partial or absent clinical recovery, further suggesting the crucial role of LTP taking place in surviving neurons to compensate coexisting neuronal loss (Mori et al., 2014). Overall, these studies suggest that CNS inflammation in MS patients negatively influences pathways involved in LTP induction and maintenance (Tongiorgi et al., 2012; Stampanoni Bassi et al., 2017a). In addition, some studies suggest that negative impact of acute inflammation on LTP may be reduced by immune-modulating therapies (Mori et al., 2012; Di Filippo et al., 2016). In MS, it is likely that inflammation-induced LTP alterations could lessen brain network reorganization influencing clinical recovery after a relapse and disease progression and that resolving inflammation could positively influence clinical recovery.

NIBS AND SYMPTOMS RECOVERY IN MS

NIBS has been used in healthy subjects for enhancing motor skills and cognitive functions, and in neurological and psychiatric patients for therapeutic purposes (Hummel et al., 2005; Miniussi et al., 2008). Different studies showed that focal perturbation of neural activity by NIBS selectively modulates functional and effective connectivity in different connected networks (Grefkes et al., 2010; Eldaief et al., 2011; Grefkes and Fink, 2011; Cocchi et al., 2016). Furthermore, as inflammation alters synaptic plasticity, boosting LTP through NIBS could help to improve recovery in MS patients.

rTMS and tDCS represent the most commonly used NIBS techniques able to induce LTP-like plasticity (Ziemann et al., 2008). In M1, this plastic effect can be generally measured as an increase of the peak-to-peak amplitude of the motor evoked potentials (MEPs) after the plasticity-inducing protocol, likely coming from enhanced excitability of the cortico-cortical facilitatory synaptic inputs onto the corticospinal cells (Di Lazzaro et al., 2010b). A number of rTMS protocols are able to induce persistent changes in cortical excitability depending on the intensity, frequency and number of stimuli applied, frequency playing a pivotal role. In particular, high-frequency (i.e., $\geq$5 Hz) rTMS protocols produce LTP-like plasticity (Siebner and Rothwell, 2003; Ziemann et al., 2008). Subsequently, new rTMS protocols have been introduced to modulate cortical plasticity, including TBS. In particular, iTBS produces excitatory after-effects through LTP-like plasticity (Huang et al., 2005). tDCS employs weak transcranial currents to induce changes in cortical excitability depending on stimulation polarity (Nitsche and Paulus, 2000). In particular, anodal tDCS may entail LTP-like mechanisms (Liebetanz et al., 2002; Nitsche et al., 2003).

NIBS techniques have been applied to treat different symptoms in MS patients. Spasticity is considered as the consequence of the hyperexcitability of the stretch reflex secondary to corticospinal tract lesions and reduced supraspinal inhibitory input (Young, 1994). In MS, a single session of 5 Hz rTMS over M1 reduced stretch reflex hyperexcitability (Centonze et al., 2007a). Moreover, daily application for 2 weeks of both 5 Hz rTMS and iTBS can be useful to reduce lower limb spasticity in MS (Centonze et al., 2007a; Mori et al., 2010a). Noticeably, one longitudinal study showed that repeated daily iTBS sessions associated with physical rehabilitation may induce functional reorganization of M1 connectivity. In particular, reduced spasticity was associated with both changes in local connectivity and in the inter-hemispheric balance (Boutière et al., 2017). Conversely, one study reported that anodal tDCS on M1 for 5 consecutive days had no clinical impact on spasticity in MS patients (Iodice et al., 2015).

Some studies explored the effects of both anodal tDCS and 5 Hz rTMS over M1 to reduce motor deficits in MS (Koch et al., 2008; Cuypers et al., 2013; Meesen et al., 2014; Elzamarany et al., 2016). It has been shown that 5 Hz rTMS over M1 improved hand dexterity in MS patients with cerebellar symptoms (Koch et al., 2008). Intriguingly, the beneficial effect of high frequency rTMS may have raised from enhanced M1 excitatory drive onto the pontine nuclei modulating the cerebro-pontine-cerebellar network (Schwarz and Thier, 1999) and possibly counteracting the reduced cerebellar inputs to these structures due to demyelination. Similarly, another study showed that two consecutive daily sessions of 5 Hz rTMS on M1 improved hand dexterity in a group of RR and progressive MS patients, with a more pronounced effect in RR-MS (Elzamarany et al., 2016). Of the two studies exploring the effects of anodal tDCS, one study evidenced that anodal tDCS could increase cortico-spinal output (Cuypers et al., 2013) and the other study showed that a single concurrent M1 anodal tDCS session had no beneficial effects on a unimanual motor sequence task in a group of RR-MS and progressive MS (Meesen et al., 2014). In addition, repeated 5 Hz rTMS on M1 for 5 consecutive days over 2 weeks may induce beneficial effects also in other dysfunctions, such as lower urinary tract involvement (Centonze et al., 2007b). Notably, other motor symptoms including gait disturbances may respond to NIBS, as five consecutive sessions of high frequency rTMS over the left dorsolateral prefrontal cortex (DLPFC) improved gait in a RR-MS patient (Burhan et al., 2015).

In MS, neuropathic pain and both positive and negative sensory symptoms, including paresthesia and hypoanestesia, are frequently observed and scarcely responsive to pharmacological treatment. It has been reported that 5 consecutive days of anodal tDCS on M1 may improve neuropathic pain in MS (Mori et al., 2010b). In addition, another study reported that 3 consecutive days of anodal tDCS over the DLPFC reduced neuropathic pain in MS (Ayache et al., 2016). Finally, tactile hypoanesthesia improved in RR-MS after 5 consecutive days of anodal tDCS over the somatosensory cortex (Mori et al., 2013).

Fatigue represents another disabling symptom frequently observed in MS patients, occurring in all disease stages (Krupp and Pollina, 1996; Kos et al., 2004; Lerdal et al., 2007). The nature of fatigue in MS is multifactorial and it has been related to different pathophysiological mechanisms, including structural or functional brain alterations (Ayache and Chalah, 2017). Different studies explored the effects of anodal tDCS on fatigue in MS. The available studies differ in terms of parameters and stimulation sites, including M1 (Ferrucci et al., 2014), somatosensory cortex (Tecchio et al., 2014), left DLPFC (Saiote et al., 2014; Chalah et al., 2015, 2017), and right posterior parietal cortex (Chalah et al., 2017). Overall, whereas the results suggest that tDCS may represent a promising approach to treat fatigue, further studies are needed to define the optimal stimulation parameters and site (Lefaucheur et al., 2017).

Finally, only few studies explored the use of NIBS for treating cognitive deficits associated with MS. One study showed that 10 daily sessions of anodal tDCS over the left DLPFC significantly improved concurrent cognitive training (Mattioli et al., 2016). Another study explored the effects of 5 Hz rTMS over the right DLPFC on working memory deficits (Hulst et al., 2016). In that study, cognitive performance improvement was associated with a reduced aberrant hyperactivation of the prefrontal areas observed in MS patients. It is worth noting that although cognitive activities are subserved by diffuse networks, focal modulation of a node may induce functional changes in remote regions (Siebner et al., 2009).

CONCLUSIONS

Improved understanding of features inducing brain disconnection in MS (i.e., demyelination, neurodegeneration, inflammation) and those influencing recovery (i.e., plasticity) may help to characterize the underlying pathophysiology. As neuroinflammation could induce brain connectivity dysfunction and impair network reorganization, contrasting inflammation may hinder connectivity disruption in MS. Furthermore, strategies aimed at promoting plasticity could be particularly relevant in MS, as plasticity reserve is reduced in these patients. Although NIBS could represent a promising approach for treating different symptoms in MS, it will be useful to identify the brain areas that should be stimulated and relate the lesion site to therapeutic response, establish the need to perform consecutive stimulation sessions and better predict the individual response to NIBS, also considering that in MS plasticity is altered in response to inflammation. It is therefore crucial to understand how focal modulation of brain activity by NIBS can enhance network efficiency. In particular, identifying anatomical and functional principles determining how local perturbations affect large-scale neural activity (Sale et al., 2015) may help to predict the impact of NIBS on brain network reorganization (Gollo et al., 2017). This could help to define whether restoring the original networks or promoting alternative circuits could be the best strategy for recovery, and therefore to use NIBS with an increasingly tailored approach.

AUTHOR CONTRIBUTIONS

MS and EI: work conception and design, drafting the work, work revision, final approval and global agreement; LG: work conception and design, work revision, final approval and global agreement; FB, PM, GM, and DR: work revision, final approval and global agreement; DC: work conception and design, guarantor of integrity of entire study, manuscript revision for important intellectual content, final approval.

REFERENCES

Achard, S., and Bullmore, E. (2007). Efficiency and cost of economical brain functional networks. *PLoS Comput. Biol.* 3:e17. doi: 10.1371/journal.pcbi.0030017

Achard, S., Salvador, R., Whitcher, B., Suckling, J., and Bullmore, E. D. (2006). A resilient, low-frequency, small-world human brain functional network with highly connected association cortical hubs. *J. Neurosci.* 26, 63–72. doi: 10.1523/JNEUROSCI.3874-05.2006

d'Ambrosio, A., Hidalgo de la Cruz, M., Valsasina, P., Pagani, E., Colombo, B., Rodegher, M., et al. (2017). Structural connectivity-defined thalamic subregions have different functional connectivity abnormalities in multiple sclerosis patients: implications for clinical correlations. *Hum. Brain Mapp.* 38, 6005–6018. doi: 10.1002/hbm.23805

Alstott, J., Breakspear, M., Hagmann, P., Cammoun, L., and Sporns, O. (2009). Modeling the impact of lesions in the human brain. *PLoS Comput. Biol.* 5:e1000408. doi: 10.1371/journal.pcbi.1000408

Ayache, S. S., and Chalah, M. A. (2017). Fatigue in multiple sclerosis– Insights into evaluation and management. *Neurophysiol. Clin.* 47, 139–171. doi: 10.1016/j.neucli.2017.02.004

Ayache, S. S., Palm, U., Chalah, M. A., Al-Ani, T., Brignol, A., Abdellaoui, M., et al. (2016). Prefrontal tDCS decreases pain in patients with multiple sclerosis. *Front. Neurosci.* 10:147. doi: 10.3389/fnins.2016.00147

Baltruschat, S. A., Ventura-Campos, N., Cruz-Gómez, Á. J., Belenguer, A., and Forn, C. (2015). Gray matter atrophy is associated with functional connectivity reorganization during the Paced Auditory Serial Addition Test (PASAT) execution in Multiple Sclerosis (MS). *J. Neuroradiol.* 42, 141–149. doi: 10.1016/j.neurad.2015.02.006

Barkhof, F. (2002). The clinico-radiological paradox in multiple sclerosis revisited. *Curr. Opin. Neurol.* 15, 239–245. doi: 10.1097/00019052-200206000-00003

Biswal, B., Yetkin, F. Z., Haughton, V. M., and Hyde, J. S. (1995). Functional connectivity in the motor cortex of resting human brain using echo-planar MRI. *Magn. Reson. Med.* 34, 537–541. doi: 10.1002/mrm.1910340409

Bliss, T. V., and Gardner-Medwin, A. R. (1973). Long-lasting potentiation of synaptic transmission in the dentate area of the unanaesthetized rabbit following stimulation of the perforant path, *J. Physiol.* 232, 357–374. doi: 10.1113/jphysiol.1973.sp010274

Bonavita, S., Gallo, A., Sacco, R., Corte, M. D., Bisecco, A., Docimo, R., et al. (2011). Distributed changes in default-mode resting-state connectivity in multiple sclerosis. *Mult. Scler.* 17, 411–422. doi: 10.1177/1352458510394609

Boroojerdi, B., Hungs, M., Mull, M., Töpper, R., and Noth, J. (1998). Interhemispheric inhibition in patients with multiple sclerosis. *Electroencephalogr. Clin. Neurophysiol.* 109, 230–237. doi: 10.1016/S0924-980X(98)00013-7

Boutière, C., Rey, C., Zaaraoui, W., Le Troter, A., Rico, A., Crespy, L., et al. (2017). Improvement of spasticity following intermittent theta burst stimulation in multiple sclerosis is associated with modulation of resting-state functional connectivity of the primary motor cortices. *Mult. Scler.* 23, 855–863. doi: 10.1177/1352458516661640

Bullmore, E. T., and Bassett, D. S. (2011). Brain graphs: graphical models of the human brain connectome. *Annu. Rev. Clin. Psychol.* 7, 113–140. doi: 10.1146/annurev-clinpsy-040510-143934

Burhan, A. M., Subramanian, P., Pallaveshi, L., Barnes, B., and Montero-Odasso, M. (2015). Modulation of the left prefrontal cortex with high frequency repetitive transcranial magnetic stimulation facilitates gait in multiple sclerosis. *Case Rep. Neurol. Med.* 2015:251829. doi: 10.1155/2015/251829

Capuron, L., Pagnoni, G., Demetrashvili, M., Woolwine, B. J., Nemeroff, C. B., Berns, G. S., et al. (2005). Anterior cingulate activation and error processing during interferon-alpha treatment. *Biol. Psychiatry* 58, 190–196. doi: 10.1016/j.biopsych.2005.03.033

Caramia, M. D., Palmieri, M. G., Desiato, M. T., Boffa, L., Galizia, P., Rossini, P. M., et al. (2004). Brain excitability changes in the relapsing and remitting phases of multiple sclerosis: a study with transcranial magnetic stimulation. *Clin. Neurophysiol.* 115, 956–965. doi: 10.1016/j.clinph.2003.11.024

Carrera, E., and Tononi, G. (2014). Diaschisis: past, present, future. *Brain* 137, 2408–2422. doi: 10.1093/brain/awu101

Centonze, D., Koch, G., Versace, V., Mori, F., Rossi, S., Brusa, L., et al. (2007a). Repetitive transcranial magnetic stimulation of the motor cortex ameliorates spasticity in multiple sclerosis. *Neurology* 68, 1045–1050. doi: 10.1212/01.wnl.0000257818.16952.62

Centonze, D., Petta, F., Versace, V., Rossi, S., Torelli, F., Prosperetti, C., et al. (2007b). Effects of motor cortex rTMS on lower urinary tract dysfunction in multiple sclerosis. *Mult. Scler.* 13, 269–271. doi: 10.1177/1352458506070729

Centonze, D., Rossi, S., Tortiglione, A., Picconi, B., Prosperetti, C., De Chiara, V., et al. (2007c). Synaptic plasticity during recovery from permanent occlusion of the middle cerebral artery. *Neurobiol. Dis.* 27, 44–53. doi: 10.1016/j.nbd.2007.03.012

Chalah, M. A., Riachi, N., Ahdab, R., Créange, A., Lefaucheur, J. P., and Ayache, S. S. (2015). Fatigue in multiple sclerosis: neural correlates and the role of non-invasive brain stimulation. *Front. Cell. Neurosci.* 9:460. doi: 10.3389/fncel.2015.00460

Chalah, M. A., Riachi, N., Ahdab, R., Mhalla, A., Abdellaoui, M., Créange, A., et al. (2017). Effects of left DLPFC vs. right PPC tDCS on multiple sclerosis fatigue. *J. Neurol. Sci.* 372, 131–137. doi: 10.1016/j.jns.2016.11.015

Cocchi, L., Sale, M. V., Gollo, L. L., Bell, P. T., Nguyen, V. T., Zalesky, A., et al. (2016). A hierarchy of timescales explains distinct effects of local inhibition of primary visual cortex and frontal eye fields. *Elife* 5:e15252. doi: 10.7554/eLife.15252

Codecà, C., Mori, F., Kusayanagi, H., Monteleone, F., Boffa, L., Paolillo, A., et al. (2010). Differential patterns of interhemispheric functional disconnection in mild and advanced multiple sclerosis. *Mult. Scler.* 16, 1308–1316. doi: 10.1177/1352458510376957

Cruz-Gómez, Á. J., Ventura-Campos, N., Belenguer, A., Ávila, C., and Forn, C. (2014). The link between resting-state functional connectivity and cognition in MS patients. *Mult. Scler.* 20, 338–348. doi: 10.1177/1352458513495584

Cuypers, K., Leenus, D. J., Van Wijmeersch, B., Thijs, H., Levin, O., Swinnen, S. P., et al. (2013). Anodal tDCS increases corticospinal output and projection strength in multiple sclerosis. *Neurosci. Lett.* 554, 151–155. doi: 10.1016/j.neulet.2013.09.004

Di Filippo, M., Chiasserini, D., Gardoni, F., Viviani, B., Tozzi, A., Giampà, C., et al. (2013). Effects of central and peripheral inflammation on hippocampal synaptic plasticity. *Neurobiol. Dis.* 52, 229–236. doi: 10.1016/j.nbd.2012.12.009

Di Filippo, M., de Iure, A., Giampà, C., Chiasserini, D., Tozzi, A., Orvietani, P. L., et al. (2016). Persistent activation of microglia and NADPH oxidase drive hippocampal dysfunction in experimental multiple sclerosis. *Sci. Rep.* 18:20926. doi: 10.1038/srep20926

Di Lazzaro, V., Profice, P., Pilato, F., Capone, F., Ranieri, F., Pasqualetti, P., et al. (2010a). Motor cortex plasticity predicts recovery in acute stroke. *Cereb. Cortex* 20, 1523–1528. doi: 10.1093/cercor/bhp216

Di Lazzaro, V., Profice, P., Pilato, F., Dileone, M., Oliviero, A., and Ziemann, U. (2010b). The effects of motor cortex rTMS on corticospinal descending activity. *Clin. Neurophysiol.* 121, 464–473. doi: 10.1016/j.clinph.2009.11.007

Dipasquale, O., Cooper, E. A., Tibble, J., Voon, V., Baglio, F., Baselli, G., et al. (2016). Interferon-α acutely impairs whole-brain functional connectivity network architecture–A preliminary study. *Brain Behav. Immun.* 58, 31–39. doi: 10.1016/j.bbi.2015.12.011

Eldaief, M. C., Halko, M. A., Buckner, R. L., and Pascual-Leone, A. (2011). Transcranial magnetic stimulation modulates the brain's intrinsic activity in a frequency-dependent manner. *Proc. Natl. Acad. Sci. U.S.A.* 108, 21229–21234. doi: 10.1073/pnas.1113103109

Elzamarany, E., Afifi, L., El-Fayoumy, N. M., Salah, H., and Nada, M. (2016). Motor cortex rTMS improves dexterity in relapsing-remitting and secondary progressive multiple sclerosis. *Acta Neurol. Belg.* 116, 145–150. doi: 10.1007/s13760-015-0540-y

Faivre, A., Rico, A., Zaaraoui, W., Crespy, L., Reuter, F., Wybrecht, D., et al. (2012). Assessing brain connectivity at rest is clinically relevant in early multiple sclerosis. *Mult. Scler.* 18, 1251–1258. doi: 10.1177/1352458511435930

Feeney, D. M., and Baron, J. C. (1986). Diaschisis. *Stroke* 17, 817–830. doi: 10.1161/01.STR.17.5.817

Ferbert, A., Priori, A., Rothwell, J. C., Day, B. L., Colebatch, J. G., and Marsden, C. D. (1992). Interhemispheric inhibition of the human motor cortex. *J. Physiol.* 453, 525–546. doi: 10.1113/jphysiol.1992.sp019243

Ferrucci, R., Vergari, M., Cogiamanian, F., Bocci, T., Ciocca, M., Tomasini, E., et al. (2014). Transcranial direct current stimulation (tDCS) for fatigue in multiple sclerosis. *Neuro Rehabil.* 34, 121–127. doi: 10.3233/NRE-131019.

Filippi, M., and Rocca, M. A. (2013). Present and future of fMRI in multiple sclerosis. *Expert Rev. Neurother.* 13, 27–31. doi: 10.1586/14737175.2013.865871

Floel, A., and Cohen, L. G. (2006). Translational studies in neurorehabilitation: from bench to bedside. *Cogn. Behav. Neurol.* 19, 1–10. doi: 10.1097/00146965-200603000-00001

Fox, M. D., and Raichle, M. E. (2007). Spontaneous fluctuations in brain activity observed with functional magnetic resonance imaging. *Nat. Rev. Neurosci.* 8, 700–711. doi: 10.1038/nrn2201

Friston, K. J., Frith, C. D., and Frackowiak, R. S. J. (1993). Time-dependent changes in effective connectivity measured with PET. *Hum. Brain Mapp.* 1, 69–79. doi: 10.1002/hbm.460010108

Gerstein, G. L., and Aertsen, A. M. (1985). Representation of cooperative firing activity among simultaneously recorded neurons. *J. Neurophysiol.* 54, 1513–1528.

Gollo, L. L., Roberts, J. A., and Cocchi, L. (2017). Mapping how local perturbations influence systems-level brain dynamics. *Neuroimage* 160, 97–112. doi: 10.1016/j.neuroimage.2017.01.057

Grefkes, C., and Fink, G. R. (2011). Reorganization of cerebral networks after stroke: new insights from neuroimaging with connectivity approaches. *Brain* 134, 1264–1276. doi: 10.1093/brain/awr033

Grefkes, C., Nowak, D. A., Wang, L. E., Dafotakis, M., Eickhoff, S. B., and Fink, G. R. (2010). Modulating cortical connectivity in stroke patients by rTMS assessed with fMRI and dynamic causal modeling. *Neuroimage* 50, 233–242. doi: 10.1016/j.neuroimage.2009.12.029

Hannestad, J., Gallezot, J. D., Schafbauer, T., Lim, K., Kloczynski, T., Morris, E. D., et al. (2012). Endotoxin-induced systemic inflammation activates microglia:[11C] PBR28 positron emission tomography in nonhuman primates. *Neuroimage* 63, 232–239. doi: 10.1016/j.neuroimage.2012.06.055

Harrison, N. A., Brydon, L., Walker, C., Gray, M. A., Steptoe, A., Dolan, R. J., et al. (2009). Neural origins of human sickness in interoceptive responses to inflammation. *Biol. Psychiatry* 66, 415–422. doi: 10.1016/j.biopsych.2009.03.007

Hermundstad, A. M., Bassett, D. S., Brown, K. S., Aminoff, E. M., Clewett, D., Freeman, S., et al. (2013). Structural foundations of resting-state and task-based functional connectivity in the human brain. *Proc. Natl. Acad. Sci. U.S.A.* 110, 6169–6174. doi: 10.1073/pnas.1219562110

Honey, C. J., Kötter, R., Breakspear, M., and Sporns, O. (2007). Network structure of cerebral cortex shapes functional connectivity on multiple time scales. *Proc. Natl. Acad. Sci. U.S.A.* 104, 10240–10245. doi: 10.1073/pnas.0701519104

Honey, C. J., and Sporns, O. (2008). Dynamical consequences of lesions in cortical networks. *Hum. Brain Mapp.* 29, 802–809. doi: 10.1002/hbm.20579

Honey, C. J., Sporns, O., Cammoun, L., Gigandet, X., Thiran, J. P., Meuli, R., et al. (2009). Predicting human resting-state functional connectivity from structural connectivity. *Proc. Natl. Acad. Sci. U.S.A.* 106, 2035–2040. doi: 10.1073/pnas.0811168106

Honey, C. J., Thivierge, J. P., and Sporns, O. (2010). Can structure predict function in the human brain? *Neuroimage* 52, 766–776. doi: 10.1016/j.neuroimage.2010.01.071

Huang, Y. Z., Edwards, M. J., Rounis, E., Bhatia, K. P., and Rothwell, J. C. (2005). Theta burst stimulation of the human motor cortex. *Neuron* 45, 201–206. doi: 10.1016/j.neuron.2004.12.033

Hulst, H. E., Goldschmidt, T., Nitsche, M. A., de Wit, S. J., van den Heuvel, O. A., Barkhof, F., et al. (2016). rTMS affects working memory performance, brain activation and functional connectivity in patients with multiple sclerosis. *J. Neurol. Neurosurg. Psychiatr.* 88, 386–394. doi: 10.1136/jnnp-2016-314224

Hummel, F., Celnik, P., Giraux, P., Floel, A., Wu, W. H., Gerloff, C., et al. (2005). Effects of non-invasive cortical stimulation on skilled motor function in chronic stroke. *Brain* 128, 490–499. doi: 10.1093/brain/awh369

Iodice, R., Dubbioso, R., Ruggiero, L., Santoro, L., and Manganelli, F. (2015). Anodal transcranial direct current stimulation of motor cortex does not ameliorate spasticity in multiple sclerosis. *Restor. Neurol. Neurosci.* 33, 487–492. doi: 10.3233/RNN-150495

Joyce, K. E., Hayasaka, S., and Laurienti, P. J. (2013). The human functional brain network demonstrates structural and dynamical resilience to targeted attack. *PLoS Comput. Biol.* 9:e1002885. doi: 10.1371/journal.pcbi.1002885

Jung, P., Beyerle, A., Humpich, M., Neumann-Haefelin, T., Lanfermann, H., and Ziemann, U. (2006). Ipsilateral silent period: a marker of callosal conduction abnormality in early relapsing–remitting multiple sclerosis? *J. Neurol. Sci.* 250, 133–139. doi: 10.1016/j.jns.2006.08.008

Kaiser, M. (2013). The potential of the human connectome as a biomarker of brain disease. *Front. Hum. Neurosci.* 7:484. doi: 10.3389/fnhum.2013.00484

Koch, G., Rossi, S., Prosperetti, C., Codecà, C., Monteleone, F., Petrosini, L., et al. (2008). Improvement of hand dexterity following motor cortex rTMS in multiple sclerosis patients with cerebellar impairment. *Mult. Scler.* 14, 995–998. doi: 10.1177/1352458508088710

Kos, D., Kerckhofs, E., Ketelaer, P., Duportail, M., Nagels, G., D'Hooghe, M., et al. (2004). Self-report assessment of fatigue in multiple sclerosis: a critical evaluation. *Occup. Ther. Health Care* 17, 45–62. doi: 10.1080/J003v17n03_04

Krupp, L. B., and Pollina, D. A. (1996). Mechanisms and management of fatigue in progressive neurological disorders. *Curr. Opin. Neurol.* 9, 456–460. doi: 10.1097/00019052-199612000-00011

Kukaswadia, S., Wagle-Shukla, A., Morgante, F., Gunraj, C., and Chen, R. (2005). Interactions between long latency afferent inhibition and interhemispheric inhibitions in the human motor cortex. *J. Physiol.* 563, 915–924. doi: 10.1113/jphysiol.2004.080010

Labrenz, F., Wrede, K., Forsting, M., Engler, H., Schedlowski, M., Elsenbruch, S., et al. (2016). Alterations in functional connectivity of resting state networks during experimental endotoxemia–an exploratory study in healthy men. *Brain Behav. Immun.* 54, 17–26. doi: 10.1016/j.bbi.2015.11.010

Lefaucheur, J. P., Chalah, M. A., Mhalla, A., Palm, U., Ayache, S. S., and Mylius, V. (2017). The treatment of fatigue by non-invasive brain stimulation. *Neurophysiol. Clin.* 47, 173–184. doi: 10.1016/j.neucli.2017.03.003

Lenzi, D., Conte, A., Mainero, C., Frasca, V., Fubelli, F., Totaro, P., et al. (2007). Effect of corpus callosum damage on ipsilateral motor activation in patients with multiple sclerosis: a functional and anatomical study. *Hum. Brain Mapp.* 28, 636–644. doi: 10.1002/hbm.20305

Lerdal, A., Celius, E. G., Krupp, L., and Dahl, A. A. (2007). A prospective study of patterns of fatigue in multiple sclerosis. *Eur. J. Neurol.* 14, 1338–1343. doi: 10.1111/j.1468-1331.2007.01974.x

Liebetanz, D., Nitsche, M. A., Tergau, F., and Paulus, W. (2002). Pharmacological approach to the mechanisms of transcranial DC-stimulation-induced after-effects of human motor cortex excitability. *Brain* 125, 2238–2247. doi: 10.1093/brain/awf238

Liu, Y., Dai, Z., Duan, Y., Huang, J., Ren, Z., Liu, Z., et al. (2016). Whole brain functional connectivity in clinically isolated syndrome without conventional brain MRI lesions. *Eur. Radiol.* 26, 2982–2991. doi: 10.1007/s00330-015-4147-8

Liu, Y., Liang, P., Duan, Y., Huang, J., Ren, Z., Jia, X., et al. (2015). Altered thalamic functional connectivity in multiple sclerosis. *Eur. J. Radiol.* 84, 703–708. doi: 10.1016/j.ejrad.2015.01.001

Liu, Y., Wang, H., Duan, Y., Huang, J., Ren, Z., Ye, J., et al. (2017). Functional brain network alterations in clinically isolated syndrome and multiple sclerosis: a graph-based connectome study. *Radiology* 282, 534–541. doi: 10.1148/radiol.2016152843

Llufriu, S., Blanco, Y., Martinez-Heras, E., Casanova-Molla, J., Gabilondo, I., Sepulveda, M., et al. (2012). Influence of corpus callosum damage on cognition and physical disability in multiple sclerosis: a multimodal study. *PLoS ONE* 7:e37167. doi: 10.1371/journal.pone.0037167

Louapre, C., Perlbarg, V., García-Lorenzo, D., Urbanski, M., Benali, H., Assouad, R., et al. (2014). Brain networks disconnection in early multiple sclerosis cognitive deficits: an anatomofunctional study. *Hum. Brain Mapp.* 35, 4706–4717. doi: 10.1002/hbm.22505

Mandolesi, G., Musella, A., Gentile, A., Grasselli, G., Haji, N., Sepman, H., et al. (2013). Interleukin-1β alters glutamate transmission at purkinje cell synapses in a mouse model of multiple sclerosis. *J. Neurosci.* 33, 12105–12121. doi: 10.1523/JNEUROSCI.5369-12.2013

Marsland, A. L., Kuan, D. C. H., Sheu, L. K., Krajina, K., Kraynak, T. E., Manuck, S. B., et al. (2017). Systemic inflammation and resting state connectivity of the default mode network. *Brain Behav. Immun.* 62, 162–170. doi: 10.1016/j.bbi.2017.01.013

Mattioli, F., Bellomi, F., Stampatori, C., Capra, R., and Miniussi, C. (2016). Neuroenhancement through cognitive training and anodal tDCS in multiple sclerosis. *Mult. Scler.* 22, 222–2230. doi: 10.1177/1352458515587597

Meesen, R. L., Thijs, H., Leenus, D. J., and Cuypers, K. (2014). A single session of 1 mA anodal tDCS-supported motor training does not improve motor performance in patients with multiple sclerosis. *Restor. Neurol. Neurosci.* 32, 293–300. doi: 10.3233/RNN-130348

Miniussi, C., Cappa, S. F., Cohen, L. G., Floel, A., Fregni, F., Nitsche, M. A., et al. (2008). Efficacy of repetitive transcranial magnetic stimulation/transcranial direct current stimulation in cognitive neurorehabilitation. *Brain Stimul.* 1, 326–336. doi: 10.1016/j.brs.2008.07.002

Mori, F., Codecà, C., Kusayanagi, H., Monteleone, F., Boffa, L., Rimano, A., et al. (2010a). Effects of intermittent theta burst stimulation on spasticity in patients with multiple sclerosis. *Eur. J. Neurol.* 17, 295–300. doi: 10.1111/j.1468-1331.2009.02806.x

Mori, F., Codecà, C., Kusayanagi, H., Monteleone, F., Buttari, F., Fiore, S., et al. (2010b). Effects of anodal transcranial direct current stimulation on chronic neuropathic pain in patients with multiple sclerosis. *J. Pain.* 11, 436–442. doi: 10.1016/j.jpain.2009.08.011

Mori, F., Kusayanagi, H., Buttari, F., Centini, B., Monteleone, F., Nicoletti, C. G., et al. (2012). Early treatment with high-dose interferon beta-1a reverses cognitive and cortical plasticity deficits in multiple sclerosis. *Funct. Neurol.* 27, 163–168.

Mori, F., Kusayanagi, H., Nicoletti, C. G., Weiss, S., Marciani, M. G., and Centonze, D. (2014). Cortical plasticity predicts recovery from relapse in multiple sclerosis. *Mult. Scler.* 20, 451–457. doi: 10.1177/1352458513512541

Mori, F., Nicoletti, C. G., Kusayanagi, H., Foti, C., Restivo, D. A., Marciani, M. G., et al. (2013). Transcranial direct current stimulation ameliorates tactile sensory deficit in multiple sclerosis. *Brain Stimul.* 6, 654–659. doi: 10.1016/j.brs.2012.10.003

Mori, F., Rossi, S., Sancesario, G., Codecà, C., Mataluni, G., Monteleone, F., et al. (2011). Cognitive and cortical plasticity deficits correlate with altered amyloid-β CSF levels in multiple sclerosis. *Neuropsychopharmacology* 36, 559–568. doi: 10.1038/npp.2010.187

Morreale, M., Marchione, P., Pili, A., Lauta, A., Castiglia, S. F., Spallone, A., et al. (2016). Early vs. delayed rehabilitation treatment in hemiplegic patients with ischemic stroke: proprioceptive or cognitive approach? *Eur. J. Phys. Rehabil. Med.* 52, 81–89.

Muellbacher, W., Ziemann, U., Boroojerdi, B., Cohen, L., and Hallett, M. (2001). Role of the human motor cortex in rapid motor learning. *Exp. Brain Res.*136, 431–438. doi: 10.1007/s002210000614

Murase, N., Duque, J., Mazzocchio, R., and Cohen, L. G. (2004). Influence of interhemispheric interactions on motor function in chronic stroke. *Ann. Neurol.* 55, 400–409. doi: 10.1002/ana.10848

Neva, J. L., Lakhani, B., Brown, K. E., Wadden, K. P., Mang, C. S., Ledwell, N. H. M., et al. (2016). Multiple measures of corticospinal excitability are associated with clinical features of multiple sclerosis. *Behav. Brain Res.* 297, 187–195. doi: 10.1016/j.bbr.2015.10.015

Ni, Z., Gunraj, C., Nelson, A. J., Yeh, I. J., Castillo, G., Hoque, T., et al. (2009). Two phases of interhemispheric inhibition between motor related cortical areas and the primary motor cortex in human. *Cereb. Cortex* 19, 1654–1665. doi: 10.1093/cercor/bhn201

Nisticò, R., Mango, D., Mandolesi, G., Piccinin, S., Berretta, N., Pignatelli, M., et al. (2013). Inflammation subverts hippocampal synaptic plasticity in experimental multiple sclerosis. *PLoS ONE* 8:e54666. doi: 10.1371/journal.pone.0054666

Nitsche, M. A., Fricke, K., Henschke, U., Schlitterlau, A., Liebetanz, D., Lang, N., et al. (2003). Pharmacological modulation of cortical excitability shifts induced by transcranial direct current stimulation in humans. *J. Physiol.* 553, 293–301. doi: 10.1113/jphysiol.2003.049916

Nitsche, M. A., and Paulus, W. (2000). Excitability changes induced in the human motor cortex by weak transcranial direct current stimulation. *J. Physiol.* 527, 633–639. doi: 10.1111/j.1469-7793.2000.t01-1-00633.x

Pantano, P., Mainero, C., and Caramia, F. (2006). Functional brain reorganization in multiple sclerosis: evidence from fMRI studies. *J. Neuroimaging* 16, 104–114. doi: 10.1111/j.1552-6569.2006.00029.x

Ponten, S. C., Daffertshofer, A., Hillebrand, A., and Stam, C. J. (2010). The relationship between structural and functional connectivity: graph theoretical analysis of an EEG neural mass model. *Neuroimage* 52, 985–994. doi: 10.1016/j.neuroimage.2009.10.049

Radhu, N., Ravindran, L. N., Levinson, A. J., and Daskalakis, Z. J. (2012). Inhibition of the cortex using transcranial magnetic stimulation in psychiatric populations: current and future directions. *J. Psychiatry Neurosci.* 37, 369–378. doi: 10.1503/jpn.120003

Rioult-Pedotti, M. S., Friedman, D., and Donoghue, J. P. (2000). Learning-induced LTP in neocortex. *Science* 290, 533–536. doi: 10.1126/science.290.5491.533

Rocca, M. A., Colombo, B., Falini, A., Ghezzi, A., Martinelli, V., Scotti, G., et al. (2005). Cortical adaptation in patients with MS: a cross-sectional functional MRI study of disease phenotypes. *Lancet Neurol.* 4, 618–626. doi: 10.1016/S1474-4422(05)70171-X

Rocca, M. A., Falini, A., Colombo, B., Scotti, G., Comi, G., and Filippi, M. (2002). Adaptive functional changes in the cerebral cortex of patients with non-disabling multiple sclerosis correlate with the extent of brain structural damage. *Ann. Neurol.* 51, 330–339. doi: 10.1002/ana.10120

Rocca, M. A., Pravatà, E., Valsasina, P., Radaelli, M., Colombo, B., Vacchi, L., et al. (2015). Hippocampal-DMN disconnectivity in MS is related to WM lesions and depression. *Hum. Brain Mapp.* 36, 5051–5063. doi: 10.1002/hbm.22992

Rocca, M. A., Valsasina, P., Absinta, M., Riccitelli, G., Rodegher, M. E., Misci, P., et al. (2010). Default-mode network dysfunction and cognitive impairment in progressive MS. *Neurology* 74, 1252–1259. doi: 10.1212/WNL.0b013e3181d9ed91

Rocca, M. A., Valsasina, P., Martinelli, V., Misci, P., Falini, A., Comi, G., et al. (2012). Large-scale neuronal network dysfunction in relapsing-remitting multiple sclerosis. *Neurology* 79, 1449–1457. doi: 10.1212/WNL.0b013e31826d5f10

Rocca, M. A., Valsasina, P., Meani, A., Falini, A., Comi, G., and Filippi, M. (2016). Impaired functional integration in multiple sclerosis: a graph theory study. *Brain Struct. Funct.* 221, 115–131. doi: 10.1007/s00429-014-0896-4

Roosendaal, S. D., Schoonheim, M. M., Hulst, H. E., Sanz-Arigita, E. J., Smith, S. M., Geurts, J. J., et al. (2010). Resting state networks change in clinically isolated syndrome. *Brain* 133, 1612–1621. doi: 10.1093/brain/awq058

Rossi, S., Furlan, R., De Chiara, V., Motta, C., Studer, V., Mori, F., et al. (2012a). Interleukin-1β causes synaptic hyperexcitability in multiple sclerosis. *Ann. Neurol.* 71, 76–83. doi: 10.1002/ana.22512

Rossi, S., Muzio, L., De Chiara, V., Grasselli, G., Musella, A., Musumeci, G., et al. (2011). Impaired striatal GABA transmission in experimental autoimmune encephalomyelitis. *Brain Behav. Immun.* 25, 947–956. doi: 10.1016/j.bbi.2010.10.004

Rossi, S., Studer, V., Motta, C., De Chiara, V., Barbieri, F., Bernanrdi, G., et al. (2012b). Inflammation inhibits GABA transmission in multiple sclerosis. *Mult. Scler.* 18, 1633–1635. doi: 10.1177/1352458512440207

Rossini, P. M., Burke, D., Chen, R., Cohen, L. G., Daskalakis, Z., Di Iorio, R., et al. (2015). Non-invasive electrical and magnetic stimulation of the brain, spinal cord, roots and peripheral nerves: basic principles and procedures for routine clinical and research application. An updated report from an IFCN Committee. *Clin. Neurophysiol.* 126, 1071–1107. doi: 10.1016/j.clinph.2015.02.001

Rubinov, M., Sporns, O., van Leeuwen, C., and Breakspear, M. (2009). Symbiotic relationship between brain structure and dynamics. *BMC Neurosci.* 10:55. doi: 10.1186/1471-2202-10-55

Saiote, C., Goldschmidt, T., Timäus, C., Steenwijk, M. D., Opitz, A., Antal, A., et al. (2014). Impact of transcranial direct current stimulation on fatigue in multiple sclerosis. *Restor. Neurol. Neurosci.* 32, 423–436. doi: 10.3233/RNN-130372

Sale, M. V., Mattingley, J. B., Zalesky, A., and Cocchi, L. (2015). Imaging human brain networks to improve the clinical efficacy of non-invasive brain stimulation. *Neurosci. Biobehav. Rev.* 57, 187–198. doi: 10.1016/j.neubiorev.2015.09.010

Sbardella, E., Tona, F., Petsas, N., Upadhyay, N., Piattella, M. C., Filippini, N., et al. (2015). Functional connectivity changes and their relationship with clinical disability and white matter integrity in patients with relapsing-remitting multiple sclerosis. *Mult. Scler.* 21, 1681–1692. doi: 10.1177/1352458514568826

Schmierer, K., Irlbacher, K., Grosse, P., Röricht, S., and Meyer, B. U. (2002). Correlates of disability in multiple sclerosis detected by transcranial magnetic stimulation. *Neurology* 59, 1218–1224. doi: 10.1212/WNL.59.8.1218

Schmierer, K., Niehaus, L., Röricht, S., and Meyer, B. U. (2000). Conduction deficits of callosal fibres in early multiple sclerosis. *J. Neurol. Neurosurg. Psychiatr.* 68, 633–638. doi: 10.1136/jnnp.68.5.633

Schoonheim, M. M., Meijer, K. A., and Geurts, J. J. (2015). Network collapse and cognitive impairment in multiple sclerosis. *Front. Neurol.* 6:82. doi: 10.3389/fneur.2015.00082.

Schwarz, C., and Thier, P. (1999). Binding of signals relevant for action: towards a hypothesis of the functional role of the pontine nuclei. *Trends Neurosci.* 22, 443–451. doi: 10.1016/S0166-2236(99)01446-0

Shafi, M. M., Westover, M. B., Fox, M. D., and Pascual-Leone, A. (2012). Exploration and modulation of brain network interactions with noninvasive brain stimulation in combination with neuroimaging. *Eur. J. Neurosci.* 35, 805–825. doi: 10.1111/j.1460-9568.2012.08035.x

Siebner, H. R., Hartwigsen, G., Kassuba, T., and Rothwell, J. C. (2009). How does transcranial magnetic stimulation modify neuronal activity in the brain? Implications for studies of cognition *Cortex* 45, 1035–1042. doi: 10.1016/j.cortex.2009.02.007

Siebner, H., and Rothwell, J. (2003). Transcranial magnetic stimulation: new insights into representational cortical plasticity. *Exp. Brain Res.* 148, 1–16. doi: 10.1007/s00221-002-1234-2

Sporns, O., Tononi, G., and Kötter, R. (2005). The human connectome: a structural description of the human brain. *PLoS Comput. Biol.* 1:e42. doi: 10.1371/journal.pcbi.0010042

Stampanoni Bassi, M., Leocani, L., Comi, G., Iezzi, E., and Centonze, D. (2017a). Can pharmacological manipulation of LTP favor the effects of motor rehabilitation in multiple sclerosis? *Mult. Scler.* doi: 10.1177/1352458517721358. [Epub ahead of print].

Stampanoni Bassi, M., Mori, F., Buttari, F., Marfia, G. A., Sancesario, A., Centonze, D., et al. (2017b). Neurophysiology of synaptic functioning in multiple sclerosis. *Clin. Neurophysiol.* 128, 1148–1157 doi: 10.1016/j.clinph.2017.04.006

Tecchio, F., Cancelli, A., Cottone, C., Zito, G., Pasqualetti, P., Ghazaryan, A., et al. (2014). Multiple sclerosis fatigue relief by bilateral somatosensory cortex neuromodulation. *J. Neurol.* 261, 1552–1558. doi: 10.1007/s00415-014-7377-9

Tona, F., Petsas, N., Sbardella, E., Prosperini, L., Carmellini, M., Pozzilli, C., et al. (2014). Multiple sclerosis: altered thalamic resting-state functional connectivity and its effect on cognitive function. *Radiology* 271, 814–821. doi: 10.1148/radiol.14131688

Tongiorgi, E., Sartori, A., Baj, G., Bratina, A., Di Cola, F., Zorzon, M., et al. (2012). Altered serum content of brain-derived neurotrophic factor isoforms in multiple sclerosis. *J. Neurol. Sci.* 320, 161–165. doi: 10.1016/j.jns.2012.07.016

Uehara, K., Morishita, T., Kubota, S., and Funase, K. (2013). Neural mechanisms underlying the changes in ipsilateral primary motor cortex excitability during unilateral rhythmic muscle contraction. *Behav. Brain Res.* 240, 33–45. doi: 10.1016/j.bbr.2012.10.053

van Dellen, E., Hillebrand, A., Douw, L., Heimans, J. J., Reijneveld, J. C., and Stam, C. J. (2013). Local polymorphic delta activity in cortical lesions causes global decreases in functional connectivity. *Neuroimage* 83, 524–532. doi: 10.1016/j.neuroimage.2013.06.009

van den Heuvel, M. P., and Hulshoff Pol, H. E. (2010). Exploring the brain network: a review on resting-state fMRI functional connectivity. *Eur. Neuropsychopharmacol.* 20, 519–534. doi: 10.1016/j.euroneuro.2010.03.008

von Monakow, C. (1914). *Die Localization im Grosshirn und der Abbau der Funktion Durch Korticale Herde.* Wiesbaden: JF Bergmann.

Wahl, M., Hübers, A., Lauterbach-Soon, B., Hattingen, E., Jung, P., Cohen, L. G., et al. (2011). Motor callosal disconnection in early relapsing-remitting multiple sclerosis. *Hum. Brain Mapp.* 32, 846–855. doi: 10.1002/hbm.21071

Wassermann, E. M., Fuhr, P., Cohen, L. G., and Hallett, M. (1991). Effects of transcranial magnetic stimulation on ipsilateral muscles. *Neurology* 41, 1795–1799. doi: 10.1212/WNL.41.11.1795

Wu, G. F., Matthew, R., Parks, C. A. L., Ances, B. M., and Van Stavern, G. P. (2015). An eye on brain integrity: acute optic neuritis affects resting state functional connectivity impact of acute on on rs-fcMRI. *Invest. Ophthalmol. Vis. Sci.* 56, 2541–2546. doi: 10.1167/iovs.14-16315

Young, R. R. (1994). Spasticity: a review. *Neurology* 44, 12–20.

Zhou, F., Zhuang, Y., Gong, H., Wang, B., Wang, X., Chen, Q., et al. (2014). Altered inter-subregion connectivity of the default mode network in relapsing remitting multiple sclerosis: a functional and structural connectivity study. *PLoS ONE* 9:e101198. doi: 10.1371/journal.pone.0101198

Ziemann, U., Iliać, T. V., Pauli, C., Meintzschel, F., and Ruge, D. (2004). Learning modifies subsequent induction of long-term potentiation-like and long-term depression-like plasticity in human motor cortex. *J. Neurosci.* 24, 1666–1672. doi: 10.1523/JNEUROSCI.5016-03.2004

Ziemann, U., Paulus, W., Nitsche, M. A., Pascual-Leone, A., Byblow, W. D., Berardelli, A., et al. (2008). Consensus: motor cortex plasticity protocols. *Brain Stimul.* 1, 164–182. doi: 10.1016/j.brs.2008.06.006

11

Exposure of BALB/c Mice to Diesel Engine Exhaust Origin Secondary Organic Aerosol (DE-SOA) during the Developmental Stages Impairs the Social Behavior in Adult Life of the Males

Tin-Tin Win-Shwe[1], Chaw Kyi-Tha-Thu[2], Yadanar Moe[2], Yuji Fujitani[3], Shinji Tsukahara[2] and Seishiro Hirano[3]*

[1] Center for Environmental Health Sciences, National Institute for Environmental Studies, Tsukuba, Japan, [2] Division of Life Science, Graduate School of Science and Engineering, Saitama University, Saitama City, Japan, [3] Center for Environmental Risk Research, National Institute for Environmental Studies, Tsukuba, Japan

Edited by:
Kazuaki Nakamura,
National Research Institute for Child Health and Development, Japan

Reviewed by:
Tatsushi Onaka,
Jichi Medical University, Japan
Chunmei Li,
Nanjing Agricultural University, China
Sohel Ahmed,
Jahangirnagar University, Bangladesh

***Correspondence:**
Tin-Tin Win-Shwe
tin.tin.win.shwe@nies.go.jp

Secondary organic aerosol (SOA) is a component of particulate matter (PM) 2.5 and formed in the atmosphere by oxidation of volatile organic compounds. Recently, we have reported that inhalation exposure to diesel engine exhaust (DE) originated SOA (DE-SOA) affect novel object recognition ability and impair maternal behavior in adult mice. However, it is not clear whether early life exposure to SOA during the developmental stages affect social behavior in adult life or not. In the present study, to investigate the effects of early life exposure to DE-SOA during the gestational and lactation stages on the social behavior in the adult life, BALB/c mice were exposed to clean air (control), DE, DE-SOA and gas without any PM in the inhalation chambers from gestational day 14 to postnatal day 21 for 5 h a day and 5 days per week. Then adult mice were examined for changes in their social behavior at the age of 13 week by a sociability and social novelty preference, social interaction with a juvenile mouse and light-dark transition test, hypothalamic mRNA expression levels of social behavior-related genes, estrogen receptor-alpha and oxytocin receptor as well as of the oxidative stress marker gene, heme oxygenase (HO)-1 by real-time RT-PCR method. In addition, hypothalamic level of neuronal excitatory marker, glutamate was determined by ELISA method. We observed that sociability and social novelty preference as well as social interaction were remarkably impaired, expression levels of estrogen receptor-alpha, oxytocin receptor mRNAs were significantly decreased, expression levels of HO-1 mRNAs and glutamate levels were significantly increased in adult male mice exposed to DE-SOA compared to the control ones. Findings of this study indicate early life exposure of BALB/c mice to DE-SOA may affect their late-onset hypothalamic expression of social behavior related genes, trigger neurotoxicity and impair social behavior in the males.

Keywords: diesel exhaust, secondary organic aerosol, brain, social behavior, mice

INTRODUCTION

Current epidemiological studies have indicated that inhalation of high levels of particulate matter (PM) is associated with damage to the central nervous system (Block and Calderón-Garcidueñas, 2009; Win-Shwe and Fujimaki, 2011; Block et al., 2012; Genc et al., 2012; Weisskopf et al., 2015). Ambient PM consists of primary particles emitted directly from sources, and secondary particles formed by photo-oxidation reactions of volatile organic compounds and gases in the atmosphere, which are known as secondary organic aerosols (SOAs) (Robinson et al., 2007). Diesel exhaust (DE) is a major component of PM and a major precursor of SOA (Kanakidou et al., 2005; Virtanen et al., 2012). Nowadays, the importance of SOA formation in urban areas is well-recognized, not only in the atmosphere but also in indoor environments (Wang et al., 2012; Youssefi and Waring, 2012). It has been reported that exposure to SOA emitted from coal-fired power plants may be associated with an increased risk of heart disease in susceptible animals (Wellenius et al., 2011). However, data showing the effects of SOA on central nervous system and neurobehavioral functions are very limited.

Human epidemiological studies and animal studies suggest that exposure to air pollution may lead to neurotoxicity (Costa et al., 2014). Recent review report indicates that the constituents of air fresheners can react with ozone to produce SOA and these pollutants adversely affect human health such as damage to the central nervous system and respiratory system and alteration of hormone secretion and immune responses (Kim et al., 2015). Previously, our research group has shown that the effects of primary particles such as carbon black nanoparticles and nanoparticle-rich diesel exhaust on brain inflammatory mediators, neurotransmitter system, memory function-related gene expression and learning performance in adult mice (Win-Shwe and Fujimaki, 2011). We have demonstrated that neuroinflammatory effects and neurotoxic effects of carbon black nanoparticle exposure by measuring inflammatory mediators and excitatory amino acid neurotransmitter levels in the hippocampus of BALB/c adult mice (Win-Shwe et al., 2006, 2008a). Furthermore, we have also shown that the effects of nanoparticle-rich diesel exhaust exposure on brain neurotransmitter, inflammatory biomarkers and learning ability in adult mice (Win-Shwe et al., 2008a,b, 2009, 2012a,b). We have generated SOA by adding ozone to diesel exhaust particles and established SOA inhalation chamber in our Research Institute. Using SOA inhalation chambers, we have shown that exposure to SOA for 3 months caused learning and memory impairment in adult male mice and SOA exposure for 1 month in female mice may cause changes in maternal behavior (Win-Shwe et al., 2014). Moreover, we have established the neonatal animal model for early detection of environmental pollutant-induced learning disability and reported that the diesel engine exhaust-derived secondary organic aerosol (DE-SOA) impairs olfactory-based spatial learning activity in preweaning mice (Win-Shwe et al., 2015). In that study, we have also shown that learning impairment was associated with modulation of N-methyl-D-aspartate (NMDA) receptor, signaling pathway gene CaMKII and inflammatory markers in the hippocampi of preweaning mice.

The purpose of the study was to investigate the early life exposure to DE-SOA during the gestational stages and lactation impairs the hypothalamic expression of social behavior-related genes and social behavior in adult life using a mouse model. We hypothesized that the potential toxic substances contained in DE-SOA may reach the brain via the olfactory nerve route or via the systemic circulation and cause social behavioral impairment in later life. Our study is the first report to show that exposure to DE-SOA during the developmental stage affects social performance and the related gene expressions in the hypothalamus of mature mice.

MATERIALS AND METHODS

Animals

Timed pregnant BALB/c mice (gestational day; GD 13) purchased from SLC Japan, Inc. (Tokyo, Japan) were exposed to clean air, diesel engine exhaust (DE), diesel engine exhaust origin secondary organic aerosol (DE-SOA) and gas only without diesel exhaust particles (Gas) from GD 14 to postnatal day (PND) 21 in the whole body exposure chambers. Food and water were given *ad libitum*. The day of the birth was recorded as PND 0 and the offspring were housed in cages with mothers under controlled environmental condition (temperature, 22 ± 0.5°C; humidity, 50 ± 5%; lights on 07:00–19:00 h). The pups were weaned at PND 21 and 5~6 pups of same sex were housed in a plastic cage. Social behavioral tests were started at approximately 13-week-old. Our social behavioral test consisted of sociability and social novelty preference task, social interaction with a juvenile mouse, and light-dark test. Behavioral testing was performed between 09:00 and 17:00 h. Before performing each test, the apparatus to be used was cleaned with 50% ethanol. After completing social behavioral test, these mice were sacrificed for brain sampling. The experimental protocols were approved by the Ethics Committee of the Animal Care and Experimentation Council of the National Institute for Environmental Studies (NIES), Japan.

Generation of DE-SOA

DE-SOA was generated at the National Institute for Environmental Studies, Japan as described previously (Fujitani et al., 2009; Win-Shwe et al., 2014). An 81-diesel engine (J08C; Hino Motors Ltd., Hino, Japan) was used to generate diesel exhaust. The engine was operated under a steady-state condition for 5 h per day. In the present study, our driving condition of diesel engine was not simulated to any special condition as in the real world. The engine operating condition (2000 rpm engine speed and 0 Nm engine torque) in this study permits suppression of the generation of soot particles of relatively large size as well as the generation of high concentrations of nanoparticles. There are four chambers: a control chamber receiving clean air filtered through a HEPA filter and a charcoal filter (referred to as "clean air"), the diluted exhaust (DE which was without mixing O_3), DE-SOA which was generated by mixing DE with ozone at 0.6 ppm after secondary dilution and gas without diesel exhaust particles. Secondary dilution ratio in DE and DE-SOA chambers were the same which resulted in the same particle and gaseous concentrations when O_3 was not mixed. Actually, the concentrations of particles in DE-SOA was higher when O_3 was mixed and concentrations of DE and DE-SOA were 113.19 ± 19.5 μg/m^3 and 130.90 ± 31.2 μg/m^3, respectively. The increased mass concentration was due to the generation of secondary particles. The temperature and relative humidity inside each chamber were adjusted to approximately 22 ± 0.5°C and 50 ± 5%, respectively. The particle characteristics were evaluated from the sample air taken from inside of the exposure chamber and presented in **Table 1**. In detail, sample air was taken from the breeding space of the inhalation chamber (2.25 m^3) using stainless steel tubing. The gas concentrations (CO, CO_2, NO, NO_2, and SO_2) were monitored using a gas analyzer (Horiba, Kyoto, Japan). CO and NOx concentrations in both chambers were similar, but NO and NO_2 are different each other because NO was oxidized to NO_2 by reacted with O_3. The particle size distributions were measured using a scanning mobility particle sizer (SMPS 3034; TSI, MN). The sizes of the particles used in the present study were 25.42 ± 1.6 nm for DE and 28.30 ± 1.3 nm for DE-SOA. The particles were collected using a Teflon filter (FP-500; Sumitomo Electric, Osaka, Japan) and a Quartz fiber filter (2500 QAT-UP; Pall, Pine Bush, NY, USA), and the particle mass concentrations were measured using a Teflon filter. The particle weights were measured using an electrical microbalance (UMX 2, Mettler- Toledo, Columbus; OH, USA; readability 0.1 μg) in an air-conditioned chamber (CHAM-1000; Horiba) under constant temperature and relative humidity conditions (21.5°C, 35%). For the Quartz fiber filter, the quantities of elemental carbon (EC) and organic carbon (OC) were determined using a carbon analyzer (Desert Research Institute, NV, USA). EC to OC ratio in the present study were 0.14 ± 0.05 for the control chamber, 0.33 ± 0.02 for DE-SOA chamber and 0.32 ± 0.03 for DE exposure chamber. An analysis of the particle composition (DE and DE-SOA) showed that the percentage of OC relative to the total carbon in diluted exhaust was about 60% and the DE and DE-SOA was nearly same carbon composition.

Experimental Schedule

Pregnant mice were exposed to clean air, DE, DE-SOA or gas in the whole-body exposure chamber (Shibata) for 5 h per day (from 22:00 h to 03:00 h) on 5 days of the week till PND 21. The male offspring mice at PND 21 were allocated into four different groups (n = 12 per group) as follows: (1) mice exposed to clean filtered air; (2) mice exposed to DE; (3) mice exposed to DE-SOA, and (4) mice exposed to gas only without diesel exhaust particles. On the day after the final exposure, the social performance of each mouse was examined using a three chamber sociability and social novelty preference performance, social interaction and

TABLE 1 | Characteristics of diesel exhaust particles and gaseous compounds in the exposure chambers.

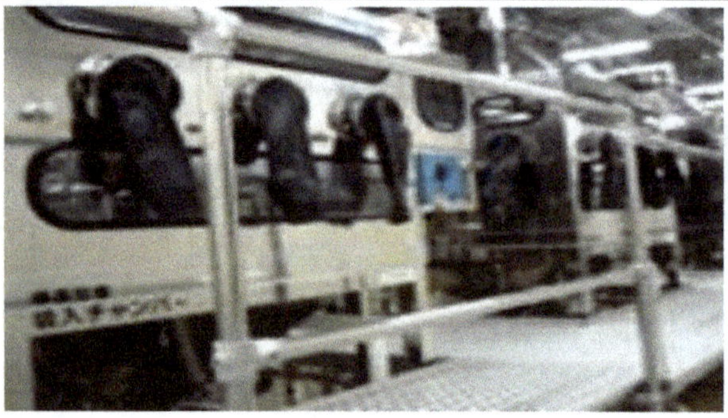

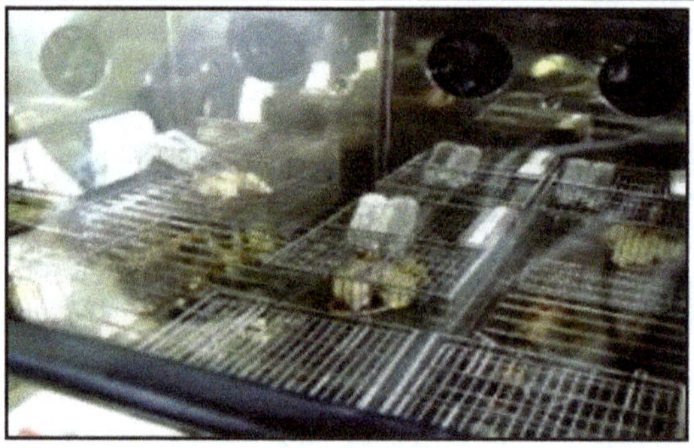

	Diesel exhaust particles			Temperature	Relative humidity		
	Size (nm)	Particle number (cm^{-3})	Concentration (μg/m^3)	(°C)	(%)	EC/OC	WSOC/OC
Clean air	–	0.87 ± 0.57	13.20 ± 2.78	23.58 ± 0.27	48.07 ± 0.77	0.14 ± 0.05	0.03 ± 0.04
DE-SOA	28.30 ± 1.28	2.74 × 10^6 ± 8.69 × 10^4	130.90 ± 31.17	23.76 ± 0.19	48.40 ± 0.85	0.33 ± 0.02	0.11 ± 0.05
DE	25.42 ± 1.63	2.85 × 10^6 ± 6.10 × 10^4	113.19 ± 19.46	22.97 ± 0.21	49.32 ± 0.87	0.32 ± 0.03	0.17 ± 0.11
Gas	–	5.55 ± 1.12	13.30 ± 1.45	23.67 ± 0.24	48.56 ± 1.08	0.14 ± 0.04	0.12 ± 0.06
GASEOUS COMPOUNDS							
	CO (ppm)	SO_2 (ppm)	NO_x (ppm)	NO_2 (ppm)	NO (ppm)	O_3 (ppm)	CO_2 (%)
Clean air	0.21 ± 0.04	0.00 ± 0.00	0.00 ± 0.00	0.00 ± 0.00	0.00 ± 0.00	–	0.05 ± 0.00
DE-SOA	2.51 ± 0.07	0.00 ± 0.00	1.14 ± 0.03	0.99 ± 0.03	0.15 ± 0.03	0.07 ± 0.00	0.07 ± 0.00
DE	2.52 ± 0.07	0.01 ± 0.00	1.21 ± 0.03	0.43 ± 0.02	0.78 ± 0.02	–	0.07 ± 0.00
Gas	2.50 ± 0.06	0.00 ± 0.00	1.14 ± 0.03	0.99 ± 0.03	0.14 ± 0.03	0.06 ± 0.00	0.07 ± 0.00

Data were expressed as mean ± SD.

light-dark test with Any-maze software video-assisted tracking system (Muromachi Kikai Co. Ltd., Japan).

Behavioral Tasks

All behavioral procedures were video-recorded, and data were analyzed by an experimental blind to the conditions.

Sociability and Social Novelty Preference

The apparatus is a Plexiglas rectangular, three-chambered box (60 × 40 × 22 cm). The size of three chambers is equal. Dividing partition was made by clear Plexiglas, with small doorways (5 × 8 cm) allowing free access to each chamber. Small Plexiglas cups (diameter 8 cm; height, 10 cm) were used to house strangers and placed in each side chamber. Stranger mouse was placed on the left or right side. For habituation, subject mice from four different groups were first placed in center of the middle chamber and allowed to explore for 5 min. During habituation phase, each of two side chambers contained an empty Plexiglas cup. Following habituation, for the sociability test, a novel mouse (stranger 1, age-matched male) was enclosed in one of the cup and placed in one of the side chambers; the subject mice were allowed to explore for 10 min. The social novelty preference test was performed immediately after the sociability test. Another novel mouse (stranger 2, age-matched mouse) was enclosed in the other cup. And the subject mice were allowed to explore the two strangers for 10 min. The time spent in each Plexiglas cup was measured. The subject mouse was considered to be spent in cup when its head was facing the cup from a distance of within 3 cm.

Social Interaction with a Juvenile Mouse

Male juvenile mice were used instead of adults to avoid any effect of mutual aggression (Moretti et al., 2005; Jung et al., 2013). A single male subject mouse was placed in a new cage which was identical to those in which the mice were normally housed and allowed to free for 10 min (habituation phase). Three to four week-old juvenile male mouse was introduced to the new cage and then allowed for 5 min (Test phase). Nose-to-nose sniffing, direct contact and close following (within <1 cm) were recorded as social interaction parameters (Jung et al., 2013). The total time of social interaction with juvenile mouse was measured.

Light-Dark Test

The test apparatus consisted of a clear plastic box (40 × 20 × 25 cm) with a dark compartment (20 × 25 × 25 cm) and a light compartment (20 × 25 × 25 cm). The dark compartment had an open doorway (2 × 5 cm) that led to the light side of the apparatus, which was illuminated by a 40-W bulb (about 350 lux on the floor). Mice were moved from the living room to the testing room at least 1 h before the test. At the beginning of the tests, mice were removed from their cages, gently placed to the corner of the dark side of black box away from the doorway. Any-maze software were used to collect and store data. For each mouse, the following measurements were recorded for 10 min: total moving time, total time spent in the dark compartment, total time in the light compartment, number of transitions between the dark and light compartments, and the latency to the first emergence from the dark to the light compartment. Between the tests, the apparatus was thoroughly wiped to clean with 50% alcohol.

Quantification of the Expression Levels of mRNAs

Twenty-four hours after the completion of the social behavioral tests, the mice from each group were sacrificed under deep pentobarbital anesthesia and the hypothalami were collected for mRNA analyses. Hypothalami samples were frozen quickly in liquid nitrogen then stored at –80°C until the total RNA was extracted. Briefly, total RNA extraction from the hypothalami samples was performed using the BioRobot EZ-1 and EZ-1 RNA tissue mini kits (Qiagen GmbH, Hilden, Germany). Then, the purity of the total RNA was examined, and the quantity was estimated using the ND-1000 NanoDrop RNA Assay protocol (NanoDrop, USA), as described previously (Win-Shwe et al., 2006, 2008a,b). Next, we performed first-strand cDNA synthesis from the total RNA using SuperScript RNase H^- Reverse Transcriptase II (Invitrogen, Carlsbad, USA), according to the Manufacturer's protocol. Next, we examined the expression levels of 18S, estrogen receptor (ER) α and oxytocin receptor (OTR), cyclo-oxygenase (COX)-2, heme-oxygenase (HO)-1, interleukin (IL)1 β, tumor necrosis factor (TNF) α mRNAs by a quantitative real-time RT-PCR method using the Applied Biosystems (ABI) Prism 7000 Sequence Detection System (Applied Biosystems Inc., Foskr City, CA, USA). The tissue 18S rRNA level was used as an internal control. Primers (ER-α, NM_007956; OTR, NM_001081147, IL-1β NM_008361; COX2, NM_011198; HO1, NM_010442) were purchased from Qiagen, Sample & Assay Technologies. TNF-α primer (forward: 5′-GGTTCCTTTGTGGCACTTG-3′, reverse: 5′-TTCTCTTGGTGACCGGGAG-3′) was purchased from Hokkaido System Science (Hokkaido System Science, Hokkaido, Japan). Data were analyzed using the comparative threshold cycle method. Then, the relative expression levels of memory function-related genes and the related transduction pathway molecule mRNAs were individually normalized to the 18S rRNA content in the respective samples and expressed as mRNA signals per unit of 18S rRNA expression.

Measurement of Glutamate Concentration

Glutamate concentration in the right hypothalamus of mice was measured using glutamate research ELISA assay kit (Ref: BA E-2300, Neuroscience. Inc., Tokyo, Japan) according to the manufacturer's instructions.

Statistical Analysis

All the data were expressed as the mean ± standard error (S.E.). The statistical analysis was performed using the StatMate II statistical analysis system for Microsoft Excel, Version 5.0 (Nankodo Inc., Tokyo, Japan). Paired *t* test was used to analyze the time approach to the empty cup and stranger 1, then stranger 1 and stranger 2. Messenger RNA data and glutamate concentration were analyzed by a one-way analysis of variance with a *post-hoc* analysis using the Bonferroni/Dunn method. Differences were considered significant at $P < 0.05$.

RESULTS

Body and Brain Weight of Adult Mice Exposed to Clean Air, DE, DE-SOA and Gas during Developmental Period

To detect the general toxicity, body and brain weight were measured in adult male mice exposed to clean air, DE, DE-SOA and gas without particles at the time of sampling (**Table 2**). We did not find any significant changes between the control and exposure groups.

Effects of DE or DE-SOA on Social Behavior

Sociability

The control mice spent more exploring time with the stranger 1 than the empty cup (**Figure 1A**, $*P < 0.05$). In contrast, DE, DE-SOA, or gas exposed mice showed no preference for stranger 1, which could reflect decreased sociability.

Social Novelty Preference

The control mice spent more exploring time with the stranger 2 than the known mouse (stranger 1) (**Figure 1B**, $*P < 0.05$). However, DE, DE-SOA or gas exposed mice showed no preference for novel one (stranger 2). DE-SOA exposed mice preferred old one (stranger 1) significantly compared to the novel one (stranger 2) (**Figure 1B**, $*P < 0.05$), which may indicate that they may have poor social novelty preference.

Social Interaction with a Juvenile Mouse

Nose-to-nose sniffing, direct contact and close following (within <1 cm) were recorded as social interaction parameters. The total time of social interaction with juvenile mouse was measured. We found that DE or DE-SOA exposed mice showed significantly decreased interaction time with juvenile mouse compared to the control mice (**Figure 1C**, $*P < 0.05$).

Light-Dark Test

Light-dark box is a characteristic tool used in the assessment of anxiety. In the present study, total moving time, total time spent in the dark compartment, total time in the light compartment, number of transitions between the dark and light compartments, and the latency to the first emergence from the dark to the light compartment. However, we did not find any significant difference between the control and exposure groups. Time spent in the light compartment was shown in **Figure 1D**.

TABLE 2 | Body and brain weight of adult mice exposed to clean air, DE, DE-SOA, and gas during developmental period.

Exposure groups	Control	DE	DE-SOA	Gas
Body weight (g)	28.22 ± 0.39	28.99 ± 0.97	28.03 ± 0.57	29.07 ± 0.53
Whole brain (mg)	462.11 ± 5.19	469.75 ± 5.14	468.67 ± 4.57	472.33 ± 4.90

Effects of DE or DE-SOA on the Hypothalamic Expression of Social Behavior-Related Genes

Recently, Ervin and colleagues have demonstrated that estrogens are involved in various social behavior such as social preferences, aggression and dominance, and learning and memory (Ervin et al., 2015). Moreover, it was reported that the ERα in the medial amygdala and ventromedial nucleus of the hypothalamus palys a role in social recognition, anxiety and aggression (Spiteri et al., 2010). Our present study has shown that expression of ERα was decreased significantly in DE-SOA exposed group compared to the control group (**Figure 2A**, $*P < 0.05$).

The role of the OT in the normal processing of socially relevant clues has been extensively investigated in genetically-modified rodent models. Social deficit has been observed in OT receptor knockout mice (Winslow and Insel, 2002; Crawley et al., 2007). In the present study, expression level of OTR in the hypothalamus was examined and found that OTR mRNA was decreased significantly in mouse exposed to DE-SOA compared to DE group (**Figure 2B**, $*P < 0.05$) and tended to decrease compared to the control group.

Effects of DE or DE-SOA on the Hypothalamic Expression of Inflammatory and Oxidative Stress Marker Genes

To detect the inflammatory response in the brain, we investigated the expression level of potent inflammatory cytokines such as IL-1 β, TNF-α and potent inflammatory marker COX2. The expression levels of IL-1 β and TNF-α were not different between the control and the exposure groups (data not shown). COX is the enzyme responsible for the conversion of arachidonic acid to prostaglandin, which is involved in the inflammatory response. COX2 is an inducible form and is released at the site of inflammation. In the present study, COX2 mRNA was tended to increase in the DE-SOA-exposed group compared with the control ones (**Figure 3A**). To understand the mechanism underlying the inflammatory response in the hypothalamus of mice exposed to DE-SOA, we also examined the expression of the oxidative stress marker HO1 and found that HO1 mRNA was significantly upregulated in the DE-SOA-exposed group compared with the control group (**Figure 3B**, $*P < 0.05$).

Effects of DE or DE-SOA on the Hypothalamic Level of Neuronal Excitatory Marker

Glutamate is the major excitatory neurotransmitter in the mammalian central nervous system (Fonnum, 1984) and the excessive increase in extracellular glutamate level, known as excitotoxicity, triggers the death of neurons (Choi and Rothman, 1990). We detected glutamate concentration in the mouse hypothalamus and found that glutamate secretion was increased remarkably in mice exposed to DE or DE-SOA during fetal and neonatal developmental period (**Figure 4**, $**P < 0.01$).

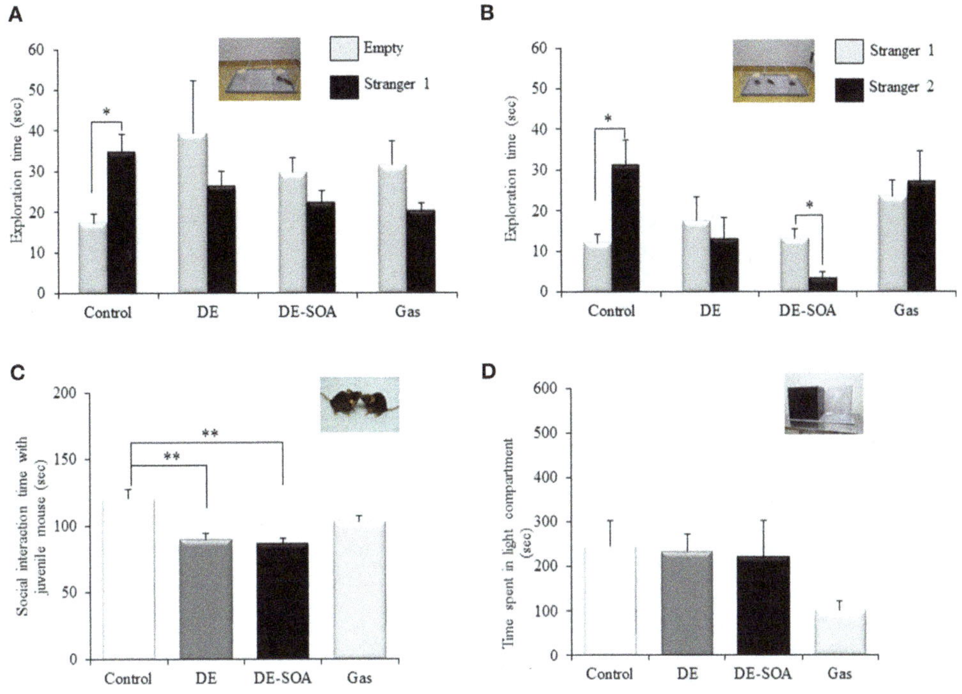

FIGURE 1 | Scores of the social behavioral tests. (A) sociability test, **(B)** social novelty preference test, **(C)** social interaction test with juvenile mouse and **(D)** light dark test in 13 week-old male mice after developmental period exposure to clean air, DE, DE-SOA or gas without particles. Each bar represents the mean ± SE ($n = 12$, $^{**}P < 0.01$, $^{*}P < 0.05$).

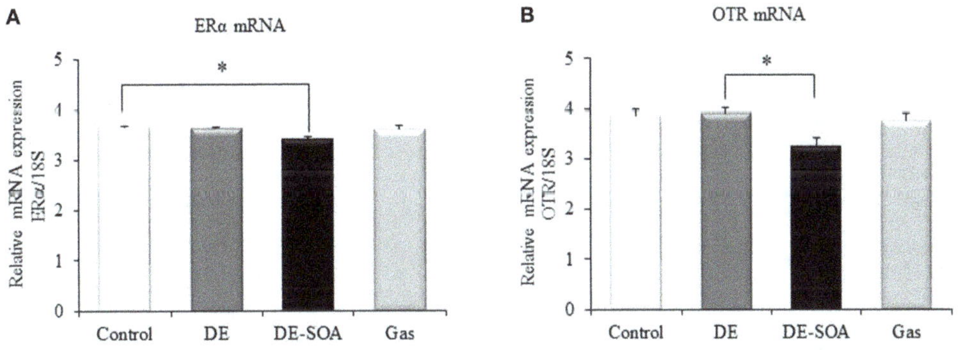

FIGURE 2 | Hypothalamic expression of social behavior-related genes. Messenger RNA expression level of **(A)** ERα and **(B)** OTR in the hypothalami of 13 week-old male mice after developmental period exposure to clean air, DE, DE-SOA or gas without particles. Each bar represents the mean ± SE ($n = 12$, $^{*}P < 0.05$).

DISCUSSION

The major findings in the present study indicate that exposure to DE-SOA during brain developmental period may impair some social behaviors in adult male BALB/c mice accompanied with modulation of expression of ERα and OTR, inflammatory mediator COX2 and oxidative stress marker HO1 in the hypothalamus. We suggest that, although the potential toxic substances contained in DE-SOA have not yet been identified, they may reach the brain via placenta of pregnant mice during fetal period and via the olfactory nerve route or systemic circulation during neonatal period and induce neurotoxicity. These effects may be persistent because we exposed the mice during early brain developmental period and investigated the social behavior and related gene expression in later age.

Previous epidemiological evidences have shown the existence of positive associations between the inhalation of elevated levels of PM and pulmonary and cardiovascular morbidities and mortality in susceptible populations (Dockery, 1993; Peters et al., 1997; Penttinen et al., 2001; Pope et al., 2002). Recent reports indicate that the central nervous system is an important target for air pollution to cause adverse health effects such as neurodevelopmental and neurodegenerative disorders like autism spectrum disorder (ASD) and Alzheimer's disease

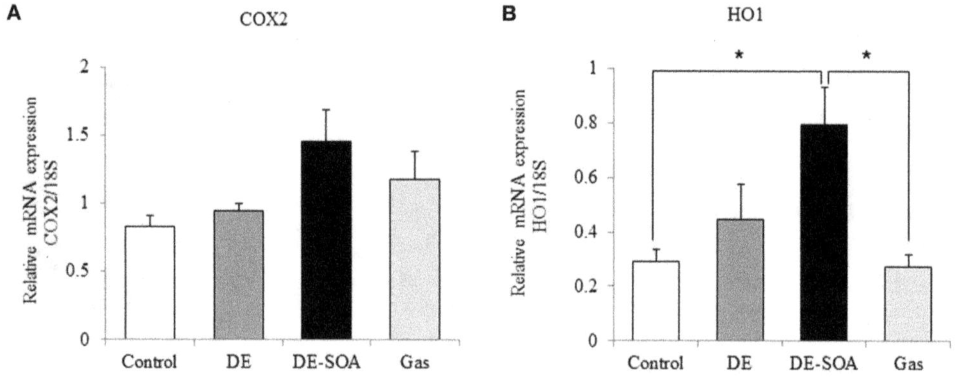

FIGURE 3 | Hypothalamic expression of inflammatory and oxidative stress markers. (A) COX2 and **(B)** HO1 mRNAs in 13 week-old male mice after developmental period exposure to clean air, DE, DE-SOA or gas without particles. Each bar represents the mean ± SE (n = 12, *P < 0.05).

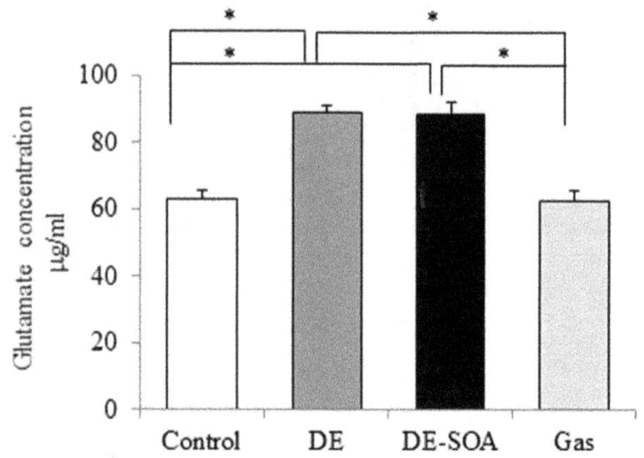

FIGURE 4 | Hypothalamic levels of neuronal excitatory marker. Glutamate concentration in the hypothalami of 13 week-old male mice after developmental period exposure to clean air, DE, DE-SOA or gas without particles. Each bar represents the mean ± SE (n = 12, *P < 0.05).

(Calderón-Garcidueñas et al., 2004; Deth et al., 2008; Lee et al., 2010; Landrigan et al., 2012). DE is a major source of ambient PM and one of the major precursors for SOA formation. SOAs are formed in the atmosphere by oxidation of products originating from anthropogenic and biogenic volatile organic compounds (Virtanen et al., 2012). SOA formation may occur not only in the atmosphere, but also in indoor environments where laser printer, copiers were used (Wang et al., 2012; Youssefi and Waring, 2012).

First, we have shown that a single intranasal administration of SOA induces inflammatory responses in the lungs by modulating the expressions of proinflammatory cytokines, transcription factors, and inflammation-responsive neurotrophins (Win-Shwe et al., 2013). Currently, we have generated SOA by adding ozone to diesel exhaust particles and establish SOA inhalation chamber in our Research Institute. Using SOA inhalation chambers, we have shown that exposure to SOA for 3 months caused learning and memory impairment in adult male mice and SOA exposure for 1 month in female mice may cause changes in maternal behavior (Win-Shwe et al., 2014). Recently, we have established the neonatal animal model for early detection of environmental pollutant-induced learning disability and reported that DE-SOA impairs olfactory-based spatial learning activity in preweaning mice (Win-Shwe et al., 2015). In that study, we have also shown that learning impairment was associated with modulation of NMDA receptor, signaling pathway gene CaMKII and inflammatory markers in the hippocampus. From these findings, we suggest that glutamate, a ligand for NMDA receptor, may involve SOA induced neurobehavioral dysfunctions.

Human studies have reported that children from Mexico City with prefrontal lesions exposed to air pollution showed cognitive deficits (Calderón-Garcidueñas et al., 2008a, 2011). An association has also been shown between air pollution and cognitive impairment in healthy individuals, including adult and elderly women (Calderón-Garcidueñas et al., 2004, 2008b). An *in vitro* study indicated that decreased phagocytic activity was found in human macrophages exposed to SOA from alpha-pinene, and IL-8 production was increased in pig explants exposed to SOA from 1,3,5-trimethlbenzene with high particle numbers (Gaschen et al., 2010). However, it is not clear whether an association may exist between exposure to SOA derived from DE and higher functions of the brain such as social behavior.

In the present study, the control group only approached longer time to stranger 1 cup compared to empty cup in sociability test. In social novelty preference test, the control group approached longer time to stranger 2 cup compared to stranger 1 cup. These findings suggests that treatment groups such as DE, DE-SOA or gas without particles groups may have poor communication with new partner. We have also examined social behavioral related genes such as ERα and OTR and proinflammatory cytokines and potent inflammatory marker and oxidative stress marker and found that the expression level of COX2 and HO1 mRNA were increased in the hypothalamus of DE-SOA exposed mice. Components of DE-SOA may exert their deleterious effects directly on the central nervous system, the possibility and the extent of a peripheral contribution to the central effects should be considered. It was reported that high levels of circulating proinflammatory cytokines may negatively affect the he central nervous system (Block and Calderón-Garcidueñas, 2009; Calderón-Garcidueñas et al., 2013), and the blood-brain barrier may represent an important site for air pollution induced neurotoxicity.

To detect the possible mechanism of the action of SOA in social impairment, we have examined glutamate concentration in hypothalamus. Glutamate is one of excitatory amino acid neurotransmitters. Neurotransmitters play many critical roles in the neuronal transmission and maintenance of many higher brain functions. Deviation of neurotransmitter from the normal physiological level may lead to certain malfunctions and pathological states of the brain. Under normal conditions, extracellular glutamate is maintained at safe physiological concentrations by a number of buffering mechanisms which include uptake of glutamate by glial cells and its conversion by glutamine synthetase or glutamate decarboxylase to the nontoxic glutamine (Bezzi et al., 1999; Rauen et al., 1999). In the present study, glutamate concentration was remarkably increased in DE or DE-SOA exposed mice. It is suggested that there may be association exists between increased glutamate neurotransmission and impaired social behavior. Amino acid transporters present in both the neurons and the glial cells are critically important for the normal function of glutamatergic transmission, as well as for the maintenance of extracellular glutamate levels below potentially excitotoxic concentrations (Kanai et al., 1993, 1995). The possible reasons for increased glutamate level in DE-SOA exposed mice are due to blockade of re-uptake by glutamate transporter in the presynaptic neurons and decreased downstream enzymes such as glutamic acid decarboxylase (GAD) 67 and GAD 65 for gamma amino butyric acid (GABA) synthesis. Further studies are needed to evaluate the role of glutamate transporters in SOA induced impaired behavior.

Recent report has indicated that estrogens are involved in various social behavior such as social preferences, aggression and dominance, and learning and memory (Ervin et al., 2015). It was also reported that the ERα in the medial amygdala and ventromedial nucleus of the hypothalamus palys a role in social recognition, anxiety and aggression. (Spiteri et al., 2010). Our present study has shown that expression of ERα was decreased in DE-SOA exposed group compared to the control group. Moreover, impaired social recognition has been observed in OT peptide and receptor knockout mice (Winslow and Insel, 2002; Takayanagi et al., 2005). Oxytocin can reduce repetitive behavior in subjects with autism (File et al., 1998) and promote social behavior in high functioning ASDs (Andari et al., 2010). Recent reports have indicated that intranasal oxytocin reduces psychotic symptoms and improves theory of mind and social performance in schizophrenia patients (Pedersen et al., 2011; Davis et al., 2013). In the present study, although statistically not significant, OTR mRNA expression tends to decrease in DE-SOA exposed mice compared to the other groups. Taken together, ERα and OTR, at least in part, may play a role in DE-SOA induced social behavioral disturbance.

Our present results indicate that brain developmental period exposure to diesel exhaust origin SOA may impair some social behavior in adult BALB/c mice. In the present study, not only the offspring, but also the dam were exposed to DE-SOA during gestational and lactational periods. Normal maternal behaviors such as nesting, licking, crouching and retrieving were observed during exposure period. Therefore, impairment of social behavior in adult male mice might not due to abnormal maternal caring during brain developing periods. Glutamate neurotransmission and ERα-OTR signaling pathway in the hypothalamus may take part in DE-SOA induced social behavioral impairment. Further studies are needed to explore the effects of DE-SOA on other brain targets such as amygdala and hippocampus and other social behavior such as sexual, aggressive or anxiety after early life exposure. Furthermore, animal experiments showed the same pattern of neurotoxic effects such as increased oxidative stress markers, increased neuroinflammatory mediators and age factor, as in humans, suggesting that animal studies would be useful predictors of human outcomes (Costa et al., 2014). Finally, *in vitro* studies are needed for better understanding of air pollution induced neurotoxicity and their consequences.

AUTHOR CONTRIBUTIONS

TW and SH designed this research; YF, arranged the exposure system; CK and YM performed the behavioral tests and molecular analyses; TW wrote the article; SH and ST critically revised the article.

ACKNOWLEDGMENTS

This research was supported by a Research fund from The Ministry of Environment, Japan (36007) to SH, a Grant-in-Aid for Scientific Research (C) JSPS KAKENHI (25340066) and a research fund from the National Institute for Environmental Studies (1416AT001) to TW.

REFERENCES

Andari, E., Duhamel, J. R., Zalla, T., Herbrecht, E., Leboyer, M., and Sirigu, A. (2010). Promoting social behavior with oxytocin in high functioning autism spectrum disorders. *Proc. Natl. Acad. Sci. U.S.A.* 107, 4389–4394. doi: 10.1073/pnas.0910249107

Bezzi, P., Vesce, S., Panzarasa, P., and Volterra, A. (1999). Astrocytes as active participants of glutamatergic function and regulators of its homeostasis. *Adv. Exp. Med. Biol.* 468, 69–80. doi: 10.1007/978-1-4615-4685-6_6

Block, M. L., and Calderón-Garcidueñas, L. (2009). Air pollution: mechanisms of neuroinflammation and CNS disease. *Trends Neurosci.* 32, 506–516. doi: 10.1016/j.tins.2009.05.009

Block, M. L., Elder, A., Auten, R. L., Bilbo, S. D., Chen, H., Chen, J. C., et al. (2012). The outdoor air pollution and brain health workshop. *Neurotoxicology* 33, 972–984. doi: 10.1016/j.neuro.2012.08.014

Calderón-Garcidueñas, L., Cross, J. V., Franco-Lira, M., Aragón-Flores, M., Kavanaugh, M., Torres-Jardón, R., et al. (2013). Brain immune interactions and air pollution: macrophage inhibitory factor (MIF), prion cellular protein (PrP(C)), Interleukin-6 (IL-6), interleukin 1 receptor antagonist (IL-1Ra), and interleukin-2 (IL-2) in cerebrospinal fluid and MIF in serum differentiate urban children exposed to severe vs. low air pollution. *Front. Neurosci.* 7:183. doi: 10.3389/fnins.2013.00183

Calderón-Garcidueñas, L., Engle, R., Mora-Tiscareño, A., Styner, M., Gómez-Garza, G., Zhu, H., et al. (2011). Exposure to severe urban air pollution influences cognitive outcomes, brain volume and systemic inflammation in clinically healthy children. *Brain Cogn.* 77, 345–355. doi: 10.1016/j.bandc.2011.09.006

Calderón-Garcidueñas, L., Mora-Tiscareño, A., Ontiveros, E., Gomez-Garza, G., Barragán-Mejía, G., Broadway, J., et al. (2008a). Air pollution, cognitive deficits and brain abnormalities: a pilot study with children and dogs. *Brain Cogn.* 68, 117–127. doi: 10.1016/j.bandc.2008.04.008

Calderón-Garcidueñas, L., Reed, W., Maronpot, R. R., Henríquez-Roldán, C., Delgado-Chavez, R., Calderón-Garcidueñas, A., et al. (2004). Brain inflammation and Alzheimer's-like pathology in individuals exposed to severe air pollution. *Toxicol. Pathol.* 32, 650–658. doi: 10.1080/01926230490520232

Calderón-Garcidueñas, L., Solt, A. C., Henríquez-Roldán, C., Torres-Jardón, R., Nuse, B., Herritt, L., et al. (2008b). Long-term air pollution exposure is associated with neuroinflammation, an altered innate immune response, disruption of the blood-brain barrier, ultrafine particulate deposition, and accumulation of amyloid beta-42 and alpha-synuclein in children and young adults. *Toxicol. Pathol.* 36, 289–310. doi: 10.1177/0192623307313011

Choi, D. W., and Rothman, S. M. (1990). The role of glutamate neurotoxicity in hypoxic-ischemic neuronal death. *Annu. Rev. Neurosci.* 13, 171–182. doi: 10.1146/annurev.ne.13.030190.001131

Costa, L. G., Cole, T. B., Coburn, J., Chang, Y. C., Dao, K., and Roque, P. (2014). Neurotoxicants are in the air: convergence of human, animal, and *in vitro* studies on the effects of air pollution on the brain. *Biomed Res. Int.* 2014:736385. doi: 10.1155/2014/736385

Crawley, J. N., Chen, T., Puri, A., Washburn, R., Sullivan, T. L., Hill, J. M., et al. (2007). Social approach behaviors in oxytocin knockout mice: comparison of two independent lines tested in different laboratory environments. *Neuropeptides* 41, 145–163. doi: 10.1016/j.npep.2007.02.002

Davis, M. C., Lee, J., Horan, W. P., Clarke, A. D., McGee, M. R., Green, M. F., et al. (2013). Effects of single dose intranasal oxytocin on social cognition in schizophrenia. *Schizophr. Res.* 147, 393–397. doi: 10.1016/j.schres.2013.04.023

Deth, R., Muratore, C., Benzecry, J., Power-Charnitsky, V. A., and Waly, M. (2008). How environmental and genetic factors combine to cause autism: a redox/methylation hypothesis. *Neurotoxicology* 29, 190–201. doi: 10.1016/j.neuro.2007.09.010

Dockery, D. W. (1993). Epidemiologic study design for investigating respiratory health effects of complex air pollution mixtures. *Environ. Health Perspect.* 101, 187–191. doi: 10.1289/ehp.93101s4187

Ervin, K. S., Lymer, J. M., Matta, R., Clipperton-Allen, A. E., Kavaliers, M., and Choleris, E. (2015). Estrogen involvement in social behavior in rodents: rapid and long-term actions. *Horm. Behav.* 74, 53–76. doi: 10.1016/j.yhbeh.2015.05.023

File, S. E., Mahal, A., Mangiarini, L., and Bates, G. P. (1998). Striking changes in anxiety in Huntington's disease transgenic mice. *Brain Res.* 2, 234–240. doi: 10.1016/S0006-8993(98)00736-7

Fonnum, F. (1984). Glutamate: a neurotransmitter in mammalian brain. *J. Neurochem.* 42, 1–11. doi: 10.1111/j.1471-4159.1984.tb09689.x

Fujitani, Y., Hirano, S., Kobayashi, S., Tanabe, K., Suzuki, A., Furuyama, A., et al. (2009). Characterization of dilution conditions for diesel nanoparticle inhalation studies. *Inhal. Toxicol.* 21, 200–209. doi: 10.1080/08958370802339491

Gaschen, A., Lang, D., Kalberer, M., Savi, M., Geiser, T., Gazdhar, A., et al. (2010). Cellular responses after exposure of lung cell cultures to secondary organic aerosol particles. *Environ. Sci. Technol.* 44, 1424–1430. doi: 10.1021/es902261m

Genc, S., Zadeoglulari, Z., Fuss, S. H., and Genc, K. (2012). The adverse effects of air pollution on the nervous system. *J. Toxicol.* 2012:782462. doi: 10.1155/2012/782462

Jung, S., Seo, J. S., Kim, B. S., Lee, D., Jung, K. H., Chu, K., et al. (2013). Social deficits in the AY-9944 mouse model of atypical absence epilepsy. *Behav. Brain Res.* 236, 23–29. doi: 10.1016/j.bbr.2012.08.029

Kanai, Y., Bhide, P. G., DiFiglia, M., and Hediger, M. A. (1995). Neuronal high-affinity glutamate transport in the rat central nervous system. *Neuroreport* 27, 2357–2362. doi: 10.1097/00001756-199511270-00020

Kanai, Y., Smith, C. P., and Hediger, M. A. (1993). A new family of neurotransmitter transporters: the high-affinity glutamate transporters. *FASEB J.* 7, 1450–1459.

Kanakidou, M., Seinfeld, J. H., Pandis, S. N., Barnes, I., Dentener, F. J., Facchini, M. C., et al. (2005). Organic aerosol and global climate modelling: a review. *Atmos. Chem. Phys.* 5, 1053–1123. doi: 10.5194/acp-5-1053-2005

Kim, S., Hong, S. H., Bong, C. K., and Cho, M. H. (2015). Characterization of air freshener emission: the potential health effects. *J. Toxicol. Sci.* 40, 535–550. doi: 10.2131/jts.40.535

Landrigan, P. J., Lambertini, L., and Birnbaum, L. S. (2012). A research strategy to discover the environmental causes of autism and neurodevelopmental disabilities. *Environ. Health Perspect.* 120, a258–a260. doi: 10.1289/ehp.1104285

Lee, Y. J., Han, S. B., Nam, S. Y., Oh, K. W., and Hong, J. T. (2010). Inflammation and Alzheimer's disease. *Arch. Pharm. Res.* 33, 1539–1556. doi: 10.1007/s12272-010-1006-7

Moretti, P., Bouwknecht, J. A., Teague, R., Paylor, R., and Zoghbi, H. Y. (2005). Abnormalities of social interactions and home-cage behavior in a mouse model of Rett syndrome. *Hum. Mol. Genet.* 14, 205–220. doi: 10.1093/hmg/ddi016

Pedersen, C. A., Gibson, C. M., Rau, S. W., Salimi, K., Smedley, K. L., Casey, R. L., et al. (2011). Intranasal oxytocin reduces psychotic symptoms and improves Theory of Mind and social perception in schizophrenia. *Schizophr. Res.* 132, 50–53. doi: 10.1016/j.schres.2011.07.027

Penttinen, P., Timonen, K. L., Tittanen, P., Mirme, A., Ruuskanen, J., and Pekkanen, J. (2001). Ultrafine particles in urban air and respiratory health among adult asthmatics. *Eur. Respir. J.* 17, 428–435. doi: 10.1183/09031936.01.17304280

Peters, A., Döring, A., Wichmann, H. E., and Koenig, W. (1997). Increased plasma viscosity during an air pollution episode: a link to mortality? *Lancet* 349, 1582–1587.

Pope, C. A. III, Burnett, R. T., Thun, M. J., Calle, E. E., Krewski, D., Ito, K., et al. (2002). Lung cancer, cardiopulmonary mortality, and long-term exposure to fine particulate air pollution. *J. Am. Med. Assoc.* 287, 1132–1141. doi: 10.1001/jama.287.9.1132

Rauen, T., Fischer, F., and Wiessner, M. (1999). Glia-neuron interaction by high-affinity glutamate transporters in neurotransmission. *Adv. Exp. Med. Biol.* 468, 81–95. doi: 10.1007/978-1-4615-4685-6_7

Robinson, A. L., Donahue, N. M., Shrivastava, M. K., Weitkamp, E. A., Sage, A. M., Grieshop, A. P., et al. (2007). Rethinking organic aerosols: semivolatile emissions and photochemical aging. *Science* 315, 1259–1262. doi: 10.1126/science.1133061

Spiteri, T., Musatov, S., Ogawa, S., Ribeiro, A., Pfaff, D. W., and Agmo, A. (2010). The role of the estrogen receptor alpha in the medial amygdala and ventromedial nucleus of the hypothalamus in social recognition, anxiety and aggression. *Behav. Brain Res.* 210, 211–220. doi: 10.1016/j.bbr.2010.02.033

Takayanagi, Y., Yoshida, M., Bielsky, I. F., Ross, H. E., Kawamata, M., Onaka, T., et al. (2005). Pervasive social deficits, but normal parturition, in oxytocin receptor-deficient mice. *Proc. Natl. Acad. Sci. U.S.A.* 102, 16096–16101. doi: 10.1073/pnas.0505312102

Virtanen, A., Joutsensaari, J., Koop, T., Kannosto, J., Yli-Pirilä, P., Leskinen, J., et al. (2012). An amorphous solid state of biogenic secondary organic aerosol particles. *Nature* 467, 824–827. doi: 10.1038/nature09455

Wang, H., He, C., Morawska, L., McGarry, P., and Johnson, G. (2012). Ozone-initiated particle formation, particle aging, and precursors in a laser printer. *Environ. Sci. Technol.* 46, 704–712. doi: 10.1021/es203066k

Weisskopf, M. G., Kioumourtzoglou, M. A., and Roberts, A. L. (2015). Air pollution and autism spectrum disorders: causal or confounded? *Curr. Environ. Health Rep.* 2, 340–349. doi: 10.1007/s40572-015-0073-9

Wellenius, G. A., Diaz, E. A., Gupta, T., Ruiz, P. A., Long, M., Kang, C. M., et al. (2011). Electrocardiographic and respiratory responses to coal-fired power plant emissions in a rat model of acute myocardial infarction: Results from the toxicological evaluation of realistic emissions of source aerosols study. *Inhal. Toxicol.* 23, 84–94. doi: 10.3109/08958378.2010.554461

Win-Shwe, T. T., and Fujimaki, H. (2011). Nanoparticles and neurotoxicity. *Int. J. Mol. Sci.* 12, 6267–6280. doi: 10.3390/ijms12096267

Win-Shwe, T. T., Fujimaki, H., Fujitani, Y., and Hirano, S. (2012b). Novel object recognition ability in female mice following exposure to nanoparticle-rich diesel exhaust. *Toxicol. Appl. Pharmacol.* 262, 355–362. doi: 10.1016/j.taap.2012.05.015

Win-Shwe, T. T., Fujitani, Y., Kyi-Tha-Thu, C., Furuyama, A., Michikawa, T., Tsukahara, S., et al. (2014). Effects of diesel engine exhaust origin secondary organic aerosols on novel object recognition ability and maternal behavior in BALB/c mice. *Int. J. Environ. Res. Public Health* 11, 11286–11307. doi: 10.3390/ijerph111111286

Win-Shwe, T. T., Fujitani, Y., Sone, H., Furuyama, A., Nitta, H., and Hirano, S. (2013). Effects of acute single intranasal instillation of secondary organic aerosol on neurological and immunological biomarkers in the brain and lung of BALB/c mice. *J. Toxicol. Sci.* 38, 71–82. doi: 10.2131/jts.38.71

Win-Shwe, T. T., Kyi-Tha-Thu, C., Moe, Y., Maekawa, F., Yanagisawa, R., Furuyama, A., et al. (2015). Nano-sized secondary organic aerosol of diesel engine exhaust origin impairs olfactory-based spatial learning performance in preweaning mice. *Nanomaterials* 2015, 1147–1162. doi: 10.3390/nano5031147

Win-Shwe, T. T., Mitsushima, D., Yamamoto, S., Fujitani, Y., Funabashi, T., Hirano, S., et al. (2009). Extracellular glutamate level and NMDA receptor subunit expression in mouse olfactory bulb following nanoparticle-rich diesel exhaust exposure. *Inhal. Toxicol.* 21, 828–836. doi: 10.1080/08958370802538068

Win-Shwe, T. T., Mitsushima, D., Yamamoto, S., Fukushima, A., Funabashi, T., Kobayashi, T., et al. (2008a). Changes in neurotransmitter levels and proinflammatory cytokine mRNA expressions in the mice olfactory bulb following nanoparticle exposure. *Toxicol. Appl. Pharmacol.* 226, 192–198. doi: 10.1016/j.taap.2007.09.009

Win-Shwe, T. T., Yamamoto, S., Ahmed, S., Kakeyama, M., Kobayashi, T., and Fujimaki, H. (2006). Brain cytokine and chemokine mRNA expression in mice induced by intranasal instillation with ultrafine carbon black. *Toxicol. Lett.* 163, 153–160. doi: 10.1016/j.toxlet.2005.10.006

Win-Shwe, T. T., Yamamoto, S., Fujitani, Y., Hirano, S., and Fujimaki, H. (2008b). Spatial learning and memory function-related gene expression in the hippocampus of mouse exposed to nanoparticle-rich diesel exhaust. *Neurotoxicology* 29, 940–947. doi: 10.1016/j.neuro.2008.09.007

Win-Shwe, T. T., Yamamoto, S., Fujitani, Y., Hirano, S., and Fujimaki, H. (2012a). Nanoparticle-rich diesel exhaust affects hippocampal-dependent spatial learning and NMDA receptor subunit expression in female mice. *Nanotoxicology* 6, 543–553. doi: 10.3109/17435390.2011.590904

Winslow, J. T., and Insel, T. R. (2002). The social deficits of the oxytocin knockout mouse. *Neuropeptides* 36, 221–229. doi: 10.1054/npep.2002.0909

Youssefi, S., and Waring, M. S. (2012). Predicting secondary organic aerosol formation from terpenoid ozonolysis with varying yields in indoor environments. *Indoor Air* 22, 415–426. doi: 10.1111/j.1600-0668.2012.00776.x

12

Galvanic Vestibular Stimulation (GVS) Augments Deficient Pedunculopontine Nucleus (PPN) Connectivity in Mild Parkinson's Disease: fMRI Effects of Different Stimuli

Jiayue Cai[1], Soojin Lee[2,3], Fang Ba[4], Saurabh Garg[3], Laura J. Kim[3], Aiping Liu[3,5], Diana Kim[6], Z. Jane Wang[1] and Martin J. McKeown[1,3,6]*

[1] Department of Electrical and Computer Engineering, University of British Columbia, Vancouver, BC, Canada, [2] School of Biomedical Engineering, University of British Columbia, Vancouver, BC, Canada, [3] Pacific Parkinson's Research Centre, Vancouver, BC, Canada, [4] Division of Neurology, Department of Medicine, University of Alberta, Edmonton, AB, Canada, [5] School of Electronics and Applied Physics, Hefei University of Technology, Hefei, China, [6] Department of Medicine (Neurology), University of British Columbia, Vancouver, BC, Canada

Edited by:
Takashi Hanakawa, National Center of Neurology and Psychiatry, Japan

Reviewed by:
Martijn Müller, University of Michigan, United States
Antonio Currà, Sapienza Università di Roma, Italy
Kazumi Iseki, Sakakibara Hakuho Hospital, Japan

***Correspondence:**
Aiping Liu
aipingl@ece.ubc.ca

Falls and balance difficulties remain a major source of morbidity in Parkinson's Disease (PD) and are stubbornly resistant to therapeutic interventions. The mechanisms of gait impairment in PD are incompletely understood but may involve changes in the Pedunculopontine Nucleus (PPN) and its associated connections. We utilized fMRI to explore the modulation of PPN connectivity by Galvanic Vestibular Stimulation (GVS) in healthy controls ($n = 12$) and PD subjects even without overt evidence of Freezing of Gait (FOG) while on medication ($n = 23$). We also investigated if the type of GVS stimuli (i.e., sinusoidal or stochastic) differentially affected connectivity. Approximate PPN regions were manually drawn on T1 weighted images and 58 other cortical and subcortical Regions of Interest (ROI) were obtained by automatic segmentation. All analyses were done in the native subject's space without spatial transformation to a common template. We first used Partial Least Squares (PLS) on a subject-by-subject basis to determine ROIs across subjects that covaried significantly with the voxels within the PPN ROI. We then performed functional connectivity analysis on the PPN-ROI connections. In control subjects, GVS did not have a significant effect on PPN connectivity. In PD subjects, baseline overall magnitude of PPN connectivity was negatively correlated with UPDRS scores ($p < 0.05$). Both noisy and sinusoidal GVS increased the overall magnitude of PPN connectivity ($p = 6 \times 10^{-5}$, 3×10^{-4}, respectively) in PD, and increased connectivity with the left inferior parietal region, but had opposite effects on amygdala connectivity. Noisy stimuli selectively decreased connectivity with basal ganglia and cerebellar regions.

Our results suggest that GVS can enhance deficient PPN connectivity seen in PD in a stimulus-dependent manner. This may provide a mechanism through which GVS assists balance in PD, and may provide a biomarker to develop individualized stimulus parameters.

Keywords: vestibular stimulation, pedunculopontine nucleus, functional connectivity, Parkinson's Disease, non-invasive neuromodulation, fMRI

INTRODUCTION

Falls in older adult populations are a significant cause of morbidity and mortality (Cameron et al., 2012) with non-fatal injuries initiating a vicious cycle leading to a fear of falling, social isolation, loss of independence, deconditioning, and a significantly greater use of health care services (Stevens et al., 2006; Williams et al., 2006).

In Parkinson's Disease (PD), gait disturbances such as decreased stride length and gait variability are associated with increased risk of falls. Balance and gait deficits in PD are frequently refractory to therapy (Azevedo Coste et al., 2014; Perez-Lloret et al., 2014) and may be actually worsened by pharmacological and surgical interventions (Bloem et al., 1996), making falls a significant source of morbidity in PD (Schaafsma et al., 2003). Freezing of gait (FOG) is a syndrome normally seen in advanced PD and can occur when subjects are either on or off medication. FOG may be partly due to a failure to adequately scale amplitudes for the intended movement (Chee et al., 2009) and/or defective motor programming setting by the Supplemental Motor Area (SMA) and its maintenance by the basal ganglia, leading to a mismatch between intention and automation (Chee et al., 2009).

Cognitive and motor function must be carefully integrated to execute gait. Dysfunction of the basal ganglia in PD results in impaired motor control of skilled voluntary movements (Magrinelli et al., 2016) and movements become excessively slow and underscaled in size (Benecke et al., 1987). Biochemically, imbalance in multiple neurotransmitters (including but not limited to dopamine, acetylcholine, and GABA) is seen not only in basal ganglia and motor structures, but also limbic circuitries (Ondo and Hunter, 2003; Perez-Lloret and Barrantes, 2016). Balance disturbance and falls in PD may be more related to disruption in cholinergic rather than dopaminergic neurotransmission (Bohnen et al., 2009).

A key part of the subcortical cholinergic system is the pedunculopontine nucleus (PPN), which appears critically involved in gait disturbances in PD (Mazzone et al., 2005; Androulidakis et al., 2008; Acar et al., 2011), as PPN neuronal loss is evident in PD (Rinne et al., 2008) (Note that although we refer to the "PPN" throughout this manuscript, at the resolution of the imaging used here, it would perhaps be more accurate to refer to this region as the "mesencephalic locomotor region" as it likely includes the cuneiform nucleus—however, we use PPN as this terminology is consistent with much prior literature (e.g., Mazzone et al., 2005; Androulidakis et al., 2008; Acar et al., 2011).

Connectivity to/from the PPN appears critical for FOG in PD (Fling et al., 2014). Structural deficits in connectivity are evident between basal ganglia-PPN and other tracts in FOG (Fling et al., 2014; Vercruysse et al., 2015). DTI tractography obtained with 3T MR imaging in PD patients with FOG has demonstrated asymmetrically decreased connectivity between the PPN and the SMA, compared to PD subjects without FOG (Fling et al., 2014). FOG is also associated with diffuse white matter damage involving major cortico-cortical, corticofugal motor, and several striatofrontal tracts with DTI (Vercruysse et al., 2015). In addition to structural/anatomical connectivity, advanced neuroimaging techniques have enabled the studies of functional connectivity, which refers to the statistical temporal dependences between anatomically separated brain regions, to reveal the functional communication in the brain. Functional imaging studies (e.g., fMRI) have reported increased activity or altered connectivity during gait visualization in the midbrain locomotion centers between FOG episodes (Hanakawa et al., 1999), possibly reflecting compensatory mechanisms which might be overwhelmed with stress by turning or multitasking (Shine et al., 2013). Moreover, resting state functional magnetic resonance imaging (rs-fMRI) has allowed the inference of functional connectivity by measuring the level of spontaneous co-activation between fMRI time courses of brain regions recorded during rest. *In vivo* functional connectivity studies with rs-fMRI suggest that FOG patients may have significantly altered connectivity between PPN-SMA (Fling et al., 2014), which might reflect a maladaptive compensatory mechanism.

While the PPN has most often been investigated in PD in the context of FOG, it is unclear if altered PPN activity is present in non-FOG PD patients. Surgical targeting of the PPN is usually reserved for people with FOG resulting in significant impairment. Yet, even in early stages of the disease, there are a number of ways in which Parkinsonian gait is different from controls. While mildly affected PD patients can usually perform simple straight-line walk tasks without difficulty, they experience difficulties with turning, and when performing simultaneous motor or cognitive tasks (dual tasks), and/or crossing obstacles (Camicioli et al., 1998; Bond and Morris, 2000). They may have an abnormal gait pattern characterized by a shortened stride length, increased stride variability, and reduced walking speed (Morris et al., 2001; Buckley et al., 2008).

Ways to modulate PPN activity and connectivity have proven elusive. Acetylcholinesterase inhibitors may affect the PPN but such effects are likely to be modest. PPN Deep Brain Stimulation (DBS) has been shown to (inconsistently) improve gait difficulties in PD (Mazzone et al., 2005; Peppe et al., 2010; Acar et al., 2011; Hamani et al., 2011; Tykocki et al., 2011; Wilcox et al., 2011). However, the PPN tends to be spatially diffuse and is difficult to visualize on standard T1-weighted images, making electrode placement for DBS therapy difficult. Another potential way to modulate PPN is through the vestibular system, as PPN neurons tend to be highly vestibular-responsive (Aravamuthan and Angelaki, 2012). Galvanic vestibular stimulation (GVS) is a non-invasive technique that activates vestibular afferents to the thalamus and also the basal ganglia (Stiles and Smith, 2015) which in turn are directed to the PPN (Visser and Bloem, 2005), possibly explaining why GVS may positively impact posture/standing balance in PD (Kataoka et al., 2016). A few studies have demonstrated that noisy GVS improved postural and balance responses (Pal et al., 2009; Samoudi et al., 2015) as well as motor deficits in PD (Yamamoto et al., 2005; Pan et al., 2008; Lee et al., 2015a,b). These studies have speculated that noisy vestibular input may have improved information flow through the basal ganglia via *stochastic facilitation* (SF). SF is a phenomenon observed in a non-linear system where stochastic biological noise paradoxically increases sensitivity of a system to detect a weak stimulus possibly resulting in functional benefits (Mcdonnell and Ward, 2011). In addition to noisy stimuli, sinusoidal stimuli have been suggested as a means to activate steady-state, as opposed to transient balance responses that would be induced with pulsed stimuli (Latt et al., 2003). Sinusoidally oscillating stimuli may also activate irregular vestibular afferents (Gensberger et al., 2016) relying on voltage dependent K-channels (Eatock and Songer, 2011). While a couple of fMRI studies have shown sinusoidal GVS modulated activations in various brain regions (Della-Justina et al., 2014; Lee et al., 2016), GVS's influence on the PPN has not yet been investigated. A recent study in healthy older adults ($n = 20$) found that noisy GVS resulted in sustained reduction in Centre of Pressure (COP) parameters, such as velocity, and Root Mean Square (RMS) (Fujimoto et al., 2016). The mechanisms of this reduction was speculated to be on the basis of induced synaptic plasticity in the vestibular nuclei and the flocculus of the cerebellum, but effects on the PPN were not considered (Fujimoto et al., 2016).

Given the non-invasive, and potentially portable nature of GVS, we wished to determine if PPN connectivity could be modulated in mildly-affected PD subjects who may demonstrate reduced stride length for example, and thus may be at increased risk for falls, but did not exhibit FOG. Thus, in this study, we investigated whether or not functional connectivity between the PPN and other brain regions could be reliably assessed, whether or not these connections were significantly modulated by GVS, and if the connectivity was modulated in a stimulus-specific manner. Since *a priori* knowledge about functional connectivity to/from the PPN at the spatial and temporal resolution afforded by fMRI is unknown, this was essentially an exploratory approach. Careful care was taken to detect robust activation from PPN structures by analyzing the data in native space (without registration to a template) and utilizing subject-specific weightings of voxels within the PPN region. We demonstrated that PPN connectivity is sensitive to vestibular stimulation in PD in a stimulus-dependent manner.

METHODS

Subjects

Twenty three PD patients (see **Table 1** for the clinical information) and 12 age-matched healthy controls [5 females; age: 63.3 ± 10.4 (mean ± standard deviation)] participated in the study. The PD patients had mild to moderate PD (Hoehn and Yahr stage I–III) (see **Table 1**) and were scanned at the on-medication state. All participants were recruited from the Pacific Parkinson's Research Centre (PPRC) at the University of British Columbia (UBC) and provided written, informed consent prior to participation. All studies were approved by the UBC Ethics Review Board. The data were collected in two experiments: in the first group GVS was assessed both ON and OFF L-dopa medication and has been partially reported in a separate short report (Lee et al., 2016), and the second group were only assessed in the ON medication state. Only the ON medication studies from the first group are reported here. In the first group, UPDRS scores Part III were assessed in the OFF medication state, while in the second group UPDRS scores were assessed in the ON medication state. A regression model was used to control for these differences (described below).

GVS

Digital signals of the GVS stimuli were first generated on a PC with MATLAB (MathWorks, MA, USA) and were converted to analog signals via a NI USB-6221 BNC digital acquisition module (National Instruments, TX, USA). The analog command voltage signals were then subsequently passed to a bipolar, constant current stimulator (DS5 model, Digitimer Ltd., U.K.). The DS5 constant current stimulator was isolated in the console room with the output cable leading into the scanning room through a waveguide. Along the twisted coaxial output cable, four inductance capacity filters spaced 20 cm apart and tuned for the Larmor frequency (128 MHz) were custom-built. Near the subject, high-resistance radiotranslucent carbon-fiber leads (Biopac Inc., Montreal, Canada) were connected to pre-gelled Ag/AgCl electrodes that were MR-compatible (Biopac Inc., Montreal, Canada). For bilateral stimulation, an electrode was placed over the mastoid process behind each ear. Since the GVS stimuli are alternating current (AC), the anode and cathode are not fixed on one side (as for DC) but they are alternating.

TABLE 1 | Clinical information on PD patients.

Characteristics	Statistics (mean ± standard deviation)
Age	66.4 ± 7.0
Sex	17 males, 6 females
UPDRS motor score	22.3 ± 12.4
UPDRS assessed during on/off medication	13 on-medication, 10 off-medication
Hoehn and Yahr stage	1.9 ± 1.0
L-dopa equivalent daily dose (LEDD)	988.8 ± 798.9

The order of GVS condition was kept consistent to be rest, noisy GVS, and sinusoidal GVS across all the participants. The potential caveat of keeping the sequence the same is the case where there are any post-stimulation effects. To avoid such confounding effects, we allowed a 2-min break between the two GVS conditions. To the best of our knowledge, after-effects of GVS on cortical activation have not yet been investigated. However, we think that the break time was sufficient to avoid after effects based on literature on after-effects of transcranial alternating current stimulation (Strüber et al., 2015).

Since individuals have an inherently subjective perception of GVS, prior to scanning, we determined the individual sensory threshold level (cutaneous sensation at the electrode site) utilizing systematic procedures used in prior GVS studies (Hummel et al., 2005; Wilkinson et al., 2008; Utz et al., 2011). We delivered two different types of stimuli at 90% of the individual threshold level: noisy and sinusoidal. The noisy stimulus was zero-mean with 1/f-type power spectrum between 0.1 and 10 Hz and the sinusoidal stimulus was a 1 Hz sine wave.

MRI

Resting state data were collected on a 3 Tesla scanner (Philips Achieva 3.0T R3.2; Philips Medical Systems, Netherlands) equipped with a head-coil. During the scanning, all the subjects were instructed to be awake with eyes closed. Blood oxygenation level-dependent (BOLD) contrast echo-planar (EPI) T2*-weighted images were taken with the following specifications with a repetition time of 1,985 ms, echo time of 37 ms, flip angle 90°, field of view 240.00 mm, matrix size 128 × 128, and with pixel size 1.9 × 1.9 mm. The duration of each functional run was 8 min for rest condition and 5 min for GVS condition with noisy and sinusoidal stimulus, respectively. As stated above, the order of functional runs was rest, noisy GVS and sinusoidal GVS, and it was kept consistent across all subjects. We allowed 2 min gaps after the noisy stimulus to account for possible post-stimulation effects.

An ROI presumed to include the PPN and cuneiform nucleus was drawn manually on the T1 sequence at the level of the superior cerebellar decussation between medial lemniscus and superior cerebellar peduncle (Aravamuthan et al., 2007; Zrinzo et al., 2008) (**Figure 1**). T1 and the fMRI data were registered via FLIRT (with "Boundary-Based Registration" option) in FSL (Smith et al., 2004). The PPN voxels drawn on the T1 were then registered to the fMRI data by applying the inverse transformation calculated by registering the fMRI to the T1 weighted image. After registration, we included neighboring voxels around PPN voxels in our analysis to account for possible partial volume effects.

Resting State Functional MRI (rs-fMRI) Preprocessing

The acquired fMRI data were preprocessed using both AFNI and SPM8 software packages. On the whole brain, several preprocessing steps from the AFNI software package were performed. These included despiking, slice timing correction, and 3D isotropic correction (3 mm in each dimension). While the subjects were asked to keep the head still during the scanning session, some head movements occurred during the acquisition process. Motion correction using rigid body alignment was performed to correct for any major head motion during the scan. Besides the fMRI scans, we also collected a T1-weighted structural scan of each of the participants. FreeSurfer was performed on the T1-weighted scans to get the different ROI masks in the T1 space. Each of the subjects' structural scans was then registered to the fMRI scan using rigid registration. This registration step provided us with the FreeSurfer segmented ROI mask in the fMRI space. All analysis was done in the individual fMRI space rather than transforming all fMRI data to a common template. This was done to prevent introducing any unwanted distortions in the fMRI data by registering it to a common template. In the next step, several sources of variance such as head-motion parameters, their temporal derivatives and their squares, white-matter signal, CSF signal were removed using nuisance regression. The fMRI signal was then detrended, and any linear or quadratic trends in the fMRI signal were removed. The signal was then iteratively smoothed until it reached 6 FWHM of smoothness. Finally, bandpass filtering was performed to retain the signal between the recommended frequencies of interest (0.01–0.08 Hz).

Since the brainstem can move independently from the rest of the brain, motion correction on the whole brain motion estimates may not be ideal. Therefore, a separate motion correction of the brainstem was performed. First, the brainstem mask was generated using FreeSurfer on the T1-weighted image of the same subject. The mask was then transferred over to the fMRI using registration as mentioned before. The registered mask was then dilated using a spherical structuring element of radius 3 to incorporate for any errors in the segmentation and registration process. The motion within the brainstem was then corrected independently using the SPM toolbox.

Brain Region Selection

In this study, we included 58 ROIs automatically segmented by FreeSurfer as shown in **Table 2**. Two PPN ROIs were manually drawn on the T1-weighted images to include the PPN on each side, namely left PPN, and right PPN, respectively. When assessing the functional connectivity between PPN and other brain regions, we first utilized Partial Least Squares (PLS) to initially select candidate brain regions that significantly covaried with PPN voxels.

PLS is a statistical method that explores the predictive models between predictor variables and response variables (Wold, 1985). It constructs a linear regression model by projecting the predictor variables and response variables to a new set of latent variables the covariance of which is maximized. PLS is particularly useful when the predictor variables are highly collinear, or when the number of predictor variables is larger than that of observations, while classical multiple linear regression models will fail in these cases. PLS has been widely used in various fields of chemometrics, social science, bioinformatics, and neuroscience (e.g., Ziegler et al., 2013; Chen et al., 2016).

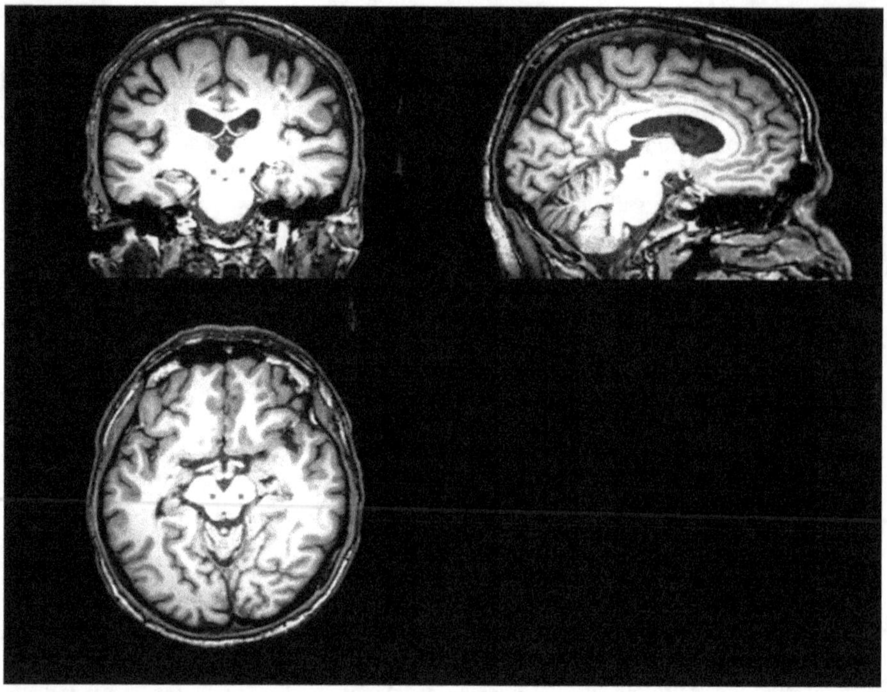

FIGURE 1 | The placement of the PPN VOI on the T1 sequence. The red area represents where the PPN VOI is placed.

When applying PLS, we used the 58-ROI dataset as predictor variables, X, and the PPN voxels as response variables, Y, and then tried to predict PPN activity from those 58-ROI time courses.

The general model for PLS is

$$X = TP^T + E \quad (1)$$

$$Y = UQ^T + F \quad (2)$$

where X is a *t*-by-*m* matrix of ROI data (predictor variables), with *t* corresponding to the number of time points, and *m* (= 58) representing the number of subject-independent (non-PPN) ROIs; Y is a *t*-by-*n* matrix of PPN voxel time courses (response variables), where *n* is the number of PPN voxels (which was subject-dependent); T and U are, respectively, *t*-by-*c* component matrices decomposed from X and Y (T and U are also called X Score and Y Score, respectively), where *c* is the number of components; P is an *m*-by-*c* loading matrix of ROI dataset, and Q is an *n*-by-*c* loading matrix of PPN voxels; and E, F are the *t*-by-*m* and *t*-by-*n* matrices, respectively, representing error terms. Essentially, PLS performs the decompositions of X and Y to maximize the covariance between T and U.

We then interrogated the loadings of the X components (i.e., the columns of P) to determine if they were significantly different from zero across subjects. The same procedure was conducted for both left PPN and right PPN, respectively, and then the union set of the selected regions from left PPN and right PPN was used as the final candidate set of brain regions. In addition, we used the first component of Y (i.e., the first column of Y Score) to represent the PPN signal in the subsequent functional connectivity analyses.

Functional Connectivity Analyses

We further performed functional connectivity analyses between the PPN and PLS-derived regions. Functional connectivity measures were obtained by computing the partial correlation coefficients between the represented PPN signal, which was obtained by the PLS analysis, and the averaged time courses of each PLS-derived region. We conducted the functional connectivity analyses on a subject-by-subject and task-by-task basis. Specifically, for each subject, functional connectivity was assessed for each of the three conditions, i.e., rest, noisy and sinusoidal GVS conditions, by taking the time courses for each condition time segment of interest from the PPN and PLS-derived regions and computing the partial correlation coefficients between them. For simplicity, we summed the absolute values of the significant connectivity coefficients from both left and right PPN to get an overall PPN connectivity.

To investigate whether or not functional connectivity between the PPN nuclei and PLS-derived regions was significantly affected by GVS, we calculated overall PPN connectivity differences between GVS on (i.e., noisy/sinusoidal GVS condition) and GVS off (i.e., rest condition). An independent one-sample *t*-test was then performed on the calculated connection coefficient *differences* across subjects, with the null hypothesis that the difference was zero, to determine if significant connectivity changes were induced by GVS.

TABLE 2 | The 58 ROIs (in addition to the 2 PPN ROIs) used in the analysis.

1	Left-Cerebellum-Cortex
2	Left-Thalamus-Proper
3	Left-Caudate
4	Left-Putamen
5	Left-Pallidum
6	Left-Hippocampus
7	Left-Amygdala
8	Left-Accumbens-area
9	ctx-lh-caudalanteriorcingulate
10	ctx-lh-caudalmiddlefrontal
11	ctx-lh-cuneus
12	ctx-lh-entorhinal
13	ctx-lh-inferiorparietal
14	ctx-lh-inferiortemporal
15	ctx-lh-lateralorbitofrontal
16	ctx-lh-medialorbitofrontal
17	ctx-lh-middletemporal
18	ctx-lh-parahippocampal
19	ctx-lh-paracentral
20	ctx-lh-postcentral
21	ctx-lh-posteriorcingulate
22	ctx-lh-precentral
23	ctx-lh-precuneus
24	ctx-lh-rostralanteriorcingulate
25	ctx-lh-rostralmiddlefrontal
26	ctx-lh-superiorfrontal
27	ctx-lh-superiorparietal
28	ctx-lh-superiortemporal
29	ctx-lh-insula
30	Right-Cerebellum-Cortex
31	Right-Thalamus-Proper
32	Right-Caudate
33	Right-Putamen
34	Right-Pallidum
35	Right-Hippocampus
36	Right-Amygdala
37	Right-Accumbens-area
38	ctx-rh-caudalanteriorcingulate
39	ctx-rh-caudalmiddlefrontal
40	ctx-rh-cuneus
41	ctx-rh-entorhinal
42	ctx-rh-inferiorparietal
43	ctx-rh-inferiortemporal
44	ctx-rh-lateralorbitofrontal
45	ctx-rh-medialorbitofrontal
46	ctx-rh-middletemporal
47	ctx-rh-parahippocampal
48	ctx-rh-paracentral
49	ctx-rh-postcentral
50	ctx-rh-posteriorcingulate
51	ctx-rh-precentral
52	ctx-rh-precuneus
53	ctx-rh-rostralanteriorcingulate
54	ctx-rh-rostralmiddlefrontal
55	ctx-rh-superiorfrontal
56	ctx-rh-superiorparietal
57	ctx-rh-superiortemporal
58	ctx-rh-insula

RESULTS

Brain Region Selection

The PLS analysis results found 10 ROIs in the PD group and 5 ROIs in the control group that significantly covaried with PPN voxels ($p < 0.05$). In the PD group, the ROIs included the cerebellum cortex, hippocampus, amygdala, inferior parietal, middle temporal, and precuneus regions on the left, and the pallidum, hippocampus, amygdala, and middle temporal on the right (**Figure 2**). In the control group, the caudate on the left, and the caudate, entorhinal cortex, inferior temporal, and parahippocampal regions on the right were associated with PPN activity (**Figure 3**).

Functional Connectivity Analyses

To determine the effect of the L-dopa equivalent daily dose (LEDD) on connectivity and to correct for the fact that some subjects had their UPDRS assessed off medication, we performed a regression analysis where connection strengths across subjects was the dependent variable, and LEDD, UPDRS score, whether or not the UPDRS was done on or off medication were independent variables. We then evaluated the regression coefficients for the LEDD to determine if it had a significant effect on overall PPN connectivity, which it did not ($p > 0.05$).

The functional analysis results demonstrated that GVS differently affected overall PPN connectivity in PD and control groups. In the control group, no significant differences in overall PPN connectivity were found between GVS on (i.e., noisy/sinusoidal GVS condition) and GVS off (i.e., rest condition). In the PD group, the overall magnitude of PPN connectivity correlated negatively with UPDRS scores ($r = -0.39$, $p = 0.035$, **Figure 4**). Both noisy and sinusoidal GVS increased the magnitude of overall PPN connectivity ($p = 6 \times 10^{-5}$ and 3×10^{-4}, respectively, **Figure 5**). Furthermore, in order to determine if overall connectivity of the PPN was particularly related to postural instability, we also compared the connectivity to the retropulsion test score from the UPDRS (**Figure 4**, inset). Since our emphasis was on early patients, we could not perform a statistical analysis, as there was only 1 subject with a score of 2 and 1 subject with a score of 4. However, as shown in **Figure 4**, and consistent with overall UPDRS scores, there was a trend toward decreased connectivity with higher retropulsion test scores.

Although both types of stimuli augmented overall PPN connectivity (both positive and negative connectivity as shown in **Figure 5**), in order to determine if there are differences between the types of stimuli, we performed a *post-hoc* analysis to determine which PPN connections were most influential in

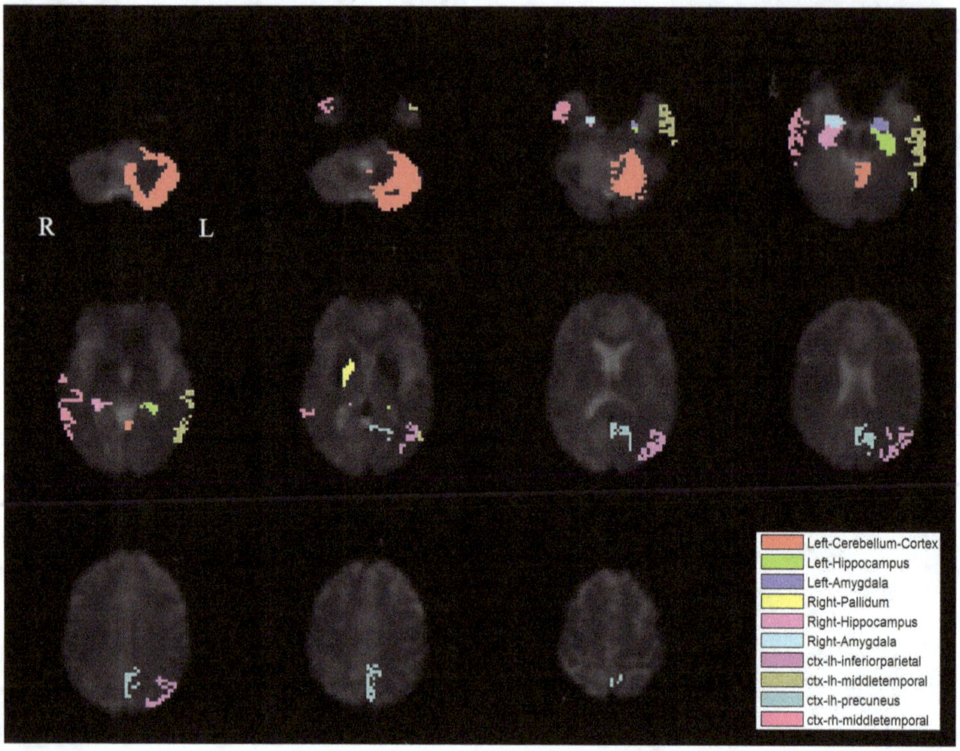

FIGURE 2 | PLS-derived ROIs in the PD group that significantly covaried with PPN voxels. The detected 10 regions, including cerebellum cortex, hippocampus, amygdala, inferior parietal, middle temporal, and precuneus regions on the left, and the pallidum, hippocampus, amygdala, and middle temporal on the right, are marked with different colors.

determining changes in overall connectivity. Specifically, we performed t-tests on each connection to determine if the different types of GVS stimuli increased or decreased connectivity between the PPN and other brain regions.

For the left PPN, noisy GVS decreased connectivity with the right pallidum and sinusoidal GVS increased connectivity with the left inferior parietal region (**Table 3** and **Figure 6**). For the right PPN, noisy GVS decreased connectivity with the left cerebellar cortex, increased connectivity with the right amygdala and increased connectivity with the left inferior parietal region; sinusoidal GVS decreased connectivity with the left amygdala (**Table 4** and **Figure 7**). Note that only the connection between left PPN and left inferior parietal region would survive multiple comparisons.

DISCUSSION

Balance impairment remains a vexing problem in PD and is associated with considerable morbidity. Pharmacological (particularly dopaminergic) and surgical interventions have had varying degrees of success. Development of novel therapies has also been challenging because the pathophysiology and neuropathological substrates underlying gait disturbances are incompletely known.

To the best of our knowledge, we have shown for the first time that is possible with GVS to non-invasively modulate the functional connectivity in PD subjects between cortical/subcortical ROIs and the PPN—a structure critical for normal supraspinal control of locomotion. This demonstrated alteration in functional connectivity complements previous work examining anatomic connectivity patterns. Anatomically, the PPN has been shown to have connections with various areas such as the vestibular nuclei (Aravamuthan and Angelaki, 2012), deep cerebellar nuclei (Hazrati and Parent, 1992), premotor, supplemental motor (SMA) and primary motor cortices (Aravamuthan et al., 2007), frontal eye fields (Matsumura et al., 2000), thalamic nuclei and basal ganglia nuclei (Charara et al., 1996). Widespread projections involving the PPN include direct glutamatergic inputs from the motor cortex, and GABAergic inputs from substantia nigra pars reticulata (SNr), globus pallidus internus (GPi), subthalamic nucleus (STN), and deep nuclei of cerebellum. Ascending efferent projections target GPi, substantia nigra pars compacta (SNc), and thalamus. Descending efferent projections connect to pontine, medullary reticular formation, and the spinal cord vital for control of muscle tone and locomotion. Additionally, the PPN appears to be important in the initiation, acceleration, deceleration, and termination of locomotion through connections to the basal ganglia and higher cortical regions (Lee et al., 2000).

Our results indicate significant differences in the PPN functional connectivity between PD subjects and controls. This is particularly relevant when noting that none of our PD subjects

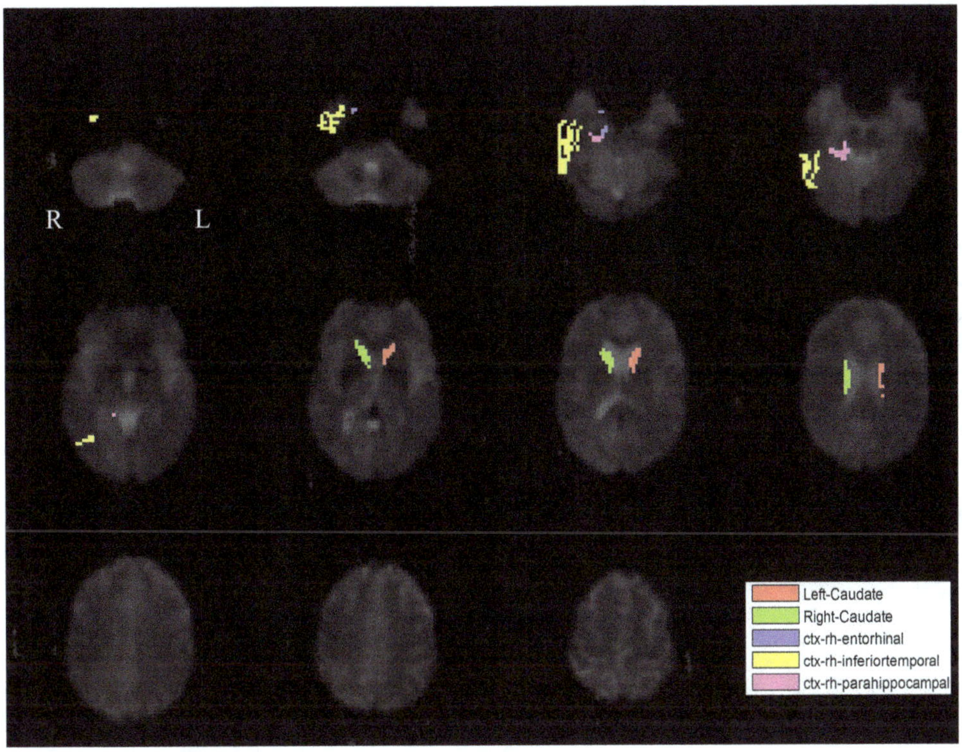

FIGURE 3 | PLS-derived ROIs in the control group that significantly covaried with PPN voxels. The detected five regions, including the caudate on the left, and the caudate, entorhinal cortex, inferior temporal, and parahippocampal regions on the right, are marked with different colors.

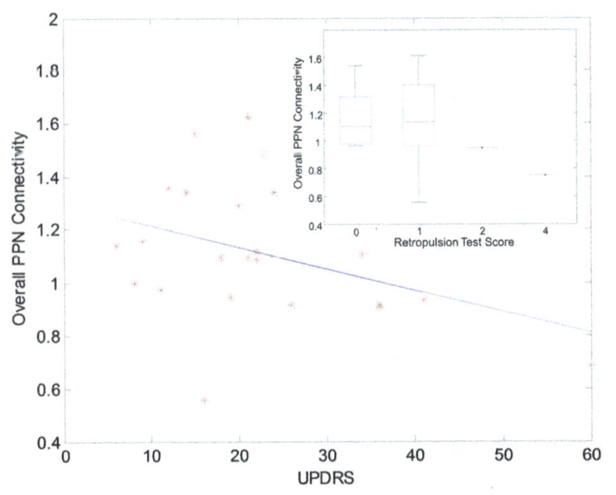

FIGURE 4 | The correlation relationship between the overall PPN connectivity and UPDRS scores in the PD group. The inset shows the relationship between the overall PPN connectivity and the retropulsion test scores from the UPDRS.

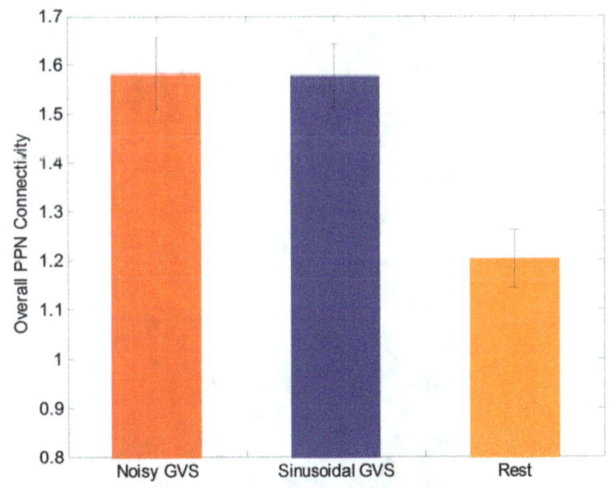

FIGURE 5 | The overall PPN connectivity differences between GVS on (i.e., noisy and sinusoidal GVS condition) and GVS off (i.e., rest condition) in the PD group.

had FOG, given their relatively mild disease. However, even mild disease is associated with altered gait and our results suggest that PPN functional connectivity patterns change even in the early stages of disease course.

We have shown that both GVS stimuli patterns (noisy and sinusoidal) augment overall deficient PPN connectivity in PD. Our results are consistent with previous studies demonstrating GVS activation of vestibular afferents to basal ganglia (Visser and Bloem, 2005; Stiles and Smith, 2015), which are also directed to the midbrain locomotion network (Peppe et al., 2010). PET studies in humans have also shown activation in the putamen in response to vestibular stimulation (Bottini et al., 1994).

We found differences in PPN network connectivity depending upon the type of stimulus used. Noisy GVS significantly decreased the functional connectivity between the left PPN and right-pallidum in PD. The PPN receives strong inhibitory, GABAergic inputs from the BG nuclei (GPi, STN, and SNr), which have disrupted connectivity in PD (Pahapill and Lozano, 2000). In particular, previous studies suggest that the PPN may be the principal target of pallidal outflow, since more than 80% GPi neurons were found to send axonal branches to both the PPN and thalamus in monkeys (Harnois and Filion, 1982). In PD, the inhibitory GABAergic synaptic activities from the GPi to the PPN is abnormally overactive, which may underlie the akinesia and the gait problems seen in the PD (Pahapill and Lozano, 2000). Taken together, these studies demonstrate the important role of the PPN and pallidal connectivity in motor and gait dysfunctions of PD. We demonstrated that noisy GVS significantly decreased connectivity between the left PPN and right-pallidum in PD (but not normal controls), which suggests that potential benefits of GVS on balance in PD may be partly mediated through attenuation of overactive pallidal inputs to the PPN.

Noisy GVS also decreased connectivity between the right PPN and the left cerebellar cortex. A DWI study found the connectivity of the PPN region with the cerebellum, thalamus, pallidum, and STN (Muthusamy et al., 2007). The cerebellum functions that help control of movement, coordination, and posture (Saab and Willis, 2003) are speculated to be associated with the existence of the pathway with the PPN (Muthusamy et al., 2007). The fact that prior studies have suggested a beneficial effect of noisy GVS (Fujimoto et al., 2016) may indicate that hyperactive PPN-cerebellar connections are partly "normalized" with GVS.

TABLE 3 | Statistics on significant left PPN connectivity changes induced by GVS stimuli in the PD group.

Connectivity	Type of Stimuli	*t*-value	*p*-value
Right pallidum	Noisy GVS	−2.32	0.015
Left inferior parietal	Sinusoidal GVS	2.81	0.005

TABLE 4 | Statistics on significant right PPN connectivity changes induced by GVS stimuli in the PD group.

Connectivity	Type of Stimuli	*t*-value	*p*-value
Left cerebellum cortex	Noisy GVS	−1.89	0.036
Right amygdala	Noisy GVS	1.90	0.035
Left inferior parietal	Noisy GVS	2.05	0.026
Left amygdala	Sinusoidal GVS	−2.09	0.024

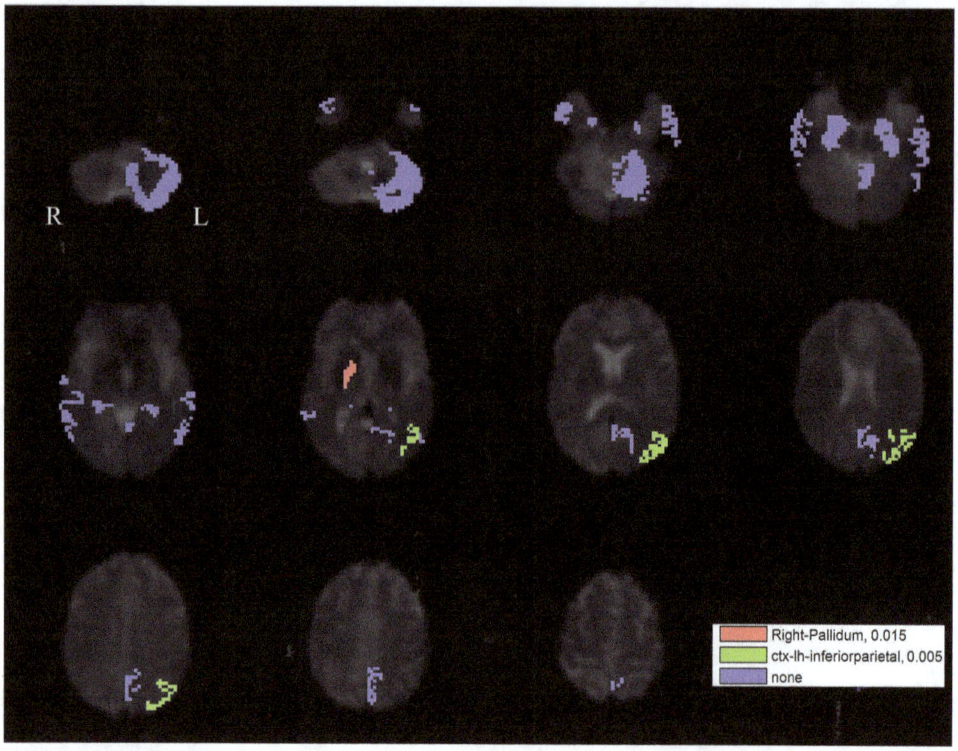

FIGURE 6 | The GVS impact on the connectivity between the left PPN and PLS-derived regions in the PD group. The red areas represent the regions significantly affected by noisy GVS. The green areas represent the regions significantly affected by sinusoidal GVS. The blue areas represent the regions with no significant changes. The corresponding ROI names and significance values are labeled in the figure.

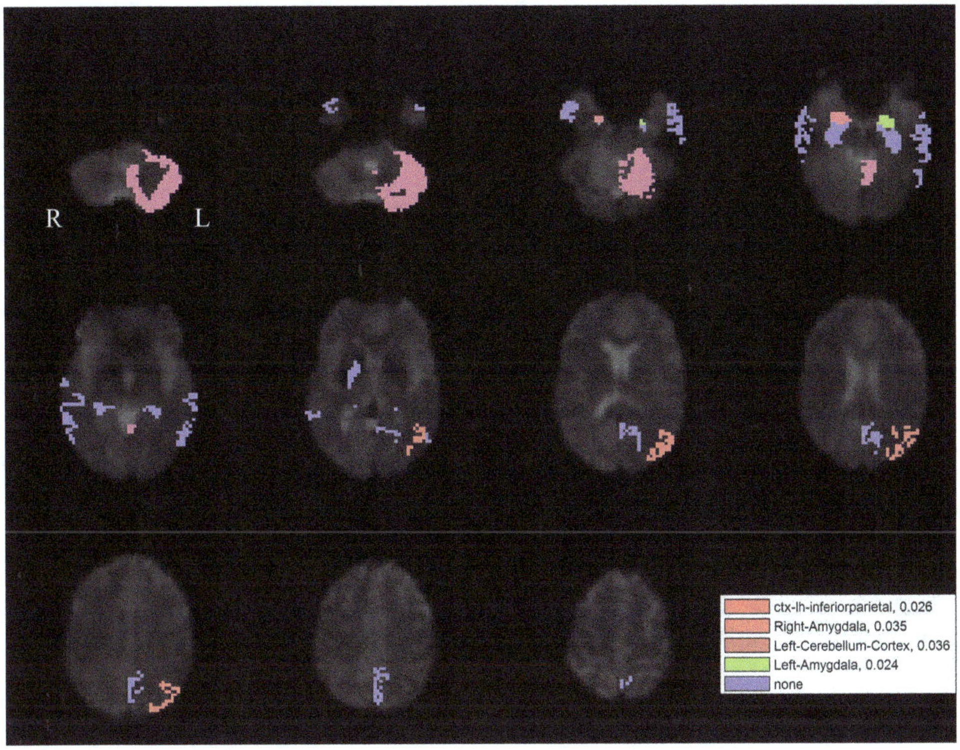

FIGURE 7 | The GVS impact on the connectivity between the right PPN and PLS-derived regions in the PD group. The red areas (with three different color levels indicating the different levels of significance values) represent the regions significantly affected by noisy GVS. The green areas represent the regions significantly affected by sinusoidal GVS. The blue areas represent the regions with no significant changes. The corresponding ROI names and significance values are labeled in the figure.

We also found that GVS increased the functional connectivity between the left inferior parietal cortex and the right PPN (with noisy stimuli) and left PPN (with sinusoidal stimuli). Previous studies in non-human primates examining cortical inputs to the pontine nuclei have supported the anatomical and functional relationships between the PPN and the inferior parietal cortex (May and Andersen, 1986; Martinez-Gonzalez et al., 2011). Like the PPN, the left inferior parietal cortex is involved in gait as well as visuospatial information processing, motor planning, and preparation (Caspers et al., 2012). Imagining normal gait activates the left inferior parietal lobule, in addition to the precuneus and bilateral dorsal premotor cortex, the left dorsolateral prefrontal cortex, and the right posterior cingulate cortex (Malouin et al., 2003). The left inferior parietal cortex appears to be especially related to FOG. Gray matter volume in the left inferior parietal region is significantly reduced in PD subjects with FOG patients compared to both PD subjects without FOG and healthy controls (Kostić et al., 2012). Thus, our result that noisy GVS increased the connectivity between the PPN and the left inferior parietal cortex might suggest GVS could improve gait difficulties in PD by augmenting the connectivity.

In the current study, one of the advantages is that we performed analyses keeping each subject's data in their original space without warping the data to a common template. We are frankly skeptical of fMRI studies suggesting robust activation from brainstem structures (e.g., PPN) when data are spatially transformed to a template, given the significant registration errors that can occur to small brainstem nuclei during whole-brain registration (Ng et al., 2009). In addition, we utilized PLS to find the combination of PPN voxels on a subject-by-subject basis that maximally corresponded with other ROIs. In effect, the first column of Q in Equation (2) represents a subject-specific spatial filter to "focus" the activity that maximally covaried with other ROIs.

It is interesting that many of the abnormal connectivities that we detected are lateralized, when balance might be considered a "midline" function. Balance control and gait are asymmetrical in patients with PD, and gait asymmetries have been linked to the pathophysiology of FOG (Boonstra et al., 2014). The symptoms of PD generally show an asymmetric onset and progression and it has been proposed that this may lead to a degree of "unbalanced" motor function, such that FOG is triggered by a breakdown in the bilateral co-ordination underlying the normal timing of gait (Plotnik et al., 2005).

There are a few limitations in our study. We examined a relatively small number of PD patients. However, by carefully selecting the PPN voxels via PLS on a subject-by-subject basis, we expect that we have significantly enhanced our effect size, and thus increasing our statistical power and thus increasing our statistical power. PLS is one of the most widely used blind source separation (BSS) approaches which have largely benefited the neuroscience studies (Ziegler et al., 2013; Chen et al., 2016, 2018; Smith and Nichols, 2018). In the future studies, we are interested to further explore the effective voxel selections using such data-driven approaches. We have shown GVS induced changes in PPN connectivity in people with mild to moderate PD but not in healthy controls. We speculate an "inverted-U" shape of effectiveness of GVS as a function of disease severity: in controls, GVS had minimal effect, in early/moderate PD, it had some effect (shown here), and in severe disease, degeneration in the PPN itself may prevent modulation of its connectivity. Future work is required to further investigate the relationship between disease severity and PPN connectivity and determine the behavioral significance of this altered PPN connectivity. We do note that we found a negative correlation between UPDRS scores and overall PPN connectivity, yet still found robust modulation of connectivity across all of our subjects.

The relation between behavioral gait measures (e.g., gait variability) and ultimate falls risk—the most important issue for people with PD—is an active area of research. Conceivably, previously-described GVS improvements in balance may not ultimately translate into reduced fall risk but such determination would require a prospective trial in the future. We have focused on the PPN because of its possible therapeutic implications, but gait disturbances in PD likely involve several cortical and subcortical structures. For example, PD patients have decreased activity of the SMA during gait (Hanakawa et al., 1999), and PD individuals have diminished pre-movement electroencephalographic potentials originating from the SMA prior to step initiation (Smith et al., 2012). Future studies to assess connectivity changes modified by GVS in other supra-spinal locomotion centers including SMA/pre-SMA may help to guide the development of optimal stimuli on a subject-specific basis.

ETHICS STATEMENT

This study was carried out in accordance with the recommendations of TCPS2, UBC Clinical Research Ethics Board with written informed consent from all subjects. All subjects gave written informed consent in accordance with the Declaration of Helsinki. The protocol was approved by the UBC Clinical Research Ethics Board.

AUTHOR CONTRIBUTIONS

This study is ideated by MM. SL, LK, and DK conducted the experiment and data acquisition. SG and FB contributed to the data preprocessing. JC performed data analysis and manuscript writing. Interpretation of the results was performed by SL, JC, AL, FB, and MM. MM, ZW, and AL contributed to the project supervision and manuscript finalization. All authors have approved the final manuscript.

ACKNOWLEDGMENTS

This work was partly supported by the National Key R&D Program of China (2017YFB1300301), NSFC (61701158), PPRI/UBC Chair in Parkinson's Research (MM) and a generous grant from the Mottershead Foundation.

REFERENCES

Acar, F., Acar, G., Bir, L. S., Gedik, B., and Oguzhanoglu, A. (2011). Deep brain stimulation of the pedunculopontine nucleus in a patient with freezing of gait. *Stereotact. Funct. Neurosurg.* 89, 214–219. doi: 10.1159/0003 26617

Androulidakis, A. G., Mazzone, P., Litvak, V., Penny, W., Dileone, M., Gaynor, L. M., et al. (2008). Oscillatory activity in the pedunculopontine area of patients with Parkinson's disease. *Exp. Neurol.* 211, 59–66. doi: 10.1016/j.expneurol.2008.01.002

Aravamuthan, B., Muthusamy, K., Stein, J., Aziz, T., and Johansen-Berg, H. (2007). Topography of cortical and subcortical connections of the human pedunculopontine and subthalamic nuclei. *Neuroimage* 37, 694–705. doi: 10.1016/j.neuroimage.2007.05.050

Aravamuthan, B. R., and Angelaki, D. E. (2012). Vestibular responses in the macaque pedunculopontine nucleus and central mesencephalic reticular formation. *Neuroscience* 223, 183–199. doi: 10.1016/j.neuroscience.2012.07.054

Azevedo Coste, C., Sijobert, B., Pissard-Gibollet, R., Pasquier, M., Espiau, B., and Geny, C. (2014). Detection of freezing of gait in Parkinson disease: preliminary results. *Sensors* 14, 6819–6827. doi: 10.3390/s140406819

Benecke, R., Rothwell, J., Dick, J., Day, B., and Marsden, C. (1987). Disturbance of sequential movements in patients with Parkinson's disease. *Brain* 110:361. doi: 10.1093/brain/110.2.361

Bloem, B. R., Beckley, D. J., Van Dijk, J. G., Zwinderman, A. H., Remler, M. P., and Roos, R. A. (1996). Influence of dopaminergic medication on automatic postural responses and balance impairment in Parkinson's disease. *Mov. Disord.* 11, 509–521. doi: 10.1002/mds.870110506

Bohnen, N., Muller, M., Koeppe, R., Studenski, S., Kilbourn, M., Frey, K., et al. (2009). History of falls in Parkinson disease is associated with reduced cholinergic activity. *Neurology* 73, 1670–1676. doi: 10.1212/WNL.0b013e3181c1ded6

Bond, J. M., and Morris, M. (2000). Goal-directed secondary motor tasks: their effects on gait in subjects with Parkinson disease. *Arch. Phys. Med. Rehabil.* 81, 110–116. doi: 10.1016/S0003-9993(00)90230-2

Boonstra, T. A., van Vugt, J. P. P., van der Kooij, H., and Bloem, B. R. (2014). Balance asymmetry in Parkinson's disease and its contribution to freezing of gait. *PLoS ONE* 9:e102493. doi: 10.1371/journal.pone.0102493

Bottini, G., Sterzi, R., Paulesu, E., Vallar, G., Cappa, S. F., Erminio, F., et al. (1994). Identification of the central vestibular projections in man: a positron emission tomography activation study. *Exp. Brain Res.* 99, 164–169. doi: 10.1007/BF00241421

Buckley, T. A., Pitsikoulis, C., and Hass, C. J. (2008). Dynamic postural stability during sit-to-walk transitions in Parkinson disease patients. *Mov. Disord.* 23, 1274–1280. doi: 10.1002/mds.22079

Cameron, I. D., Gillespie, L. D., Robertson, M. C., Murray, G. R., Hill, K. D., Cumming, R. G., et al. (2012). Interventions for preventing falls in older people in care facilities and hospitals. *Cochrane Database Syst. Rev.* 12:CD005465. doi: 10.1002/14651858.CD005465.pub3

Camicioli, R., Howieson, D., Oken, B., Sexton, G., and Kaye, J. (1998). Motor slowing precedes cognitive impairment in the oldest old. *Neurology* 50, 1496–1498. doi: 10.1212/WNL.50.5.1496

Caspers, S., Schleicher, A., Bacha-Trams, M., Palomero-Gallagher, N., Amunts, K., and Zilles, K. (2012). Organization of the human inferior parietal lobule based on receptor architectonics. *Cerebral Cortex* 23, 615–628. doi: 10.1093/cercor/bhs048

Charara, A., Smith, Y., and Parent, A. (1996). Glutamatergic inputs from the pedunculopontine nucleus to midbrain dopaminergic neurons in primates: *Phaseolus vulgaris*-leucoagglutinin anterograde labeling combined with

postembedding glutamate and GABA immunohistochemistry. *J. Comp. Neurol.* 364, 254–266. doi: 10.1002/(SICI)1096-9861(19960108)364:2<254::AID-CNE5>3.0.CO;2-4

Chee, R., Murphy, A., Danoudis, M., Georgiou-Karistianis, N., and Iansek, R. (2009). Gait freezing in Parkinson's disease and the stride length sequence effect interaction. *Brain* 132, 2151–2160. doi: 10.1093/brain/awp053

Chen, X., Wang, Z. J., and Mckeown, M. (2016). Joint blind source separation for neurophysiological data analysis: Multiset and multimodal methods. *IEEE Signal Process. Mag.* 33, 86–107. doi: 10.1109/MSP.2016.2521870

Chen, X., Xu, X., Liu, A., McKeown, M. J., and Wang, Z. J. (2018). The use of multivariate EMD and CCA for denoising muscle artifacts from few-channel EEG recordings. *IEEE Trans. Instrum. Meas.* 67, 359–370. doi: 10.1109/TIM.2017.2759398

Della-Justina, H. M., Manczak, T., Winkler, A. M., de Araújo, D. B. D., de Souza, M. A., Amaro Junior, E., et al. (2014). Galvanic vestibular stimulator for fMRI studies. *Rev. Bras. Eng. Bioméd.* 30, 70–82. doi: 10.4322/rbeb.2013.046

Eatock, R. A., and Songer, J. E. (2011). Vestibular hair cells and afferents: two channels for head motion signals. *Annu. Rev. Neurosci.* 34, 501–534. doi: 10.1146/annurev-neuro-061010-113710

Fling, B. W., Cohen, R. G., Mancini, M., Carpenter, S. D., Fair, D. A., Nutt, J. G., et al. (2014). Functional reorganization of the locomotor network in Parkinson patients with freezing of gait. *PLoS ONE* 9:e100291. doi: 10.1371/journal.pone.0100291

Fujimoto, C., Yamamoto, Y., Kamogashira, T., Kinoshita, M., Egami, N., Uemura, Y., et al. (2016). Noisy galvanic vestibular stimulation induces a sustained improvement in body balance in elderly adults. *Sci. Rep.* 6:37575. doi: 10.1038/srep37575

Gensberger, K. D., Kaufmann, A.-K., Dietrich, H., Branoner, F., Banchi, R., Chagnaud, B. P., et al. (2016). Galvanic vestibular stimulation: cellular substrates and response patterns of neurons in the vestibulo-ocular network. *J. Neurosci.* 36, 9097–9110. doi: 10.1523/JNEUROSCI.4239-15.2016

Hamani, C., Moro, E., and Lozano, A. M. (2011). The pedunculopontine nucleus as a target for deep brain stimulation. *J. Neural Transm.* 118, 1461–1468. doi: 10.1007/s00702-010-0547-8

Hanakawa, T., Fukuyama, H., Katsumi, Y., Honda, M., and Shibasaki, H. (1999). Enhanced lateral premotor activity during paradoxical gait in Parkinson's disease. *Ann. Neurol.* 45, 329–336. doi: 10.1002/1531-8249(199903)45:3<329::AID-ANA8>3.0.CO;2-S

Harnois, C., and Filion, M. (1982). Pallidofugal projections to thalamus and midbrain: a quantitative antidromic activation study in monkeys and cats. *Exp. Brain Res.* 47, 277–285. doi: 10.1007/BF00239387

Hazrati, L.-N., and Parent, A. (1992). Projection from the deep cerebellar nuclei to the pedunculopontine nucleus in the squirrel monkey. *Brain Res.* 585, 267–271. doi: 10.1016/0006-8993(92)91216-2

Hummel, F., Celnik, P., Giraux, P., Floel, A., Wu, W.-H., Gerloff, C., et al. (2005). Effects of non-invasive cortical stimulation on skilled motor function in chronic stroke. *Brain* 128, 490–499. doi: 10.1093/brain/awh369

Kataoka, H., Okada, Y., Kiriyama, T., Kita, Y., Nakamura, J., Morioka, S., et al. (2016). Can postural instability respond to galvanic vestibular stimulation in patients with Parkinson's disease? *J. Mov. Disord.* 9, 40–43. doi: 10.14802/jmd.15030

Kostić, V., Agosta, F., Pievani, M., Stefanova, E., Ječmenica-Lukić, M., Scarale, A., et al. (2012). Pattern of brain tissue loss associated with freezing of gait in Parkinson disease. *Neurology* 78, 409–416. doi: 10.1212/WNL.0b013e318245d23c

Latt, L., Sparto, P., Furman, J., and Redfern, M. (2003). The steady-state postural response to continuous sinusoidal galvanic vestibular stimulation. *Gait Posture* 18, 64–72. doi: 10.1016/S0966-6362(02)00195-9

Lee, M. S., Rinne, J. O., and Marsden, C. D. (2000). The pedunculopontine nucleus: Its role in the genesis of movement. *Yonsei Med. J.* 41 167–184. doi: 10.3349/ymj.2000.41.2.167

Lee, S., Cai, J., Kim, D., Wang, Z., and Mckeown, M. (2016). "Differential effects of noisy and sinusoidal galvanic vestibular stimulation on resting state functional connectivity," in *4th Annual Minnesota Neuromodulation Symposium* (Minneapolis, MN).

Lee, S., Kim, D. J., Svenkeson, D., Parras, G., Oishi, M. M. K., and Mckeown, M. J. (2015a). Multifaceted effects of noisy galvanic vestibular stimulation on manual tracking behavior in Parkinson's disease. *Front. Syst. Neurosci.* 9:5. doi: 10.3389/fnsys.2015.00005

Lee, S., Kim, D., Svenkeson, D., Oishi, M. M. K., and Mckeown, M. J. (2015b). Synergistic effects of noisy galvanic vestibular stimulation and oral L-dopa in improving manual tracking performance in Parkinson's disease. *Brain Stimul.* 8:368. doi: 10.1016/j.brs.2015.01.184

Magrinelli, F., Picelli, A., Tocco, P., Federico, A., Roncari, L., Smania, N., et al. (2016). Pathophysiology of motor dysfunction in Parkinson's disease as the rationale for drug treatment and rehabilitation. *Parkinson Dis.* 2016:9832839. doi: 10.1155/2016/9832839

Malouin, F., Richards, C. L., Jackson, P. L., Dumas, F., and Doyon, J. (2003). Brain activations during motor imagery of locomotor-related tasks: a PET study. *Hum. Brain Mapp.* 19, 47–62. doi: 10.1002/hbm.10103

Martinez-Gonzalez, C., Bolam, J. P., and Mena-Segovia, J. (2011). Topographical organization of the pedunculopontine nucleus. *Front. Neuroanat.* 5:22. doi: 10.3389/fnana.2011.00022

Matsumura, M., Nambu, A., Yamaji, Y., Watanabe, K., Imai, H., Inase, M., et al. (2000). Organization of somatic motor inputs from the frontal lobe to the pedunculopontine tegmental nucleus in the macaque monkey. *Neuroscience* 98, 97–110. doi: 10.1016/S0306-4522(00)00099-3

May, J., and Andersen, R. (1986). Different patterns of corticopontine projections from separate cortical fields within the inferior parietal lobule and dorsal prelunate gyrus of the macaque. *Exp. Brain Res.* 63, 265–278. doi: 10.1007/BF00236844

Mazzone, P., Lozano, A., Stanzione, P., Galati, S., Scarnati, E., Peppe, A., et al. (2005). Implantation of human pedunculopontine nucleus: a safe and clinically relevant target in Parkinson's disease. *Neuroreport* 16, 1877–1881. doi: 10.1097/01.wnr.0000187629.38010.12

Mcdonnell, M. D., and Ward, L. M. (2011). The benefits of noise in neural systems: bridging theory and experiment. *Nat. Rev. Neurosci.* 12, 415–426. doi: 10.1038/nrn3061

Morris, S., Morris, M. E., and Iansek, R. (2001). Reliability of measurements obtained with the Timed "Up & Go" test in people with Parkinson disease. *Phys. Ther.* 81, 810–818. doi: 10.1093/ptj/81.2.810

Muthusamy, K., Aravamuthan, B., Kringelbach, M., Jenkinson, N., Voets, N., Johansen-Berg, H., et al. (2007). Connectivity of the human pedunculopontine nucleus region and diffusion tensor imaging in surgical targeting. *J. Neurosurg.* 107, 814–820. doi: 10.3171/JNS-07/10/0814

Ng, B., Abu-Gharbieh, R., and Mckeown, M. J. (2009). "Adverse effects of template-based warping on spatial fMRI analysis," in *SPIE Medical Imaging* (Lake Buena Vista, FL).

Ondo, W. G., and Hunter, C. (2003). Flumazenil, a GABA antagonist, may improve features of Parkinson's disease. *Mov. Disord.* 18, 683–685. doi: 10.1002/mds.10426

Pahapill, P. A., and Lozano, A. M. (2000). The pedunculopontine nucleus and Parkinson's disease. *Brain* 123, 1767–1783. doi: 10.1093/brain/123.9.1767

Pal, S., Rosengren, S. M., and Colebatch, J. G. (2009). Stochastic galvanic vestibular stimulation produces a small reduction in sway in Parkinson's disease. *J. Ves. Res.* 19, 137–142. doi: 10.3233/VES-2009-0360

Pan, W., Soma, R., Kwak, S., and Yamamoto, Y. (2008). Improvement of motor functions by noisy vestibular stimulation in central neurodegenerative disorders. *J. Neurol.* 255, 1657–1661. doi: 10.1007/s00415-008-0950-3

Peppe, A., Pierantozzi, M., Chiavalon, C., Marchetti, F., Caltagirone, C., Musicco, M., et al. (2010). Deep brain stimulation of the pedunculopontine tegmentum and subthalamic nucleus: effects on gait in Parkinson's disease. *Gait Posture* 32, 512–518. doi: 10.1016/j.gaitpost.2010.07.012

Perez-Lloret, S., and Barrantes, F. J. (2016). Deficits in cholinergic neurotransmission and their clinical correlates in Parkinson's disease. *NPJ Parkinson Dis.* 2:16001. doi: 10.1038/npjparkd.2016.1

Perez-Lloret, S., Negre-Pages, L., Damier, P., Delval, A., Derkinderen, P., Destée, A., et al. (2014). Prevalence, determinants, and effect on quality of life of freezing of gait in Parkinson disease. *JAMA Neurol.* 71, 884–890. doi: 10.1001/jamaneurol.2014.753

Plotnik, M., Giladi, N., Balash, Y., Peretz, C., and Hausdorff, J. M. (2005). Is freezing of gait in Parkinson's disease related to asymmetric motor function? *Ann. Neurol.* 57, 656–663. doi: 10.1002/ana.20452

Rinne, J. O., Ma, S. Y., Lee, M. S., Collan, Y., and Röyttä, M. (2008). Loss of cholinergic neurons in the pedunculopontine nucleus in Parkinson's disease is related to disability of the patients. *Parkinsonism Relat. Disord.* 14, 553–557. doi: 10.1016/j.parkreldis.2008.01.006

Saab, C. Y., and Willis, W. D. (2003). The cerebellum: organization, functions and its role in nociception. *Brain Res. Rev.* 42, 85–95. doi: 10.1016/S0165-0173(03)00151-6

Samoudi, G., Jivegård, M., Mulavara, A. P., and Bergquist, F. (2015). Effects of stochastic vestibular galvanic stimulation and LDOPA on balance and motor symptoms in patients with Parkinson's disease. *Brain Stimul.* 8, 474–480. doi: 10.1016/j.brs.2014.11.019

Schaafsma, J., Balash, Y., Gurevich, T., Bartels, A., Hausdorff, J. M., and Giladi, N. (2003). Characterization of freezing of gait subtypes and the response of each to levodopa in Parkinson's disease. *Eur. J. Neurol.* 10, 391–398. doi: 10.1046/j.1468-1331.2003.00611.x

Shine, J. M., Matar, E., Ward, P. B., Bolitho, S. J., Gilat, M., Pearson, M., et al. (2013). Exploring the cortical and subcortical functional magnetic resonance imaging changes associated with freezing in Parkinson's disease. *Brain* 136, 1204–1215. doi: 10.1093/brain/awt049

Smith, B. A., Jacobs, J. V., and Horak, F. B. (2012). Effects of magnitude and magnitude predictability of postural perturbations on preparatory cortical activity in older adults with and without Parkinson's disease. *Exp. Brain Res.* 222, 455–470. doi: 10.1007/s00221-012-3232-3

Smith, S. M., and Nichols, T. E. (2018). Statistical challenges in "Big Data" human neuroimaging. *Neuron* 97, 263–268. doi: 10.1016/j.neuron.2017.12.018

Smith, S. M., Jenkinson, M., Woolrich, M. W., Beckmann, C. F., Behrens, T. E., Johansen-Berg, H., et al. (2004). Advances in functional and structural MR image analysis and implementation as FSL. *Neuroimage* 23, S208–S219. doi: 10.1016/j.neuroimage.2004.07.051

Stevens, J. A., Corso, P. S., Finkelstein, E. A., and Miller, T. R. (2006). The costs of fatal and non-fatal falls among older adults. *Inj. Prev.* 12, 290–295. doi: 10.1136/ip.2005.011015

Stiles, L., and Smith, P. F. (2015). The vestibular-basal ganglia connection: balancing motor control. *Brain Res.* 1597, 180–188. doi: 10.1016/j.brainres.2014.11.063

Strüber, D., Rach, S., Neuling, T., and Herrmann, C. S. (2015). On the possible role of stimulation duration for after-effects of transcranial alternating current stimulation. *Front. Cell. Neurosci.* 9:311. doi: 10.3389/fncel.2015.00311

Tykocki, T., Mandat, T., and Nauman, P. (2011). Pedunculopontine nucleus deep brain stimulation in Parkinson's disease. *Arch. Med. Sci.* 7, 555–564. doi: 10.5114/aoms.2011.24119

Utz, K. S., Korluss, K., Schmidt, L., Rosenthal, A., Oppenländer, K., Keller, I., et al. (2011). Minor adverse effects of galvanic vestibular stimulation in persons with stroke and healthy individuals. *Brain Inj.* 25, 1058–1069. doi: 10.3109/02699052.2011.607789

Vercruysse, S., Leunissen, I., Vervoort, G., Vandenberghe, W., Swinnen, S., and Nieuwboer, A. (2015). Microstructural changes in white matter associated with freezing of gait in Parkinson's disease. *Mov. Dis.* 30, 567–576. doi: 10.1002/mds.26130

Visser, J. E., and Bloem, B. R. (2005). Role of the basal ganglia in balance control. *Neural Plast.* 12, 161–174. doi: 10.1155/NP.2005.161

Wilcox, R. A., Cole, M. H., Wong, D., Coyne, T., Silburn, P., and Kerr, G. (2011). Pedunculopontine nucleus deep brain stimulation produces sustained improvement in primary progressive freezing of gait. *J. Neurol. Neurosurg. Psychiatry* 82, 1256–1259. doi: 10.1136/jnnp.2010.213462

Wilkinson, D., Nicholls, S., Pattenden, C., Kilduff, P., and Milberg, W. (2008). Galvanic vestibular stimulation speeds visual memory recall. *Exp. Brain Res.* 189, 243–248. doi: 10.1007/s00221-008-1463-0

Williams, D., Watt, H., and Lees, A. (2006). Predictors of falls and fractures in bradykinetic rigid syndromes: a retrospective study. *J. Neurol. Neurosurg. Psychiatry* 77, 468–473. doi: 10.1136/jnnp.2005.074070

Wold, H. (1985). *Partial Least Squares. Encyclopedia of Statistical Sciences.* New York, NY: John Wiley & Sons.

Yamamoto, Y., Struzik, Z., Soma, R., Ohashi, K., and Kwak, S. (2005). Noisy vestibular stimulation improves autonomic and motor responsiveness in central neurodegenerative disorders. *Ann. Neurol.* 58, 175–181. doi: 10.1002/ana.20574

Ziegler, G., Dahnke, R., Winkler, A., and Gaser, C. (2013). Partial least squares correlation of multivariate cognitive abilities and local brain structure in children and adolescents. *Neuroimage* 82, 284–294. doi: 10.1016/j.neuroimage.2013.05.088

Zrinzo, L., Zrinzo, L. V., Tisch, S., Limousin, P. D., Yousry, T. A., Afshar, F., et al. (2008). Stereotactic localization of the human pedunculopontine nucleus: atlas-based coordinates and validation of a magnetic resonance imaging protocol for direct localization. *Brain* 131, 1588–1598. doi: 10.1093/brain/awn075

13

In utero and Lactational Exposure to Acetamiprid Induces Abnormalities in Socio-Sexual and Anxiety-Related Behaviors of Male Mice

Kazuhiro Sano[1], *Tomohiko Isobe*[1], *Jiaxin Yang*[1], *Tin-Tin Win-Shwe*[1], *Mitsuha Yoshikane*[1], *Shoji F. Nakayama*[1], *Takaharu Kawashima*[2], *Go Suzuki*[1,3], *Shunji Hashimoto*[4], *Keiko Nohara*[1], *Chiharu Tohyama*[5] *and Fumihiko Maekawa*[1*]

[1] Center for Health and Environmental Risk Research, National Institute for Environmental Studies, Tsukuba, Japan, [2] Center for Environmental Biology and Ecosystem Studies, National Institute for Environmental Studies, Tsukuba, Japan, [3] Center for Material Cycles and Waste Management Research, National Institute for Environmental Studies, Tsukuba, Japan, [4] Center for Environmental Measurement and Analysis, National Institute for Environmental Studies, Tsukuba, Japan, [5] Faculty of Medicine, University of Tsukuba, Tsukuba, Japan

Edited by:
Pierrette Gaudreau,
Centre hospitalier de l'Université de Montréal, Canada

Reviewed by:
Caroline Menard,
Icahn School of Medicine at Mount Sinai, USA
Cathy Vaillancourt,
INRS-Institut Armand Frappier, Canada

***Correspondence:**
Fumihiko Maekawa
fmaekawa@nies.go.jp

Neonicotinoids, a widely used group of pesticides designed to selectively bind to insect nicotinic acetylcholine receptors, were considered relatively safe for mammalian species. However, they have been found to activate vertebrate nicotinic acetylcholine receptors and could be toxic to the mammalian brain. In the present study, we evaluated the developmental neurotoxicity of acetamiprid (ACE), one of the most widely used neonicotinoids, in C57BL/6J mice whose mothers were administered ACE via gavage at doses of either 0 mg/kg (control group), 1.0 mg/kg (low-dose group), or 10.0 mg/kg (high-dose group) from gestational day 6 to lactation day 21. The results of a battery of behavior tests for socio-sexual and anxiety-related behaviors, the numbers of vasopressin-immunoreactive cells in the paraventricular nucleus of the hypothalamus, and testosterone levels were used as endpoints. In addition, behavioral flexibility in mice was assessed in a group-housed environment using the IntelliCage, a fully automated mouse behavioral analysis system. In adult male mice exposed to ACE at both low and high doses, a significant reduction of anxiety level was found in the light-dark transition test. Males in the low-dose group also showed a significant increase in sexual and aggressive behaviors. In contrast, neither the anxiety levels nor the sexual behaviors of females were altered. No reductions in the testosterone level, the number of vasopressin-immunoreactive cells, or behavioral flexibility were detected in either sex. These results suggest the possibility that *in utero* and lactational ACE exposure interferes with the development of the neural circuits required for executing socio-sexual and anxiety-related behaviors in male mice specifically.

Keywords: neonicotinoids, acetamiprid, *In utero* and lactational exposure, sociosexual behavior, anxiety-related behavior

INTRODUCTION

There is a growing concern that exposure to environmental chemicals in early life may interfere with brain development (Júlvez et al., 2016). In particular, neonicotinoid pesticides have drawn considerable attention. As a pesticide class, neonicotinoids are designed to overstimulate insect nicotinic acetylcholine receptors (nAChRs). These pesticides were previously thought to be relatively harmless to mammalian species because of their low binding affinities to mammalian nAChRs (Tomizawa and Casida, 1999, 2005). However, recent *in vivo* and *in vitro* studies have reported that neonicotinoids possess sufficient binding affinity and agonistic potential for mammalian nAChRs to exert nicotine-like effects that are stronger than originally believed (de Oliveira et al., 2010; Rodrigues et al., 2010; Li et al., 2011; Kimura-Kuroda et al., 2012). Neonicotinoids such as acetamiprid (ACE), imidacloprid, and clothianidin can bind to the α_4 and β_2 subunits of mammalian nAChRs (Tomizawa and Casida, 1999; Li et al., 2011; Kimura-Kuroda et al., 2012). The $\alpha_4\beta_2$ nAChRs are present in various brain regions such as the amygdala, hypothalamus, substantia nigra, ventral tegmental area, raphe nuclei, hippocampus, and medial habenula (Cimino et al., 1995; Millar and Gotti, 2009), and regulate the development and functions of these regions (Dwyer et al., 2009; Takarada et al., 2012). These brain regions are involved in the regulation of socio-sexual behaviors, anxiety, depression, memory, and learning (Pfaff, 1989; Newman, 1999; Nelson and Trainor, 2007; Drevets et al., 2008; Gaskin and White, 2013; Russo and Nestler, 2013). Therefore, perinatal exposure to neonicotinoids is thought to impair specific behaviors by affecting the formation of neuronal circuits, including circuits involving these areas.

Since ACE has a higher affinity and potency for mammalian nAChRs compared to those of other neonicotinoids (Tomizawa and Casida, 1999; Kimura-Kuroda et al., 2012), we here studied effects of perinatal exposure to ACE on murine behaviors later in adulthood, focusing on socio-sexual and anxiety-related behaviors and behavioral flexibility. In addition to examining these adult behaviors, we evaluated the blood testosterone levels and the numbers of cells expressing arginine-vasopressin (AVP) in the hypothalamus because they are closely associated with socio-sexual and anxiety-related behaviors (Hull and Dominguez, 2007; Nelson and Trainor, 2007; Ho et al., 2010; Stevenson and Caldwell, 2012).

MATERIALS AND METHODS

Animals

Male and female C57BL/6J mice were purchased from CLEA Japan (Tokyo, Japan) and mated at the National Institute for Environmental Studies (NIES). Mice were housed in a room that was maintained at a constant temperature (24 ± 1°C) and humidity (50 ± 10%) with a 12/12-h light/dark cycle. Food and water were provided *ad libitum* unless otherwise specified. The presence of vaginal plugs was checked daily; gestational day (GD) 0 was defined as the day on which a vaginal plug was detected. The dams were administered ACE (Sigma-Aldrich, St. Louis, MO), dissolved in H_2O, at doses of 0 mg/kg (control group), 1.0 mg/kg (low-dose group), or 10.0 mg/kg (high-dose group) by oral gavage from GD 6 to postnatal day (PND) 21. The litters were weaned from their mothers 2–3 h after the last ACE administration on PND 21 and housed with same-sex littermates. All procedures were approved by the Animal Care and Use Committee at the NIES and were conducted strictly in accordance with the NIES guidelines.

Body Weights

The body weight (BW) was measured at birth, at weaning (PND 21), and at 23–26 weeks of age, and the average body weight within a litter (BW/litter) was compared between treatment groups.

Brain Weights

At the time of weaning (PND 21), randomly selected mice that would not be used for behavioral testing were deeply anesthetized with isoflurane and decapitated. The brains were rapidly removed and weighed.

ACE Analysis in the Brain

An ACE standard was obtained from Sigma-Aldrich. Acetamiprid-d3 (Fluka, Sigma-Aldrich, St. Louis, MO, USA) was used as an internal standard (IS). The standard and IS were diluted with acetonitrile and stored at −20°C. Acetonitrile, acetic acid (LC-MS grade), and ammonium acetate (JIS Special Grade) were purchased from Wako Pure Chemical. Purified water was prepared by MilliQ filtration (Millipore, Billerica, MA, USA). The brain levels of ACE were analyzed using previously reported analytical methods with some modifications (Seccia et al., 2008; Xiao et al., 2011; Zhang et al., 2012; Ueyama et al., 2014; Gbylik-Sikorska et al., 2015). A whole brain (0.34–0.49 g) was transferred to a 15 mL polypropylene (PP) tube and mixed with 500 μL of purified water and 50 μL of 50 ng/mL IS solution. The solution was homogenized using a Handy Ultrasonic Homogenizer (Microtec, Funabashi, Chiba, Japan) for 2 min. After adding 2 mL of acetonitrile, the sample solution was vortexed and ultrasonically extracted for 5 min. The extract was centrifuged at 3500 rpm for 5 min (Centrifugator, H-36, Kokusan, Saitama, Japan,), transferred to another 15 mL PP tube, and the solvent was evaporated with a centrifugal evaporator (CentriVap, Asahi Life Science, Saitama, Japan) for 90 min. The residue was re-dissolved in 0.1 mL of acetonitrile and diluted with purified water, up to 1 mL. The sample solution was passed through an Oasis HLB cartridge (1 mL/30 mg, Waters) that was pre-conditioned with 1 mL of acetonitrile and 1 mL of purified water. After rinsing with 1 mL of purified water, the ACE was eluted with 1 mL of acetonitrile/purified water (1:1, v/v). The eluates were evaporated with a centrifugal evaporator for 60 min and re-dissolved in 0.5 mL of acetonitrile/purified water (1:9, v/v) prior to the analysis. Quantification was performed using an ultra-high performance liquid chromatography (Nexera UHPLC, Shimadzu, Kyoto, Japan) coupled to a tandem mass spectrometry (LCMS8050, Shimadzu). The analytical column was Kinetex C18 (100 × 2.1 mm, 2.6 μm, Phenomenex, Torrance, CA, USA), and the injection volume was 10 μL. The mobile phase was (a) 17 mmol/L acetic acid and 5 mmol ammonium acetate in acetonitrile and (b) 17 mmol/L acetic acid and 5 mmol ammonium acetate in purified water; the flow rate was maintained at 0.4 mL/min. The gradient parameters were as follows: the initial condition (phase ratio a:b = 10:90) for 5 min, 40:60 for 5.5 min, 100:0 for 1 min, the initial condition for 6 min. A multiple reaction monitoring (MRM; precursor ion: m/z = 222.7 and product ion: m/z = 126.0) transition was used for the ACE quantification, and another MRM transition (precursor ion: m/z = 222.7 and product ion: m/z = 56.2) was used for confirmation. Quantification was performed using the relative response to IS. The linearity of the calibration curve of the ACE standard solution was confirmed from 0.1 to 100 ng/mL, with $r^2 > 0.998$. The instrumental detection limit (IDL) of ACE was 0.024 ng/mL, which was calculated from the results of 7 replicate analyses of the standard solution. To calculate the method detection limit (MDL), 7 replicated analyses of a fortified blank sample were performed. The blank sample (0.4 mL of purified water) was spiked with 0.05 mL of 0.1 ng/mL standard solution and processed throughout the analytical procedure. The MDL was calculated to be 0.032 ng/g. The IS recovery during the sample analysis ranged from 63 to 98%. The extraction efficiency was evaluated by repeated extraction; the detected ACE level were below the IDL in the second and third extractions.

General Test Procedure

When the offspring were 9–12 weeks old, 1 or 2 mice of both sexes were randomly selected from each litter for a behavioral test battery for socio-sexual and anxiety-related behaviors, consisting of tests for male and female sexual behaviors, aggressive behaviors, and the light-dark transition (LDT) test. The behavioral tests were performed during the dark phase (starting more than 2 h after lights off) of the light/dark cycle under red light. After completing the behavioral tests, the mice were sacrificed, and blood and brain samples were collected for the enzyme immunoassays and immunohistochemistry.

Another 1–2 mice of both sexes from each litter (males: 13–20 weeks of age; females: 23–32 weeks of age) were assigned to the behavioral flexibility test using the IntelliCage apparatus (NewBehavior AG, Zurich, Switzerland). The experimental design for the tests and the number of animals for each group are shown in **Figure 1**.

Male Sexual Behavior

The male mice were separated from their littermates and individually housed in plastic cages (5 × 22 × 12 cm). Starting 12–14 days later, each mouse was tested in its home cage for sexual behavior toward ovariectomized and sex-hormone-treated C57BL/6J female mice once weekly for 3 weeks. The duration of each trial was 30 min. All female stimulus mice were primed with subcutaneous injections of estradiol benzoate (EB) in sesame oil (10 μg/0.1 mL) twice before testing (at 24 and 48 h). The mice were also administered progesterone (P) in sesame oil (500 μg/0.1 mL) 4–6 h before testing to ensure high sexual receptivity. All tests were video-recorded; the numbers of attempted mounts, successful mounts, intromissions, and ejaculations were scored for each mouse.

Male Aggressive Behavior

Five to Seven days after the last sexual behavior test, each male mouse was tested for its aggressive behavior against a gonadally intact, olfactory-bulbectomized C57BL/6J male intruder mouse using a resident-intruder paradigm. This test was performed weekly for 3 consecutive days, for a total of 9 trials. The duration of each trial was 15 min. All tests were video-recorded; the duration and number of aggressive bouts toward the intruder were scored for each mouse. The data for the 3 trials obtained each week were averaged for each mouse and used for statistical analysis. An aggressive bout was defined as a set of behavioral interactions that included at least one of the following behavioral actions toward the intruder: chasing, boxing, wrestling, biting, tail rattling, and offensive lateral attack. If the interval between 2 aggressive bouts did not exceed 3 s, the 2 bouts were considered to be continuous and scored as 1 bout.

Female Sexual Behavior

At 10–12 weeks of age, the female mice were separated from their littermates and housed individually in plastic cages (5 × 22 × 12 cm). Fourteen to Sixteen days after the isolation, all mice were ovariectomized under isoflurane inhalation anesthesia. Fourteen to Sixteen days after the ovariectomy, each female mouse was tested for sexual behavior toward a sexually experienced ICR/JCL male mouse (CLEA Japan, Tokyo, Japan) in the male's home cage. This test was performed weekly, for a total of 3 trials. The female mice were subcutaneously injected with EB (5 μg/0.1 mL dissolved in sesame oil) at 24 and 48 h before testing, and P (250 μg/0.1 mL dissolved in sesame oil) at 4–6 h before testing. Each test lasted until females received 15 mounts or intromissions. The number of lordosis responses to the male mounts or intromissions was scored for each mouse. A lordosis quotient was calculated by dividing the number of lordosis responses by 15 mounts or intromissions (Ogawa et al., 1999).

The LDT Test

Each mouse was tested once for its emotional behaviors in the LDT apparatus for 10 min. The test apparatus consisted of enclosed dark and open-top light compartments (30 × 30 × 30 cm each) connected by an inner door way (3 × 3 cm) located in the center of the partition at the floor level. The open-top light compartment was brightly illuminated with a white light (350 lux). The latency to enter the light compartment, the cumulative time spent in the light compartment, and the total distance traveled in the light compartment were measured by an automated video tracking system (ANY-maze, Stoelting, USA). The data from 2 male mice (1 in the control group and 1 in the low-dose group) were excluded from the analysis because of recording errors.

Sample Collection

After completing the behavioral tests, mice were deeply anesthetized with sodium pentobarbital (60 mg/kg), and blood was collected from the left ventricle of each mouse. The mice were subjected to transcardial perfusion with 0.1 M phosphate-buffered saline (PBS; pH 7.2), followed by 4% paraformaldehyde (PFA) in 0.1 M PBS. Brains were removed, post-fixed overnight

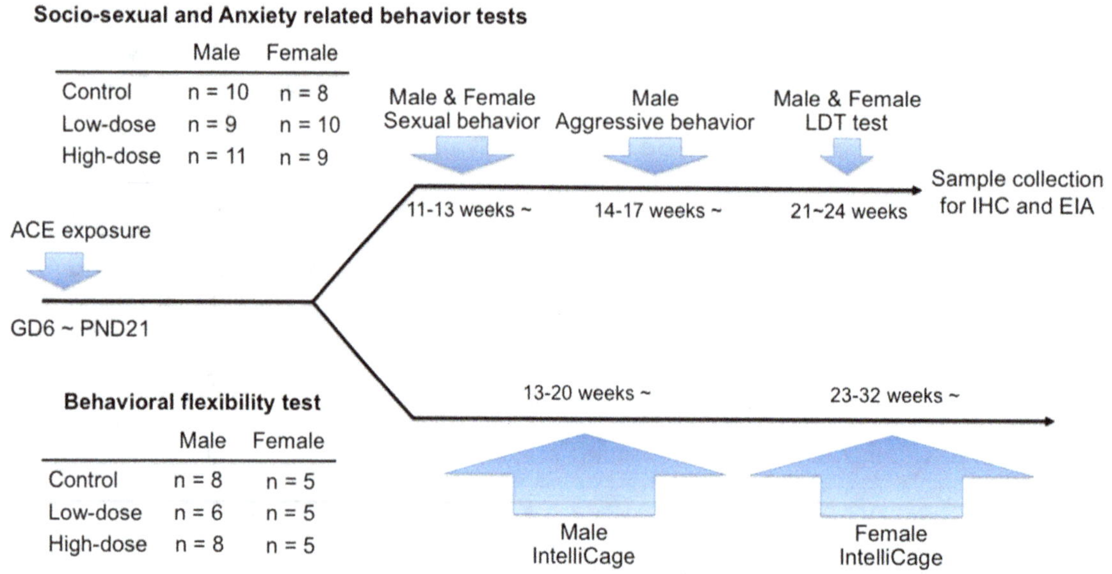

FIGURE 1 | Timeline of the behavioral tests in the study and information of the numbers of animals used in each cohort.

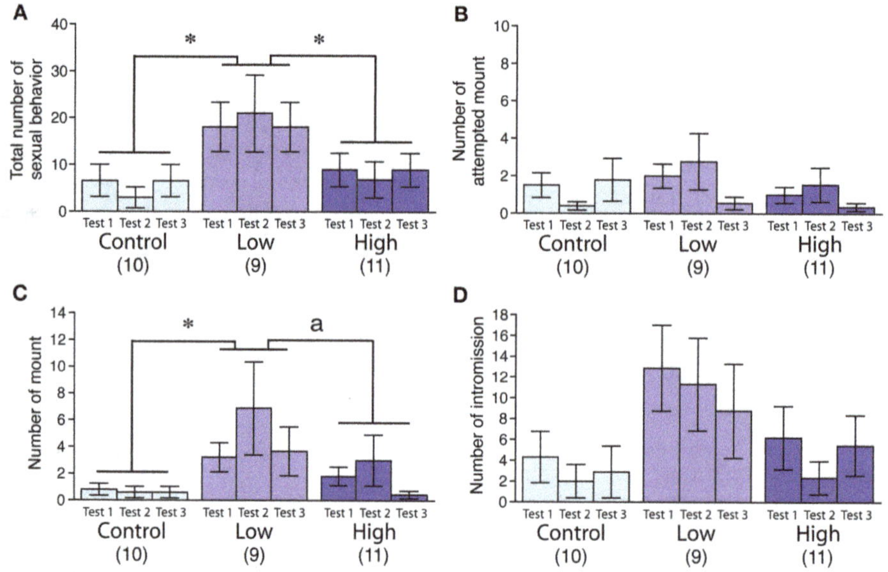

FIGURE 2 | Effects of developmental ACE exposure on male sexual behavior. Comparison of **(A)** the total number of sexual behaviors, as well as the numbers for each male sexual behavior component, including **(B)** attempted mounts, **(C)** mounts, and **(D)** intromissions across the treatment groups. The numbers of animals used are indicated in parentheses. The data are presented as the mean ± SEM. $^{*}P < 0.05$, $^{a}P < 0.1$.

at 4°C with 4% PFA in 0.1 M PBS, and cryoprotected in 0.1M PBS containing 30% sucrose.

Enzyme Immunoassay for Plasma Testosterone

Samples were extracted from plasma (100 μl) with ethyl acetate, and testosterone concentrations were determined using a testosterone enzyme immunoassay kit (Cayman Chemicals, Ann Arbor, MI, USA), according to the manufacturer's instructions. All male samples and randomly selected samples from females (5 for each treatment group) subjected to the socio-sexual and anxiety behavior tests were analyzed.

Immunohistochemistry

The brain samples were coronally sectioned at 30 μm thickness with 90 μm intervals on a freezing microtome. Sections were incubated in PBS-X (0.1 M PBS, pH 7.2 and 0.2% Triton X-100), containing 0.5% hydrogen peroxide for 20 min to

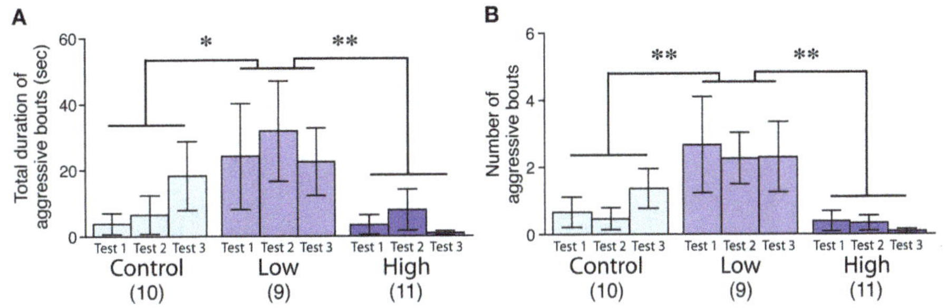

FIGURE 3 | Effects of developmental ACE exposure on male aggressive behavior. (A) The total duration and **(B)** the number of aggressive bouts toward the intruder stimuli. The numbers of animals used are indicated in parentheses. The data are presented as the mean ± SEM. $^{**}P < 0.01$, $^{*}P < 0.05$.

inhibit the endogenous peroxidase activity, and then blocked in an incubation buffer (1% casein in PBS-X) for 2 h at room temperature. Tissue sections were then incubated with a rabbit polyclonal anti-vasopressin antiserum (1:4000; Immunostar Cat. #20069, Hudson, NY, USA) in incubation buffer for 24 h at 4°C. After the completion of the incubation process, the staining was visualized using the DAKO EnVision™ Detection System (Peroxidase/DAB+, K5007). Three anatomically matched sections (30 μm thickness, 90 μm intervals) containing the paraventricular nucleus (PVN, bregma 0.70–0.94 mm) were selected for each mouse. PVN images were photographed at a 10x magnification with a digital camera mounted on a light microscope (Leica DFC290 HD; Leica Microsystems, Wetzlar, Hesse, Germany). The total number of immunoreactive cells was bilaterally counted for each animal. Because of technical issues with the sample preservation and tissue preparation, only the number of samples denoted in **Figure 7** were used for the analysis.

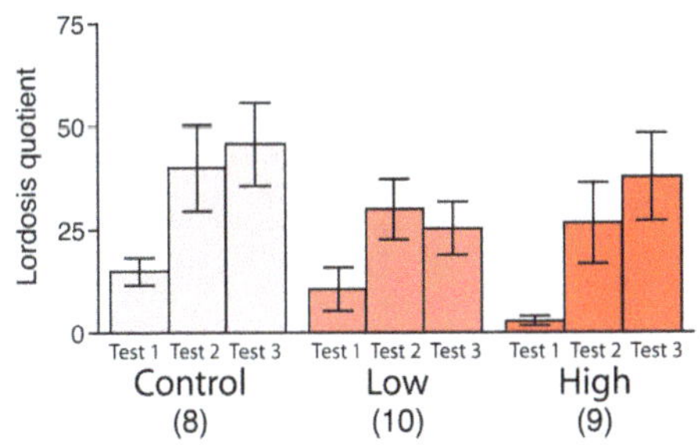

FIGURE 4 | Effects of developmental ACE exposure on female sexual behavior. The comparison of the lordosis quotient [(the number of lordosis responses/15 mounts or intromissions) * 100]. The numbers of animals used are indicated in parentheses. The data are presented as the mean ± SEM.

Evaluation of Behavioral Flexibility Using the IntelliCage

Male and female mice were tested separately for their behavioral flexibility using the IntelliCage, a fully automated testing apparatus consisting of a large plastic cage (55 × 37.5 × 20.5 cm) equipped with 4 corner chambers (15 × 15 × 21 cm each). Male mice at the age of 13–20 weeks were introduced to the IntelliCage apparatus and housed for 57 days. The female mice were housed in the apparatus for 56 days, starting at the age of 23–32 weeks. The difference in test timing of test was due to the limited capacity of the IntelliCage. Two to Three days before being introduced to the apparatus, the mice were anesthetized with isoflurane and subcutaneously implanted a glass-covered transponder having a unique ID code for radiofrequency identification (Datamars, Temple, TX, USA).

The behavioral flexibility test paradigm was composed of an acquisition phase and serial reversal phases. Prior to the behavioral flexibility test, the mice were allowed to acclimatize to the IntelliCage for 9 days. In the acquisition phase after acclimatization, mice were allowed to learn the two rewarded corners and shuttle between them. Subsequently, the mice were subjected to serial reversal tasks, in which the diagonal spatial patterns of the rewarded corners was repetitively reversed every 4–7 sessions. In total, there were 57 sessions for the male mice and 56 sessions for the female mice, including the first 14 sessions of the acquisition phase. Additional sessions were conducted with 10 serial reversals for the male mice and 9 serial reversals for the female mice. The percentage of visits to the non-rewarded corners within the first 100 visits was defined as the discrimination error rate and used to analyze the inter-session comparisons of learning performance. Additionally, the nose-poke frequency per visit within the first 100 visits was calculated for each mouse as an index of compulsive repetitive behavior. The IntelliCage apparatus and behavioral flexibility test paradigm are described in details elsewhere (Endo et al., 2011, 2012). The data from session 38–41 (6th reversal phase) and session 46–53 (8th and 9th reversal phases) in the male mice were excluded from analysis because of a mechanical malfunction of the IntelliCage apparatus. Thus, in the **Figure 8A**, the sessions 42–45, which were the 7th reversal phase, are denoted as Rev 6 and sessions 54–57, which were the 10th reversal phase, are denoted as Rev 7.

Statistical Analyses

All data are presented as mean ± standard error of the mean (SEM). All data, except the comparison of the numbers of ejaculating males, were analyzed using an ANOVA, followed by a Fisher's PLSD *post hoc* test. The incidence of ejaculation during the male sexual behavior test was compared using χ^2 tests. The differences were considered statistically significant when *P*

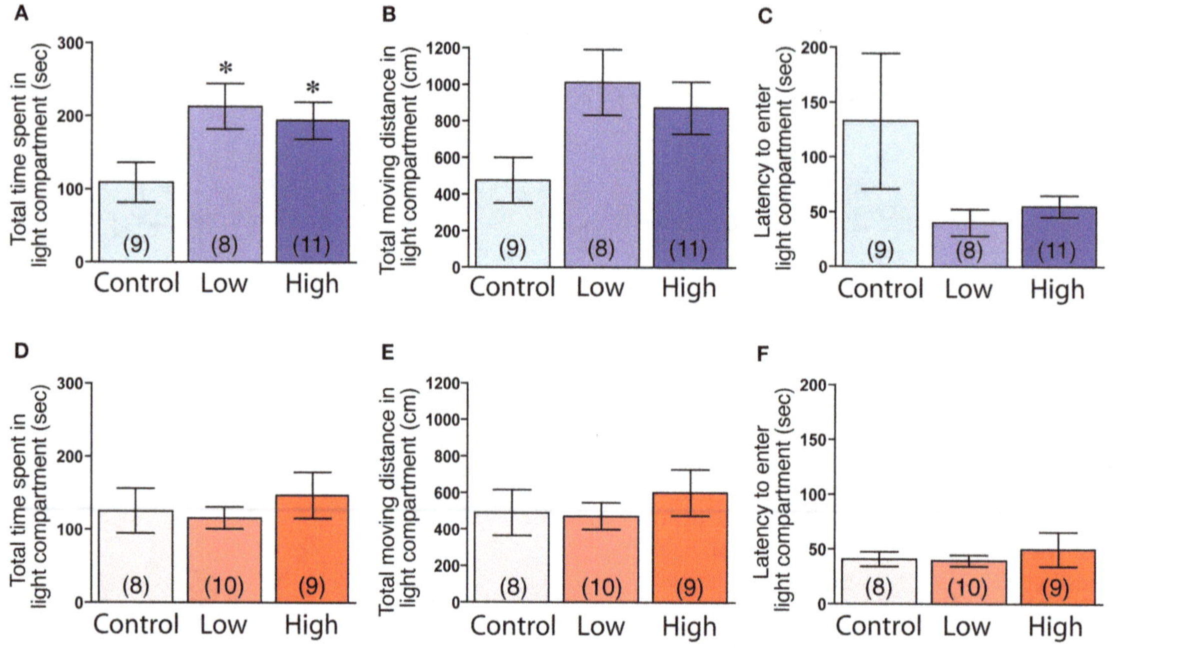

FIGURE 5 | Effects of developmental ACE exposure on anxiety-related behaviors, as measured in the light-dark transition test. (A–C) Male and **(D–F)** female mice of each treatment group. The comparison of **(A,D)** the total time spent in, **(B,E)** the total moving distance in, and **(C,F)** the latency to enter the light compartment of the light-dark transition apparatus. The numbers of animals used are indicated in parentheses. The data are presented as the mean ± SEM. $^*P < 0.05$ vs. control.

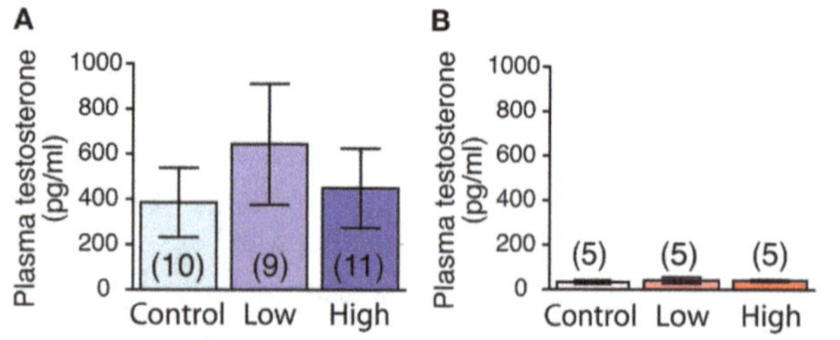

FIGURE 6 | Effects of developmental ACE exposure on plasma testosterone levels. (A) Male and **(B)** female mice of each treatment group. The numbers of animals used are indicated in parentheses. The data are presented as the mean ± SEM.

< 0.05. All data were analyzed using the SPSS 19.0 statistical package (SPSS Inc., Chicago, IL, USA) or R software (The R Foundation for Statistical Computing, Vienna, Austria).

RESULTS

Body Weight/Litter

In the male and female mice, no differences were found in BW/litter among the groups at birth, PND 21, or 23–26 weeks of age (**Table 1**).

Brain Weight

No differences were found in the brain weights of either male or female mice at PND 21 (**Table 2**). There were no differences in the brain-to-body weight ratio either [data not shown].

Brain Residual Concentration Analysis

The brain residual concentration of ACE was measured in 6 mice (3 male and 3 female) from the control group and 6 mice (3 male and 3 female) from the high-dose group. The concentrations in the high-dose group were 1.29 ± 0.46 and 1.23 ± 0.20 ng/g in males and females, respectively (**Table 3**). In contrast, the concentrations were below the MDL in the control group for both sexes.

Male Sexual Behavior

In the male sexual behavior test (**Figures 2A–D**), the total number of sexual behaviors was significantly increased in the low-dose group [$F_{(2, 27)} = 3.72, P < 0.05$; Fisher's PLSD, $P < 0.05$, low-dose group vs. control and high-dose groups; **Figure 2A**], particularly for the mean number of mounts [$F_{(2, 27)} = 3.77, P < 0.05$; Fisher's PLSD, $P < 0.05$, low-dose group vs. control group; **Figure 2C**]. We found no significant difference in the incidence of ejaculation during the tests (**Table 4**).

Male Aggressive Behavior

The aggression level in the low-dose group was significantly increased compared to that of the control and high-dose groups, as measured by the total duration [$F_{(2, 27)} = 4.44, P < 0.05$; Fisher's PLSD, $P < 0.05$, low-dose group vs. control; $P < 0.01$, low-dose group vs. high-dose group; **Figure 3A**] and the number of bouts [$F_{(2, 27)} = 6.24, P < 0.01$; Fisher's PLSD, $P < 0.01$, low-dose group vs. control and high-dose groups; **Figure 3B**].

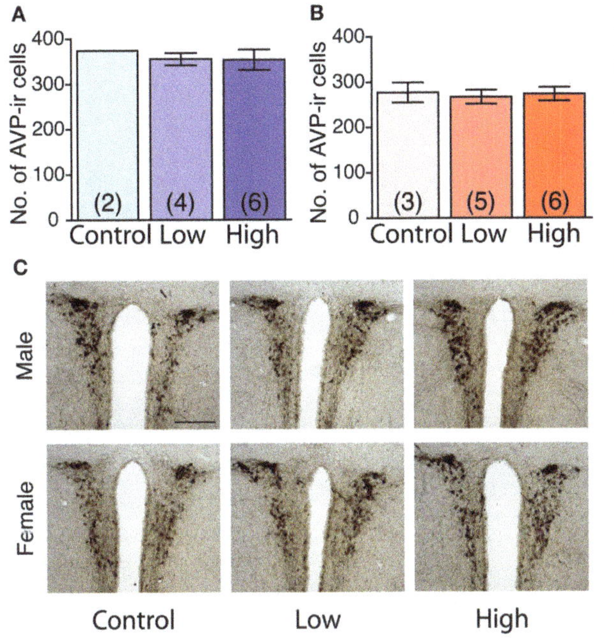

FIGURE 7 | Effects of developmental ACE exposure on the number of vasopressin (AVP) immunoreactive (ir) cells in the paraventricular nucleus (PVN). (A) Male and **(B)** female mice of each treatment group. The data are presented as the mean ± SEM. **(C)** Representative photomicrographs of AVP-ir cells in brain sections from males (top panels) and females (bottom panels) of each treatment group. The numbers of animals used are indicated in parentheses **(A,B)**. The scale bar represents 200 μm.

Female Sexual Behavior

No significant differences were found in the lordosis quotient among the groups, whereas the lordosis quotient increased with repeated testing in all groups [$F_{(2, 48)} = 12.83$, $P < 0.001$; **Figure 4**].

The LDT Test

The male mice in both the low-dose and high-dose groups spent significantly more time in the light compartment compared to the control group [$F_{(2, 25)} = 3.83$, $P < 0.05$; Fisher's PLSD, $P < 0.05$, low-dose and high-dose groups vs. control group; **Figure 5A**]. The male mice in the low-dose and high-dose groups tended to travel longer distances in the light compartment compared to the control group [$F_{(2, 25)} = 3.27$, $P = 0.055$; **Figure 5B**]. We found no significant differences in the latency to enter the light compartment (**Figure 5C**). In contrast to the males, there were no significant group differences in the females in the time spent in the light compartment (**Figure 5D**), the total distance traveled in the light compartment (**Figure 5E**) and the latency to enter the light compartment (**Figure 5F**).

Plasma Testosterone Levels

The plasma testosterone levels were significantly higher in the males compared to those of the females, regardless of treatment [$F_{(1, 39)} = 7.48$, $P < 0.01$; **Figures 6A,B**]. No main effect of ACE exposure was found on the plasma testosterone levels in either the males (**Figure 6A**) or females (**Figure 6B**).

AVP Immunoreactivity in the PVN

No main effect of ACE exposure was found on the number of AVP immunoreactive cells in either the males (**Figure 7A**) or females (**Figure 7B**). The number of AVP-immunoreactive cells was significantly higher in the males than in the females, regardless of treatment [$F_{(1, 20)} = 26.7$, $P < 0.01$; **Figures 7A,B**] as shown in representative photomicrographs (**Figure 7C**).

Behavioral Flexibility Test

During the acclimatization period, the number of corner visits per week in the IntelliCage did not differ between the groups in both males and females (Supplementary Figure 1), indicating the possibility that the developmental exposure to ACE does not affect home cage activity. In the acquisition phase, the male and female mice in all groups showed a decrease in the discrimination error rate with repeated sessions. No statistical differences were found between the groups, indicating that all groups could acquire the first task (**Figures 8A,B**). In the serial reversal phase, the male and female mice in all groups showed a similar pattern in the discrimination error rate in the reversal stage (Rev), indicating that the developmental ACE exposure had no effect on the spatial learning ability and behavioral flexibility during adulthood. We measured the nose-poke/visit ratio, which is an index of behavioral impulsivity, against rewards in the home cage, but found no significant group differences.

DISCUSSION

We evaluated the general physiological parameters, such as body and brain weights, during the developmental period of mice exposed to ACE *in utero* and via lactation, as well as a battery of socio-sexual and anxiety-related behaviors during their adulthood. ACE was found in the brains of pups of the high-dose group at PND 21, using a residual concentration analysis. These data showed that absorbed ACE was transferred into the developing brain. The ACE exposure at the used doses did not alter the body and brain weights. In addition, no impairments in behavioral flexibility were found in the *in utero* and lactational ACE-exposed adult mice. On the other hand, *in utero* and lactational ACE exposure altered socio-sexual and anxiety-related behaviors in males.

Although, the binding affinity of ACE to nAChRs is approximately 70–80 times lower than that of nicotine (Tomizawa and Casida, 1999; Picciotto et al., 2001), ACE can be bound to nAChRs containing α_4 and β_2 subunits, which are known to mediate the effects of nicotine. Based on this binding affinity difference, we propose that the effect of ACE on certain behaviors may correspond to the effect of nicotine at lower doses. Therefore, in our discussion below, we attempt to compare the present results to previous reports demonstrating the effects of developmental nicotine exposure at relatively low doses, when possible.

We found significant changes in the socio-sexual and anxiety-related behaviors in male mice exposed to ACE *in utero* and via lactation. The most significant change was found by the LDT test. ACE exposure at low or high doses prolonged the time spent in the light compartment, indicating reduction of

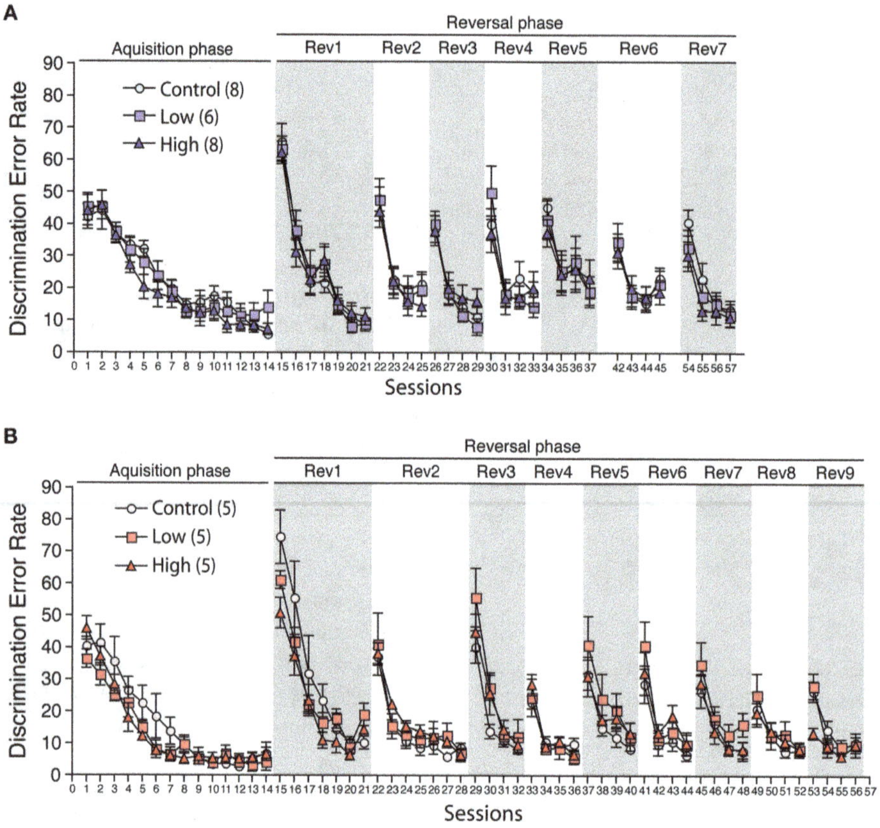

FIGURE 8 | Effects of developmental ACE exposure on behavioral flexibility. The comparison of the discrimination error rates (the number of discrimination errors in the first 100 corner visits in the session) in **(A)** male and **(B)** female mice. The numbers of animals used are indicated in parentheses. The data are presented as the mean ± SEM. The data for session 38–41 (6th reversal phase) and session 46–53 (8th and 9th reversal phases) in male were omitted due to the technical issues with the IntelliCage apparatus. Thus, the session 42 to 45 is denoted as Rev 6 and the session 54–57 is denoted as Rev 7 on **(A)**.

anxiety. This result suggests that there may be altered emotional responses in the ACE-exposed male mice. There have been many reports regarding the effects of nicotine exposure on anxiety-related behaviors during the developmental period. However, the effects of perinatal nicotine exposure reported in these studies are bidirectional, positive or negative, depending on the experimental conditions such as the dose, time of administration, and the behavioral test paradigm. Maternal nicotine exposure at a dose of 0.5 mg/kg BW from GD 10 to delivery in mice is reported to decrease anxiety-related parameters measured in the elevated plus-maze test in male offspring (Ajarem and Ahmad, 1998). In contrast, male mice whose mothers were exposed to nicotine (0.2 mg/ml) in drinking water throughout gestation or from GD 14 to delivery have been reported to exhibit increased anxiety-related responses in both the elevated plus-maze and LDT tests (Alkam et al., 2013). Vaglenova et al. (2004) reported that nicotine exposure in pregnant rats at a daily dose of 6.0 mg/kg BW from GD 3 to delivery also causes increased anxiety-related responses in their offspring as assessed in the elevated plus-maze test. The relationship between developmental nicotine exposure and anxiety shown by many studies allows us to speculate that the neural circuitry responsible for anxiety is vulnerable to cholinergic agents, although reservation is warranted because of inconsistencies among previous studies. In addition, perinatal nicotine exposure is reported to cause hyperactivity in rodents (Ajarem and Ahmad, 1998; Thomas et al., 2000; Pauly et al., 2004; Vaglenova et al., 2004; Paz et al., 2007; Heath et al., 2010; Alkam et al., 2013). We did not find any differences between the groups in corner visits in the IntelliCage, demonstrating no differences in home cage activity between the groups. However, mice exposed to ACE at both the low and high doses tended to travel longer distances in the light compartment, suggesting the possibility that ACE exposure may have induced hyperactivity under specific stressful conditions. Therefore, the longer times spent in the light compartment in the LDT test may reflect not only decreased anxiety, but also hyperactivity under specific stressful conditions. Future experiments measuring locomotor activity with or without stress are necessary to clarify whether ACE exposure decreases low anxiety, induces hyperactivity, or both under stressful conditions.

On socio-sexual behaviors, the effect of ACE appeared to be dose-specific. ACE exposure at the low dose, but not at the high dose, significantly increased male sexual and aggressive behaviors. Socio-sexual behaviors are governed by neural circuits

TABLE 1 | Body weight per litter (BW/litter) at birth, weaning (PND21), and 23–26 weeks of age.

	Groups	Birth (g)	PND21 (g)	23–26 weeks (g)
Male	Control	1.27 ± 0.02 (7)	7.85 ± 0.12 (6)	28.28 ± 0.57 (5)
	Low	1.30 ± 0.02 (6)	8.01 ± 0.37 (6)	30.09 ± 0.68 (5)
	High	1.31 ± 0.04 (9)	7.72 ± 0.39 (9)	28.08 ± 0.66 (6)
Female	Control	1.22 ± 0.02 (7)	7.38 ± 0.14 (6)	25.63 ± 0.72 (4)
	Low	1.29 ± 0.03 (6)	7.76 ± 0.27 (5)	25.82 ± 0.50 (5)
	High	1.31 ± 0.03 (9)	7.43 ± 0.31 (9)	24.85 ± 0.33 (5)

Data presented as mean ± SEM.
Number of dam is given in parentheses.

TABLE 2 | Brain weight at PND 21.

	Groups	Brain weight (g)
Male	Control ($n = 6$)	0.41 ± 0.007
	Low ($n = 2$)	0.44
	High ($n = 4$)	0.41 ± 0.008
Female	Control ($n = 6$)	0.40 ± 0.003
	Low ($n = 4$)	0.41 ± 0.003
	High ($n = 6$)	0.39 ± 0.013

Data presented as mean ± SEM.

TABLE 3 | Residual concentration of ACE in the brains of offspring at PND 21.

	Groups	Brain residual concentration (ng/mg tissue)
Male	Control ($n = 3$)	<MDL
	High dose group ($n = 3$)	1.29 ± 0.46
Female	Control ($n = 3$)	<MDL
	High dose group ($n = 3$)	1.23 ± 0.20

MDL: The method detection limit.
Data presented as mean ± SEM.

TABLE 4 | Number of male mice demonstrated ejaculation in each test.

Groups	Test 1	Test 2	Test 3
Control	2/10 (20%)	2/10 (20%)	2/10 (20%)
Low	3/9 (33.3%)	2/9 (22.2%)	5/9 (55.6%)
High	2/11 (18.2%)	2/11 (18.2%)	4/11 (36.4%)

Number of mice ejaculated/total number of mice tested; the percentage is given in parentheses.

involving various brain regions (Newman, 1999). Peripheral sex steroid hormones play an essential role in the formation of these neural circuits during the critical period. Generally in mammals, the critical period can extend from late gestational period to the early life (Hull and Dominguez, 2007; Nelson and Trainor, 2007). The cholinergic system is also thought to play a role in the formation of the neural bases of these behaviors (Dwyer et al., 2009; Blood-Siegfried and Rende, 2010). Any agents that block or enhance acetylcholine transmission may interfere with this formation.

The idea that low-dose chemical exposure alters specific behaviors has been proposed in previous studies. Dioxin and bisphenol A induce their toxicities in a non-monotonic manner (Endo et al., 2012; Vandenberg, 2014). The actions of nicotine also appear to be complex and non-monotonic, especially when given *in vivo* (Anderson and Brunzell, 2012, 2015; Alkam et al., 2013; Abreu-Villaça et al., 2015). Behaviors as well as specific neural circuit formation may potentially be dysregulated by nicotine in a non-monotonic manner. For example, the effect of developmental nicotine exposure on the development of the vasopressinergic system is complex. Prenatal nicotine exposure at a relatively high dose (6 mg/kg/day throughout the gestational period) greatly reduced vasopressin production and release in the hypothalamus of male rats (Zbuzek and Zbuzek, 1992). Although, the species difference must be taken into consideration, prenatal nicotine exposure at a relatively low dose (total amount of 1.05 mg throughout the gestational period) has been reported to increase the number of vasopressin cell bodies and fibers in the hypothalamus of the golden hamster (Rossi et al., 2003). Since vasopressinergic systems regulate both sexual and aggressive behaviors in a facilitative manner (Ho et al., 2010; Stevenson and Caldwell, 2012), we speculated that ACE exposure specifically at the low dose enhanced the development of neural networks involved in vasopressinergic systems. However, we did not find any differences in the number of AVP-immunoreactive cells in the PVN. Therefore, it is unlikely that *in utero* and lactational ACE exposure at the low dose increased aggression and sexuality in adulthood through alterations of the vasopressinergic system in the PVN. We could not examine the numbers of AVP-immunoreactive cells in areas outside the PVN, such as the bed nucleus of the stria terminalis (BNST), a region known to be critically involved in the facilitation of male socio-sexual behaviors (Newman, 1999; Nelson and Trainor, 2007). Further studies are needed to clarify whether ACE affects AVP immunoreactive cells in brain regions other than the PVN.

There have been several reports regarding the effects of in utero nicotine exposure on plasma testosterone levels in animal models, but these reports are also inconsistent with each other, presumably due to differing exposure conditions. On one hand, the plasma testosterone levels decreased in 10-week-old male rat offspring born to dams that had been administered nicotine at a dose of 0.5 mg/kg throughout gestation (Segarra and Strand, 1989). In contrast, the plasma testosterone levels increased in 13-week-old male rat offspring born to dams that had been given nicotine at a dose of 2 mg/kg throughout gestation increased (Paccola et al., 2014). In our study, we did not find any differences in plasma testosterone levels measured at 23–26 weeks of age, which excludes the possibility that increased testosterone levels in adult males caused the abnormalities in the socio-sexual and emotional behaviors. However, we did not determine plasma testosterone levels during the perinatal period, which is a critical period for the testosterone-induced masculinization of socio-sexual behaviors. Therefore, we cannot exclude the possibility that developmental ACE exposure altered the testosterone levels during the perinatal periods, resulting in the impaired sexual differentiation of socio-sexual behaviors.

Behavioral flexibility was unaffected by developmental ACE exposure under our exposure conditions. Behavioral flexibility is considered a part of executive function, which is dependent on hippocampal and prefrontal cortical function (Kosaki and Watanabe, 2012; Malá et al., 2015). Various studies have reported the negative effects of developmental nicotine exposure at relatively high doses on the cognitive performance of offspring (Yanai et al., 1992; Wickström, 2007; Parameshwaran et al., 2012). However, the effects of developmental nicotine exposure to neonicotinoids or lower doses of nicotine have not been clarified for cognitive functions. Our study demonstrated that the developmental ACE exposure did not affect the cognitive functions, at least at the ACE doses and animal ages tested in this study. However, we cannot exclude the possibility that late-onset impairment of cognitive function occurs in mice exposed to ACE. Since malfunction of the cholinergic system is associated with cognitive deficits such as those in Alzheimer's disease (Schliebs and Arendt, 2011), examining behavioral flexibility in aged mice exposed to ACE perinatally would be an interesting avenue of our research.

Sex differences in the effects of ACE exposure on socio-sexual and emotional behaviors should also be addressed since *in utero* and lactational ACE exposure at either dose had no effect on female sexual behavior and anxiety. The present study was unable to elucidate the neuropathologies underlying the sex-specific effect of ACE. Several lines of evidence suggest that the male is more susceptible to developmental nicotine exposure than the female (Fung and Lau, 1989; Ribary and Lichtensteiger, 1989; von Ziegler et al., 1991; Pauly et al., 2004). The sex-specific effect of ACE observed in this study is consistent with the reported male-biased effects of nicotine, possibly suggesting that nicotine and ACE elicit toxic effects through a common sex-specific pathway.

It is also important to mention that ACE was administered to mice throughout the gestational and lactational periods in this study. The effect of developmental nicotine exposure has been reported to vary depending on the timing of exposure (Alkam et al., 2013). Therefore, if ACE shares a common toxic pathway with nicotine, it is highly likely that the effect of ACE also varies depending on the timing of exposure. The developmental action of ACE in different time-windows should be further examined in future studies.

CONCLUSION

Our results suggest the possibility that ACE affects socio-sexual and anxiety-related behaviors in a male-specific manner. Further experiments are needed to understand the behavioral alterations and examine the mechanisms underlying the ACE-induced impairments in brain function. The action of ACE appears to be non-monotonic for the socio-sexual behaviors, as the effects were only found in mice exposed to ACE at low doses. Further empirical studies using mouse models are required to evaluate whether ACE doses equivalent to the human exposure level have detrimental effects.

AUTHOR CONTRIBUTIONS

KS, TI, TW, SN, TK, GS, SH, and FM designed the experiment. KS, TI, JY, TW, MY, TK, and FM performed the experiment. KS, TI, JY, MY, and FM analyzed the data. KS wrote the manuscript. KN, CT, and FM critically revised the manuscript.

ACKNOWLEDGMENTS

This work was supported by JSPS KAKENHI 24590307, 15K08223, and 15K14556 to FM, and 24221003 to CT, by the National Institute for Environmental Studies [1011AF005, 1416AT001] and The Grant of National Center for Child Health and Development (25-3) to FM.

REFERENCES

Abreu-Villaça, Y., Filgueiras, C. C., Correa-Santos, M., Cavina, C. C., Naiff, V. F., Krahe, T. E., et al. (2015). Tobacco smoke containing high or low levels of nicotine during adolescence: effects on novelty-seeking and anxiety-like behaviors in mice. *Psychopharmacology (Berl)* 232, 1693–1703. doi: 10.1007/s00213-014-3801-1

Ajarem, J. S., and Ahmad, M. (1998). Prenatal nicotine exposure modifies behavior of mice through early development. *Pharmacol. Biochem. Behav.* 59, 313–318.

Alkam, T., Kim, H.-C., Hiramatsu, M., Mamiya, T., Aoyama, Y., Nitta, A., et al. (2013). Evaluation of emotional behaviors in young offspring of C57BL/6J mice after gestational and/or perinatal exposure to nicotine in six different time-windows. *Behav. Brain Res.* 239, 80–89. doi: 10.1016/j.bbr.2012.10.058

Anderson, S. M., and Brunzell, D. H. (2012). Low dose nicotine and antagonism of β2 subunit containing nicotinic acetylcholine receptors have similar effects on affective behavior in mice. *PLoS ONE* 7:e48665. doi: 10.1371/journal.pone.0048665

Anderson, S. M., and Brunzell, D. H. (2015). Anxiolytic-like and anxiogenic-like effects of nicotine are regulated via diverse action at β2*nicotinic acetylcholine receptors. *Br. J. Pharmacol.* 172, 2864–2877. doi: 10.1111/bph.13090

Blood-Siegfried, J., and Rende, E. K. (2010). The long-term effects of prenatal nicotine exposure on neurologic development. *J. Midwifery Womens Health* 55, 143–152. doi: 10.1016/j.jmwh.2009.05.006

Cimino, M., Marini, P., Colombo, S., Andena, M., Cattabeni, F., Fornasari, D., et al. (1995). Expression of neuronal acetylcholine nicotinic receptor α4 and β2 subunits during postnatal development of the rat brain. *J. Neural Transmission* 100, 77–92. doi: 10.1007/BF01271531

de Oliveira, I. M., Nunes, B. V. F., Barbosa, D. R., Pallares, A. M., and Faro, L. R. F. (2010). Effects of the neonicotinoids thiametoxam and clothianidin on *in vivo* dopamine release in rat striatum. *Toxicol. Lett.* 192, 294–297. doi: 10.1016/j.toxlet.2009.11.005

Drevets, W. C., Price, J. L., and Furey, M. L. (2008). Brain structural and functional abnormalities in mood disorders: implications for neurocircuitry models of depression. *Brain Struct. Funct.* 213, 93–118. doi: 10.1007/s00429-008-0189-x

Dwyer, J. B., McQuown, S. C., and Leslie, F. M. (2009). The dynamic effects of nicotine on the developing brain. *Pharmacol. Ther.* 122, 125–139. doi: 10.1016/j.pharmthera.2009.02.003

Endo, T., Kakeyama, M., Uemura, Y., Haijima, A., Okuno, H., Bito, H., et al. (2012). Executive function deficits and social-behavioral abnormality in mice exposed to a low dose of dioxin *in utero* and via lactation. *PLoS ONE* 7:e50741. doi: 10.1371/journal.pone.0050741

Endo, T., Maekawa, F., Võikar, V., Haijima, A., Uemura, Y., Zhang, Y., et al. (2011). Automated test of behavioral flexibility in mice using a behavioral sequencing task in IntelliCage. *Behav. Brain Res.* 221, 172–181. doi: 10.1016/j.bbr.2011.02.037

Fung, Y. K., and Lau, Y. S. (1989). Effects of prenatal nicotine exposure on rat striatal dopaminergic and nicotinic systems. *Pharmacol. Biochem. Behav.* 33, 1–6.

Gaskin, S., and White, N. M. (2013). Parallel processing of information about location in the amygdala, entorhinal cortex and hippocampus. *Hippocampus* 23, 1075–1083. doi: 10.1002/hipo.22179

Gbylik-Sikorska, M., Sniegocki, T., and Posyniak, A. (2015). Determination of neonicotinoid insecticides and their metabolites in honey bee and honey by liquid chromatography tandem mass spectrometry. *J. Chromatogr. B. Analyt. Technol. Biomed. Life Sci.* 990, 132–140. doi: 10.1016/j.jchromb.2015.03.016

Heath, C. J., Horst, N. K., and Picciotto, M. R. (2010). Oral nicotine consumption does not affect maternal care or early development in mice but results in modest hyperactivity in adolescence. *Physiol. Behav.* 101, 764–769. doi: 10.1016/j.physbeh.2010.08.021

Ho, J. M., Murray, J. H., Demas, G. E., and Goodson, J. L. (2010). Vasopressin cell groups exhibit strongly divergent responses to copulation and male-male interactions in mice. *Horm. Behav.* 58, 368–377. doi: 10.1016/j.yhbeh.2010.03.021

Hull, E. M., and Dominguez, J. M. (2007). Sexual behavior in male rodents. *Horm. Behav.* 52, 45–55. doi: 10.1016/j.yhbeh.2007.03.030

Júlvez, J., Paus, T., Bellinger, D., Eskenazi, B., Tiemeier, H., Pearce, N., et al. (2016). Environment and brain development: challenges in the global context. *Neuroepidemiology* 46, 79–82. doi: 10.1159/000442256

Kimura-Kuroda, J., Komuta, Y., Kuroda, Y., Hayashi, M., and Kawano, H. (2012). Nicotine-like effects of the neonicotinoid insecticides acetamiprid and imidacloprid on cerebellar neurons from neonatal rats. *PLoS ONE* 7:e32432. doi: 10.1371/journal.pone.0032432

Kosaki, Y., and Watanabe, S. (2012). Dissociable roles of the medial prefrontal cortex, the anterior cingulate cortex, and the hippocampus in behavioural flexibility revealed by serial reversal of three-choice discrimination in rats. *Behav. Brain Res.* 227, 81–90. doi: 10.1016/j.bbr.2011.10.039

Li, P., Ann, J., and Akk, G. (2011). Activation and modulation of human $\alpha4\beta2$ nicotinic acetylcholine receptors by the neonicotinoids clothianidin and imidacloprid. *J. Neurosci. Res.* 89, 1295–1301. doi: 10.1002/jnr.22644

Malá, H., Andersen, L. G., Christensen, R. F., Felbinger, A., Hagstrom, J., Meder, D., et al. (2015). Prefrontal cortex and hippocampus in behavioural flexibility and posttraumatic functional recovery: reversal learning and set-shifting in rats. *Brain Res. Bull.* 116, 34–44. doi: 10.1016/j.brainresbull.2015.05.006

Millar, N. S., and Gotti, C. (2009). Diversity of vertebrate nicotinic acetylcholine receptors. *Neuropharmacology* 56, 237–246. doi: 10.1016/j.neuropharm.2008.07.041

Nelson, R. J., and Trainor, B. C. (2007). Neural mechanisms of aggression. *Nat. Rev. Neurosci.* 8, 536–546. doi: 10.1038/nrn2174

Newman, S. W. (1999). The medial extended amygdala in male reproductive behavior. A node in the mammalian social behavior network. *Ann. N.Y. Acad. Sci.* 877, 242–257.

Ogawa, S., Chan, J., Chester, A. E., Gustafsson, J. Å., Korach, K. S., and Pfaff, D. W. (1999). Survival of reproductive behaviors in estrogen receptor β gene-deficient (βERKO) male and female mice. *Proc. Natl. Acad. Sci. U.S.A.* 96, 12887–12892.

Paccola, C. C., Neves, F. M. O., Cipriano, I., Stumpp, T., and Miraglia, S. M. (2014). Effects of prenatal and lactation nicotine exposure on rat testicular interstitial tissue. *Andrology* 2, 175–185. doi: 10.1111/j.2047-2927.2013.00168.x

Parameshwaran, K., Buabeid, M. A., Karuppagounder, S. S., Uthayathas, S., Thiruchelvam, K., Shonesy, B., et al. (2012). Developmental nicotine exposure induced alterations in behavior and glutamate receptor function in hippocampus. *Cell. Mol. Life. Sci.* 69, 829–841. doi: 10.1007/s00018-011-0805-4

Pauly, J. R., Sparks, J. A., Hauser, K. F., and Pauly, T. H. (2004). *In utero* nicotine exposure causes persistent, gender-dependant changes in locomotor activity and sensitivity to nicotine in C57Bl/6 mice. *Int. J. Dev. Neurosci.* 22, 329–337. doi: 10.1016/j.ijdevneu.2004.05.009

Paz, R., Barsness, B., Martenson, T., Tanner, D., and Allan, A. M. (2007). Behavioral teratogenicity induced by nonforced maternal nicotine consumption. *Neuropsychopharmacology* 32, 693–699. doi: 10.1038/sj.npp.1301066

Pfaff, D. W. (1989). Features of a hormone-driven defined neural circuit for a mammalian behavior. Principles illustrated, neuroendocrine syllogisms, and multiplicative steroid effects. *Ann. N.Y. Acad. Sci.* 563, 131–147.

Picciotto, M. R., Caldarone, B. J., Brunzell, D. H., Zachariou, V., Stevens, T. R., and King, S. L. (2001). Neuronal nicotinic acetylcholine receptor subunit knockout mice: physiological and behavioral phenotypes and possible clinical implications. *Pharmacol. Ther.* 92, 89–108. doi: 10.1016/S0163-7258(01)00161-9

Ribary, U., and Lichtensteiger, W. (1989). Effects of acute and chronic prenatal nicotine treatment on central catecholamine systems of male and female rat fetuses and offspring. *J. Pharmacol. Exp. Ther.* 248, 786–792.

Rodrigues, K. J. A., Santana, M. B., Do Nascimento, J. L. M., Picanço-Diniz, D. L. W., Maués, L. A. L., Santos, S. N., et al. (2010). Behavioral and biochemical effects of neonicotinoid thiamethoxam on the cholinergic system in rats. *Ecotoxicol. Environ. Saf.* 73, 101–107. doi: 10.1016/j.ecoenv.2009.04.021

Rossi, V., Messenger, T., Peters, D., Ferris, C., and King, J. (2003). Prenatal nicotine exposure and behavior. *Ann. N.Y. Acad. Sci.* 1008, 289–292. doi: 10.1196/annals.1301.034

Russo, S. J., and Nestler, E. J. (2013). The brain reward circuitry in mood disorders. *Nat. Rev. Neurosci.* 14, 609–625. doi: 10.1038/nrn3381

Schliebs, R., and Arendt, T. (2011). The cholinergic system in aging and neuronal degeneration. *Behav. Brain Res.* 221, 555–563. doi: 10.1016/j.bbr.2010.11.058

Seccia, S., Fidente, P., Montesano, D., and Morrica, P. (2008). Determination of neonicotinoid insecticides residues in bovine milk samples by solid-phase extraction clean-up and liquid chromatography with diode-array detection. *J. Chromatogr. A.* 1214, 115–120. doi: 10.1016/j.chroma.2008.10.088

Segarra, A. C., and Strand, F. L. (1989). Perinatal administration of nicotine alters subsequent sexual behavior and testosterone levels of male rats. *Brain Res.* 480, 151–159.

Stevenson, E. L., and Caldwell, H. K. (2012). The vasopressin 1b receptor and the neural regulation of social behavior. *Horm. Behav.* 61, 277–282. doi: 10.1016/j.yhbeh.2011.11.009

Takarada, T., Nakamichi, N., Kitajima, S., Fukumori, R., Nakazato, R., Le, N. Q., et al. (2012). Promoted neuronal differentiation after activation of alpha4/beta2 nicotinic acetylcholine receptors in undifferentiated neural progenitors. *PLoS ONE* 7:e46177. doi: 10.1371/journal.pone.0046177

Thomas, J. D., Garrison, M. E., Slawecki, C. J., Ehlers, C. L., and Riley, E. P. (2000). Nicotine exposure during the neonatal brain growth spurt produces hyperactivity in preweanling rats. *Neurotoxicol. Teratol.* 22, 695–701. doi: 10.1016/S0892-0362(00)00096-9

Tomizawa, M., and Casida, J. E. (1999). Minor structural changes in nicotinoid insecticides confer differential subtype selectivity for mammalian nicotinic acetylcholine receptors. *Br. J. Pharmacol.* 127, 115–122. doi: 10.1038/sj.bjp.0702526

Tomizawa, M., and Casida, J. E. (2005). Neonicotinoid insecticide toxicology: mechanisms of selective action. *Annu. Rev. Pharmacol. Toxicol.* 45, 247–268. doi: 10.1146/annurev.pharmtox.45.120403.095930

Ueyama, J., Nomura, H., Kondo, T., Saito, I., Ito, Y., Osaka, A., et al. (2014). Biological monitoring method for urinary neonicotinoid insecticides using LC-MS/MS and its application to Japanese adults. *J. Occup. Health* 56, 461–468. doi: 10.1539/joh.14-0077-OA

Vaglenova, J., Birru, S., Pandiella, N. M., and Breese, C. R. (2004). An assessment of the long-term developmental and behavioral teratogenicity of prenatal nicotine exposure. *Behav. Brain Res.* 150, 159–170. doi: 10.1016/j.bbr.2003.07.005

Vandenberg, L. N. (2014). Non-monotonic dose responses in studies of endocrine disrupting chemicals: bisphenol a as a case study. *Dose Response* 12, 259–276. doi: 10.2203/dose-response.13-020.Vandenberg von Ziegler, N. I., Schlumpf, M., and Lichtensteiger, W. (1991). Prenatal nicotine exposure selectively affects perinatal forebrain aromatase activity and fetal adrenal function in male rats. *Brain Res. Dev. Brain Res.* 62, 23–31.

Wickström, R. (2007). Effects of nicotine during pregnancy: human and experimental evidence. *Curr. Neuropharmacol.* 5, 213–222. doi: 10.2174/157015907781695955

Xiao, Z., Li, X., Wang, X., Shen, J., and Ding, S. (2011). Determination of neonicotinoid insecticides residues in bovine tissues by pressurized solvent extraction and liquid chromatography–tandem mass spectrometry. *J. Chromatogr. B. Analyt. Technol. Biomed. Life Sci.* 879, 117–122. doi: 10.1016/j.jchromb.2010.11.008

Yanai, J., Pick, C. G., Rogel-Fuchs, Y., and Zahalka, E. A. (1992). Alterations in hippocampal cholinergic receptors and hippocampal behaviors after early exposure to nicotine. *Brain Res. Bull.* 29, 363–368.

Zbuzek, V. K., and Zbuzek, V. (1992). Vasopressin system is impaired in rat offspring prenatally exposed to chronic nicotine. *Ann. N.Y. Acad. Sci.* 654, 540–541.

Zhang, F., Li, Y., Yu, C., and Pan, C. (2012). Determination of six neonicotinoid insecticides residues in spinach, cucumber, apple and pomelo by QuEChERS method and LC-MS/MS. *Bull. Environ. Contam. Toxicol.* 88, 885–890. doi: 10.1007/s00128-012-0579-x

14

Gliotransmitter Release from Astrocytes: Functional, Developmental, and Pathological Implications in the Brain

Kazuki Harada, Taichi Kamiya and Takashi Tsuboi *

Department of Life Sciences, Graduate School of Arts and Sciences, The University of Tokyo, Tokyo, Japan

Edited by:
Fumihiko Maekawa,
National Institute for Environmental Studies, Japan

Reviewed by:
Robert Pawlak,
University of Exeter, UK
Nobuo Nagai,
Nagahama Institute of Bio-Science and Technology, Japan

***Correspondence:**
Takashi Tsuboi
takatsuboi@bio.c.u-tokyo.ac.jp

Astrocytes comprise a large population of cells in the brain and are important partners to neighboring neurons, vascular cells, and other glial cells. Astrocytes not only form a scaffold for other cells, but also extend foot processes around the capillaries to maintain the blood–brain barrier. Thus, environmental chemicals that exist in the blood stream could have potentially harmful effects on the physiological function of astrocytes. Although astrocytes are not electrically excitable, they have been shown to function as active participants in the development of neural circuits and synaptic activity. Astrocytes respond to neurotransmitters and contribute to synaptic information processing by releasing chemical transmitters called "gliotransmitters." State-of-the-art optical imaging techniques enable us to clarify how neurotransmitters elicit the release of various gliotransmitters, including glutamate, D-serine, and ATP. Moreover, recent studies have demonstrated that the disruption of gliotransmission results in neuronal dysfunction and abnormal behaviors in animal models. In this review, we focus on the latest technical approaches to clarify the molecular mechanisms of gliotransmitter exocytosis, and discuss the possibility that exposure to environmental chemicals could alter gliotransmission and cause neurodevelopmental disorders.

Keywords: astrocytes, exocytosis, glial cell, gliotransmitter, neurodevelopmental disorders, optical imaging, synaptic activity

INTRODUCTION

Astrocytes are the most abundant glial cells in the central nervous system (CNS) of mammals (Ventura and Harris, 1999). Based on electron microscopic analyses, astrocytes are located near to neurons and blood vessels (**Figure 1A**). Regarding vasculature, capillary endothelial cells are surrounded by pericytes and basal lamina, and astrocytes tightly wrap these microvascular structures (Abbott et al., 2006). Together with pericytes, astrocytes are an essential component of the blood–brain barrier (BBB), which selects and transports molecules from the bloodstream, and allows for the transfer of nutrients to neurons (**Figure 1B**). Regarding their relationship with neurons, astrocytic foot processes make close contact with pre- and post-synaptic areas, forming structures called "tripartite synapses" (Araque et al., 1999; Halassa et al., 2007). Indeed, in the hippocampus, 57% of synapses are associated with astrocytes (Ventura and Harris, 1999), suggesting that astrocytes might contribute to neural information processing in the CNS.

Despite their morphological characteristics described above, astrocytes have long been considered as mere metabolic supporters that nurture adjacent neurons (Halassa et al., 2007; Wang and Bordey, 2008; Calì et al., 2009). However, recent electrophysiology and optical imaging analyses have provided strong evidence that astrocytes respond to neurotransmitters and release chemical transmitters called "gliotransmitters" (Li et al., 2013). Gliotransmitters, including glutamate, D-serine, and ATP, bind to their respective receptors on neurons to modulate their firing frequency and/or synaptic transmission (**Figure 1C**; Halassa et al., 2007; Koizumi, 2010). In fact, the dysfunction of gliotransmitter release-related proteins (e.g., vesicular transporters and vesicle-associated membrane proteins) in astrocytes can cause serious brain disorders and abnormal behaviors (Rossi et al., 2011; Verkhratsky et al., 2014). At the same time, traumatic injury, stroke, or infection-induced astrogliosis (also known as reactive astrocytes). These reactive astrocytes produce and release neurotoxic levels of glutamate (Rossi et al., 2011; Verkhratsky et al., 2014). Astrocytes also contribute to proper development of the BBB by aligning endothelial cells and pericytes, transporting molecules selected from the bloodstream to neurons (Abbott et al., 2006), and providing a protective barrier against toxic substances (Pentreath and Slamon, 2000; Calabrese, 2008). Thus, chronic exposure to environmental chemicals, or inflammatory molecules from vasculature, may potentially affect the function of astrocytes and gliotransmitter release (Kim et al., 2014; Orellana et al., 2014; Avendano et al., 2015).

In this review, we present the latest methods that enable scientists to decipher the molecular mechanisms of gliotransmitter secretion. In particular, we focus on the vesicular exocytosis of gliotransmitters from astrocytes using optical microscopic imaging. We further discuss how genetic alterations, acute injuries, and chronically toxic conditions (including exposure to stress *in utero*) could impair gliotransmission and consequently lead to neuronal and behavioral disorders.

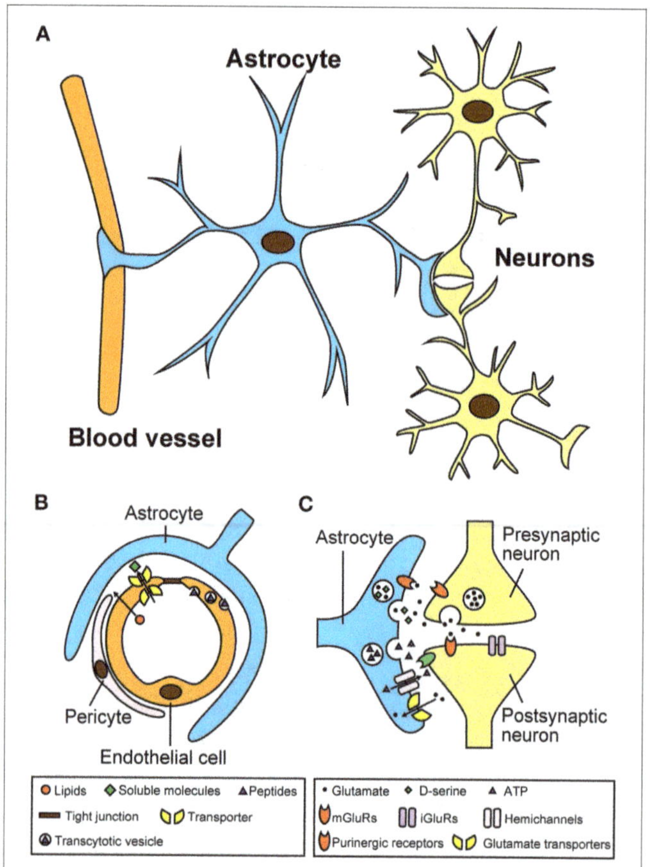

FIGURE 1 | Astrocytes have close morphological and functional associations with microvasculature and neurons. (A) Location of astrocytes around blood vessels and neurons in the central nervous system. Note that single astrocytes make contact with a large number of blood vessels and neurons through their numerous processes. **(B)** Schematic diagram showing the blood–brain barrier and its functions in selecting and transporting various molecules from the blood stream. Although, vascular endothelial cells form robust tight junctions that prevent infiltration of most soluble molecules, hydrophobic lipids can penetrate across the plasma membrane. In addition, certain soluble molecules such as glucose are actively transported across the endothelial cells via their specific transporters, and some peptides are taken up by selective vesicular transcytosis. **(C)** Schematic diagram showing the tripartite synapse and complex signaling interactions mediated by neurotransmitters and gliotransmitters. Neurotransmitters released from presynaptic terminals such as glutamate act not only on postsynapses but also on astrocytes. Activated astrocytes release gliotransmitters including glutamate, D-serine, and ATP, via vesicular exocytosis (and also possibly via hemichannels for ATP). Released gliotransmitters bind to presynaptic and postsynaptic receptors to regulate synaptic transmission. Astrocytes also take part in clearance of extracellular glutamate via glutamate transporters.

MOLECULAR MECHANISMS UNDERLYING THE RELEASE OF GLIOTRANSMITTERS

There have been two major methodological breakthroughs that have allowed for profound understanding of astrocytic activities including gliotransmission: calcium imaging and advanced optical microscopy (Li et al., 2013). The initial discovery made by using chemical calcium indicators was that astrocytes exhibit increased intracellular calcium concentration ($[Ca^{2+}]_i$), which spreads to adjacent astrocytes. This phenomenon is called Ca^{2+} waves (Cornell-Bell et al., 1990; Charles et al., 1991; Rusakov et al., 2014). Genetically encoded calcium indicators have enabled more detailed analysis of astrocyte functions (Shigetomi et al., 2013).

Two-photon microscopy enabled scientists to observe fluorescence with superior penetration depth. Thus, studies on astrocytes have been expanded to experiments using brain slices and *in vivo* models (Nimmerjahn et al., 2004; Nishida and Okabe, 2007). Moreover, thanks to total internal reflection fluorescence microscopy, which can visualize fluorescent molecule behaviors beneath the plasma membrane, the interaction between $[Ca^{2+}]_i$ elevation and subsequent vesicular trafficking became precisely clarified (Bezzi et al., 2004; Shigetomi et al., 2012; Oya et al., 2013).

Because of these experimental advancements, accumulating evidence suggests the paradigm that: (1) inositol 1,4,5-trisphosphate-mediated Ca^{2+} release from endoplasmic reticulum causes $[Ca^{2+}]_i$ increases in astrocytes in response to the activity of adjacent astrocytes and neurons; (2) elicited $[Ca^{2+}]_i$ elevation induces release of gliotransmitters (Halassa et al., 2007; Oya et al., 2013; Khakh and McCarthy, 2015). Although the exact mechanisms of gliotransmission are unclear, recent studies have partially revealed the release mechanisms of glutamate, D-serine, and ATP in astrocytes (**Figure 2**; Gucek et al., 2012; Li et al., 2013).

GLUTAMATE

Although, glutamate is well-known as a neurotransmitter, it also acts as a gliotransmitter. Application of bradykinin to cultured astrocytes induces glutamate release and influences adjacent neurons through N-methyl-D-aspartate (NMDA) receptors (Parpura et al., 1994). In contrast, application of clostridium, tetanus, and botulinum neurotoxins, which differentially cleave the exocytosis-regulating soluble N-ethylmaleimide-sensitive factor attachment protein receptor (SNARE) proteins, reduces Ca^{2+}-dependent glutamate release. These findings suggest that the SNARE proteins, including vesicle-associated membrane protein-2 (VAMP2), syntaxin-1, and synaptosome-associated protein-23, mediate Ca^{2+}-dependent glutamate release (Montana et al., 2006; Parpura and Zorec, 2010).

The uptake of cytoplasmic glutamate into exocytotic vesicles is mediated by vesicular glutamate transporters (VGLUTs), which are driven by a proton gradient produced by vacuolar-type H^+ ATPases (V-ATPases; Takamori et al., 2000; Gucek et al., 2012). Inhibition of V-ATPases blocks Ca^{2+}-dependent glutamate release (Parpura and Zorec, 2010). Furthermore,

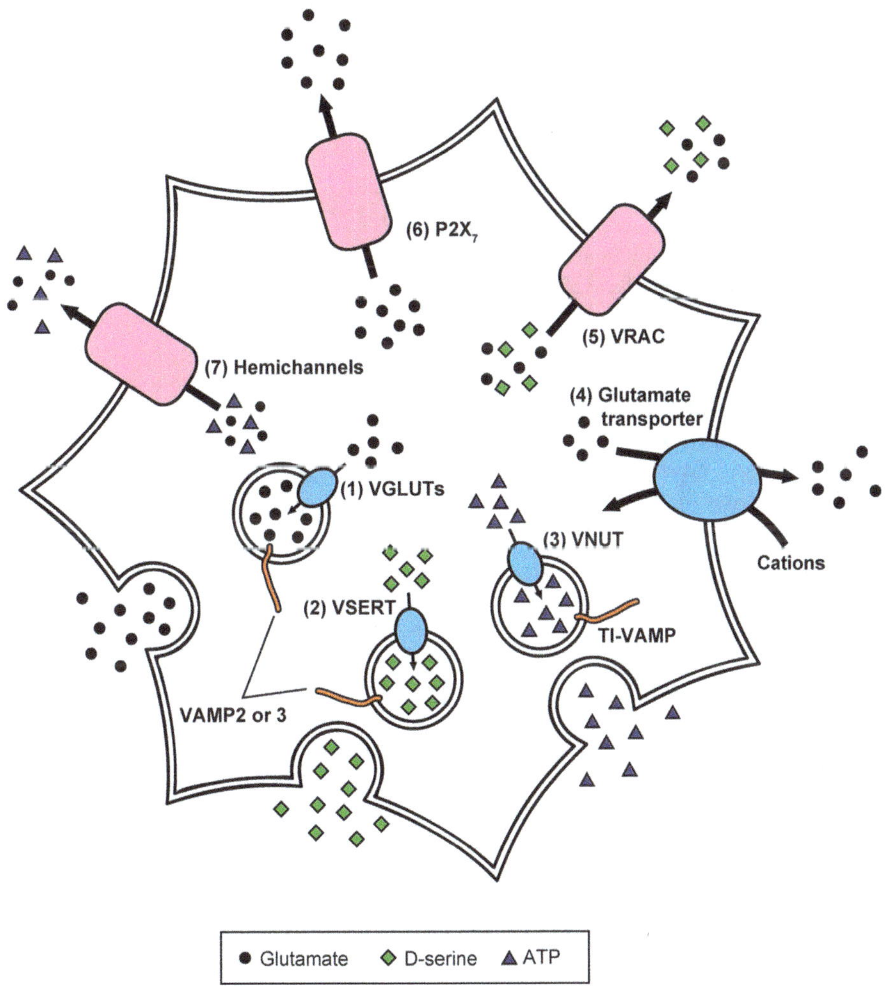

FIGURE 2 | Precise intracellular machinery involved in the release of glutamate, D-serine, and ATP from astrocytes. Glutamate and D-serine are taken up into synaptic-like vesicles through (1) VGLUT and (2) vesicular D-serine transporters (VSERT), respectively. These synaptic-like vesicles fuse to the plasma membrane, mediated by SNARE proteins including VAMP2 or VAMP3, in response to $[Ca^{2+}]_i$ increase. In contrast, ATP is released through secretory lysosomes. Storage of ATP into secretory lysosomes is achieved by (3) VNUT. Through the interaction of SNARE proteins including TI-VAMP, ATP-containing secretory lysosomes are Ca^{2+}-dependently exocytosed. Moreover, the existence of other release mechanisms has been discovered: (4) reverse operation of plasma membrane glutamate transporters, (5) cell swelling-induced anion transporter (VRAC) opening, (6) release via $P2X_7$ receptors, and (7) gap junction channels (hemichannels) on the cell surface of astrocytes.

VGLUT1 and 2 are colocalized with synaptic-like vesicles (Bezzi et al., 2004), suggesting that glutamate is packaged into synaptic-like vesicles and released from astrocytes in a Ca^{2+}-dependent manner.

Meanwhile, other release mechanisms have been identified: (1) reverse operation of plasma membrane glutamate transporters (Longuemare and Swanson, 1995); (2) cell swelling-induced anion transporter opening (Kimelberg et al., 1990); (3) release via $P2X_7$ receptors (Duan et al., 2003); (4) gap junction channels (i.e., hemichannels) on the cell surface of astrocytes (Ye et al., 2003). However, it is not clear how often and to what extent astrocytes employ these different mechanisms. Further studies will be needed to clarify whether there are specific release mechanisms that operate under particular conditions.

D-SERINE

The discovery of D-serine as a gliotransmitter was remarkable because it was long thought that mammalian tissues only produced L-isomers of amino acids (Oliet and Mothet, 2006; Henneberger et al., 2012). D-serine is thought to be produced from L-serine by serine racemase (de Miranda et al., 2002). In cultured astrocytes, application of glutamate enhanced Ca^{2+}-dependent secretion of D-serine via the activation of α-amino-3-hydroxy-5-methyl-4-isoxazolepropionic acid (AMPA)/kainate receptors (AMPA/KARs) and metabotropic glutamate receptors (Mothet et al., 2005). Correspondingly, agonists for AMPA/KARs and metabotropic glutamate receptors were found to increase $[Ca^{2+}]_i$ as well as subsequent secretion of D-serine, which is reduced by inhibition of these receptors. Furthermore, tetanus neurotoxins and V-ATPase inhibitors suppress agonist-evoked secretion of D-serine, and VAMP2/3 and VGLUT2-containing vesicles that are colocalized with D-serine. These results suggest that D-serine is stored in the synaptic-like vesicles and released from the vesicles in a Ca^{2+}-dependent manner (Martineau et al., 2013).

ATP

Although ATP is the primary energy currency of the cells, ATP can also act as a signaling molecule through purinergic receptors. A recent study showed that culture medium from cultured astrocytes exhibiting Ca^{2+} waves contained more ATP than control culture medium. Interestingly, the addition of collected culture medium to astrocytes induced Ca^{2+} waves that were inhibited by purinergic receptor antagonists (Guthrie et al., 1999). Thus, the ATP released from astrocytes induces Ca^{2+} waves, which astrocytes use to communicate with each other. However, the ATP release mechanisms still remain controversial; several lines of investigation have suggested various putative models for ATP release from astrocytes (Koizumi, 2010).

Connexin 43 (Cx43) assembles into a hemichannel which constitutes gap junctions in astrocytes, and exchanges signaling molecules, including Ca^{2+} and inositol 1,4,5-trisphosphate,between adjacent astrocytes (Orellana and Stehberg, 2014). Bioluminescence imaging of ATP combined with single channel recording showed that Cx43 hemichannels in rat glioma C6 cells and CA1 hippocampal astrocytes are permeable to ATP (Kang et al., 2008). Consistent with this finding, glutamate evoked $[Ca^{2+}]_i$ increase and ATP release in astrocytes of hippocampal slices, which were inhibited by application of a hemichannel blocker and in Cx43/Cx30 knockout mice (Torres et al., 2012), suggesting that ATP is released extracellularly through Cx43 hemichannels.

However, some studies have shown the involvement of secretory lysosomes in ATP release from astrocytes. In fact, primary cultured astrocytes express a secretory lysosome marker called vesicle-associated membrane protein-7 (also called TI-VAMP), and TI-VAMP-positive secretory lysosomes contain ATP which is Ca^{2+}-dependently released (Verderio et al., 2012). In an experiment using primary cultured astrocytes and C6 cells, vesicular nucleotide transporter (VNUT)-positive lysosomes were labeled with fluorescent ATP, and application of VNUT inhibitor reduced the number of fluorescent ATP-containing vesicles. Observation by total internal reflection fluorescence microscopy revealed exocytotic events of secretory lysosomes in the cells following the application of a calcium ionophore, ATP, and glutamate. Thus, ATP is stored in lysosomes and released from lysosomes in a Ca^{2+}-dependent manner (Oya et al., 2013).

CONTRIBUTION OF GLIOTRANSMITTER RELEASE TO DEVELOPMENT AND DISEASE

Release of gliotransmitters regulates synaptic transmission between neurons and the extracellular environment in the brain. It is known that glutamate and D-serine excite synaptic transmission. However, whether ATP potentiates or inhibits synaptic transmission is still under debate because adenosine, a metabolite synthesized from ATP, usually inhibits synaptic activity via adenosine A_1 receptors (Koizumi, 2010; Nam et al., 2012; Delekate et al., 2014). It is therefore reasonable to speculate that imbalance in the release of these gliotransmitters could result in altered neuronal activity. Various pathological conditions, including CNS diseases, traumatic brain injuries, developmental disorders, and prenatal exposure to deleterious molecules have been reported to be closely associated with impairment of gliotransmission.

CNS DISEASES

Many CNS diseases are attributed to hyperactivity of neurons or unregulated neuronal cell death. Although such conditions have long been the focus of "neurocentric" studies, recent progress in the study of astrocytic gliotransmission has provided accumulating evidence for the contribution of astrocytes (Rossi et al., 2011; Verkhratsky et al., 2014).

Epilepsy is one of the most common CNS diseases, and is characterized by sudden and frequent seizures resulting from excessive firings by neurons (Wetherington et al., 2008). In slices from epilepsy model mice, astrocytic glutamate release was found to cause abnormal and prolonged depolarization in neurons (Tian et al., 2005). Furthermore, tumor necrosis factor-α (TNFα) and prostaglandins (PGs), released from astrocytes under traumatic events, can reactivate their calcium signaling, and can cause increased glutamate release (Bezzi et al., 1998, 2001; Domercq et al., 2006).

Reactive astrocytes are also involved in the pathogenesis of other neuronal disorders. In a mouse model of Huntington's disease, cultured astrocytes exhibited hyperactivated Ca^{2+}-dependent glutamate release. This activity was owing to increased expression of pyruvate carboxylase (Lee et al., 2013), or reduced expression of glutamate transporter-1 and $K_{ir}4.1$ K^+ channels, which are key regulators for the clearance of extracellular glutamate and maintenance of membrane potentials, respectively (Behrens et al., 2002; Tong et al., 2014). In addition to overpotentiating neuronal activity, excessive accumulation of extracellular glutamate causes cytotoxicity. For instance, mice with genetic deletion in glutamate transporter-1 exhibit reduced glutamate clearance, and consequently display abnormal cell death in motor neurons, reminiscent of amyotrophic lateral sclerosis (Staats and Van Den Bosch, 2009).

In Alzheimer's disease (AD) mouse models, reactive astrocytes are detected near β-amyloid plaques (Nagele et al., 2004). Although chronic rise in $[Ca^{2+}]_i$ is a well-known phenomenon in reactive astrocytes in AD, its underlying mechanisms remain unclear. A recent study demonstrated that purinergic signaling through Cx43 hemichannels and P2Y1 receptors mediated the hyperactivity of astrocytes in AD (Delekate et al., 2014). Consistent with this finding, upregulation of Cx43 hemichannels was observed in an AD mouse model (Mei et al., 2010), and AD patients displayed higher levels of ATP in brain regions surrounding β-amyloid plaques (Mecheri et al., 1997; Mandal et al., 2012).

Gliotransmitter release from astrocytes is also required for correct development of neuronal circuits. In particular, glial-neuronal communication through NMDA receptors is an essential process for proper dendritic morphogenesis and establishment of synaptic connections (Rabacchi et al., 1992; Sin et al., 2002; Espinosa et al., 2009). Although NMDA receptors are activated by both glutamate and D-serine, recent discoveries suggest that D-serine plays an important role in dendritic development and long-term potentiation (Henneberger et al., 2010; Devito et al., 2011; Balu and Coyle, 2012; Diniz et al., 2012). Mice with a deletion of serine racemase showed reduced levels of brain D-serine and brain-derived neurotrophic factor, and loss of glutamatergic neurotransmission, and consequently had less complex dendrites (Morita et al., 2007; Balu and Coyle, 2012). Because NMDA receptor malfunction has been considered to be responsible for schizophrenia, deficiency in D-serine secretion from astrocytes can be a potent schizophrenia risk factor (Van Horn et al., 2013). Indeed, association studies of schizophrenia patients revealed several mutations in genes for serine racemase, as well as D-amino acid oxidase and its interacting protein G72 (Boks et al., 2007; Morita et al., 2007; Muller et al., 2011; Caldinelli et al., 2013).

INJURY AND INFECTION

Acute brain insults, caused by ischemia or infection, affect neuronal circuitry through direct inflammatory responses in neurons and through signals from glial cells (Vesce et al., 2007; Calì et al., 2009). Astrocytes under acute inflammatory conditions undergo reactive astrogliosis similarly to those in CNS diseases, albeit with differences in gene expression and cell structure (Khakh and Sofroniew, 2015). Upon injury or ischemia, damaged neurons, endothelial cells and glial cells are known to release considerable amounts of ATP (Cook and McCleskey, 2002; Wang et al., 2004; Davalos et al., 2005; Nedergaard et al., 2010). Increased levels of extracellular ATP activate purinergic receptors on astrocytes, particularly P2Y1 (Domercq et al., 2006), thereby inducing $[Ca^{2+}]_i$ elevation and release of glutamate, as well as ATP (Domercq et al., 2006; Nedergaard et al., 2010). Furthermore, inflammatory molecules including TNFα, interleukin-1β, and PGs, are profoundly engaged in these responses. Not only the activated microglia converge to the site of injury and secrete cytokines; astrocytes themselves synthesize TNFα and PGs (Domercq et al., 2006; Santello et al., 2011). TNFα and PGs either interact with certain processes in the stimulus–secretion coupling machinery within astrocytes (Domercq et al., 2006; Santello et al., 2011), or bind to TNFα and PGs receptors on astrocytes after secretion (Bezzi et al., 2001; Vesce et al., 2007).

CHRONIC AND PRENATAL EXPOSURE TO CHEMICALS

Increasing evidence shows significant correlations between environmentally deleterious chemicals and the risk of neurodevelopmental disorders (Feng et al., 1990; Leonardsson and Ny, 1997). Previous studies have focused on the effects of toxic substances on neurons, but recently it was suggested that astrocytes are also involved in the pathogenesis of those conditions.

Owing to their close connections with microvascular units via BBB, astrocytes tend to be chronically exposed to noxious molecules in circulation. Probably because of their interactions with environmental toxins, astrocytes possess more resilient and adaptive machinery against toxic molecules compared with neurons (Pentreath and Slamon, 2000; Calabrese, 2008). These protective systems include the glutathione system, superoxide dismutase, and hemeoxygenase (Dwyer et al., 1995; Huang and Philbert, 1995; Blaauwgeers et al., 1996; Pentreath and Slamon, 2000). Nevertheless, excessive passage of harmful substances across the BBB seriously affects astrocyte homeostasis and functionality.

The toxicological effects of heavy metals (e.g., mercury, zinc, manganese, and aluminum) on neurons and glial cells have been studied for decades (Calabrese, 2008; De Keyser et al., 2008). However, it is unclear how these metals affect gliotransmitter release. Some studies have shown that lead and manganese induce cytotoxic cell death by impairing glutamate uptake in astrocytes (Normandin and Hazell, 2002; Struzynska et al., 2005). However, pathological effects on gliotransmission by lifestyle associated factors, such as smoking, drinking, and insufficient sleep, are becoming the focus of growing interest. Because nicotinic acetylcholine receptors are expressed on astrocytes, they exhibit nicotine sensitivity and $[Ca^{2+}]_i$ increase (Oikawa et al., 2005; Delbro et al., 2009). Ethanol causes reactive oxygen species production, and $[Ca^{2+}]_i$ increase and glutamate secretion from astrocytes (Salazar et al., 2008). Astrocytes exposed to ethanol also exhibit alterations in Golgi complex morphology, secretory vesicle biogenesis, and expression levels of Rab GTPases and motor proteins (Tomas et al., 2005), which may be an additional factor for the dysfunction of brain development caused by ethanol.

Because adenosine plays a critical role in the control of sleep-wakefulness (Thakkar et al., 2003), and chronic alcoholism is frequently accompanied by sleep disorders (Brower, 2001), changes in sleep pattern may also induce alteration in gliotransmitter release. Interestingly, hypothalamic astrocytes from rats following sleep deprivation exhibited different proteome profiles, and the expression of VAMP2, which is an essential protein for vesicular exocytosis (Kim et al., 2014), was significantly increased. These findings suggest a strong association between alcohol intake, sleep disorders, and astrocytic gliotransmission.

Additionally, certain ambient ultrafine particles, which are defined as particulate substances with a diameter less than 100 nm, are emerging as another toxic substance that may deleteriously affect brain function (Block and Calderón-Garcidueñas, 2009; Loane et al., 2013). In a recent study, ultrafine carbon black, a surrogate for ultrafine particles, was shown to induce the release of glutamate and ATP from astrocytes by activating Cx43 and pannexin-1 hemichannels (Wei et al., 2014).

Recent epidemiological and experimental studies have demonstrated that children born from mothers who are exposed to infections or are addicted to alcohol or drugs have a higher risk of neuronal disorders and abnormal behaviors (Jacobsen et al., 2006; Stringari et al., 2008; Boksa, 2010; Brolese et al., 2015). However, the effects of these agents on astrocytes still remain largely unknown. Some studies have shown that prenatal exposure to lipopolysaccharides or nicotine together with postnatal high-fat/cholesterol diet result in enhancement of Cx43 hemichannel activity, and consequently increases the release of glutamate and ATP (Orellana et al., 2014; Avendano et al., 2015).

CONCLUSIONS

Over several decades, researchers have attempted to understand the properties and pathologies of the CNS by focusing solely on neurons; however, recent improvements in molecular and cellular imaging techniques are increasingly indicating that this neurocentric approach needs to be revised. In addition to neurons, glial cells including astrocytes are important elements for brain functions. Astrocytes are located in close morphological and functional relationships with blood vessels and neurons, and various genetic or environmental factors are implicated in gliotransmission impairment. Considering these characteristics of astrocytes, further studies will provide new insight on the significance of gliotransmitter release for fetal neurodevelopment. Thus, new therapies can be developed to overcome environmental chemical-induced neurodevelopmental disorders.

AUTHOR CONTRIBUTIONS

KH, TK, and TT wrote the paper.

ACKNOWLEDGMENTS

The authors thank Dr. Fumihiko Maekawa, Dr. Kazuaki Nakamura, and Dr Manami Oya for their helpful discussion and comments.

REFERENCES

Abbott, N. J., Rönnback, L., and Hänsson, E. (2006). Astrocyte-endothelial interactions at the blood-brain barrier. *Nat. Rev. Neurosci.* 7, 41–53. doi: 10.1038/nrn.1824

Araque, A., Parpura, V., Sanzgiri, R. P., and Haydon, P. G. (1999). Tripartite synapses: glia, the unacknowledged partner. *Trends Neurosci.* 22, 208–215. doi: 10.1016/S0166-2236(98)01349-6

Avendaño, B. C., Montero, T. D., Chávez, C. E., Von Bernhardi, R., and Orellana, J. A. (2015). Prenatal exposure to inflammatory conditions increases Cx43 and Panx1 unopposed channel opening and activation of astrocytes in the offspring effect on neuronal survival. *Glia.* 63, 2058–2072. doi: 10.1002/glia.22877

Balu, D. T., and Coyle, J. T. (2012). Neuronal D-serine regulates dendritic architecture in the somatosensory cortex. *Neurosci. Lett.* 517, 77–81. doi: 10.1016/j.neulet.2012.04.020

Behrens, P. F., Franz, P., Woodman, B., Lindenberg, K. S., and Landwehrmeyer, G. B. (2002). Impaired glutamate transport and glutamate-glutamine cycling: downstream effects of the Huntington mutation. *Brain* 125, 1908–1922. doi: 10.1093/brain/awf180

Bezzi, P., Carmignoto, G., Pasti, L., Vesce, S., Rossi, D., Rizzini, B. L., et al. (1998). Prostaglandins stimulate calcium-dependent glutamate release in astrocytes. *Nature* 391, 281–285. doi: 10.1038/34651

Bezzi, P., Domercq, M., Brambilla, L., Galli, R., Schols, D., De Clercq, E., et al. (2001). CXCR4-activated astrocyte glutamate release via TNFalpha: amplification by microglia triggers neurotoxicity. *Nat. Neurosci.* 4, 702–710. doi: 10.1038/89490

Bezzi, P., Gundersen, V., Galbete, J. L., Seifert, G., Steinhäuser, C., Pilati, E., et al. (2004). Astrocytes contain a vesicular compartment that is competent for regulated exocytosis of glutamate. *Nat. Neurosci.* 7, 613–620. doi: 10.1038/nn1246

Blaauwgeers, H. G., Vianney De Jong, J. M., Verspaget, H. W., Van Den Berg, F. M., and Troost, D. (1996). Enhanced superoxide dismutase-2 immunoreactivity of astrocytes and occasional neurons in amyotrophic lateral sclerosis. *J. Neurol. Sci.* 140, 21–29. doi: 10.1016/0022-510X(96)00110-4

Block, M. L., and Calderon-Garciduenas, L. (2009). Air pollution: mechanisms of neuroinflammation and CNS disease. *Trends Neurosci.* 32, 506–516. doi: 10.1016/j.tins.2009.05.009

Boks, M. P., Rietkerk, T., Van De Beek, M. H., Sommer, I. E., De Koning, T. J., and Kahn, R. S. (2007). Reviewing the role of the genes G72 and DAAO in glutamate neurotransmission in schizophrenia. *Eur. Neuropsychopharmacol.* 17, 567–572. doi: 10.1016/j.euroneuro.2006.12.003

Boksa, P. (2010). Effects of prenatal infection on brain development and behavior: a review of findings from animal models. *Brain Behav. Immun.* 24, 881–897. doi: 10.1016/j.bbi.2010.03.005

Brolese, G., Lunardi, P., De Souza, D. F., Lopes, F. M., Leite, M. C., and Goncalves, C. A. (2015). Pre- and postnatal exposure to moderate levels of ethanol can have long-lasting effects on hippocampal glutamate uptake in adolescent offspring. *PLoS ONE* 10:e0127845. doi: 10.1371/journal.pone.0127845

Brower, K. J. (2001). Alcohol's effects on sleep in alcoholics. *Alcohol Res. Health* 25, 110–125.

Calabrese, E. J. (2008). Astrocytes: adaptive responses to low doses of neurotoxins. *Crit. Rev. Toxicol.* 38, 463–471. doi: 10.1080/10408440802004023

Caldinelli, L., Sacchi, S., Molla, G., Nardini, M., and Pollegioni, L. (2013). Characterization of human DAAO variants potentially related to an increased risk of schizophrenia. *Biochim. Biophys. Acta* 1832, 400–410. doi: 10.1016/j.bbadis.2012.11.019

Calì, C., Marchaland, J., Spagnuolo, P., Gremion, J., and Bezzi, P. (2009). Regulated exocytosis from astrocytes physiological and pathological related aspects. *Int. Rev. Neurobiol.* 85, 261–293. doi: 10.1016/S0074-7742(09)85020-4

Charles, A. C., Merrill, J. E., Dirksen, E. R., and Sanderson, M. J. (1991). Intercellular signaling in glial cells: calcium waves and oscillations in response to mechanical stimulation and glutamate. *Neuron* 6, 983–992. doi: 10.1016/0896-6273(91)90238-U

Cook, S. P., and McCleskey, E. W. (2002). Cell damage excites nociceptors through release of cytosolic ATP. *Pain* 95, 41–47. doi: 10.1016/S0304-3959(01)00372-4

Cornell-Bell, A. H., Finkbeiner, S. M., Cooper, M. S., and Smith, S. J. (1990). Glutamate induces calcium waves in cultured astrocytes: long-range glial signaling. *Science* 247, 470–473. doi: 10.1126/science.1967852

Davalos, D., Grutzendler, J., Yang, G., Kim, J. V., Zuo, Y., Jung, S., et al. (2005). ATP mediates rapid microglial response to local brain injury *in vivo*. *Nat. Neurosci.* 8, 752–758. doi: 10.1038/nn1472

De Keyser, J., Mostert, J. P., and Koch, M. W. (2008). Dysfunctional astrocytes as key players in the pathogenesis of central nervous system disorders. *J. Neurol. Sci.* 267, 3–16. doi: 10.1016/j.jns.2007.08.044

Delbro, D., Westerlund, A., Björklund, U., and Hansson, E. (2009). In inflammatory reactive astrocytes co-cultured with brain endothelial cells nicotine-evoked Ca(2+) transients are attenuated due to interleukin-1beta release and rearrangement of actin filaments. *Neuroscience* 159, 770–779. doi: 10.1016/j.neuroscience.2009.01.005

Delekate, A., Füchtemeier, M., Schumacher, T., Ulbrich, C., Foddis, M., and Petzold, G. C. (2014). Metabotropic P2Y1 receptor signalling mediates astrocytic hyperactivity *in vivo* in an Alzheimer's disease mouse model. *Nat. Commun.* 5, 5422. doi: 10.1038/ncomms6422

de Miranda, J., Panizzutti, R., Foltyn, V. N., and Wolosker, H. (2002). Cofactors of serine racemase that physiologically stimulate the synthesis of the N-methyl-D-aspartate (NMDA) receptor coagonist D-serine. *Proc. Natl. Acad. Sci. U.S.A.* 99, 14542–14547. doi: 10.1073/pnas.222421299

Devito, L. M., Balu, D. T., Kanter, B. R., Lykken, C., Basu, A. C., Coyle, J. T., et al. (2011). Serine racemase deletion disrupts memory for order and alters cortical dendritic morphology. *Genes Brain Behav.* 10, 210–222. doi: 10.1111/j.1601-183X.2010.00656.x

Diniz, L. P., Almeida, J. C., Tortelli, V., Vargas Lopes, C., Setti-Perdigão, P., Stipursky, J., et al. (2012). Astrocyte-induced synaptogenesis is mediated by transforming growth factor beta signaling through modulation of D-serine levels in cerebral cortex neurons. *J. Biol. Chem.* 287, 41432–41445. doi: 10.1074/jbc.M112.380824

Domercq, M., Brambilla, L., Pilati, E., Marchaland, J., Volterra, A., and Bezzi, P. (2006). P2Y1 receptor-evoked glutamate exocytosis from astrocytes: control by tumor necrosis factor-alpha and prostaglandins. *J. Biol. Chem.* 281, 30684–30696. doi: 10.1074/jbc.M606429200

Duan, S., Anderson, C. M., Keung, E. C., Chen, Y., and Swanson, R. A. (2003). P2X7 receptor-mediated release of excitatory amino acids from astrocytes. *J. Neurosci.* 23, 1320–1328.

Dwyer, B. E., Nishimura, R. N., and Lu, S. Y. (1995). Differential expression of heme oxygenase-1 in cultured cortical neurons and astrocytes determined by the aid of a new heme oxygenase antibody. Response to oxidative stress. *Brain Res. Mol. Brain Res.* 30, 37–47. doi: 10.1016/0169-328X(94)00273-H

Espinosa, J. S., Wheeler, D. G., Tsien, R. W., and Luo, L. (2009). Uncoupling dendrite growth and patterning: single-cell knockout analysis of NMDA receptor 2B. *Neuron* 62, 205–217. doi: 10.1016/j.neuron.2009.03.006

Feng, P., Ohlsson, M., and Ny, T. (1990). The structure of the TATA-less rat tissue-type plasminogen activator gene. Species-specific sequence divergences in the promoter predict differences in regulation of gene expression. *J. Biol. Chem.* 265, 2022–2027.

Gucek, A., Vardjan, N., and Zorec, R. (2012). Exocytosis in astrocytes: transmitter release and membrane signal regulation. *Neurochem. Res.* 37, 2351–2363. doi: 10.1007/s11064-012-0773-6

Guthrie, P. B., Knappenberger, J., Segal, M., Bennett, M. V., Charles, A. C., and Kater, S. B. (1999). ATP released from astrocytes mediates glial calcium waves. *J. Neurosci.* 19, 520–528.

Halassa, M. M., Fellin, T., and Haydon, P. G. (2007). The tripartite synapse: roles for gliotransmission in health and disease. *Trends Mol. Med.* 13, 54–63. doi: 10.1016/j.molmed.2006.12.005

Henneberger, C., Bard, L., and Rusakov, D. A. (2012). D-Serine: a key to synaptic plasticity? *Int. J. Biochem. Cell Biol.* 44, 587–590. doi: 10.1016/j.biocel.2012.01.005

Henneberger, C., Papouin, T., Oliet, S. H., and Rusakov, D. A. (2010). Long-term potentiation depends on release of D-serine from astrocytes. *Nature* 463, 232–236. doi: 10.1038/nature.08673

Huang, J., and Philbert, M. A. (1995). Distribution of glutathione and glutathione-related enzyme systems in mitochondria and cytosol of cultured cerebellar astrocytes and granule cells. *Brain Res.* 680, 16–22. doi: 10.1016/0006-8993(95)00209-9

Jacobsen, L. K., Slotkin, T. A., Westerveld, M., Mencl, W. E., and Pugh, K. R. (2006). Visuospatial memory deficits emerging during nicotine withdrawal in adolescents with prenatal exposure to active maternal smoking. *Neuropsychopharmacology* 31, 1550–1561. doi: 10.1038/sj.npp.1300981

Kang, J., Kang, N., Lovatt, D., Torres, A., Zhao, Z., Lin, J., et al. (2008). Connexin 43 hemichannels are permeable to ATP. *J. Neurosci.* 28, 4702–4711. doi: 10.1523/JNEUROSCI.5048-07.2008

Khakh, B. S., and McCarthy, K. D. (2015). Astrocyte Calcium Signaling: from observations to functions and the challenges therein. *Cold Spring Harb. Perspect. Biol.* 7:a020404. doi: 10.1101/cshperspect.a020404

Khakh, B. S., and Sofroniew, M. V. (2015). Diversity of astrocyte functions and phenotypes in neural circuits. *Nat. Neurosci.* 18, 942–952. doi: 10.1038/nn.4043

Kim, J. H., Cho, Y. E., Baek, M. C., Jung, J. Y., Lee, M. G., Jang, I. S., et al. (2014). Chronic sleep deprivation-induced proteome changes in astrocytes of the rat hypothalamus. *J. Proteome Res.* 13, 4047–4061. doi: 10.1021/pr.500431j

Kimelberg, H. K., Goderie, S. K., Higman, S., Pang, S., and Waniewski, R. A. (1990). Swelling-induced release of glutamate, aspartate, and taurine from astrocyte cultures. *J. Neurosci.* 10, 1583–1591.

Koizumi, S. (2010). Synchronization of Ca2+ oscillations: involvement of ATP release in astrocytes. *FEBS J.* 277, 286–292. doi: 10.1111/j.1742-4658.2009.07438.x

Lee, W., Reyes, R. C., Gottipati, M. K., Lewis, K., Lesort, M., Parpura, V., et al. (2013). Enhanced Ca(2+)-dependent glutamate release from astrocytes of the BACHD Huntington's disease mouse model. *Neurobiol. Dis.* 58, 192–199. doi: 10.1016/j.nbd.2013.06.002

Leonardsson, G., and Ny, T. (1997). Characterisation of the rat tissue-type plasminogen activator gene promoter – identification of a TAAT-containing promoter element. *Eur. J. Biochem.* 248, 676–683. doi: 10.1111/j.1432-1033.1997.t01-1-00676.x

Li, D., Agulhon, C., Schmidt, E., Oheim, M., and Ropert, N. (2013). New tools for investigating astrocyte-to-neuron communication. *Front. Cell. Neurosci.* 7:193. doi: 10.3389/fncel.2013.00193

Loane, C., Pilinis, C., Lekkas, T. D., and Politis, M. (2013). Ambient particulate matter and its potential neurological consequences. *Rev. Neurosci.* 24, 323–335. doi: 10.1515/revneuro-2013-0001

Longuemare, M. C., and Swanson, R. A. (1995). Excitatory amino acid release from astrocytes during energy failure by reversal of sodium-dependent uptake. *J. Neurosci. Res.* 40, 379–386. doi: 10.1002/jnr.490400312

Mandal, P. K., Akolkar, H., and Tripathi, M. (2012). Mapping of hippocampal pH and neurochemicals from *in vivo* multi-voxel 31P study in healthy normal young male/female, mild cognitive impairment, and Alzheimer's disease. *J. Alzheimers. Dis.* 31(Suppl. 3), S75–S86. doi: 10.3233/JAD-2012-1 20166

Martineau, M., Shi, T., Puyal, J., Knolhoff, A. M., Dulong, J., Gasnier, B., et al. (2013). Storage and uptake of D-serine into astrocytic synaptic-like vesicles specify gliotransmission. *J. Neurosci.* 33, U3413–U3605. doi: 10.1523/jneurosci.3497-12.2013

Mecheri, G., Marie-Cardine, M., Sappey-Marinier, D., Bonmartin, H., Albrand, G., Ferry, G., et al. (1997). *In vivo* hippocampal (31)P NMR metabolites in Alzheimer's disease and ageing. *Eur. Psychiatry* 12, 140–148. doi: 10.1016/S0924-9338(97)80203-9

Mei, X., Ezan, P., Giaume, C., and Koulakoff, A. (2010). Astroglial connexin immunoreactivity is specifically altered at beta-amyloid plaques in beta-amyloid precursor protein/presenilin1 mice. *Neuroscience* 171, 92–105. doi: 10.1016/j.neuroscience.2010.08.001

Montana, V., Malarkey, E. B., Verderio, C., Matteoli, M., and Parpura, V. (2006). Vesicular transmitter release from astrocytes. *Glia* 54, 700–715. doi: 10.1002/glia.20367

Morita, Y., Ujike, H., Tanaka, Y., Otani, K., Kishimoto, M., Morio, A., et al. (2007). A genetic variant of the serine racemase gene is associated with schizophrenia. *Biol. Psychiatry* 61, 1200–1203. doi: 10.1016/j.biopsych.2006.07.025

Mothet, J. P., Pollegioni, L., Ouanounou, G., Martineau, M., Fossier, P., and Baux, G. (2005). Glutamate receptor activation triggers a calcium-dependent and SNARE protein-dependent release of the gliotransmitter D-serine. *Proc. Natl. Acad. Sci. U.S.A.* 102, 5606–5611. doi: 10.1073/pnas.0408483102

Müller, D. J., Zai, C. C., Shinkai, T., Strauss, J., and Kennedy, J. L. (2011). Association between the DAOA/G72 gene and bipolar disorder and meta-analyses in bipolar disorder and schizophrenia. *Bipolar Disord.* 13, 198–207. doi: 10.1111/j.1399-5618.2011.00905.x

Nagele, R. G., Wegiel, J., Venkataraman, V., Imaki, H., and Wang, K. C. (2004). Contribution of glial cells to the development of amyloid plaques in Alzheimer's disease. *Neurobiol. Aging* 25, 663–674. doi: 10.1016/j.neurobiolaging.2004.01.007

Nam, H. W., Mciver, S. R., Hinton, D. J., Thakkar, M. M., Sari, Y., Parkinson, F. E., et al. (2012). Adenosine and glutamate signaling in neuron-glial interactions: implications in alcoholism and sleep disorders. *Alcohol. Clin. Exp. Res.* 36, 1117–1125. doi: 10.1111/j.1530-0277.2011.01722.x

Nedergaard, M., Rodríguez, J. J., and Verkhratsky, A. (2010). Glial calcium and diseases of the nervous system. *Cell Calcium* 47, 140–149. doi: 10.1016/j.ceca.2009.11.010

Nimmerjahn, A., Kirchhoff, F., Kerr, J. N. D., and Helmchen, F. (2004). Sulforhodamine 101 as a specific marker of astroglia in the neocortex *in vivo*. *Nat. Methods* 1, 31–37. doi: 10.1038/nmeth.706

Nishida, H., and Okabe, S. (2007). Direct astrocytic contacts regulate local maturation of dendritic spines. *J. Neurosci.* 27, 331–340. doi: 10.1523/JNEUROSCI.4466-06.2007

Normandin, L., and Hazell, A. S. (2002). Manganese neurotoxicity: an update of pathophysiologic mechanisms. *Metab. Brain Dis.* 17, 375–387. doi: 10.1023/A:1021970120965

Oikawa, H., Nakamichi, N., Kambe, Y., Ogura, M., and Yoneda, Y. (2005). An increase in intracellular free calcium ions by nicotinic acetylcholine receptors in a single cultured rat cortical astrocyte. *J. Neurosci. Res.* 79, 535–544. doi: 10.1002/jnr.20398

Oliet, S. H., and Mothet, J. P. (2006). Molecular determinants of D-serine-mediated gliotransmission: from release to function. *Glia* 54, 726–737. doi: 10.1002/glia.20356

Orellana, J. A., Busso, D., Ramírez, G., Campos, M., Rigotti, A., Eugenín, J., et al. (2014). Prenatal nicotine exposure enhances Cx43 and Panx1 unopposed channel activity in brain cells of adult offspring mice fed a high-fat/cholesterol diet. *Front. Cell. Neurosci.* 8:403. doi: 10.3389/fncel.2014.00403

Orellana, J. A., and Stehberg, J. (2014). Hemichannels: new roles in astroglial function. *Front. Physiol.* 5:193. doi: 10.3389/fphys.2014.00193

Oya, M., Kitaguchi, T., Pais, R., Reimann, F., Gribble, F., and Tsuboi, T. (2013). The G protein-coupled receptor family C group 6 subtype A (GPRC6A) receptor is involved in amino acid-induced glucagon-like peptide-1 secretion from GLUTag cells. *J. Biol. Chem.* 288, 4513–4521. doi: 10.1074/jbc.M112.402677

Parpura, V., Basarsky, T. A., Liu, F., Jeftinija, K., Jeftinija, S., and Haydon, P. G. (1994). Glutamate-mediated astrocyte-neuron signalling. *Nature* 369, 744–747. doi: 10.1038/369744a0

Parpura, V., and Zorec, R. (2010). Gliotransmission: exocytotic release from astrocytes. *Brain Res. Rev.* 63, 83–92. doi: 10.1016/j.brainresrev.2009.11.008

Pentreath, V. W., and Slamon, N. D. (2000). Astrocyte phenotype and prevention against oxidative damage in neurotoxicity. *Hum. Exp. Toxicol.* 19, 641–649. doi: 10.1191/096032700676221595

Rabacchi, S., Bailly, Y., Delhaye-Bouchaud, N., and Mariani, J. (1992). Involvement of the N-methyl D-aspartate (NMDA) receptor in synapse elimination during cerebellar development. *Science* 256, 1823–1825. doi: 10.1126/science.1352066

Rossi, D., Martorana, F., and Brambilla, L. (2011). Implications of gliotransmission for the pharmacotherapy of CNS disorders. *CNS Drugs* 25, 641–658. doi: 10.2165/11593090-000000000-00000

Rusakov, D. A., Bard, L., Stewart, M. G., and Henneberger, C. (2014). Diversity of astroglial functions alludes to subcellular specialisation. *Trends Neurosci.* 37, 228–242. doi: 10.1016/j.tins.2014.02.008

Salazar, M., Pariente, J. A., Salido, G. M., and González, A. (2008). Ethanol induces glutamate secretion by Ca2+ mobilization and ROS generation in rat hippocampal astrocytes. *Neurochem. Int.* 52, 1061–1067. doi: 10.1016/j.neuint.2007.11.001

Santello, M., Bezzi, P., and Volterra, A. (2011). TNFalpha controls glutamatergic gliotransmission in the hippocampal dentate gyrus. *Neuron* 69, 988–1001. doi: 10.1016/j.neuron.2011.02.003

Shigetomi, E., Bushong, E. A., Haustein, M. D., Tong, X. P., Jackson-Weaver, O., Kracun, S., et al. (2013). Imaging calcium microdomains within entire astrocyte territories and endfeet with GCaMPs expressed using adeno-associated viruses. *J. Gen. Physiol.* 141, 633–647. doi: 10.1085/jgp.201210949

Shigetomi, E., Tong, X., Kwan, K. Y., Corey, D. P., and Khakh, B. S. (2012). TRPA1 channels regulate astrocyte resting calcium and inhibitory synapse efficacy through GAT-3. *Nat. Neurosci.* 15, 70–80. doi: 10.1038/nn.3000

Sin, W. C., Haas, K., Ruthazer, E. S., and Cline, H. T. (2002). Dendrite growth increased by visual activity requires NMDA receptor and Rho GTPases. *Nature* 419, 475–480. doi: 10.1038/nature00987

Staats, K. A., and Van Den Bosch, L. (2009). Astrocytes in amyotrophic lateral sclerosis: direct effects on motor neuron survival. *J. Biol. Phys.* 35, 337–346. doi: 10.1007/s10867-009-9141-4

Stringari, J., Nunes, A. K., Franco, J. L., Bohrer, D., Garcia, S. C., Dafre, A. L., et al. (2008). Prenatal methylmercury exposure hampers glutathione antioxidant system ontogenesis and causes long-lasting oxidative stress in the mouse brain. *Toxicol. Appl. Pharmacol.* 227, 147–154. doi: 10.1016/j.taap.2007.10.010

Struzynska, L., Chalimoniuk, M., and Sulkowski, G. (2005). The role of astroglia in Pb-exposed adult rat brain with respect to glutamate toxicity. *Toxicology* 212, 185–194. doi: 10.1016/j.tox.2005.04.013

Takamori, S., Rhee, J. S., Rosenmund, C., and Jahn, R. (2000). Identification of a vesicular glutamate transporter that defines a glutamatergic phenotype in neurons. *Nature* 407, 189–194. doi: 10.1038/35025070

Thakkar, M. M., Winston, S., and McCarley, R. W. (2003). A1 receptor and adenosinergic homeostatic regulation of sleep-wakefulness: effects of antisense to the A1 receptor in the cholinergic basal forebrain. *J. Neurosci.* 23, 4278–4287.

Tian, G. F., Azmi, H., Takano, T., Xu, Q., Peng, W., Lin, J., et al. (2005). An astrocytic basis of epilepsy. *Nat. Med.* 11, 973–981. doi: 10.1038/nm.1277

Tomás, M., Marín, P., Megías, L., Egea, G., and Renau-Piqueras, J. (2005). Ethanol perturbs the secretory pathway in astrocytes. *Neurobiol. Dis.* 20, 773–784. doi: 10.1016/j.nbd.2005.05.012

Tong, X., Ao, Y., Faas, G. C., Nwaobi, S. E., Xu, J., Haustein, M. D., et al. (2014). Astrocyte Kir4.1 ion channel deficits contribute to neuronal dysfunction in Huntington's disease model mice. *Nat. Neurosci.* 17, 694–703. doi: 10.1038/nn.3691

Torres, A., Wang, F. S., Xu, Q. W., Fujita, T., Dobrowolski, R., Willecke, K., et al. (2012). Extracellular Ca^{2+} acts as a mediator of communication from neurons to glia. *Sci. Signal.* 5:ra8. doi: 10.1126/scisignal.2002160

Van Horn, M. R., Sild, M., and Ruthazer, E. S. (2013). D-serine as a gliotransmitter and its roles in brain development and disease. *Front. Cell. Neurosci.* 7:39. doi: 10.3389/fncel.2013.00039

Ventura, R., and Harris, K. M. (1999). Three-dimensional relationships between hippocampal synapses and astrocytes. *J. Neurosci.* 19, 6897–6906.

Verderio, C., Cagnoli, C., Bergami, M., Francolini, M., Schenk, U., Colombo, A., et al. (2012). TI-VAMP/VAMP7 is the SNARE of secretory lysosomes contributing to ATP secretion from astrocytes. *Biol. Cell* 104, 213–228. doi: 10.1111/boc.201100070

Verkhratsky, A., Parpura, V., Pekna, M., Pekny, M., and Sofroniew, M. (2014). Glia in the pathogenesis of neurodegenerative diseases. *Biochem. Soc. Trans.* 42, 1291–1301. doi: 10.1042/BST20140107

Vesce, S., Rossi, D., Brambilla, L., and Volterra, A. (2007). Glutamate release from astrocytes in physiological conditions and in neurodegenerative disorders characterized by neuroinflammation. *Int. Rev. Neurobiol.* 82, 57–71. doi: 10.1016/S0074-7742(07)82003-4

Wang, D. D., and Bordey, A. (2008). The astrocyte odyssey. *Prog. Neurobiol.* 86, 342–367. doi: 10.1016/j.pneurobio.2008.09.015

Wang, X., Arcuino, G., Takano, T., Lin, J., Peng, W. G., Wan, P., et al. (2004). P2X7 receptor inhibition improves recovery after spinal cord injury. *Nat. Med.* 10, 821–827. doi: 10.1038/nm.1082

Wei, H., Deng, F., Chen, Y., Qin, Y., Hao, Y., and Guo, X. (2014). Ultrafine carbon black induces glutamate and ATP release by activating connexin and pannexin hemichannels in cultured astrocytes. *Toxicology* 323, 32–41. doi: 10.1016/j.tox.2014.06.005

Wetherington, J., Serrano, G., and Dingledine, R. (2008). Astrocytes in the epileptic brain. *Neuron* 58, 168–178. doi: 10.1016/j.neuron.2008.04.002

Ye, Z. C., Wyeth, M. S., Baltan-Tekkok, S., and Ransom, B. R. (2003). Functional hemichannels in astrocytes: a novel mechanism of glutamate release. *J. Neurosci.* 23, 3588–3596.

15

Effect of Error Augmentation on Brain Activation and Motor Learning of a Complex Locomotor Task

Laura Marchal-Crespo[1,2*]*, Lars Michels*[3,4]*, Lukas Jaeger*[1,3]*, Jorge López-Olóriz*[1] *and Robert Riener*[1,2]

[1] Sensory-Motor Systems Lab, Department of Health Sciences and Technology, Institute of Robotics and Intelligent Systems, ETH Zurich, Zurich, Switzerland, [2] Reharobotics Group, Spinal Cord Injury Center, Balgrist University Hospital, Medical Faculty, University of Zurich, Zurich, Switzerland, [3] Clinic of Neuroradiology, University Hospital Zurich, Zurich, Switzerland, [4] MR-Center, University Children's Hospital Zurich, Zurich, Switzerland

Edited by:
Lorenzo Masia,
Nanyang Technological University,
Singapore

Reviewed by:
Marco Bove,
Università di Genova, Italy
Ryan McKendrick,
Northrop Grumman, United States

***Correspondence:**
Laura Marchal-Crespo
laura.marchal@hest.ethz.ch

Up to date, the functional gains obtained after robot-aided gait rehabilitation training are limited. Error augmenting strategies have a great potential to enhance motor learning of simple motor tasks. However, little is known about the effect of these error modulating strategies on complex tasks, such as relearning to walk after a neurologic accident. Additionally, neuroimaging evaluation of brain regions involved in learning processes could provide valuable information on behavioral outcomes. We investigated the effect of robotic training strategies that augment errors—error amplification and random force disturbance—and training without perturbations on brain activation and motor learning of a complex locomotor task. Thirty-four healthy subjects performed the experiment with a robotic stepper (MARCOS) in a 1.5 T MR scanner. The task consisted in tracking a Lissajous figure presented on a display by coordinating the legs in a gait-like movement pattern. Behavioral results showed that training without perturbations enhanced motor learning in initially less skilled subjects, while error amplification benefited better-skilled subjects. Training with error amplification, however, hampered transfer of learning. Randomly disturbing forces induced learning and promoted transfer in all subjects, probably because the unexpected forces increased subjects' attention. Functional MRI revealed main effects of training strategy and skill level during training. A main effect of training strategy was seen in brain regions typically associated with motor control and learning, such as, the basal ganglia, cerebellum, intraparietal sulcus, and angular gyrus. Especially, random disturbance and no perturbation lead to stronger brain activation in similar brain regions than error amplification. Skill-level related effects were observed in the IPS, in parts of the superior parietal lobe (SPL), i.e., precuneus, and temporal cortex. These neuroimaging findings indicate that gait-like motor learning depends on interplay between subcortical, cerebellar, and fronto-parietal brain regions. An interesting observation was the low activation observed in the brain's reward system after training with error amplification compared to training without perturbations. Our results suggest that to enhance learning of a locomotor task, errors should be augmented based on subjects' skill level. The impacts of these strategies on motor learning, brain activation, and motivation in neurological patients need further investigation.

Keywords: motor learning, error augmentation, random disturbance, error amplification, gait rehabilitation, rehabilitation robotics, MR-compatible robotics, fMRI

INTRODUCTION

Robot-aided gait rehabilitation was developed to improve rehabilitation in patients with severe gait impairments (Behrman and Harkema, 2000; Riener et al., 2005). During robotic gait training, patients are provided with body weight support while a gait orthosis moves their legs into a correct kinematic gait pattern. It is thought that by moving the limb in ways that patients are otherwise not able to move would provide novel somatosensory stimulation that helps induce brain plasticity (Poon, 2004; Rossini and Dal Forno, 2004). Furthermore, robotic guidance might motivate repetitive and intensive practice in a safe environment (Reinkensmeyer and Housman, 2007). However, robotic guidance also appears to decrease physical effort during training (Israel et al., 2006), suggesting that robotic rehabilitation could potentially decrease recovery if it encourages patient's slacking, i.e., a decrease in effort, energy consumption, or attention during repeated movements when movement errors are small (Scheidt et al., 2000; Reinkensmeyer et al., 2009).

In fact, up to date, the functional gains obtained after robotic gait training are still limited (Dobkin and Duncan, 2012). There have been several clinical studies that have compared robotic gait training to conventional therapy—see (Pennycott et al., 2012) for a review. Results from these studies suggest that robotic-aided gait rehabilitation is especially suitable in the stroke acute phase, when patients can benefit from the higher degree of support from the robotic device. In general, the best results were found when the robot was employed in combination with conventional therapy (Husemann et al., 2007; Schwartz et al., 2009). In fact, a recent report suggested that robotic therapy combined with conventional therapy was more effective than conventional therapy alone in subacute stroke patients with greater motor impairment (Morone et al., 2011). Thereby, current rehabilitation robots might be working with suboptimal training strategies—only using a fraction of the rehabilitation potential—by not considering the subjects' individual needs.

Active subject participation is vital in order to provoke motor plasticity (Lotze et al., 2003), and is therefore, an important feature of gait training, especially in patients with lower motor impairments. In order to promote higher levels of subject participation and challenge, "challenge-based" controllers have been proposed, i.e., controllers that, unlike guiding controllers, make movement tasks more challenging or difficult (Marchal-Crespo and Reinkensmeyer, 2009). Research on motor learning has emphasized that errors are needed in order to drive motor adaptation (Emken and Reinkensmeyer, 2005; Reisman et al., 2013). Experimental evidence with healthy subjects has demonstrated that adaptive processes can be accelerated when trajectory errors are amplified using robotic forces during walking (Emken and Reinkensmeyer, 2005). In post-stroke patients, increasing subjects' legs phasing error (i.e., walking asymmetry) through a split-belt treadmill that moved each leg at a different speed resulted in a long term increase in walking symmetry (Reisman et al., 2013). Error amplification training also induced more robust aftereffects after locomotion training as compared to assistive training (Yen et al., 2012). However, augmenting errors did not always benefit motor learning. In a recent experiment with healthy subjects, training a golf putting task with augmented velocity errors had no effect on task performance and resulted in a decrease in motivation that lasted even after the error augmentation was retired (Duarte and Reinkensmeyer, 2015). A possible rationale for these inconsistent results is that the motivation decrease associated with error amplification might hamper learning.

Movement errors can also be induced using unexpected randomly-varying robotic forces that disturb subjects' movements during training. Recent research has stated that motor variability exhibited before training predicts motor learning ability (i.e., subjects with more variable movements showed faster adaptation; Wu et al., 2014). Unexpected randomly-varying feedforward forces might increase movement variability, and therefore, create an excellent framework to boost motor learning. Furthermore, error exploration is an important element to enhance learning, especially during the first stages of learning (Huberdeau et al., 2015). Unexpected forces might push subjects away from their "comfort zone," and therefore, encourage them to explore and investigate the new motor tasks. In a motor learning experiment with healthy subjects, training with randomly-varying robotic forces resulted in better tracking skills than training without robotic assistance or training with repulsive forces proportional to errors (Lee and Choi, 2010). Furthermore, we found that adding random disturbing forces during training improved motor learning of a simple locomotion task, probably because the addition of unforeseen forces increased subjects' effort (muscle activation) and attention (Marchal-Crespo et al., 2014a,b).

A well-known motor learning theory, the Challenge Point Theory states that learning is maximized when the task difficulty is appropriate for the individual skill level of the performer (Guadagnoli and Lee, 2004). This is line with recent studies that found that robotic guidance seems to be especially helpful to train subjects with initial lower skill level (Marchal-Crespo et al., 2010, 2013), while error amplification was found to be more beneficial to train more skilled participants (Milot et al., 2010; Duarte and Reinkensmeyer, 2015). Additionally, error-augmenting strategies might be more suitable to enhance learning of especially simple tasks, i.e., tasks that can be learned in only one training session, since it might increase subjects' concentration (Marchal-Crespo et al., 2014b). On the other hand, in more challenging tasks, augmenting errors might decrease feelings of perceived satisfaction and competence and result in a decrease in motivation that might limit the effectiveness of error amplification on motor learning (Duarte and Reinkensmeyer, 2015).

Only few motor learning studies have compared the effectiveness of different robotic training strategies, and their relative benefits compared to unassisted practice, on motor learning. Most of these studies were performed with the upper limbs and/or using simple tasks, i.e., artificial tasks that have only one degree of freedom and can be learned in only one training session (Wulf and Shea, 2002). However, it has been shown that "*principles derived from the study of simple skills do not always generalize to complex skill learning*," such as, relearning how to walk after a neurologic accident (Wulf and Shea, 2002). The goal of robotic therapy is to develop robotic devices that promote motor recovery, i.e., that provoke participant's motor plasticity. Currently, however, there is not a solid scientific understanding of how this goal can best be achieved. Recent work has highlighted the relevance of motor learning principles in stroke recovery and neurorehabilitation (Krakauer, 2006; Shumway-Cook and Woollacott, 2007). In fact, it has been proposed that recovery after a brain injury is a form of motor learning or relearning (Dietz and Ward, 2015). Therefore, understanding the underlying mechanisms of motor learning might suggest novel training strategies to improve neurorehabilitation. Neuroimaging evaluation of brain areas involved in learning under different robotic training strategies can provide valuable insights on the observed behavioral outcomes. Furthermore, evaluation of brain areas involved in learning might also allow tailoring the best motor training strategies to the different patterns of brain damage (Burke and Cramer, 2013).

In this study, we present results of a motor learning experiment performed with thirty-four healthy subjects to evaluate the impact of three different training strategies on motor learning of a complex locomotor task: No perturbation, error amplification, and random force disturbance. The experiment was conducted while performing functional Magnetic Resonance Imaging (fMRI) employing an MRI-compatible robotic device (MARCOS). We hypothesized that training with the challenge-based strategies would result in better motor learning in initially more skilled subjects. We also expected that training with challenge-based strategies would hamper motor learning in initially less skilled subjects. To our knowledge, no studies have evaluated the brain regions activated during entire gait-like movements. Therefore, our hypothesis related to brain activation derives from studies that investigated isolated movements of ankle and knee joints (Luft et al., 2002) or imagination of walking (Miyai et al., 2003; Jahn et al., 2004; la Fougère et al., 2010). We hypothesize to find activity in somatosensory/motor related areas (S1/M1) and supplementary and pre-supplementary motor areas (SMA/pSMA). Hypothetically, during training with the challenge-based strategies, we expect more activity within all somatosensory/motor related areas, as well as in brain areas involved in error processing, such as, the anterior cingulate cortex (Mars et al., 2005), posterior medial frontal cortex (Hester et al., 2008), and cerebellum (Tseng et al., 2007; Grafton et al., 2008). Activation in the brainstem is also expected, based on animal studies.

METHODS

MARCOS

MARCOS was employed to conduct the experiment. MARCOS is an MRI-compatible robotic device pneumatically actuated and with one degree-of-freedom per leg (Hollnagel et al., 2011; **Figure 1**, left). MARCOS was built by the SMS-lab at ETH Zurich with low magnetic susceptibility materials to allow the assessment of brain activation using fMRI during gait-like stepping movements (Jaeger et al., 2014). The robot is actuated by two pneumatic cylinders (per leg), one attached to the subject's knee through a knee orthosis that can move the knee up and down, and a second one attached to the subject's foot sole using a special shoe, which can render forces that mimic ground reaction forces. The device allows hip, knee, and ankle flexion and extension movements in the sagittal plane that resemble on-the-spot stepping. The robot incorporates force sensors mounted at the orthoses-human contact points to measure the interaction forces between human and robot. The position of each cylinder piston is measured redundantly by optical encoders with a ceramic scale and a foil potentiometer. For more detailed information about the robot design, the reader is referred to (Hollnagel et al., 2011).

The Complex Locomotor Task

The experimental task consisted in tracking a white dot that moved on top of a Lissajous figure presented on a visual display (**Figure 1**, right) by coordinating the legs in a predefined gait-like pattern. The knees vertical displacements were mapped into the movement of a green dot on the visual display: The green dot moved up and down when the left leg moved up and down, and moved right and left when the right leg moved up and down. The predefined gait-like pattern to be learned consisted of moving the knees up and down following sinusoidal movements of equal frequency (0.5 Hz), but different amplitudes (left leg: 0.16 m; right leg: 0.08 m, i.e., axis ratio of 2) and with a phase difference between legs of 60°. This task was selected because it was challenging enough to observe learning in most of the subjects (Marchal-Crespo et al., 2014b). This task is also appealing because it resembles the abnormal gait pattern observed in stroke survivors with a paretic lower limb: An asymmetric pattern with the paretic leg performing shorter and faster steps.

Training Strategies

Subjects trained the gait-like task with one of three different training strategies: (i) No perturbation (NP): no disturbances were presented, (ii) Error amplification (EA): errors were amplified with repulsive forces proportional to errors, and (iii) Random force disturbance (RD): errors were induced with unexpected randomly-varying force disturbances. The design and evaluation of the training strategies was described in detail in (Marchal-Crespo et al., 2014b). Here, only a brief summary is given for completeness.

No Perturbation

When training with no perturbation, subjects are free to move without feeling any disturbance or assistance force from the robot. The control approach for the no perturbation strategy is a closed-loop zero force controller that minimizes the measured interaction forces between subjects and robot. The controller includes the compensation of the weight of the knee orthosis and the dependency of pressure build-up on chamber volume (Hollnagel et al., 2013; Marchal-Crespo et al., 2014b).

Error Amplification

In order to amplify the tracking errors (i.e., the differences between the desired and measured knee positions) created when trying to track the Lissajous figure, a proportional controller with

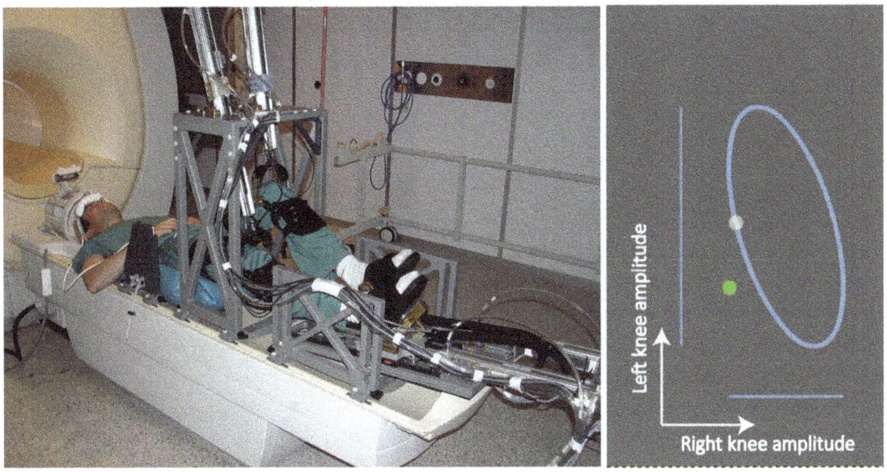

FIGURE 1 | (Left) The MRI-compatible robotic stepping actuator MARCOS in the 1.5 Tesla MR scanner (Hollnagel et al., 2011). The participant in this figure consented to the publication of his image. **(Right)** The Lissajous figure visually presented to participants. Subjects were requested to track a white dot that moved on top of a Lissajous figure by coordinating the legs in a predefined gait-like pattern. Subjects tracked the white dot with a green dot that moved up and down when the left leg moved up and down, and moved right and left when the right leg moved up and down.

negative impedance gain was developed. Therefore, the repulsive force applied by the knee cylinder is proportional to the tracking error, i.e., the force is smaller as smaller is the tracking error and increases proportional to the error. The forces from the error amplification controller were fed into a close-loop force controller. We saturated the magnitude of the error-amplification forces to guarantee the subjects' safety and to limit the difficulty of the task (Marchal-Crespo et al., 2014b).

Random Force Disturbance

The idea behind the random force disturbance strategy is to push subjects away from their "comfort zone," by forcing them to experience errors/movements that would otherwise not been created. The controller applies unpredictable random perturbing forces using the knee cylinder while subjects train the tracking task. The knee cylinder applies a disturbing force that last for 0.1 s with a random magnitude between ± 100 N, every 0.5 s. The random force disturbance controller works on top of a closed-loop force controller, therefore, the subjects are always in charge of the movement generation (Marchal-Crespo et al., 2014b).

Experimental Protocol

The study was approved by the local ethical committee (Kantonale Ethikkommission Zürich, Application Number: EK-856) and conducted in compliance with the Declaration of Helsinki. Thirty-four healthy subjects (23 male), 26.6 ± 3.5 years old, gave written consent to participate. All subjects were right footed (evaluated with the Waterloo Handedness Questionnaire, (Bryden, 1977). FMRI was recorded in the MR-Center of the University of Zurich and ETH Zurich, on a Philips Achieva (Philips Medical System, Best, The Netherlands) 1.5 T MR system equipped with an 8-channel head coil.

Subjects were supine positioned with their knees fixed to the MARCOS knee orthosis, while the feet were placed in special shoes and fixed with Velcro fasteners (**Figure 1**, left). Head motion was minimized through several solutions, such as, custom made hip-fixations and shoulder belts, a vacuum pillow at the participants' back, and an inflatable headgear (Crania, www.pearltec.ch; Hollnagel et al., 2011). The video display of the game was projected onto a screen placed in front of the scanner and viewed by the subjects through a mirror mounted on the MRI head coil (**Figure 1**, left).

A parallel design was used in order to evaluate the effects of training with the three different training strategies (**Figure 2**). The first 23 subjects were randomly assigned to one of the three training groups: No perturbation (NP), error amplification (EA), random disturbance (RD). After a preliminary evaluation of the data, we found that the tracking errors created during baseline (i.e., before training) had a significant effect on the benefits of practicing with the different training strategies (Marchal-Crespo et al., 2014b). Although it is expected that by randomizing subjects into the different training groups would result in a balanced level of tracking error across groups, it is still possible—especially in relative small sampling sizes—to end up with imbalanced groups that could bias our results. Therefore, we decided to allocate the remainder 11 subjects to one of the three training groups using adaptive randomization methods. The idea was to yield training groups whose subjects' initial errors followed normal distributions with similar means and standard distributions. To accomplish this goal, we assigned new subjects to one of the three training groups based in the visualization of the histograms of the errors created by the subjects evaluated till the moment and the error performed by the new subjects during baseline. Eleven subjects ended in the no-perturbation group, eleven in the error-amplification group, and twelve in the random-disturbance group.

In order to instruct subjects about the task to be performed, they were presented with a video, outside the scanner room,

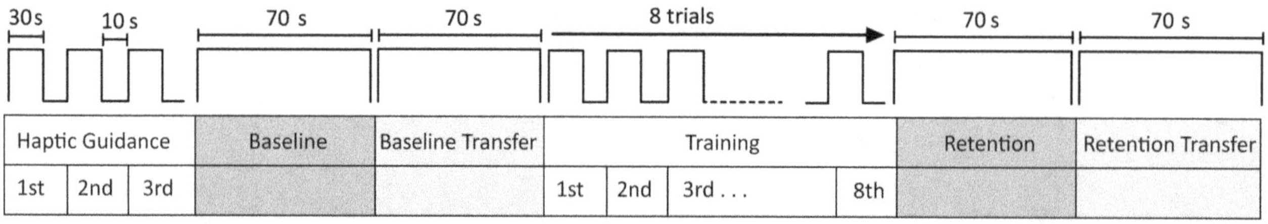

FIGURE 2 | Experimental protocol. Haptic guidance was employed to help subjects to understand the locomotor task. Three trials of 30 s with the robot passively moving the subjects' legs were employed to present the locomotor task. During baseline, subjects actively tracked the Lissajous figure during 70 s in no perturbation mode. Subjects performed a second baseline test (baseline-transfer), where they tracked a similar figure but with the left leg with the smallest amplitude. During training, subjects played with no perturbation, error amplification or random force disturbance, depending on their training group. Each training session consisted of eight trials of 30 s of movement with 10 s rest between trials. The short-term retention and transfer tests followed the same structure and order as baseline and baseline-transfer tests. Subjects were scanned by the fMRI during all phases.

that showed a subject in MARCOS moving alternatively his legs up and down and how these knee movements controlled the movement of a green dot on a screen. They were not informed about the training group they were assigned to, but were informed that during practice the robot could disturb them. The experiment started with a haptic demonstration phase, where the robot passively guided the subjects' legs in the desired gait-like pattern during three trials of 30 s, with 10 s of rest between trials in order to help subjects to understand the task to be performed (Hollnagel et al., 2013). During the haptic-guidance condition, subjects were instructed to relax and keep both legs passive while they observed the white and green dot moving on top of the Lissajous figure on the screen. After the haptic demonstration of the locomotor task, subjects performed the baseline test during 70 s. They were instructed to coordinate their legs in order to track the white dot that moved on top of the Lissajous figure in no perturbation mode. Transfer of learning, i.e., the capacity to apply an acquired skill on a task to another very similar task (Schmidt and Lee, 2010) is a crucial aspect of motor learning. Therefore, after baseline, subjects performed a second baseline test during 70 s (baseline-transfer), where they followed a similar Lissajous figure but with the left leg moving with the smallest amplitude (left leg: 0.08 m; right leg: 0.16 m). During training, subjects played without perturbation, error amplification or random force disturbance, depending on their training strategy group. Each training session consisted of eight trials of 30 s of movement with 10 s rest between trials. The challenge-based training strategies were applied to the left leg only, while the right leg was controlled in no perturbation mode in order to limit the task difficulty. The short-term retention and short-term retention transfer tests were 70 s long each and were performed in no perturbation mode. Overall, the experiment was <1 h. Subjects were actively scanned by the fMRI through the duration of the experiment.

Data Processing and Statistical Analysis

Behavioral Data

For each protocol test and training trial, we calculated the mean tracking error for each leg as the mean of the absolute value of the difference between the measured and target knee positions. We evaluated whether the challenge-based training strategies worked as expected (i.e., they increased the error during training): We compared the error of the left leg in the first training trial to the error during baseline using a repeated measures ANOVA with training strategy as a between subjects factor. To determine whether subjects increased the left leg error when training started, a paired t-test between baseline and the first training trial was performed per each training group. We further compared the tracking error during the eight training trials between training groups using ANOVAs. In order to determine whether subjects adapted to the challenged-based strategies during training—i.e., they reduced the error of the left leg during training—we performed a paired t-test between the left leg tracking error created at the first and last (eighth) training trials.

The absolute tracking error during baseline was employed as a qualitative measure of initial skill level (i.e. the larger the error during baseline, the initially less skilled a subject was). We used K-means cluster analysis to divide subjects into two skill-based groups, based on the tracking error created during baseline. Thirteen subjects who performed systematically worse during baseline (cluster center = 0.065 m) were assigned into the novice group (5 NP, 4 RD, 4 EA), and the remainder 21 subjects were classified (cluster center = 0.041 m) as skilled (6 NP, 8 RD, 7 EA). An ANOVA was used to evaluate whether the skill groups performed differently during baseline. We used repeated measures ANOVA to test the effect that training strategies [no perturbation (NP), error amplification (EA), and random force disturbance (RD) as fixed effect], initial skill level (novice and skilled as fixed effects) and their interaction had on the tracking error reduction from baseline to retention. In order to determine whether subjects learned the complex locomotor task, a paired t-test between baseline and retention was performed. To determine whether subjects in each training strategy group and skill level subgroup learned the task, a Wilcoxon test between the tracking error at baseline and retention was performed. We compared the error reduction between training groups in each skill level subgroup using Kruskal-Wallis tests. Four subjects in the skilled group (2 RD, 2 EA) who performed remarkably well during baseline (error < 0.032 m) were not considered in these Wilcoxon tests in order to avoid the negative effect of learning ceiling. To test the correlation between error reduction after the different training strategies and initial skill level, Pearson's correlation tests were performed.

We used a second performance variable in order to evaluate whether subjects learned the desired phase between legs. The period between legs at each step was calculated as the difference between the time at which the left leg is at its maximum high and the time when the right leg reaches its highest position during a step. The phase was calculated as 360° over this period. For each protocol test, the absolute mean phase error (calculated as the difference between the calculated phase and the desired one of 60°) across all steps was calculated. Data from one subject in the no-perturbation group during baseline was removed from statistical analysis, since the error reached its maximum. In order to test whether subjects learned the desired phase, a paired t-test between baseline and retention was performed. We used repeated measures ANOVA to test the effect that the training strategies, initial skill level and their interaction had on the phase error reduction from baseline to retention.

Transfer could not be evaluated in four subjects (1 NP, 2 RD, 1 EA), because data was not correctly recorded during baseline-transfer. Transfer was evaluated using repeated measures ANOVA to test the effect of the training strategy (NP, EA, and RD as fixed effects), initial skill level (novice and skilled) and their interaction on the tracking error reduction from baseline—transfer to retention-transfer. Paired t-tests between the tracking error created during baseline-transfer and retention-transfer were performed in order to evaluate whether subjects in each training group transferred the learned motor skills.

Normal distribution was checked visually using Q–Q plots. Post-hoc comparisons were performed with Tukey correction. The significance value was set to $\alpha = 0.05$. Statistical analyses were performed using IBM® SPSS® Software (version 23, Chicago, IL).

Functional MR Data

FMRI of the brain was acquired using a T2*-weighted, single-shot, echo planar imaging sequence (echo time = 50 ms, repetition time = 3.025 s, flip angle = 90°, SENSE factor = 1.6). A total of 35 interleaved, angulated, transversal slices covering the whole brain were acquired in each volume (FOV = 220 × 220 mm, acquisition voxel size: 2.75 × 2.8 × 3.8 mm, resliced to 1.72 × 1.72 × 3.8 mm).

FMRI data were analyzed using SPM8 (Wellcome Department of Cognitive Neurology, London, UK). Images were realigned to the mean image and normalized to standard MNI space using the EPI template provided by the Montreal Neurological Institute (MNI brain) and smoothed using an 8 mm full-width at half-maximum Gaussian kernel. The estimated realignment parameter data were filtered using the discrete cosine transform matrix filter incorporated in SPM8, to remove any linear drift. In order to avoid movement artifacts, FMRI data sets that after filtering showed a total head displacement above half voxel size in each dimension were excluded from the 1st-level statistical analysis. Contrast images of the motor task performed at different time points in the MR scanner (period: baseline, training, and retention) vs. an implicit rest (no movements) condition were calculated. FMRI data sets from 10 subjects during training, and data from one subject during the retention test were excluded from further analysis because the measured head motions were above the threshold. FMRI data from a total of 24 subjects (9 NP, 7 EA, and 8 RD) during training, and 33 (10 NP, 11 EA, 12 RD) during baseline and retention were employed at 2nd-level analysis. The 1st-level contrast images were then subject to a 2nd-level full factorial group analysis (2-way ANOVA). Here we computed main effects of initial skill level and training strategy for the contrasts: Training—rest, and retention—baseline. In case of significant main effect of strategy, we compared by *post-hoc* t-tests the following contrasts:

1. Error amplification vs. no perturbation (and vice versa)
2. Error amplification vs. random force disturbance (and vice versa)
3. No perturbation vs. random force disturbance (and vice versa)

In case of a significant main effect of skill level, we compared by unpaired t-tests skilled vs. novice participants (across all training strategies). We also computed strategy × initial skill-level interaction effects. However, we did not perform *post-hoc* tests on the interaction, as we had not enough subjects ($n < 10$) and, thus, lacking statistical power.

All statistical tests were thresholded at $p \leq 0.001$ (uncorrected) and were cluster-corrected ($k_E = 27$ voxels) to achieve $p < 0.05$ corrected. This cluster threshold was based on a Monte-Carlo simulation approach using a script to estimate the average size of the random clusters that can occur in our data given a $p \leq 0.001$ (Slotnick et al., 2003).

RESULTS

Behavioral Data

Performance during Training

The different training groups responded differently when training started, as suggested by a significant difference between training groups in the tracking error change from baseline to the first training trial [**Figure 3**, $F_{(2, 31)} = 9.84$, $p < 0.001$] Subjects trained with error amplification significantly increased the error from baseline to the first training trial ($p = 0.002$), while subjects trained without perturbations and with random-disturbance did not changed the errors significantly. Subjects in the error-amplification group performed systematically worse than subjects in the random-disturbance and no-perturbation groups during the first training trials, as observed in a significant greater tracking error during the first, second and fourth training trials [**Figure 3**, Trial 2, $F_{(2, 31)} = 6.62$, $p = 0.004$; Trial 3, $F_{(2, 31)} = 4.17$, $p = 0.025$; Trial 4, $F_{(2, 31)} = 2.40$, $p = 0.107$; Trial 5, $F_{(2, 31)} = 4.17$, $p = 0.025$]. The differences between groups were non-significant during the last training trials. This is due to the fact that subjects in the error-amplification group adapted to the error amplification disturbance, suggested by the significant error reduction from the first to the last (eighth) training trials (paired t-test, $p = 0.004$). This adaptation was not observed in the no-perturbation and random-disturbance groups. Both groups reduced the error from the first to the last training trials, although not significantly. The random-disturbance and no-perturbation groups performed similarly through the duration of the training.

Effect of Training Strategies and Skill Level on Learning

The performance during baseline was significantly different between skill groups. They showed significant differences in the tracking error during baseline [$F_{(1, 32)} = 52.14$, $p < 0.001$]. We examined the effect of the subjects' skill level (i.e., the tracking error during baseline) on the effectiveness of the different training strategies. We found a non-significant linear correlation between initial skill level and the error reduction from baseline to retention after training without perturbations (**Figure 4** left, Pearson's correlation, $R = 0.544$, $p = 0.083$). We also found a quadratic relationship between the initial skill level and the error reduction from baseline to retention after training with error amplification (**Figure 4** left, $R = 0.716$, $p = 0.057$).

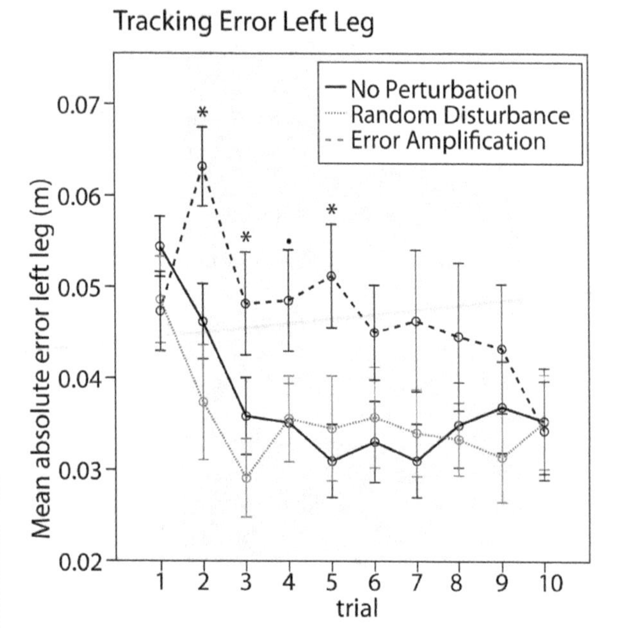

FIGURE 3 | Performance during training. Mean absolute tracking error created with the left leg during baseline (trial 1), training with the different strategies (trials 2–9, shaded area), and retention (trial 10). Error bars show ± 1 CI. *$p < 0.05$, •$p < 0.1$.

We used repeated measures ANOVA to test the effect that different training strategies [no perturbation (NP), error amplification (EA), random disturbance (RD)], initial skill level (novice, skilled), and their interaction had on the tracking error reduction from baseline to retention. We found that all subjects reduced the tracking error after training [$F_{(1, 28)} = 27.30$, $p < 0.001$]. Subjects in all training strategies learned the task (NP: $p = 0.011$; RD: $p = 0.016$; EA: $p = 0.022$). The main effect of initial skill level on the error reduction was non-significant. The main effect of training strategy was also non-significant. However, we found an interaction between the initial skill level and the training strategy that approached statistical significance [$F_{(2, 28)} = 3.22$, $p = 0.055$]. Novices only reduced the error significantly when trained without perturbation (**Figure 4** right, Wilcoxon, $p = 0.043$). In fact, novices tended to reduce the errors to a greater amount when trained without perturbation in comparison with the other training strategies (Kruskal-Wallis $p = 0.063$). The skilled group only reduced significantly the error after training with challenge-based strategies (**Figure 4** right, Wilcoxon, EA: $p = 0.043$, RD: $p = 0.075$).

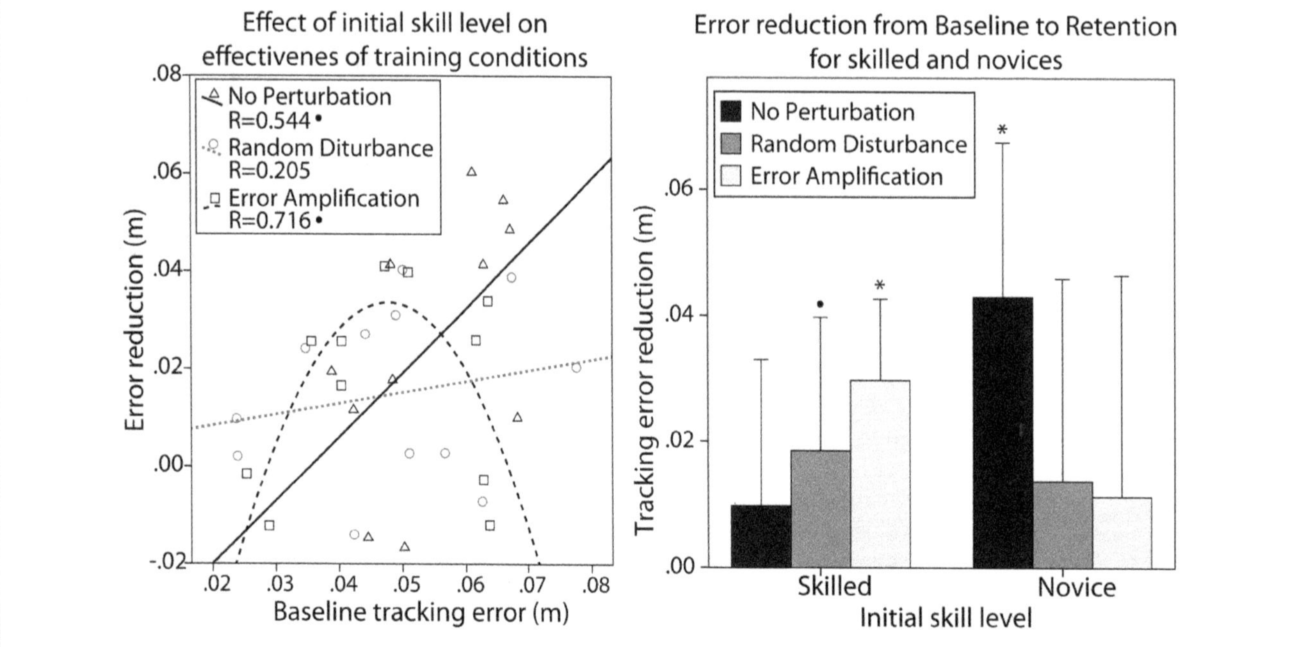

FIGURE 4 | (Left) Effect of initial skill level (i.e., tracking error during baseline) on the error reduction from baseline to retention with the different training strategies. **(Right)** Error reduction after training with the different training strategies, in the skilled and novice groups. Error bars show ± 1 CI. *$p < 0.05$, •$p < 0.1$.

In general, all subjects reduced the absolute phase error from baseline to retention [$F_{(1, 28)} = 7.50$, $p = 0.011$]. The effect of the training strategy on the phase error reduction was one-sided significant [$F_{(2, 28)} = 2.82$, $p = 0.076$]. In particular, the EA group reduced the error in a smaller amount than the NP group (**Figure 5**, $p = 0.077$). We did not find a significant effect of skill level in the error reduction, neither an interaction effect of the training strategy and the initial skill level.

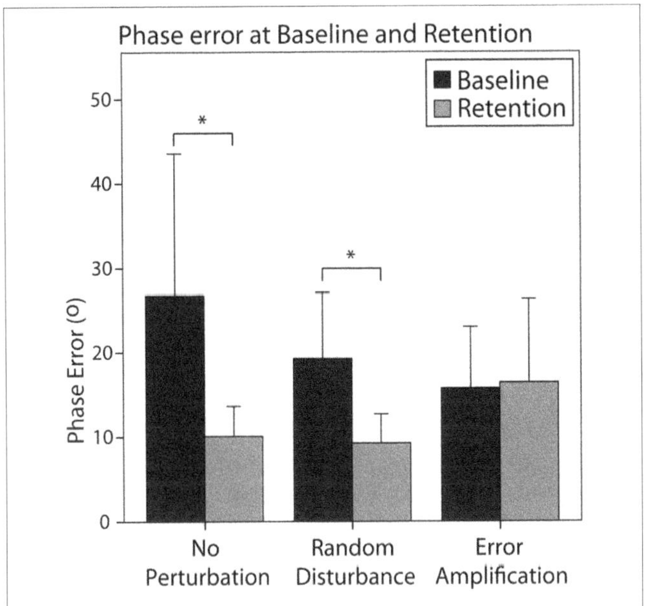

FIGURE 5 | Absolute phase error for the different training groups during baseline and retention. Error bars show ± 1 CI. *$p < 0.05$.

Effect of Training Strategy on Transfer

Subjects generalized the learning to the untrained task, i.e., they significantly reduced the errors from baseline-transfer to retention-transfer [$F_{(1, 24)} = 9.59$, $p = 0.005$]. In particular, subjects trained without perturbation reduced significantly the tracking error (**Figure 6** left, $p = 0.016$). Subjects trained with random disturbance also reduced the tracking errors significantly (**Figure 6** left, $p = 0.007$). However, subjects trained with error amplification did not reduce the error from baseline-transfer to retention-transfer. The main effect of training strategy was, however, non-significant [$F_{(2, 24)} = 1.58$, $p = 0.228$]. The main effect of initial skill level was also non-significant. The interaction effect of the skill level and training strategy did not reach significance [$F_{(2, 24)} = 2.64$, $p = 0.092$].

Subjects did not significantly reduce the phase error from baseline-transfer to retention-transfer (**Figure 6** right). The effect of the training strategy on the phase error reduction in the transfer task did not reach significance [$F_{(2, 24)} = 2.97$, $p = 0.070$]. As observed in **Figure 6** right, subjects trained without perturbation and with random disturbance reduced the errors (although not significantly), while subjects in the error-amplification group tended to increase the errors after training. The main effect of initial skill level was non-significant. The interaction effect of the skill level and training strategy almost reached significance [$F_{(2, 24)} = 3.25$, $p = 0.055$].

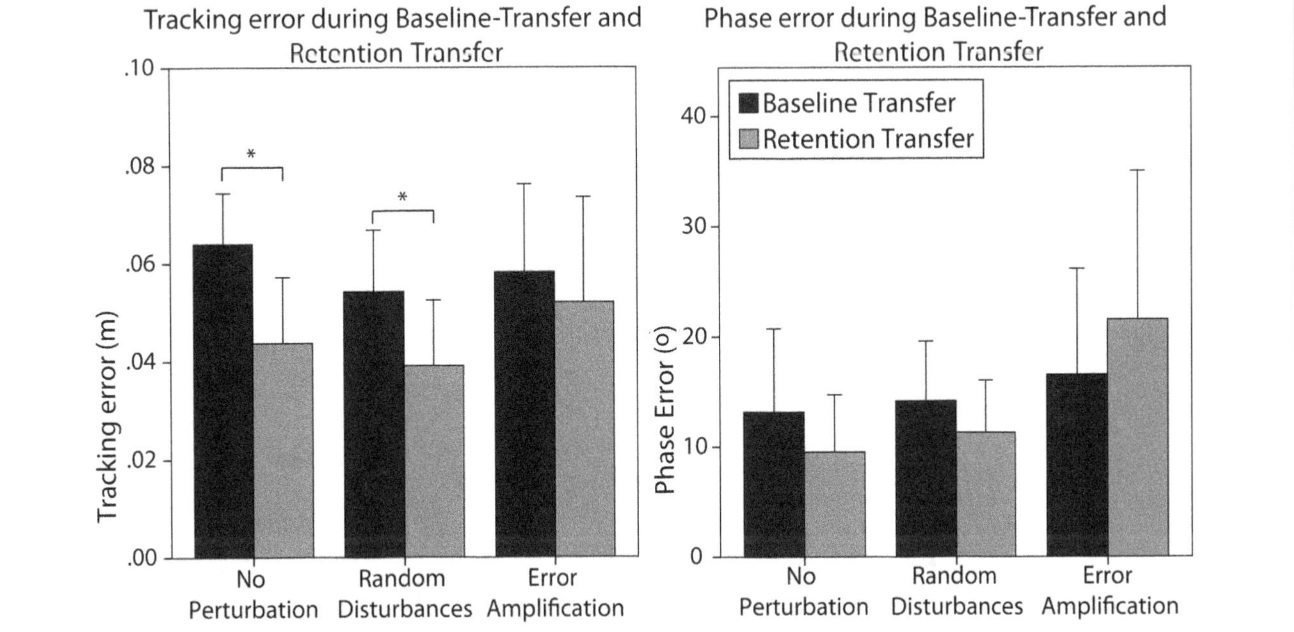

FIGURE 6 | Tracking error **(Left)** and phase error **(Right)** created by the different training groups during baseline-transfer and retention-transfer tests. Error bars show ± 1 CI. *$p < 0.05$.

Functional MRI Data

Training Period

We first visualized the general activation for the three different strategies (NP, EA, and RD) during the training period. As it can be observed in **Figure 7**, all strategies lead to significant bilateral activation ($p < 0.001$, uncorrected) in the area 4a (leg area). The activation map was most widespread for NP and activation for this strategy lead also to activation in other brain regions (results not reported).

Strategy-related main effects were seen in the basal ganglia (putamen, caudate nucleus, and pallidum), thalamus as well as in different parts of the cerebellum (**Table 1A**). In addition, fMRI signal responses were seen in the parietal cortex such as, the intraparietal sulcus (IPS)—which represented largest cluster in the activation map—the posterior cingulate cortex (PCC) and in different regions of the visual and frontal cortex.

We then asked which training strategies differed in brain activation strength (**Table 2**). Error amplification did not lead to stronger fMRI signal responses relative to no perturbation or random disturbance. On the contrary, the contrast "no perturbations vs. error amplification" revealed numerous brain activations, which are—for simplicity—reported on $p < 0.05$ (FWE-corrected, $t > 7.1$; **Table 2A**). In a similar vein, the comparison "no perturbations vs. random disturbance" showed several activated clusters ($p < 0.001$, $t > 3.6$, **Table 2B**). The contrast "random disturbance vs. error amplification" demonstrated few significant clusters ($p < 0.001$, $t > 3.6$, **Table 2C**).

Main effects of initial skill level were seen dominantly in right temporal and parietal regions, including the IPS (**Table 1B**). *Post-hoc t*-test analysis revealed that skilled subjects showed stronger activation compared to novices in the right IPS, SPL (precuneus), medial temporal lobe, and inferior temporal gyrus (**Table 3**). At the same threshold but with lower cluster-size cut-off ($k_E > 15$ voxels) we additionally observed activation in the brainstem and left cerebellum.

Similar to the main effect of training strategy, strategy × initial skill-level interaction effects were most pronounced (i.e., largest activation cluster) in the IPS (**Table 1C**). Apart from activation in frontal and visual brain regions, we noticed further activation of the basal ganglia, primary motor cortex (M1) and somatosensory regions (e.g., SMA) as well as the cerebellum.

Retention—Baseline Period

As summarized in **Table 4**, a main effect of strategy was seen in the subgenual and anterior cingulate cortex and in M1. No main effect of initial skill level was seen (also not when bi-directionally comparing skilled vs. non-skilled subjects by *t*-tests) nor a strategy × initial skill-level interaction. Post-hoc analysis on the main effect of strategy revealed significant differences for the contrasts "no perturbation vs. error amplification" and "random disturbance vs. error amplification" (see **Table 5**). The first contrast demonstrated primarily activation in the frontal cortex. Both contrasts revealed activation in orbitofrontal regions (**Figure 8**).

DISCUSSION

We evaluated the impact of three error-modulation robotic training strategies on brain activation and motor learning of a complex locomotor task: No perturbation, error amplification, and random force disturbance. The experimental task consisted in learning a complex locomotor task: Coordinating the legs in a particular gait-like pattern in order to track a Lissajous figure presented on a visual display. The MRI-compatible one degree-of-freedom steeper robot (MARCOS) developed in our institution was employed to conduct the experiment, while performing fMRI in a 1.5 Tesla MR scanner. Even though none of fMRI results survives a voxel threshold of $p < 0.05$ using familywise error correction, all fMRI results are presented at a widely accepted cluster-corrected *p*-value of $p < 0.05$.

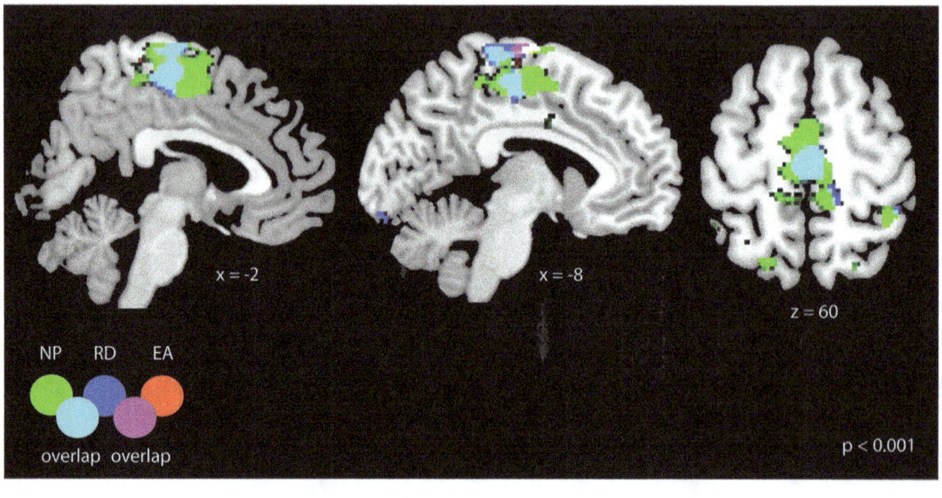

FIGURE 7 | General fMRI activation for the three training strategies: NP, RD, and EA. All results are displayed at $p < 0.001$ (uncorrected, $t > 3.6$) with a cluster-extend threshold of $k_E > 27$ voxels. The activation overlaps for all three training strategies at the somatosensory cortex (at the leg area).

TABLE 1 | Summary of brain activation during training for the main effect of training strategy, initial skill level, and its interaction in the training model.

Region	Hemisphere	MNI			Cluster-size
(A) MAIN EFFECT OF TRAINING STRATEGY					
Putamen	Left	−22	13	0	122
Middle orbital	Left	−35	47	0	225
Pallidum	Right	22	−4	0	82
Thalamus	Left	−13	−24	0	33
	Right	12	−6	12	28
Cerebellum (lobule VI)	Right	35	−41	−30	27
	Left	−20	−55	−8	52
Intraparietal sulcus (IPS)	Right	45	−55	38	934
	Left	−42	−57	39	153
Posterior cingulate cortex (PCC)	Right	1	−38	35	283
Inferior frontal gyrus (BA 44/45)	Left	−48	−13	34	326
	Right	48	23	28	45
Middle frontal gyrus	Left	−28	31	34	139
Cuneus	Right	18	−70	27	90
Amygdala	Left	−30	0	−19	61
Hippocampus	Right	40	−16	−14	59
Fusiform gyrus	Right	25	−61	5	55
(B) MAIN EFFECT OF INITIAL SKILL					
Medial temporal gyrus	Left	−40	14	−32	75
SPL (precuneus)	Right	−2	−66	60	56
IPS	Right	42	−49	36	64
Inferior temporal gyrus	Right	64	−38	−12	20
Rolandic operculum	Right	50	−1	13	16
(C) INTERACTION STRATEGY × INITIAL SKILL					
IPS	Right	42	−48	36	1595
	Left	−40	−57	39	320
Lingual/fusiform	Left	−20	−62	−6	226
Fusiform gyrus	Left	−37	−78	−12	28
Supplemtary motor area (SMA)	Right	2	−15	56	173
PCC	Right	4	−48	40	133
Primary motor cortex (area 4a/4p)	Right	28	−28	58	118
Middle frontal gyrus	Right	36	18	56	116
Postcental gyrus (area 1/2)	Right	24	−48	66	49
	Right	50	−40	58	109
Caudate nucleus	Right	18	12	10	108
Cerebellum (lobule VI)	Right	28	−36	−26	80
hOC3v	Left	−14	−92	2	70
Insula	Left	−26	19	0	56
Medial temporal gyrus	Right	56	−48	0	53
Superior orbital gyrus	Right	14	38	−14	47
Temporal pole	Left	−24	2	−28	44
Thalamus	Right	8	−2	12	41
Putamen	Right	16	8	4	107

All results are reported at $p < 0.001$ (uncorrected, $t > 3.6$), F-contrast, $k_E > 27$.

TABLE 2 | Summary of *post-hoc t*-tests on the main effect of training strategy during training.

Region	Hemisphere	MNI			Cluster-size
(A) NP−EA*					
IPS	Right	43	−50	37	72
Inferior parietal lobe	Right	42	−68	39	32
Inferior frontal gyrus	Left	−57	8	31	15
Middle orbital gyrus	Left	−36	48	0	4
(B) NP−RD**					
Angular gyrus	Right	42	−60	30	1262
Fusiform gyrus	Left	−22	−52	−8	217
	Left	−27	−77	−5	136
Thalamus	Left	−31	−27	1	161
	Right	15	−6	12	33
Superior frontal gyrus	Left	−21	18	38	92
Ant.insula/ant. putamen	Left	−28	16	1	73
Cerebellum (lobule VI)	Left	−26	−30	−26	72
Cerebellum (dentate nucleus)	Left	−22	−52	−32	32
PCC	Right	12	−50	32	68
Lingual gyrus	Right	26	−63	4	62
Pallidum	Right	17	1	6	59
Inferior frontal gyrus	Right	47	21	27	54
Caudate nucleus	Left	−14	6	9	50
Hippocampus	Right	37	−16	−14	40
Precentral gyrus	Right	64	−3	28	36
(C) RD−EA**					
IPS	Right	47	−56	39	587
Inferior frontal gyrus (BA 44/45)	Left	−54	10	34	111
Superior orbital gyrus	Left	−37	52	1	37
Calcarine gyrus (V1/V2)	Right	1	−99	9	35
Superior frontal gyrus	Left	−13	53	40	34

$^{*}p < 0.05$ (FWE corrected, $t > 7.1$).
$^{**}p < 0.001$ (uncorrected, $t > 3.6$).
The following training strategies were compared: NP−EA, NP−RD, RD−EA. For readability, results for NP−EA are shown at $p < 0.05$ (family-wise error corrected). All other contrasts are reported at $p < 0.001$ (uncorrected, $t > 3.6$), $k_E > 27$.

TABLE 3 | Brain activation differences for "skilled vs. non-skilled" participants averaged across all learning strategies during training.

Region	Hemisphere	MNI			Cluster-size
SKILLED vs. NON-SKILLED					
SPL (precuneus)	Midline	0	−68	57	94
Medial temporal pole	Left	−40	14	−32	114
IPS	Right	42	−48	36	96
Inferior temporal gyrus	Right	64	−38	−12	35

All results are reported at $p < 0.001$ (uncorrected, $t > 3.6$), F-contrast, $kE > 27$.

Effects of Training Strategies on Performance during Training

The error amplification training strategy worked as expected, i.e., it significantly increased the tracking error when firstly introduced. Training with error amplification resulted in larger tracking errors during the firsts training trials compared to training with random force disturbance and no perturbation, suggesting that error amplification was the most difficult training strategy. We did not find significant differences in subjects'

TABLE 4 | Summary of brain activation for the main effect of learning strategy for the contrast "retention−baseline".

Region	Hemisphere	MNI			Cluster-size
MAIN EFFECT OF STRATEGY					
Subgenual cingulate (BA 25)	Right	2	0	13	101
	Left	−8	−2	−12	88
Anterior cingulate cortex (BA 24/32)	Left	−13	16	−8	42
Primary motor cortex (area 4p)	Right	37	−16	38	29

Results are displayed at $p < 0.001$ (uncorrected, $t > 3.6$) with a cluster-extend threshold of $k_E > 27$ voxels. There was no significant main effect of initial skill level or an interaction effect (learning strategy × initial skill level) visible.

TABLE 5 | Summary of *post-hoc t*-tests on the main effect of learning strategy for the contrast "retention−baseline".

Region	Hemisphere	MNI			Cluster-size
(A) NP−EA					
Inferior temporal gyrus	Right	62	−42	−10	41
Frontal operculum	Right	6	0	−12	617
Superior orbital gyrus	Left	−12	16	−8	
	Right	14	2	−14	
Primary motor cortex (area 3a/4p)	Right	36	−16	38	95
	Right	48	−14	38	
Anterior temporal lobe	Left	−48	10	−16	147
	Left	−54	2	−16	
	Left	−48	−6	−16	
Middle orbital gyrus	Right	22	34	−4	34
	Right	32	36	−4	
Inferior frontal gyurs/Middle orbital gyrus	Right	34	26	−16	98
	Right	44	48	−14	
	Right	32	40	−8	
Precentral gyrus (BA 44/45)	Right	56	4	36	31
Frontal operculum (fo1)	Right	4	44	−14	29
Frontal operculum (fo3)	Left	−26	36	−2	27
(B) RD−EA					
Superior orbital gyrus	Left	−8	−2	−12	53
Superior orbital gyrus/BA 24 and BA 25	Right	6	−2	−12	33
Middle occipital gyrus (area hOC4lp)	Right	36	−86	16	34
Inferior temporal gyrus	Left	−40	−28	18	69
Supramarginal gyrus (IPL/IPS)	Left	−48	−42	34	64
OP2	Right	30	−24	22	39
OP1 (S2)	Left	−56	−30	24	58
IPL (PFm/PGa)	Left	−52	−64	42	39
	Left	−52	−54	44	
Thalamus	Right	4	−20	20	27
	Left	−4	−22	18	

Results are displayed at $p < 0.001$ (uncorrected $t > 3.6$) with a cluster-extend threshold of $k_E > 27$ voxels. NP and RD showed stronger fMRI signal changes compared to EA.

performance when training with random disturbance and no perturbation. The forces applied during random disturbance created short and fast change in the trajectory smoothness (Marchal-Crespo et al., 2011) and thereby, maybe the overall mean tracking error was not significantly affected. This is in line with a previous study we conducted using MARCOS to train a simple locomotor task with random force disturbance: The introduction of force disturbances did not increase the mean tracking error, but increased the muscle activation, suggesting that training with random disturbances was more physically demanding (Marchal-Crespo et al., 2014b). In fact, this higher muscular activity may explain why the tracking error during training with force disturbances did not differ from the mean error created when training without perturbations: Maybe subjects were able to cancel the tracking errors using muscular effort.

Subjects adapted to the error-amplification strategy during training. This is in line with previous research on motor learning that suggested that training with error-amplification promote the formation of an internal model (Emken and Reinkensmeyer, 2005). Subjects did not significantly reduce the tracking error when training with random disturbances, probably because the disturbing forces were unpredictably applied and the formation of an internal model was not possible.

The Training Strategy that Enhances Learning Depends on Subjects' Skill Level

We expected better motor learning when training with the challenge-based strategies in initially more skilled subjects. We also hypothesized that training with challenge-based strategies would hamper motor learning in initially less skilled subjects. Behavioral results confirmed our hypothesis: The training strategy that enhances learning depended on subjects' initial skill level. Training without perturbations benefited learning in novices, while amplifying tracking errors during training enhanced learning in initially more skilled subjects. This is in line with previous experiments that showed that error amplification seemed to be specifically beneficial for skilled subjects (Milot et al., 2010; Duarte and Reinkensmeyer, 2015). This can be explained by the Challenge Point Theory, which states that learning is maximized when the task difficulty is appropriate for the individual subject's level of expertise (Guadagnoli and Lee, 2004). Error amplification, on the other hand, hampered learning in initially less skilled subjects, maybe because it made the task to be learned too difficult and frustrating (Duarte and Reinkensmeyer, 2015). Indeed, our fMRI data showed an involvement of the brain reward system in the error-amplification group for the contrast NP—EA, which could support this theory.

In a previous experiment performed with MARCOS and similar error-challenging robotic strategies, we found contradictory results (Marchal-Crespo et al., 2014b). Training with error amplification was most suitable for initially less skilled subjects. This contradiction might be explained by the differences in the motor task to be learned. In the previous experiment, the task consisted in trying to synchronize the non-dominant leg with the dominant leg, passively moved by the robot. Therefore, it was a simple one degree-of-freedom locomotor task, compared to the complex two degree-of-freedom bipedal

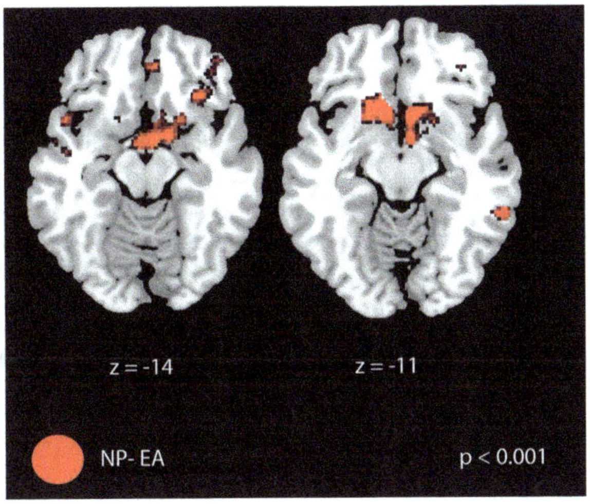

FIGURE 8 | Brain activation difference between "retention−baseline" for the contrast no perturbation−error amplification. FMRI signal changes were most pronounced in the frontal cortex including the orbitofrontal cortex (for a full list of activation see **Table 5**).

locomotor task employed in the current experiment. This is in line with previous research that found that "*principles derived from the study of simple skills do not always generalize to complex skill learning*" (Wulf and Shea, 2002). For less skilled subjects, error augmenting strategies might be more suitable to enhance learning of especially simple tasks, but might hamper learning of more complex tasks. Therefore, matching the training strategy to the relative trainee's skill level to perform a specific task, may provide the greatest opportunity for learning (Marchal-Crespo et al., 2015).

Interestingly, we found that for the error-amplification group, the relationship between error reduction after training and initial skill level was quadratic. Initially proficient subjects—i.e., subjects who performed particularly well during baseline—did not benefit from error amplification. This can be explained by the behavior of the controller. The perturbations of the error-amplification strategy depend on the subjects' performance—i.e., only existing errors are amplified, with higher amplification for larger errors. Thereby, proficient subjects may not have been sufficiently challenged during training, since they were making systematically small errors and thereby, error amplification failed to have a significant impact on their performance during training.

Random force disturbances seemed to benefit motor learning in all subjects, independently of their initial skill level. It is interesting to note that the random force disturbance did not increase the mean tracking error during training. The goal of the random force disturbance strategy is to push subjects away from their "comfort zone," so they are encouraged to examine and investigate new solutions to fulfill the motor tasks by themselves. Therefore, maybe the lack of anticipation of the random disturbing forces motivated subjects to be more concentrated and attentive during training. The random-disturbance strategy was independent of the subjects' performance, thus it might increase subjects' attention during training, even if proficient subjects created very small errors. Our fMRI data support this idea, since we found stronger activation in brain areas associated with attentional control (Shulman et al., 2003; Luks et al., 2007; such as, SPL and IPS) when training with random disturbance, compared to training with error amplification. However, we did not observe differences in brain activation between training with random force disturbances and without perturbations. This might be due to some overlapping activity in the frontal cortex (see **Tables 2A,B**) when we compare to error amplification. Alternatively, maybe the difference in the behavioral results was due to a change in the limbs' stiffness. Training in unstable environments tend to alter the effective stiffness of the limbs through co-contraction of muscles (Franklin et al., 2007; Marchal-Crespo et al., 2014b). However, this stiffness difference did not lead do detectable brain activation differences, maybe because the muscle co-contraction was not strong enough (Marchal-Crespo et al., 2014b).

Error Amplification Hampered Transfer of Learning

We confirmed our hypothesis that the training strategy that enhances learning of a complex locomotor task depends on subjects' initial skill level. However, we also found that training with error amplification limited transfer of learning, while training with no perturbation and random disturbance seemed to transfer the learning gains to a similar task. Although there was no statistical proof that the transfer was greater after training without perturbation and random noise relative to error amplification, our results suggest evidence for transfer in these conditions only. The lack of transfer observed in the error-amplification group contradicts motor learning research that found a positive effect of error amplification on transfer (Milot et al., 2010).

A possible rationale for the differences observed in transfer between the challenge-based training strategies is that subjects trained with error amplification focused mainly in reducing the tracking errors to reduce the perturbing forces, and failed to interiorized or consciously understand the desired gait-like pattern. This idea is supported by the fact that subjects trained with error amplification failed to learn the correct phase difference between legs also in the trained task, while subjects trained without perturbation and random disturbance did learn the correct diphase. Therefore, the good performance of subjects after training with error amplification might have resulted from implicit learning, i.e., subjects learned without awareness of what has been learned. On the other hand, subjects trained with random force disturbance (and without perturbation) might have experienced explicit learning, i.e. they actively searched for the gait-like pattern to correctly track the presented figure. Several studies have shown that implicit learning shows negative transfer of the acquired motor skills, whereas explicit learning showed strong positive transfer (Lee and Vakoch, 1996). Therefore, based on the transfer and phase error results, we hypothesized that for the specific complex locomotion task presented in this paper, error amplification might have promoted implicit motor learning, while random force disturbance promoted explicit motor learning. Results from fMRI data support this hypothesis, since training with random disturbance revealed stronger activation in brain areas associated with explicit learning (such as, precuneus) when compared to training with error amplification (Yang and Li, 2012).

Effects of Training Strategies and Initial Skill Level on Brain Activation during Training

During the training period, strategy and skill-level dependent effects were observed in the IPS. Human fMRI studies support a decrease in activation in pre-SMA and dorsolateral prefrontal cortex (DLPFC), but an increase in activation in the parietal lobe (especially in the IPS) as visuomotor sequence learning progresses (Hikosaka et al., 1998; Sakai et al., 1998). Grafton et al. (1998) reported that activation in the parietal lobe progressively increased with learning, whereas other groups (Seitz et al., 1990; Jenkins et al., 1994; van Mier et al., 1998) demonstrated stronger parietal activation during learning of a novel motor sequence compared to performance on a pre-learned sequence.

Our study revealed stronger activation of the SPL (precuneus) and the IPS in skilled subjects (across all training strategies) during a motor task using leg movements. Less skilled subjects did not show any significant ($p < 0.001$) activation at the pre-selected voxel-threshold relative to skilled participants. In fact, the no-perturbation and random-disturbance strategies lead stronger activation in these (but also other frontal, visual, and temporal) regions than error amplification. This could suggest that attentional control is an important factor for motor learning but in different ways. During an easy condition such as no perturbation, a high level of attention is required to maintain subjects focused on the task. In contrast, during random disturbance, subjects are disturbed in an unexpected manner (in contrast to error amplification) to perform the task and hence attentional control is required to minimize tracking errors during training.

We found main effects of strategy as well as strategy × initial skill interaction effects in different parts of the cerebellum. Some authors demonstrated a particular link between cerebellum activation and skill level (Jenkins et al., 1994; Seitz et al., 1994). For example, Toni and colleagues (Toni et al., 1998) showed a decrease in left cerebellar activation (but also in other brain regions) during a prolonged period of trial and error motor sequence learning. The right anterior cerebellum, however, showed greater activation during later learning than during initial learning. In addition, in our experiment, skilled participants showed stronger activation of the cerebellum (and brainstem) compared to novices but this was only seen at $p < 0.001$ with $k_E > 15$ voxels instead of $k_E > 27$ voxels, indicating an association between the strength of the activation in the cerebellum and the success of learning. The only region—again at $p < 0.001$ and $k_E > 15$ voxels—showing greater activation in untrained participants was the right rolandic operculum.

The basal ganglia are involved in the regulation of non-motor as well as motor sequences, and motor sequence learning (Vakil et al., 2000; Exner et al., 2002; Tzvi et al., 2014, 2015, 2016; Fermin et al., 2016). Although the activation of the basal ganglia for the training period in our study might reflect on-line learning processes, we cannot distinguish activation linked to attentional demands and on-line error correction (adaptation). The activation of the basal ganglia was evident for the contrast "no perturbation (NP)—random disturbance (RD)." This was a bit surprising, as we did not expect a particular involvement of the basal ganglia in a very simple task such as no perturbation compared to random disturbance and error-amplification strategies. We conclude that basal ganglia are rather involved in the learning of non-challenging task, in which the sequence of motor movements is not disturbed by noise or by any error amplification.

Effects of Training Strategies on Brain Activation during Learning

The contrast "retention—baseline" revealed activation within the frontal cortex but also in sensorimotor regions (e.g., M1, parietal opercular regions, i.e., OP1 and OP2, Young et al., 2004). This activation could reflect learning (as the error rates drop during retention relative to baseline) but it is difficult to differentiate between mechanisms related to attention and error correction. One interesting observation was the involvement of orbitofrontal regions during no perturbation relative to error amplification (**Table 5**, **Figure 8**). In fact, practicing with error amplification is related to a persistent lower self-reported level of enjoyment (Duarte and Reinkensmeyer, 2015). The systematic large errors experienced during training with error amplification, which made the task more challenging, resulted in unconventionally low activation of the reward system. We computed several contrasts in order to further evaluate the effect of the skill level as we found differences comparing NP—EA in the reward system: (NP—EA skilled) > (NP—EA non-skilled) and vice versa,. We also performed the contrasts "EA skilled vs. EA non-skilled" and "NP skilled vs. NP non-skilled." Yet, we did not observe any activation differences for these contrasts (at $p < 0.001$, uncorrected), suggesting that the reward system was not differently activated between skill groups. However, when we used an unconventionally low threshold of $p < 0.01$ (uncorrected), we found some differences in the reward system between skilled and non-skilled subjects comparing conditions. Of course, this needs to be examined in future studies on the role of affective components during motor learning. However, it is evident from other studies that affective control (resulting in high motivation) is an important factor during complicated motor learning tasks (McAuley et al., 1989; Duarte and Reinkensmeyer, 2015).

Implications for Robot-Aided Gait Rehabilitation

Recovery after a brain injury has been proposed to be a form of motor learning or relearning (Dietz and Ward, 2015). However, we cannot guarantee that the impact on motor learning of the training strategies here investigated do not differ in neurological patients. Patients probably have a lower initial skill level and therefore, their optimal challenge point (i.e., where subjects show the best motor learning) may be at a different level. Hypothetically, the haptic guidance mode may be especially suitable for more disabled patients, as suggested in Klamroth-Marganska et al. (2014).

Based on the results presented in this paper, we are developing new training strategies to improve rehabilitation outcomes using the Lokomat (Hocoma, Switzerland)—a commercially available robotic gait trainer that comprises two actuated leg orthoses (Riener et al., 2005). We developed a novel error-modulating robotic strategy that limits large errors that can be dangerous and frustrating with haptic guidance, while amplifies task relevant small errors. We also developed a random disturbance controller that can work together with the error-modulating controller (Rüdt et al., 2016). We hypothesize that an optimal framework for motor learning and neurorehabilitation would consist on a combination of all these strategies: Random force disturbance would increase subjects' concentration on the task, error amplification would increase subjects' active participation and awareness of small task relevant errors, and haptic guidance would limit dangerous and/or discouraging errors.

We plan to perform motor learning experiments with neurological patients employing the different controllers presented here, and the novel controllers derived from the actual findings. Results from the motor learning experiments performed with neurological patients will provide an insight into motor learning in the impaired motor system and may suggest new neurorehabilitation therapies and novel ways to use robots in rehabilitation. It has been hypothesized that in order to enhance recovery after a neurologic insult it is crucial to increase the dose and intensity of therapy (Dietz and Ward, 2015). We believe that employing a training strategy that optimizes learning based on patients' specific impairments and specific motor task to be performed would be a more effective approach than just increasing dose and intensity of raw therapy.

CONCLUSIONS

We investigated the effect of robotic training strategies that augment errors-error amplification and random force disturbance—on brain activation and learning of a complex locomotor task. We found that the most effective training strategy depends on subjects' initial skill level. Training without perturbations was especially suitable to enhance motor learning in initially less skilled subjects, while more skilled subjects benefited from error amplification. However, training with error amplification limited transfer of learning. Random disturbing forces induced learning and promoted transfer in all subjects, probably because they increased subjects' attention. A possible rationale for the differences in transfer between the challenge-based strategies is that for the specific complex locomotion task presented in this paper, error amplification might have promoted implicit motor learning, while random force disturbance promoted explicit motor learning.

FMRI analysis revealed main effects of strategy and skill level during training. These neuroimaging findings indicate that gait-like motor learning depends on interplay between subcortical, cerebellar, and fronto-parietal brain regions. An interesting observation was the low activation seen in the brain reward system after training with error amplification compared to training without perturbations.

Our results suggest that learning a complex locomotor task can be enhanced when errors are augmented based on subjects' initial skill level. The impacts of these strategies on motor learning, brain activation and motivation in neurological patients need further investigation.

AUTHOR CONTRIBUTIONS

LMC, LJ, and RR contributed to the experimental design and project supervision. LMC, LJ, and JL participated in the study design and data acquisition. LM, LJ, and JL performed the fMRI data analysis. Interpretation of the fMRI results was performed by LM. LMC performed the behavioral data analysis and interpretation of results. LMC and LM prepared the manuscript. All authors read and approved the final manuscript.

ACKNOWLEDGMENTS

The authors would like to thank the Institute for Biomedical Engineering at ETH Zurich for the allocation of scanner time. The authors gratefully acknowledge the contributions of Spyros Kollias, Peter Wolf, Christoph Hollnagel, Mike Brügger, and Andre Fisher.

REFERENCES

Behrman, A. L., and Harkema, S. J. (2000). Locomotor training after human spinal cord injury: a series of case studies. *Phys. Ther.* 80, 688–700. doi: 10.1093/ptj/80.7.688

Bryden, M. P. (1977). Measuring handedness with questionnaires. *Neuropsychologia* 15, 617–624. doi: 10.1016/0028-3932(77)90067-7

Burke, E., and Cramer, S. C. (2013). Biomarkers and predictors of restorative therapy effects after stroke. *Curr. Neurol. Neurosci. Rep.* 13:329. doi: 10.1007/s11910-012-0329-9

Dietz, V., and Ward, N. (Eds) (2015). "The applicability of motor learning to neurorehabilitation," in *Oxford Textbook of Neurorehabilitation* (Oxford University Press), 55–64. Available online at: http://www.oxfordmedicine.com/view/10.1093/med/9780199673711.001.0001/med-9780199673711-chapter-7 (Accessed September 16, 2016).

Dobkin, B. H., and Duncan, P. W. (2012). Should body weight-supported treadmill training and robotic-assistive steppers for locomotor training trot back to the starting gate? *Neurorehabil. Neural Repair* 26, 308–317. doi: 10.1177/1545968312439687

Duarte, J. E., and Reinkensmeyer, D. J. (2015). Effects of robotically modulating kinematic variability on motor skill learning and motivation. *J. Neurophysiol.* 113, 2682–2691. doi: 10.1152/jn.00163.2014

Emken, J. L., and Reinkensmeyer, D. J. (2005). Robot-enhanced motor learning: accelerating internal model formation during locomotion by transient dynamic amplification. *IEEE Trans. Neural Syst. Rehabil. Eng.* 13, 33–39. doi: 10.1109/TNSRE.2004.843173

Exner, C., Koschack, J., and Irle, E. (2002). The differential role of premotor frontal cortex and basal ganglia in motor sequence learning: evidence from focal basal ganglia lesions. *Learn. Mem.* 9, 376–386. doi: 10.1101/lm.48402

Fermin, A. S. R., Yoshida, T., Yoshimoto, J., Ito, M., Tanaka, S. C., and Doya, K. (2016). Model-based action planning involves cortico-cerebellar and basal ganglia networks. *Sci. Rep.* 6:31378. doi: 10.1038/srep31378

Franklin, D. W., Liaw, G., Milner, T. E., Osu, R., Burdet, E., and Kawato, M. (2007). Endpoint stiffness of the arm is directionally tuned to instability in the environment. *J. Neurosci.* 27, 7705–7716. doi: 10.1523/JNEUROSCI.0968-07.2007

Grafton, S. T., Hazeltine, E., and Ivry, R. B. (1998). Abstract and effector-specific representations of motor sequences identified with PET. *J. Neurosci.* 18, 9420–9428.

Grafton, S. T., Schmitt, P., Van Horn, J., and Diedrichsen, J. (2008). Neural substrates of visuomotor learning based on improved feedback control and prediction. *Neuroimage* 39, 1383–1395. doi: 10.1016/j.neuroimage.2007.09.062

Guadagnoli, M. A., and Lee, T. D. (2004). Challenge point: a framework for conceptualizing the effects of various practice conditions in motor learning. *J. Mot. Behav.* 36, 212–224. doi: 10.3200/JMBR.36.2.212-224

Hester, R., Barre, N., Murphy, K., Silk, T. J., and Mattingley, J. B. (2008). Human medial frontal cortex activity predicts learning from errors. *Cereb. Cortex N. Y.* 18, 1933–1940. doi: 10.1093/cercor/bhm219

Hikosaka, O., Miyashita, K., Miyachi, S., Sakai, K., and Lu, X. (1998). Differential roles of the frontal cortex, basal ganglia, and cerebellum in visuomotor sequence learning. *Neurobiol. Learn. Mem.* 70, 137–149. doi: 10.1006/nlme.1998.3844

Hollnagel, C., Brügger, M., Vallery, H., Wolf, P., Dietz, V., Kollias, S., et al. (2011). Brain activity during stepping: a novel MRI-compatible device. *J. Neurosci. Methods* 201, 124–130. doi: 10.1016/j.jneumeth.2011.07.022

Hollnagel, C., Vallery, H., Schädler, R., López, I. G.-L., Jaeger, L., Wolf, P., et al. (2013). Non-linear adaptive controllers for an over-actuated pneumatic MR-compatible stepper. *Med. Biol. Eng. Comput.* 51, 799–809. doi: 10.1007/s11517-013-1050-9

Huberdeau, D. M., Krakauer, J. W., and Haith, A. M. (2015). Dual-process decomposition in human sensorimotor adaptation. *Curr. Opin. Neurobiol.* 33, 71–77. doi: 10.1016/j.conb.2015.03.003

Husemann, B., Müller, F., Krewer, C., Heller, S., and Koenig, E. (2007). Effects of locomotion training with assistance of a robot-driven gait orthosis in hemiparetic patients after stroke: a randomized controlled pilot study. *Stroke* 38, 349–354. doi: 10.1161/01.STR.0000254607.48765.cb

Israel, J. F., Campbell, D. D., Kahn, J. H., and Hornby, T. G. (2006). Metabolic costs and muscle activity patterns during robotic- and therapist-assisted treadmill walking in individuals with incomplete spinal cord injury. *Phys. Ther.* 86, 1466–1478. doi: 10.2522/ptj.20050266

Jaeger, L., Marchal-Crespo, L., Wolf, P., Riener, R., Michels, L., and Kollias, S. (2014). Brain activation associated with active and passive lower limb stepping. *Front. Hum. Neurosci.* 8:828. doi: 10.3389/fnhum.2014.00828

Jahn, K., Deutschländer, A., Stephan, T., Strupp, M., Wiesmann, M., and Brandt, T. (2004). Brain activation patterns during imagined stance and locomotion in functional magnetic resonance imaging. *Neuroimage* 22, 1722–1731. doi: 10.1016/j.neuroimage.2004.05.017

Jenkins, I. H., Brooks, D. J., Nixon, P. D., Frackowiak, R. S., and Passingham, R. E. (1994). Motor sequence learning: a study with positron emission tomography. *J. Neurosci.* 14, 3775–3790.

Klamroth-Marganska, V., Blanco, J., Campen, K., Curt, A., Dietz, V., Ettlin, T., et al. (2014). Three-dimensional, task-specific robot therapy of the arm after stroke: a multicentre, parallel-group randomised trial. *Lancet Neurol.* 13, 159–166. doi: 10.1016/S1474-4422(13)70305-3

Krakauer, J. W. (2006). Motor learning: its relevance to stroke recovery and neurorehabilitation. *Curr. Opin. Neurol.* 19, 84–90. doi: 10.1097/01.wco.0000200544.29915.cc

la Fougère, C., Zwergal, A., Rominger, A., Förster, S., Fesl, G., Dieterich, M., et al. (2010). Real versus imagined locomotion: a [18F]-FDG PET-fMRI comparison. *Neuroimage* 50, 1589–1598. doi: 10.1016/j.neuroimage.2009.12.060

Lee, J., and Choi, S. (2010). "Effects of haptic guidance and disturbance on motor learning: potential advantage of haptic disturbance," in *2010 IEEE Haptics Symposium* (Waltham, MA), 335–342.

Lee, Y., and Vakoch, D. A. (1996). Transfer and retention of implicit and explicit learning. *Br. J. Psychol.* 87, 637–651. doi: 10.1111/j.2044-8295.1996.tb02613.x

Lotze, M., Braun, C., Birbaumer, N., Anders, S., and Cohen, L. G. (2003). Motor learning elicited by voluntary drive. *Brain J. Neurol.* 126, 866–872. doi: 10.1093/brain/awg079

Luft, A. R., Smith, G. V., Forrester, L., Whitall, J., Macko, R. F., Hauser, T.-K., et al. (2002). Comparing brain activation associated with isolated upper and lower limb movement across corresponding joints. *Hum. Brain Mapp.* 17, 131–140. doi: 10.1002/hbm.10058

Luks, T. L., Simpson, G. V., Dale, C. L., and Hough, M. G. (2007). Preparatory allocation of attention and adjustments in conflict processing. *Neuroimage* 35, 949–958. doi: 10.1016/j.neuroimage.2006.11.041

Marchal-Crespo, L., Hollnagel, C., Brügger, M., Kollias, S., and Riener, R. (2011). An fMRI pilot study to evaluate brain activation associated with locomotion adaptation. *IEEE Int. Conf. Rehabil. Robot. Proc.* 2011:5975371. doi: 10.1109/ICORR.2011.5975371

Marchal-Crespo, L., López-Olóriz, J., Jaeger, L., and Riener, R. (2014a). Optimizing learning of a locomotor task: amplifying errors as needed. *Conf. Proc. Annu. Int. Conf. IEEE Eng. Med. Biol. Soc.* 2014, 5304–5307. doi: 10.1109/EMBC.2014.6944823

Marchal-Crespo, L., McHughen, S., Cramer, S. C., and Reinkensmeyer, D. J. (2010). The effect of haptic guidance, aging, and initial skill level on motor learning of a steering task. *Exp. Brain Res.* 201, 209–220. doi: 10.1007/s00221-009-2026-8

Marchal-Crespo, L., and Reinkensmeyer, D. J. (2009). Review of control strategies for robotic movement training after neurologic injury. *J. Neuroeng. Rehabil.* 6:20. doi: 10.1186/1743-0003-6-20

Marchal-Crespo, L., Schneider, J., Jaeger, L., and Riener, R. (2014b). Learning a locomotor task: with or without errors? *J. Neuroeng. Rehabil.* 11:25. doi: 10.1186/1743-0003-11-25

Marchal-Crespo, L., van Raai, M., Rauter, G., Wolf, P., and Riener, R. (2013). The effect of haptic guidance and visual feedback on learning a complex tennis task. *Exp. Brain Res.* 231, 277–291. doi: 10.1007/s00221-013-3690-2

Marchal-Crespo, L., Wolf, P., Gerig, N., Rauter, G., Jaeger, L., Vallery, H., et al. (2015). "The role of skill level and motor task characteristics on the effectiveness of robotic training: first results," in *2015 IEEE International Conference on Rehabilitation Robotics (ICORR)* (Singapore), 151–156.

Mars, R. B., Coles, M. G. H., Grol, M. J., Holroyd, C. B., Nieuwenhuis, S., Hulstijn, W., et al. (2005). Neural dynamics of error processing in medial frontal cortex. *Neuroimage* 28, 1007–1013. doi: 10.1016/j.neuroimage.2005.06.041

McAuley, E., Duncan, T., and Tammen, V. V. (1989). Psychometric properties of the intrinsic motivation inventory in a competitive sport setting: a confirmatory factor analysis. *Res. Q. Exerc. Sport* 60, 48–58. doi: 10.1080/02701367.1989.10607413

Milot, M.-H., Marchal-Crespo, L., Green, C. S., Cramer, S. C., and Reinkensmeyer, D. J. (2010). Comparison of error-amplification and haptic-guidance training techniques for learning of a timing-based motor task by healthy individuals. *Exp. Brain Res.* 201, 119–131. doi: 10.1007/s00221-009-2014-z

Miyai, I., Yagura, H., Hatakenaka, M., Oda, I., Konishi, I., and Kubota, K. (2003). Longitudinal optical imaging study for locomotor recovery after stroke. *Stroke J. Cereb. Circ.* 34, 2866–2870. doi: 10.1161/01.STR.0000100166.81077.8A

Morone, G., Bragoni, M., Iosa, M., De Angelis, D., Venturiero, V., Coiro, P., et al. (2011). Who may benefit from robotic-assisted gait training? A randomized clinical trial in patients with subacute stroke. *Neurorehabil. Neural Repair* 25, 636–644. doi: 10.1177/1545968311401034

Pennycott, A., Wyss, D., Vallery, H., Klamroth-Marganska, V., and Riener, R. (2012). Towards more effective robotic gait training for stroke rehabilitation: a review. *J. Neuroeng. Rehabil.* 9:65. doi: 10.1186/1743-0003-9-65

Poon, C.-S. (2004). Sensorimotor learning and information processing by Bayesian internal models. *Conf. Proc. Annu. Int. Conf. IEEE Eng. Med. Biol. Soc.* 6, 4481–4482. doi: 10.1109/IEMBS.2004.1404245

Reinkensmeyer, D. J., Akoner, O., Ferris, D. P., and Gordon, K. E. (2009). Slacking by the human motor system: computational models and implications for robotic orthoses. *Conf. Proc. Annu. Int. Conf. IEEE Eng. Med. Biol. Soc.* 2009, 2129–2132. doi: 10.1109/IEMBS.2009.5333978

Reinkensmeyer, D. J., and Housman, S. J. (2007). "If I can't do it once, why do it a hundred times? connecting volition to movement success in a virtual environment motivates people to exercise the arm after stroke," in *2007 Virtual Rehabilitation* (Venice), 44–48.

Reisman, D. S., McLean, H., Keller, J., Danks, K. A., and Bastian, A. J. (2013). Repeated split-belt treadmill training improves poststroke step length asymmetry. *Neurorehabil. Neural Repair* 27, 460–468. doi: 10.1177/1545968312474118

Riener, R., Lünenburger, L., Jezernik, S., Anderschitz, M., Colombo, G., and Dietz, V. (2005). Patient-cooperative strategies for robot-aided treadmill training: first experimental results. *IEEE Trans. Neural Syst. Rehabil. Eng.* 13, 380–394. doi: 10.1109/TNSRE.2005.848628

Rossini, P. M., and Dal Forno, G. (2004). Integrated technology for evaluation of brain function and neural plasticity. *Phys. Med. Rehabil. Clin. N. Am.* 15, 263–306. doi: 10.1016/S1047-9651(03)00124-4

Rüdt, S., Moos, M., Seppey, S., Riener, R., and Marchal-Crespo, L. (2016). "Towards more efficient robotic gait training: A novel controller to modulate movement errors," in *2016 6th IEEE International Conference on Biomedical Robotics and Biomechatronics (BioRob)* (Singapore), 876–881.

Sakai, K., Hikosaka, O., Miyauchi, S., Takino, R., Sasaki, Y., and Pütz, B. (1998). Transition of brain activation from frontal to parietal areas in visuomotor sequence learning. *J. Neurosci.* 18, 1827–1840.

Scheidt, R. A., Reinkensmeyer, D. J., Conditt, M. A., Rymer, W. Z., and Mussa-Ivaldi, F. A. (2000). Persistence of motor adaptation during constrained, multi-joint, arm movements. *J. Neurophysiol.* 84, 853–862.

Schmidt, R., and Lee, T. (2010). *Motor Control and Learning: A Behavioral Emphasis*. Champaign, IL: Human Kinetics Publishers.

Schwartz, I., Sajin, A., Fisher, I., Neeb, M., Shochina, M., Katz-Leurer, M., et al. (2009). The effectiveness of locomotor therapy using robotic-assisted gait training in subacute stroke patients: a randomized controlled trial. *PM R* 1, 516–523. doi: 10.1016/j.pmrj.2009.03.009

Seitz, R. J., Canavan, A. G., Yágüez, L., Herzog, H., Tellmann, L., Knorr, U., et al. (1994). Successive roles of the cerebellum and premotor cortices in trajectorial learning. *Neuroreport* 5, 2541–2544. doi: 10.1097/00001756-199412000-00034

Seitz, R. J., Roland, E., Bohm, C., Greitz, T., and Stone-Elander, S. (1990). Motor learning in man: a positron emission tomographic study. *Neuroreport* 1, 57–60. doi: 10.1097/00001756-199009000-00016

Shulman, G. L., McAvoy, M. P., Cowan, M. C., Astafiev, S. V., Tansy, A. P., d'Avossa, G., et al. (2003). Quantitative analysis of attention and detection signals during visual search. *J. Neurophysiol.* 90, 3384–3397. doi: 10.1152/jn.00343.2003

Shumway-Cook, A., and Woollacott, M. H. (2007). *Motor Control: Translating Research Into Clinical Practice*. Lippincott Williams & Wilkins.

Slotnick, S. D., Moo, L. R., Segal, J. B., and Hart, J. (2003). Distinct prefrontal cortex activity associated with item memory and source memory for visual shapes. *Brain Res. Cogn. Brain Res.* 17, 75–82. doi: 10.1016/S0926-6410(03)00082-X

Toni, I., Krams, M., Turner, R., and Passingham, R. E. (1998). The time course of changes during motor sequence learning: a whole-brain fMRI study. *Neuroimage* 8, 50–61. doi: 10.1006/nimg.1998.0349

Tseng, Y.-W., Diedrichsen, J., Krakauer, J. W., Shadmehr, R., and Bastian, A. J. (2007). Sensory prediction errors drive cerebellum-dependent adaptation of reaching. *J. Neurophysiol.* 98, 54–62. doi: 10.1152/jn.00266.2007

Tzvi, E., Münte, T. F., and Krämer, U. M. (2014). Delineating the cortico-striatal-cerebellar network in implicit motor sequence learning. *Neuroimage* 94, 222–230. doi: 10.1016/j.neuroimage.2014.03.004

Tzvi, E., Stoldt, A., Witt, K., and Krämer, U. M. (2015). Striatal-cerebellar networks mediate consolidation in a motor sequence learning task: an fMRI study using dynamic causal modelling. *Neuroimage* 122, 52–64. doi: 10.1016/j.neuroimage.2015.07.077

Tzvi, E., Verleger, R., Münte, T. F., and Krämer, U. M. (2016). Reduced alpha-gamma phase amplitude coupling over right parietal cortex is associated with implicit visuomotor sequence learning. *Neuroimage* 141, 60–70. doi: 10.1016/j.neuroimage.2016.07.019

Vakil, E., Kahan, S., Huberman, M., and Osimani, A. (2000). Motor and non-motor sequence learning in patients with basal ganglia lesions: the case of serial reaction time (SRT). *Neuropsychologia* 38, 1–10. doi: 10.1016/S0028-3932(99)00058-5

van Mier, H., Tempel, L. W., Perlmutter, J. S., Raichle, M. E., and Petersen, S. E. (1998). Changes in brain activity during motor learning measured with PET: effects of hand of performance and practice. *J. Neurophysiol.* 80, 2177–2199.

Wu, H. G., Miyamoto, Y. R., Gonzalez Castro, L. N., Ölveczky, B. P., and Smith, M. A. (2014). Temporal structure of motor variability is dynamically regulated and predicts motor learning ability. *Nat. Neurosci.* 17, 312–321. doi: 10.1038/nn.3616

Wulf, G., and Shea, C. H. (2002). Principles derived from the study of simple skills do not generalize to complex skill learning. *Psychon. Bull. Rev.* 9, 185–211. doi: 10.3758/BF03196276

Yang, J., and Li, P. (2012). Brain networks of explicit and implicit learning. *PLoS ONE* 7:e42993. doi: 10.1371/journal.pone.0042993

Yen, S.-C., Schmit, B. D., Landry, J. M., Roth, H., and Wu, M. (2012). Locomotor adaptation to resistance during treadmill training transfers to overground walking in human SCI. *Exp. Brain Res.* 216, 473–482. doi: 10.1007/s00221-011-2950-2

Young, J. P., Herath, P., Eickhoff, S., Choi, J., Grefkes, C., Zilles, K., et al. (2004). Somatotopy and attentional modulation of the human parietal and opercular regions. *J. Neurosci.* 24, 5391–5399. doi: 10.1523/JNEUROSCI.4030-03.2004

16

Estrogenic Effects of Several BPA Analogs in the Developing Zebrafish Brain

*Joel Cano-Nicolau, Colette Vaillant, Elisabeth Pellegrini, Thierry D. Charlier, Olivier Kah and Pascal Coumailleau **

Research Institute in Health, Environment and Occupation, Institut National de la Santé et de la Recherche Médicale U1085, SFR Biosite, Université de Rennes 1, Rennes, France

Edited by:
Fumihiko Maekawa, National Institute for Environmental Studies, Japan

Reviewed by:
Maria Marino, University Roma Tre, Italy
Shinichi Miyagawa, National Institute for Basic Biology, Japan

***Correspondence:**
Pascal Coumailleau
pascal.coumailleau@univ-rennes1.fr

Important set of studies have demonstrated the endocrine disrupting activity of Bisphenol A (BPA). The present work aimed at defining estrogenic-like activity of several BPA structural analogs, including BPS, BPF, BPAF, and BPAP, on 4- or 7-day post-fertilization (dpf) zebrafish larva as an *in vivo* model. We measured the induction level of the estrogen-sensitive marker *cyp19a1b* gene (Aromatase B), expressed in the brain, using three different *in situ/in vivo* strategies: (1) Quantification of *cyp19a1b* transcripts using RT-qPCR in wild type 7-dpf larva brains exposed to bisphenols; (2) Detection and distribution of *cyp19a1b* transcripts using *in situ* hybridization on 7-dpf brain sections (hypothalamus); and (3) Quantification of the *cyp19a1b* promoter activity in live *cyp19a1b*-GFP transgenic zebrafish (EASZY assay) at 4-dpf larval stage. These three different experimental approaches demonstrated that BPS, BPF, or BPAF exposure, similarly to BPA, significantly activates the expression of the estrogenic marker in the brain of developing zebrafish. *In vitro* experiments using both reporter gene assay in a glial cell context and competitive ligand binding assays strongly suggested that up-regulation of *cyp19a1b* is largely mediated by the zebrafish estrogen nuclear receptor alpha (zfERα). Importantly, and in contrast to other tested bisphenol A analogs, the bisphenol AP (BPAP) did not show estrogenic activity in our model.

Keywords: 17β-estradiol, aromatase, cyp19a1b, bisphenol, BPA, hypothalamus, endocrine disruption

INTRODUCTION

Estrogens play important roles in many developmental and physiological processes (Boon et al., 2010) and references therein, including for brain development (Hojo et al., 2008; Hill and Boon, 2009; Bondesson et al., 2014; Coumailleau et al., 2015). Bisphenol A (BPA) is a well-known chemical compound that mimic and interfere with the actions of endogenous estrogens and thus act as an endocrine disruptor (Krishnan et al., 1993; Gould et al., 1998; Paris et al., 2002; Kitamura et al., 2005; Richter et al., 2007; Wetherill et al., 2007; Vogel, 2009; Grignard et al., 2012). BPA is a chemical used in many industrial and commercial applications including in the production of polycarbonate plastics and epoxy resins, present in a variety of consumer products such as food-packaging materials, toys, thermal and recycled papers, compact discs, impact-resistant safety equipment, and medical devices to name a few (Vinggaard et al., 2000; Vandenberg et al., 2010; Liao and Kannan, 2011; Staples et al., 2011; Huang et al., 2012; Liao et al., 2012a,c). BPA rapidly became one of the most produced and used chemicals worldwide (about 3.4 million tons per year).

The widespread use of BPA has resulted in its detection in environment (Huang et al., 2012; Liao et al., 2012b), in food (Schecter et al., 2010; Liao and Kannan, 2013), and in human biological sample (Sun et al., 2004; Calafat et al., 2005, 2009; Vandenberg et al., 2010; Zalko et al., 2011; Fenichel et al., 2012; Liao et al., 2012a; Vandenberg et al., 2012). Epidemiological studies, along with laboratory studies in many species including primates, provide increasing support that environmental BPA exposure can be harmful to humans and is associated with a wide range of effects in humans, rodents, and wildlife. Indeed, BPA exposure is linked to numerous adverse health concerns including development, diabetes, obesity, cardiovascular, reproductive disorders, behavioral troubles, chronic respiratory and kidney diseases, and carcinogenesis, likely linked to the endocrine disrupting effects (Vandenberg et al., 2012; Rochester, 2013; Rezg et al., 2014). Owing those potential health concerns, Canada (2009), USA (2010), and the European Union (2011) prohibited the use of BPA in the manufacture of polycarbonate feeding bootles for infants. In France, since January 2015, BPA is forbidden in any food or beverage packaging.

Such restrictions on BPA usage recently led manufactories to use alternative bisphenols. Such alternatives include among others bisphenol AF, bisphenol F, and bisphenol S (Liu et al., 2012). For instance, BPS is found in canned soft drinks, canned foods (Vinas et al., 2010; Gallart-Ayala et al., 2011) and in thermal receipt papers (Becerra and Odermatt, 2012; Liao et al., 2012c). BPAF is also incorporated into the production of fluoropolymers, fluoroelastomers, and in a variety of polymers that are used in the manufactoring of electronic devices and plastic optical fibers (Yang et al., 2012). Recent large-scale quantitative studies have identified, in addition to BPA, increasing concentrations of various bisphenols such as BPAF, BPAP, BPF, BPS, BPB, BPZ, and BPP in food products in the United States (Liao and Kannan, 2013). In addition, BPB, BPF, and BPS were also detected in indoor dust in the USA and in several Asian countries (Liao et al., 2012b). However, despite the increasing use of BPA analogs, there is limited information on potential toxicity and endocrine-disrupting activities of these molecules. However, few BPA analogs present some endocrine disrupting activity, as assessed by *in vitro* analysis. For instance, it was shown that BPS and BPAF can bind to estrogen receptors and subsequently exert estrogenic activity at the transcriptional level using cell culture and binding assays (Hashimoto et al., 2001; Kitamura et al., 2005; Kuruto-Niwa et al., 2005; Matsushima et al., 2010; Grignard et al., 2012). Although the estrogenic potential of few BPA analogs have been demonstrated *in vitro*, the *in vivo* potential endocrine-disrupting activity of these compounds remains largely unknown. Recent physiological studies suggest that at least a few BPA analogs have the potential to interfere and disrupt the normal functions of endocrine system in various organisms (Feng et al., 2012; Ji et al., 2013; Naderi et al., 2014; Yang et al., 2014; Eladak et al., 2015). A growing number of studies have shown that BPA has a negative impact on neural development and on the onset of neurological disorders, likely associated to its endocrine-disrupting activities (reviewed in Kajta and Wojtowicz, 2013; Leon-Olea et al., 2014; Negri-Cesi, 2015). To our knowledge, very limited work has assessed estrogenic activity of BPA analogs during brain development, and/or in adult brain. A recent study suggests that exposure to BPS might cause hyperactivity and brain changes in developing zebrafish (Kinch et al., 2015).

In the present study, we assessed the potential *in vivo* estrogenic activities of various BPA analogs and their effects on the central nervous system using the developing zebrafish brain. The developmental pattern of the zebrafish is particularly well-studied (Briggs, 2002) and the species is a widely used model to evaluate the potential adverse effects of chemicals present in the environment and to define the mechanisms underlying the endocrine-disrupting activities (Segner, 2009).Indeed, numerous estrogen-sensitive proteins have been identified in zebrafish, including the liver-produced yolk proteins Vitellogenin 1 and 3 (encoded by vtg1 and vtg3 genes), and the brain-specific aromatase B (AroB), encoded by the brain specific *cyp19a1b* gene, and change in their expression can be used as biomarker for estrogen or xenoestrogen exposure (Kausch et al., 2008; Ruggeri et al., 2008; Levi et al., 2009; Chung et al., 2011; Lam et al., 2011; Hao et al., 2013). We and others have shown that the *cyp19a1b* gene is specifically expressed in a very specific brain population, the radial glial cells, that serves as progenitors during embryonic and adult neurogenesis (for review see Diotel et al., 2010; Coumailleau et al., 2015; Pellegrini et al., 2015). In addition, the presence of functional estrogen response elements in *cyp19a1b* proximal promoter region allows for a strong transcriptional upregulation by estrogens (E2) and xenoestrogens such as ethinyl estradiol (EE2) and BPA (Le Page et al., 2006; Sawyer et al., 2006; Chung et al., 2011; Brion et al., 2012). Thus, the *cyp19a1b* gene can be used *in vivo* as a biomarker of xenoestrogen effects on the central nervous system in developing and adult zebrafish.

In the present work, we investigated the effects of various BPA analogs on *cyp19a1b* expression in developing zebrafish brain exposed from 0 to 1 day post-fertilization (0–1 dpf) to 4–7 dpf. We used 3 different *in situ/in vivo* approaches: (1) quantitative RT-PCR to monitor the expression levels of *cyp19a1b* in wild type larvae (7 dpf); (2) *cyp19a1b in situ* hybridization to precisely analyse the induction and distribution of *cyp19a1b* transcripts in wild type 7-dpf larvae, and (3) the quantification of the brain fluorescence of *cyp19a1b*-GFP transgenic 4-dpf larvae as an *in vivo* assay (EASZY assay). We demonstrate that the majority of the tested bisphenol A analogs (BPS, BPF, and BPAF) induces *in vivo* significant expression of *cyp19a1b* in the brain of zebrafish at early developmental stages.

MATERIALS AND METHODS

Chemicals

Bisphenol analogs, including bisphenol A [BPA; 2,2-bis(4-hydroxyphenyl)propane; 99%), bisphenol F [BPF; 4,4′-dihydroxydiphenyl methane; 98%), bisphenol AF [BPAF; 2,2-bis(4-hydroxylphenyl)hexafluoropropane; 98%), bisphenol S [BPS; bis-(4-hydroxyphenyl)sulfone; 98%), bisphenol AP [BPAP; 4,4′-(1- phenylethylidene)bisphenol; 98%], were purchased from Sigma-Aldrich (St. Louis, MO) and TCI America (Portland, OR). E2 [17β-estradiol] and EE2 [17α-ethinylestradiol] were purchased from Sigma Aldrich (St. Louis, MO, USA). ICI 182

780 was purchased from Tocris Bioscience. Stock solutions were prepared in dimethyl sulfoxide (DMSO; Sigma) and kept at −20°C. Dilution series were freshly prepared before each experiment. The maximum volume of the solvent did not exceed 0.1% (v/v).

Zebrafish Maintenance and Embryo/Larva Exposure

Animals were treated in agreement with the European Union regulations concerning the protection of experimental animals. This study was approved by the ethics committee (CREEA: Comité Rennais d'Ethique en matière d'Expérimentation Animale) under permit number EEA B-35-040. Zebrafish embryos were raised in our facilities (IFR 140, INRA SCRIBE, Rennes, France) in recirculated water kept at 28.5°C and spawned under standard conditions. Embryos were collected 2 h post-fertilization (hpf), and examined under a binoccular. Those embryos that had developed normally were selected and kept in several Petri dishes (zebra.s- c.edu/guides.html) in an incubator at 28.5°C (kept on a 14-h light, 10-h dark cycle).

For subsequent RT-qPCR and *in situ* hybridization analysis with wild type zebrafish, groups of 80 embryos (for each condition) were placed after 1 day post-fertilization (1-dpf) in a large glass flask containing 100 ml of embryonic medium (Mouriec et al., 2009b). Chemical treatments were performed by adding either DMSO alone (negative control), EE2 (positive control), or one of the tested bisphenols (BPA, BPS, BPF, BPAF, BPAP) diluted in water at indicated concentrations, thereby creating 7 experimental treatment conditions. The embryos were held in the exposure flasks until 7-dpf larva stage. For studies with the *cyp19a1b-GFP* transgenic zebrafish line (Tong et al., 2009; Brion et al., 2012), groups of 20 embryos (for each condition) were placed 2 h post-fertilization in crystallization dishes containing 25 ml medium and at indicated concentration of tested bisphenols analogs, EE2, or DMSO. Embryos were maintained in the exposure dishes until 4-dpf larva stage. During the treatment period, 100% of the exposure medium was renewed every 24 h (for both wild type and transgenic zebrafish). No mortality was observed for any treatments during the exposure period.

Quantitative Real-Time PCR

After exposure, approximately 70 wild type heads were collected at 7 dpf (i.e., 6 days of exposure) for each experimental conditions (DMSO, EE2, BPA, BPS, BPF, BPAF, and BPAP) into 1.5 ml Eppendorf tubes, and frozen in liquid nitrogen. Tissue was sonicated (10 s, 3 times) in 250 μL Trizol Reagent (Invitrogen) and RNA extractions were carried out according to the manufacturer's protocol. Reverse transcription was carried out by incubating 2μg total RNA with 1μg of random primer oligonucleotides, 2.5mM dNTPs, and 50 U MMLV-RT (Promega) in the appropriate buffer for 10 min at 65°C and 60 min at 37°C. Quantitative Polymerase chain reaction (qPCR) experiments were performed in an iCycler thermocycler coupled to the MyiQ detector (Bio-Rad. Hercules, CA, USA) using iQ SYBR-Green Supermix (Bio-Rad) according to the manufacturer's protocol. The following primers were used: *ef1* (fw) 5′-AGCAGCAGCTGAGGAGTGAT-3′; *ef1* (rev) 5′-CCGCATTTGTAGATCAGATGG-3′; *cyp19a1b* (AroB; fw) 5′-TCGGCACGGCGT- GCAACTAC-3′; *cyp19a1b* (AroB; rev) 5′-CATACCTATGCATTGCAGACC-3′. For each condition, the RT-PCR experiment was run in triplicates. Expression levels of *ef1* mRNA were used to normalize *cyp19a1b* expression levels. Melting curve and PCR efficiency analyses were performed to confirm correct amplification. For quantification of PCR results, the threshold cycle (Ct) was determined for each reaction. Ct values for each gene of interest were normalized with the housekeeping gene *ef1*, using the ΔΔCt method. Normalized values were used to calculate the degree of induction or inhibition expressed as a "fold difference" compared to normalized control values.

Brain Sections and *In situ* Hybridization

Larvae used for *in situ* hybridization experiments originated from the same exposition groups than RT-qPCR experiments. After exposure to the different conditions, 10 wild type 7-dpf larvae (for each treatment) were fixed overnight at 4°C in 4% paraformaldehyde, before embedding in parrafin. Serial thin transverse sections (8 μM) were placed on cryofrost slides and subjected to *in situ* hybridization experiments. Sense and antisense digoxigenin-labeled riboprobes for the *cyp19a1b* gene were transcribed using the Digoxigenin RNA labeling kit in accordance with the manufacturer's instructions (Roche, Mannheim, Germany) and as previously described (Menuet et al., 2005). The brain sections were processed for *in situ* hybridization using stringent conditions as previously published (D'Amico et al., 2011, 2013). After NBT/BCIP revelation, sections were counterstained with DAPI, and mounted in a drop of vectashield (Vector Laboratories). All sections were photographed with an Olympus PROVIS AX70 microscope with a digital camera (Olympus SP71), or a Nikon multizoom AZ100 macroscope with a DS-Ri1 color camera.

In vivo Imaging with the EASZY Assay

Quantification of fluorescence in transgenic *cyp19a1b*-GFP zebrafish larva brain was performed according to Brion et al. (2012). In this assay, estrogenic activity is detected in living 4 days-old larvae (treated or not with an estrogen mimic compound) from the observation of the reporter gene fluorescence in the radial glial cells. After exposure conditions (see above), live tg (*cyp19a1b*-GFP), 4 dpf larvae (20 specimens per condition) were observed in dorsal view and each specimen was photographed using a Zeiss AxioImager.Z1 fluorescence microscope equipped with a AxioCam Mrm camera (Zeiss GmbH, Göttingen, Germany). All photographs were taken using the same parameters: only the head was photographed under a X10 objective, with a 134 ms exposure time and maximal intensity. Photographs were analyzed using the Axiovision Imaging software and fluorescence quantification was performed using the ImageJ software (http://rsbweb.nih.gov/ij/). For each picture, the integrated density was measured, i.e., the sum of the gray-values of all the pixels within the region of interest. A gray-value of 290 was defined as background value. For each micrograph the fluorescence fold induction of fluorescence was calculated comparing the integrated pixel density with the average fluorescence induction obtained in the control group.

Plasmid Constructions

The zfER-α, zfER-β1, and zfER-β2 expression vectors correspond to Topo-pcDNA3 expression vector (Invitrogen, San Diego, CA, USA), containing the coding regions of each zebrafish estrogen receptor cDNA as previously described (Menuet et al., 2002). The *cyp19a1b*-Luciferase plasmid consists of 500 bp of the proximal promoter region of zebrafish *cyp19a1b* gene, containing an ERE, coupled to the luciferase reporter gene (Menuet et al., 2002).

Glial Cell Culture and Transfection Experiments

Human U251-MG glial cells were maintained in phenol red-free Dulbecco's Modified Eagle's Medium (DMEM; Life Technologies, Saint Aubin, France) supplemented with 10% fetal calf serum (Biowest, Nuaillé, France), 4 mM L-Glutamine (Gibco, Carlsbad, CA, USA) and 1 mM Na-Pyruvate (Life Technologies, Saint Aubin, France) and kept at 37°C and 5% CO_2 atmosphere (Le Page et al., 2006). The medium was also supplemented with 20 U/mL penicillin, 20 μg/mL streptomycin, and 50 ng/mL amphotericin B (Gibco). For transfections, cells were plated in 24-well plates at a density of 25,000 cells/ml in the same medium, except the fetal calf serum was charcoal-treated and used at a concentration of 2.5%. Cells were transfected with 25 ng/well either the vector expression containing or not the the zfERα, zfERβ1, zfERβ2 coding region and cytomegalovirus [CMV]−β-Galactosidase, and 150 ng/well of the *cyp19a1b*-Luciferase reporter plasmid, using JetPEI as a transfection reagent (Polyplus Transfection, Illkirch, France). One day after transfection, U251-MG cells were treated with chemicals using same concentrations as *in vivo* experiments (10–9 M and 10–6 M, for EE2 and bisphenols, respectively) and DMSO as a vehicle (1/10.000). Luciferase activity was measured 24 h later (Luciferase assay system, Promega, Madison, WI, USA). β-Galactosidase activity was used to normalize transfection efficiency. Chemicals were tested in at least 3 independent experiments and each experiment was performed in triplicate.

Zebrafish Estrogen Receptor Competitive-Binding Assays

We also performed a competitive binding assay to test the binding properties of our compounds of interest with the three zfERs (Blair et al., 2000). The three zebrafish estrogen receptor proteins were synthesized using the Topo-pcDNA3 expression vector containing the coding region of zfERα, zfERβ1, and zfERβ2 (Menuet et al., 2002). The TNT Quick Coupled Transcription/Translation Systems kit (Promega, Madison, WI, USA) was used for synthesis of zfER proteins by adding 1 μg of each ER expression vector and according to the manufacturer's protocol. Efficiency of translation was assessed by SDS-PAGE (data not shown). After *in vitro* synthesis, 5 μl of zfERα, zfERβ1, or zfERβ2 were incubated overnight at 4°C with 10^{-9} M [^{3}H]-E2 in absence or presence of increasing concentrations of radioinert E2 (10^{-11} M, 10^{-10} M, 10^{-9} M, 10^{-8} M, 10^{-7} M), BPA, BPF, BPS, BPAF, or BPAP (10^{-10} M, 10^{-9} M, 10^{-8} M, 10^{-7} M, 10^{-6} M, 10^{-5} M). The relative binding affinity for each compound was analyzed by their efficiency to move [^{3}H]-E2 from the zfER binding site. Results were expressed as a percentage of displaced [^{3}H]-E2 binding. The 10^{-7} M E2 containing 100-fold excess of radioinert E2 compared to [^{3}H]-E2 was considered as the non-specific binding (Blair et al., 2000). IC50 were calculated using GraphPad Prism, version 6.07.

RESULTS

In this study, we tested the estrogenic potentials of various bisphenols (BPA, BPS, BPAF, BPF, and BPAP) using the estrogen sensitive biomarker *cyp19a1b* gene in zebrafish brain. Three different experimental approaches were used to validate our results: RT-qPCR on whole brain extract and *in situ* hybridization on brain sections in wild type zebrafish larvae (7-dpf), and the EASZY assay on *cyp19a1b*-GFP zebrafish larvae (4-dpf). In addition, we performed two *in vitro* assays including a transfection experiment in a glial cell context and a competitive binding assay, in order to identify the nuclear estrogen receptors mediating up-regulation of the *cyp19a1b* gene.

Establishment of a Proper BPA Concentration Inducing cyp19a1b Gene in the Brain of 7-dpf Zebrafish Larvae

We first performed real-time RT-qPCR to determine the expression level of *cyp19a1b* mRNAs in the brain of 7-dpf zebrafish larvae exposed or not to bisphenol A (BPA) or ethinyl estradiol (EE2), a weak and a strong synthetic estrogenic compounds, respectively. Three different concentrations of BPA (0.1, 1, or 10 μM) were tested to identify the dose of BPA allowing the best *cyp19a1b* gene response, and compared to EE2 (1 nM) or control DMSO-treated larvae To overcome potential individual variations, we pooled 70 heads in each treatment group (DMSO, EE2, BPA 10, BPA 1, and BPA 0,1). In all treatment groups, no toxic or teratogenic effect was identified. Treated animals survived until 7-days larval stage and were identical to untreated larvae regarding morphology and motility (data not shown). After exposure, quantitative RT-PCR on brain extracts was then performed in triplicate as described in Materials and Methods. As shown in **Figure 1A**, exposure to EE2 induced a very strong overexpression (over 60-fold) of the *cyp19a1b* gene in the brain of 7-dpf larvae, in comparison to control larvae treated with DMSO only. A weaker induction, compared to EE2, was detected in larvae exposed to BPA ranging from 0.1 to 10 μM (**Figure 1A**). Interestingly, BPA concentration of 1 μM induced about 20-fold *cyp19a1b* transcripts levels, whereas 0,1, and 10 μM BPA concentrations had lower effects on *cyp19a1b* transcripts (9- and 12-fold inductions, respectively). As BPA was capable of stronger induction at a 1 μM concentration and did not caused notable toxicological effects, we therefore selected this specific concentration to analyze the effects of BPA analogs in subsequent experiments (RT-qPCR, *in situ* hybridization and EASZY assays). This concentration is also either below or similar to the bisphenols concentrations commonly used in studies on zebrafish embryos (Sun et al., 2009; Chung et al., 2011; Lam et al.,

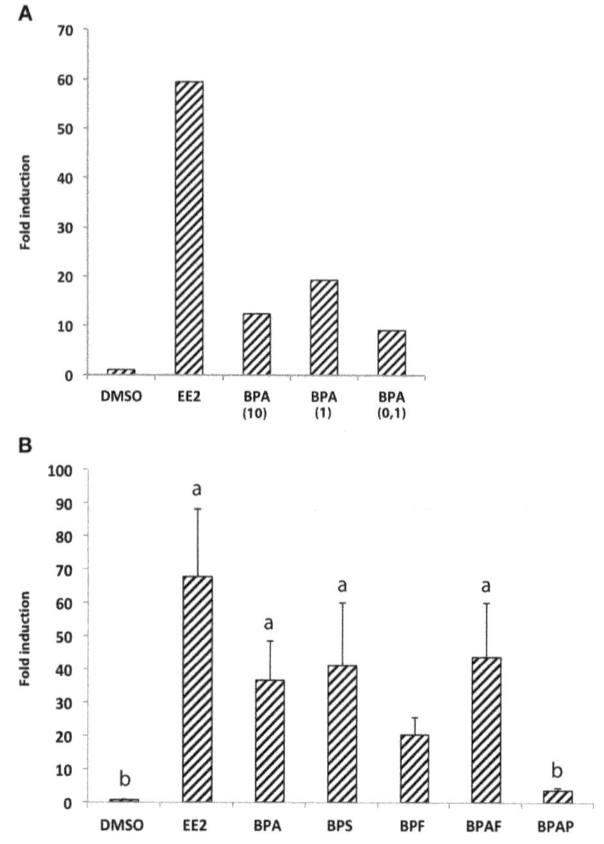

FIGURE 1 | (A) Expression of *cyp19a1b* gene in 7-dpf larvae brains upon treatments with EE2 (1 nM) and three different concentrations of BPA (0.1, 1, or 10 μM). RNA levels were measured in triplicate by real-time quantitative RT-PCR of total RNA prepared from pooled animals (70 per condition). Fold induction was expressed relative to the solvent (DMSO); **(B)** Expression of *cyp19a1b* gene in 7-dpf larvae brains upon treatments with EE2, BPA, and four individual BPA analogs (BPS, BPF, BPAF, and BPAP). For each chemical the concentration used is 1 μM excepted for EE2 (1 nM) and the vehicle (DMSO). RNA levels were measured in triplicate by real-time quantitative RT-PCR of total RNA prepared from pooled animals (70 per condition). Fold induction was expressed relative to the solvent (DMSO); Data in **(B)** are presented as mean ± SEM of six separate egg exposures derived from six independent spawns. **a**: $p < 0.05$ vs. DMSO; **b**: $p < 0.05$ vs. EE2.

2011; Staples et al., 2011; Wu et al., 2011; Keiter et al., 2012; Ji et al., 2013; Saili et al., 2013; Tse et al., 2013; Wang et al., 2013; Naderi et al., 2014).

Bisphenol A Analogs Induce cyp19a1b Gene Expression in Wild Type 7-dpf Larva Brain

The ability of BPA analogs to stimulate or not the expression of *cyp19a1b* estrogenic marker gene was then tested *in vivo* in the brain of wild type 7-dpf larvae. BPS, BPF, BPAF, and BPAP were tested at 1 μM on groups of 70 larvae. In addition, BPA (1 μM) and EE2 (1 nM) groups were used as positive controls, and a DMSO group as a negative control. Due to possible variations between egg batches, the entire experiment was repeated on six independent layings using the same standardized exposure protocols. Importantly, 1 μM treatments of BPA analogs did not affect the survival rate and the motility of exposed larvae (data not shown). In addition, no teratogenicity was observed all along the treatment and prior to the RT-qPCR analysis (data not shown). **Figure 1B** shows data obtained in the six independent experiments along with statistical analysis (Kruskal-Wallis). We found a general effect of the bisphenol analogs treatment on aromatase expression ($H = 26.95$, $p < 0.0001$). Dunn's *post-hoc* analysis showed a significant *cyp19a1b* induction by BPA, BPS, and BPAF in 7-dpf larvae (about 36-, 41-, and 43-fold induction compared to DMSO-treated larvae, respectively; **Figure 1B**). Although BPF exposure lead to an apparent increase in aromatase expression, this 20-fold up-regulation did not reach statistical significance. In contrast, BPAP had no effect on *cyp19a1b* gene.

In vivo Detection of cyp19a1b Promoter Activity Using cyp19a1b-GFP Transgenic Larvae Exposed to Bisphenols

To confirm the results obtained above, we tested the estrogenic activity of BPA analogs using the *cyp19a1b*-GFP transgenic zebrafish line, also named tg (cyp19a1b-GFP) (Tong et al., 2009). The use of tg (cyp19a1b-GFP) larvae was previously shown to be a very sensitive and fast assay (EASZY assay) to detect estrogenic activity (Brion et al., 2012; Petersen et al., 2013; Fetter et al., 2014). As described in Materials and Methods, experimental groups of 20 transgenic embryos were exposed for 4 days (from 2 h to 4 days post-fertilization) with 1 μM BPA, BPS, BPF, BPAF, or BPAP. In addition, control groups of transgenic embryos were exposed to either EE2 (1 nM) or DMSO alone. **Figure 2A** shows examples of the GFP signal generated in the whole brain by the different bisphenols together with the positive (EE2) and negative (DMSO) controls. Larvae treated only with DMSO (**Figures 2Ag,B**) show a basal GFP fluorescence, equivalent to those treated only with water (data not show). GFP induction occurs mostly in the midline of the brain, at the preoptic area level (arrow in **Figure 2Ag**). All other GFP fluorescence induction values were normalized in relation to this signal, considered as the basal activity of the *cyp19a1b* promoter (**Figure 2B**). Quantification of the signal and one-way ANOVA analysis revealed a significant overall effect of the treatment [$F_{(6, 85)} = 35.43$, $p < 0.0001$]. As expected, exposition of larvae to the synthetic estrogen EE2 (1 nM) strongly increased the GFP fluorescence intensity in the brain, attesting an important activity of the *cyp19a1b* promoter in the presence of EE2 (**Figures 2Aa,B**). An intense GFP signal is detected in the radial glial cells together with a much wider distribution from the telencephalon to the caudal hypothalamus (**Figure 2A**, compared **Figure 2Aa** and **Figure 2Ag**). As shown in **Figure 2B**, there was 31-fold induction of the GFP fluorescence in EE2-treated animals compared to DMSO-treated animals. The BPA also significantly increased the GFP fluorescence intensity (**Figures 2Ab,B**), albeit to a lower level compared to EE2 (16-fold induction compared to the DMSO control). Using this *in vivo* experiment, we also demonstrated that BPA analogs such as BPS, BPF, and BPAF also increased the GFP fluorescence in the

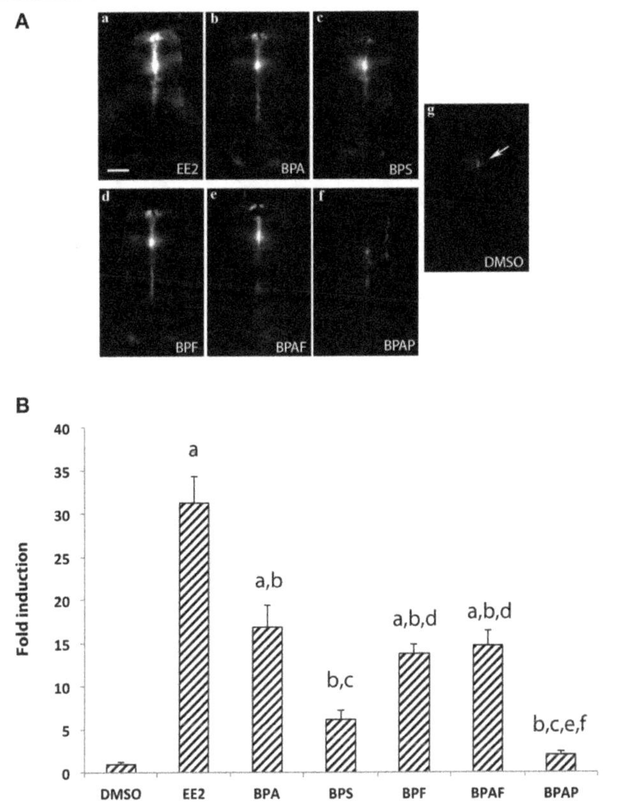

FIGURE 2 | (A) *In vivo* imaging of 4-dpf old live transgenic *cyp19a1b*-GFP zebrafish larvae exposed to EE2, BPA, and various bisphenol A analogs.For each chemical the concentration used is 1 μM excepted for EE2 (1 nM) and the vehicle (DMSO). Dorsal views of the brains. Anterior is to the top. Bar = 20 μm. **(B)** Quantification of GFP fluorescence in zebrafish larvae exposed to the various compounds. Results are expressed as fold induction above control. Data re presented as mean ± SEM of 20 specimens per condition ($n = 20$). **a**: $p < 0.05$ vs. DMSO; **b**: $p < 0.05$ vs. EE2, **c**: $p < 0.05$ vs. BPA, **d**: $p < 0.05$ vs. BPS, **e**: $p < 0.05$ vs. BPF, **f**: $p < 0.05$ vs. AF.

brain (**Figures 2Ac–e**). Quantifications of the GFP signal reveals that fluorescence intensity for BPAF and BPF (14- and 13-fold inductions, respectively) was similar to BPA and significantly higher than the control (**Figure 2B**). The 6-fold induction by BPS did not reach statistical significance (**Figure 2B**). In contrast, larvae exposed to BPAP did not affect GFP fluorescence signal (**Figures 2A,B**). Taken together, these data show a correlation between the induction of the *cyp19a1b* promoter activity in the transgenic zebrafish line (trough measuring GFP fluorescence) and the *cyp19a1b* gene expression that we observed in RT-qPCR analysis in wild type larvae with BPA, BPS, BPF, and BPAF (**Figure 1B**). In addition, we also confirm that BPAP did not significantly induce *cyp19a1b* gene expression.

Effects of Bisphenols on cyp19a1b Transcripts Distribution in the Developing Zebrafish Brain

To analyze a possible change in the distribution of *cyp19a1b* transcripts in the brain following bisphenol treatment, we performed *in situ* hybridization on serial and thin transverse sections of wild type exposed larva brains (7-dpf). We first compared *cyp19a1b* expression patterns in larvae exposed to EE2, BPA or DMSO alone. As shown in **Figures 3, 4**, *cyp19a1b* transcripts cannot be detected on thin sections along the rostral-caudal axis of brains that were only treated with DMSO (**Figures 3, 4A1-K1**). In contrast, EE2-treated larvae show a massive over-expression of the *cyp19a1b* transcripts in several and specific regions of the brain, notably in posterior telencephalon, preoptic area (arrows in **Figures 3B2–D2**) and caudal hypothalamus (lateral and posterior ventricular recesses; arrows in **Figures 4G2–J2**). Importantly, BPA-treated larvae also displayed strong presence of *cyp19a1b* transcripts in virtually identical regions than EE2-treated larvae (arrows in **Figures 3, 4A3–K3**). These *in situ* hybridization data confirm and extend previous studies showing that both estrogen and xenoestrogens increase *cyp19a1b* RNA levels in these brain regions (Menuet et al., 2005; Lassiter and Linney, 2007; Mouriec et al., 2009a; Tong et al., 2009; Chung et al., 2011).

As the strongest induction of *cyp19a1b* transcripts along the rostro-caudal axis of the brain was observed in the caudal hypothalamus, notably in the area of the nucleus recessus posterioris (nrp) (**Figures 4I2,3**), we therefore focused our analysis on this brain particular region for the assessment of estrogenic activities of BPA analogs. As shown in the **Figure 5**, we confirmed that no *cyp19a1b* transcript was detectable in the nrp of DMSO-treated larva (**Figures 5A,C**), whereas strong levels of *cyp19a1b* transcripts were found in BPA-treated larva (**Figures 5B,D**). Most importantly, a similar high detection of *cyp19a1b* transcripts was also observed in this hypothalamic region with other bisphenols such as BPS, BPAF, and BPF (**Figures 5E–H**). These *in situ* data are in perfect agreement with the above RT-qPCR and EASZY assays (**Figures 1, 2**). For BPAP-treated larva, there was also an increase in *cyp19a1b* transcripts in the nrp region (**Figure 5II**) albeit to a lower levels compared to specimens treated with other bisphenols (BPA, BPS, BPF, and BPAF). Although no significant increase of *cyp19a1b* transcripts was observed in BPAP-treated animals using RT-qPCR and EASZY assays (**Figures 1, 2**), we decided to analyze in close details the distribution of *cyp19a1b* transcripts in the whole brain of BPAP-treated larva. As clearly shown in **Figure 6**, BPAP induces expression of *cyp19a1b* transcripts in only a few (xeno) estrogen-sensitive *cyp19a1b* expression sites. In particular, *cyp19a1b* transcripts were not observed in the anterior regions of the brain, corresponding to the posterior telencephalon and the preoptic area (**Figures 6B2–E2**). For BPS-, BPF-, and BPAF-treated animals, the *cyp19a1b* transcripts distribution patterns in the whole brain were identical to EE2- and BPA-treated animals, including in brain regions other than the nrp (dat not shown). Taken together, the absence of *cyp19a1b* transcripts in anterior regions of the brain and the weak detection of *cyp19a1b* transcripts in the caudal hypothalamus argue and confirm that BPAP has almost no estrogenic activity in the brain compared to other tested bisphenols (BPA, BPF, BPAF, and BPS).

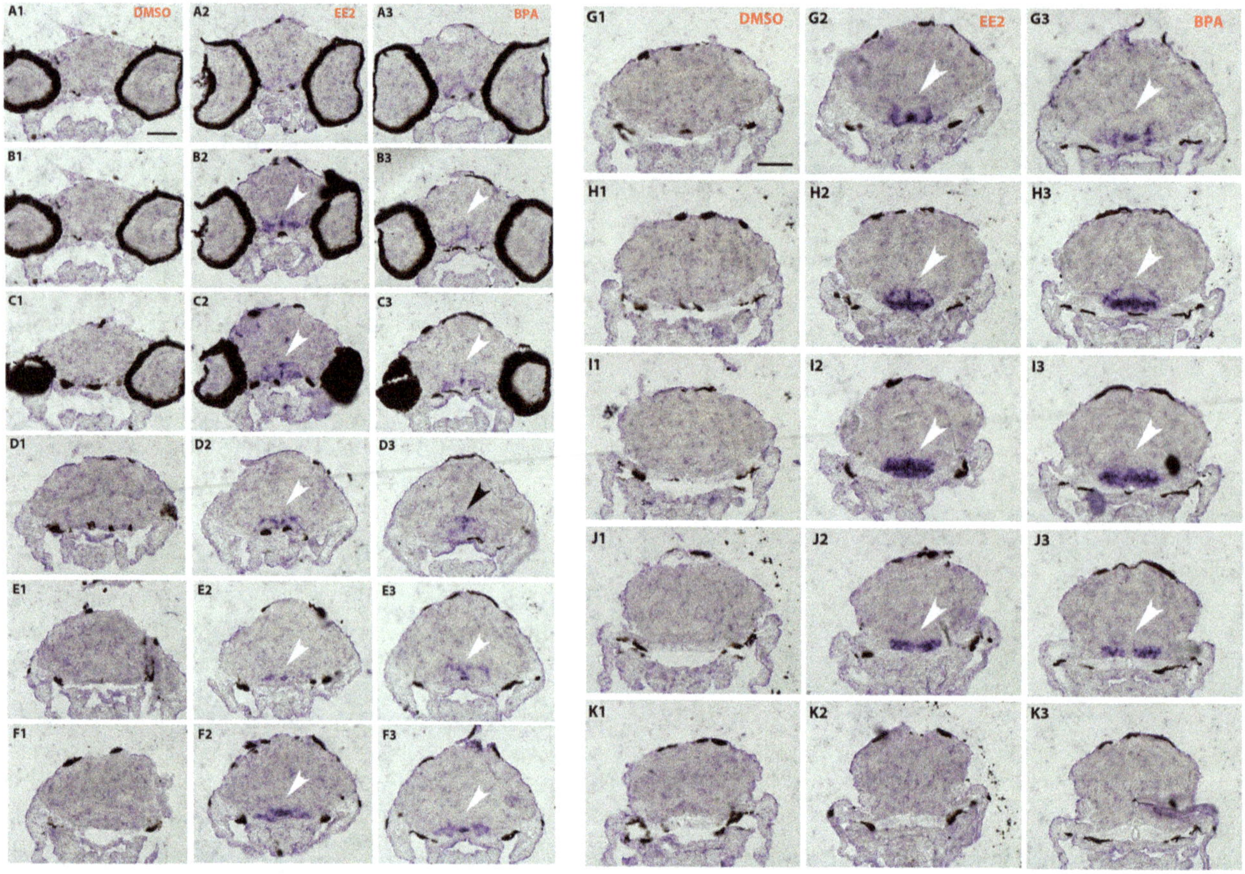

FIGURES 3, 4 | Distribution of *cyp19a1b* transcripts in 7-dpf old zebrafish brains after treatments with EE2 (A2–K2) and BPA (A3–K3) and compared to the DMSO control (A1–K1). Images of transverse sections through the rostrocaudal axis of brains. Arrowheads highlight areas of labeling. For all images, dorsal is to the top. Scale bar = 50 μm.

Bisphenols Induce cyp19a1b Activity through Estrogen Receptors in a Glial Cell Model

To investigate in more detail the mechanism of bisphenols-induced transcription of *cyp19a1b* in radial glial cells of the brain, we performed functional *cyp19a1b*-luciferase reporter gene assay in a reconstituted glial cell line model (Le Page et al., 2006). We tested the impact of each bisphenol on the transcriptional activity of the three distinct zebrafish estrogen nuclear receptors (ERα, ERβ1, and ERβ2) transfected in U251MG cells, an ER-negative human glial cell line. In this assay, the zebrafish *cyp19a1b* promoter upstream of the luciferase is used as the reporter gene. We evaluated *trans*-activation properties of the different zebrafish estrogen nuclear receptors (ERα, ERβ1, and ERβ2) upon individual bisphenol treatments (BPA, BPS, BPF, and BPAF), EE2 and DMSO in six independent transfection experiments. As shown in **Figure 7A**, a priori analysis using a one-tailed *t*-test confirmed previous studies (Le Page et al., 2010) showing a strong induction of the *cyp19a1b*-luciferase reporter gene upon EE2 treatments in cells transfected with either ERα ($t = 3.01$ $df = 10$, $p < 0.01$), ERβ1 ($t = 1.927$ $df = 10$, $p < 0.05$) or ERβ2 ($t = 2.495$, $df = 10$, $p < 0.05$) compared to DMSO treatment. EE2-dependent activation of the *cyp19a1b* promoter was about 2- to 3-fold more efficient with ERα compared to ERβ1 and ERβ2. No reporter gene activity was found in absence of estrogen receptors (**Figure 7A**; empty plasmid), confirming that the transcriptional activity detected upon EE2 treatment is mediated by the presence of an estrogen nuclear receptor. We found a significant effect of the treatment [$F_{(6,82)} = 12.69$, $p < 0.0001$], estrogen receptor subtype [$F_{(3,82)} = 24.24$, $p < 0.0001$], and an interaction [$F_{(18,82)} = 3.53$, $p < 0.0001$] on luciferase expression. More precisely, *post-hoc* analysis revealed a significant stimulation of *cyp19a1b* promoter activity by BPA and BPAF in ERα-containing cells. BPF also increased luciferase activity in ERα cells, but the stimulation did not reach statistical significance. In contrast, no significant luciferase activity was found in cell transfected with subtype receptor ERβ1 or ERβ2 upon stimulation with any bisphenols. Independently of the estrogen receptor sub-type, BPAP, and BPS did not stimulate the reporter gene (**Figure 7A**). To further confirm that stimulation of *cyp19a1b* promoter upon BPA, BPF, and BPAF treatments was mediated by ERα-dependent transcription, we repeated the transfection experiments with ERα in presence or absence of

ICI 182 780, an antagonist of estrogen nuclear receptors. As shown in **Figure 7B**, simultaneous treatment with ICI completely abolished BPA, BPF, and BPAF stimulations found in ERα-expressing cells (**Figure 7A**). Taken together, the reporter gene assays in a glial cell context provide evidence that BPA, BPF, and BPAF are ERα agonists whereas BPS is likely to work through other mechanisms.

Bisphenols Binding to Zebrafish Estrogen Nuclear Receptors

Using *in vitro* competition assays strategy, we examined the receptor-binding affinity of BPA and BPA analogs (BPS, BPA, BPF, and BPAF) relative to [3H]17beta-estradiol for the three *in vitro* translated zebrafish estrogen receptors (ERα, ERβ1, and ERβ2). As expected, E2 show a high binding activity with the three zebrafish estrogen receptors (IC50: 1.5, 1.1, and 1.2 nM for ERα, ERβ1, and ERβ2, respectively; **Figures 8A–C**). In perfect agreement with reporter gene assays, we found that BPA, BPF, and BPAF bind *in vitro* to ERα receptor (**Figure 8A**). BPAF showed the highest affinity, followed by BPA and BPF (IC50; 0.076, 2.8, 10.6 μM, respectively). In addition, these receptor-binding activities were clearly reduced with ERβ1 and ERβ2 sub-type receptors (**Figures 8B–C**). In the competition assay with BPAF, the IC50 was almost 10 times stronger for ERβ1 [IC50 = 0.66 μM] than for ERα. Importantly, BPS displayed almost no binding affinities with any ER receptors (**Figures 8A–C**). These results suggest that the weak *cyp19a1b*-luciferase activity observed in the transfection experiment for BPS was probably due to the absence of binding to ERα.

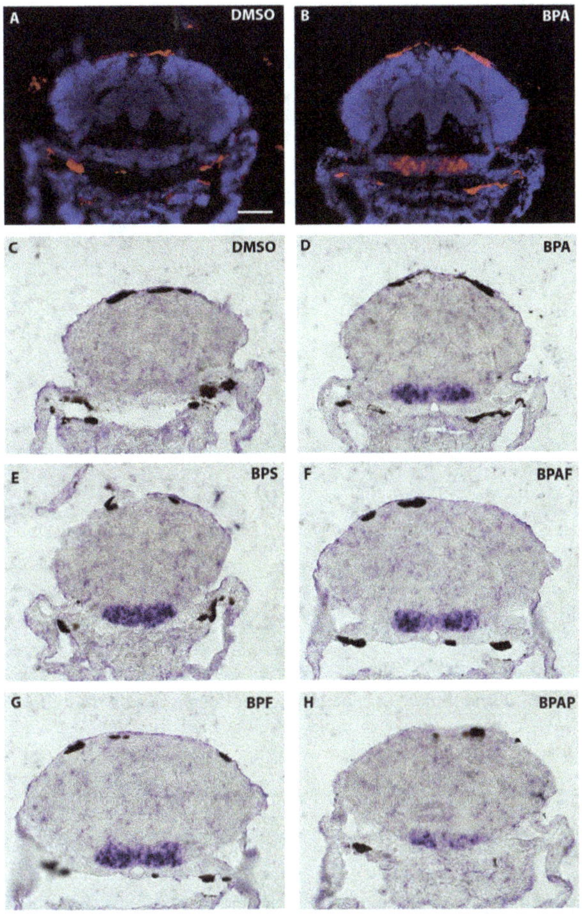

FIGURE 5 | ***In situ*** **expression of** ***cyp19a1b*** **at the level of the caudal hypothalamus (7-dpf old larvae) after treatments with various BPA analogs (E–H) and comparison with negative (A,C) and positive (B,D) controls.**

DISCUSSION

The present work investigated the effects of several bisphenol A analogs on *cyp19a1b* gene regulation, coding for aromatase B, a well-known target of (xeno) estrogen signaling pathways in the fish brain. We show here that BPA, BPS, BPF, and BPAF are able to up-regulate the aromatase B in the brain of developing zebrafish, using three different *in vivo* and *in situ* methods, i.e., RT-qPCR, *in situ* hybridization and the transgenic *cyp19a1b*-GFP.

The BPA exposure of zebrafish larvae led to a 36-fold over-expression of *cyp19a1b* gene in the brain compared to control 7-dpf larvae, as demonstrated by RT-qPCR (**Figure 1B**). This over-expression was confirmed by the EASZY assay with which we found a BPA-inducing activity of the *cyp19a1b* promoter by quantification of the GFP fluorescence in transgenic *cyp19a1b*-GFP brains in 4-dpf larvae (**Figure 2B**; 16-fold induction). The level of *cyp19a1b* induction is in agreement with previous RT-qPCR experiments carried out on whole zebrafish larvae that were exposed to BPA between 3 and 4-dpf developmental stages (Chung et al., 2011) and with previous experiments performed in our laboratory (Brion et al., 2012). Additionnally, *in situ* hybridization experiments on larva brain sections confirmed that BPA caused a strong expression of the *cyp19a1b* gene in specific areas of the brain, in particular in the hypothalamus (**Figures 3–5**). Thus, we show here that the combination of the three different techniques (RT-qPCR, EASZY assay, and *in situ* hybridization) is a valid strategy to investigate estrogenic properties of bisphenol compounds.

Our study indicates that BPA analogs, BPS, BPAF, and BPF, stimulate *cyp19a1b* expression *in vivo*. Indeed, in larvae treated with one of these three bisphenols, we observed a clear induction of the endogeneous *cyp19a1b* gene expression in the brain of wild type 7-dpf old zebrafish (**Figures 1B, 5**) and up-stimulation of the *cyp19a1b* promoter in radial glial cells of GFP transgenic zebrafish larvae (4 dpf; **Figure 2**). The pattern of up-regulation of *cyp19a1b* by the three BPA analogs is similar to the modulation observed after BPA exposure, and therefore, strongly suggest that BPS, BPAF, and BPF exert estrogenic effects on developing zebrafish brain. It is also likely that numerous other estrogen sensitive responses, in the brain but also in other tissues, will also be directly affected by the presence of the bisphenol analogs. Moreover, the up-regulation of brain aromatase will lead to an elevated local enzymatic activity and therefore,

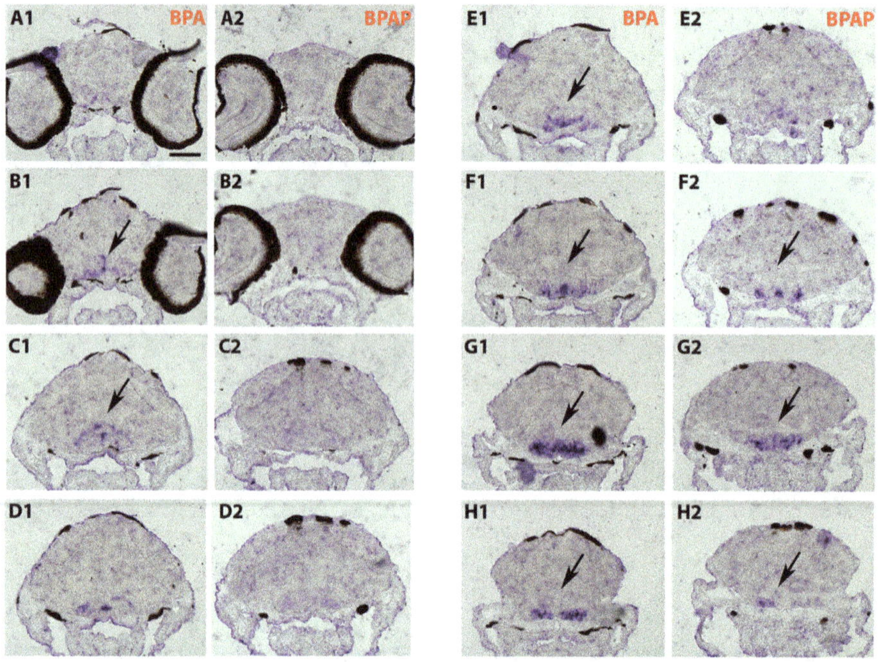

FIGURE 6 | Distribution of *cyp19a1b* transcripts in a 7-dpf old zebrafish brain after treatment with BPAP (A2–H2) and compared to a BPA-treated brain (A1–H1). Images of transverse sections through the rostrocaudal axis of brains. Arrowheads highlight areas of labeling. For all images, dorsal is to the top. Scale bar = 50 μm.

elevated levels of locally produced endogenous estrogen might be expected, adding to the direct estrogenic effect of bisphenol. This abnormal increase in estrogenic activity, considered as endocrine disrupting activity, will likely affect brain development at molecular, cellular, organ, and functional levels, as previously shown for BPA (Kajta and Wojtowicz, 2013; Rochester, 2013; Leon-Olea et al., 2014; Negri-Cesi, 2015). *In utero* or perinatal exposures to BPA in mammals leads to permanent disruptions in behavior, including increased levels of aggression and anxiety, and alterations in learning, memory, exploration, and emotional responsiveness (see for example, refereces Farabollini et al., 2002; Miyatake et al., 2006; Rubin et al., 2006; Kawai et al., 2007; Palanza et al., 2008; Tian et al., 2010; Galea and Barha, 2011; Wolstenholme et al., 2011; Xu et al., 2011). There is little information on potential *in vivo* effect of BPA analogs on brain development and function. However, studies at peripheric level provide evidence that BPA analogs can have adverse effects by interfering with the endocrine system. For instance, the balance of sex steroid hormones and normal reproduction was significantly affected in adult zebrafish following early (Naderi et al., 2014) or late (adult stage) exposure to BPS (Ji et al., 2013). In the later study, BPS exposure led to a significant increase of 17β-estradiol and decrease of testosterone in the plasma of male zebrafish, and these alterations were accompanied by an up-regulation of central and peripheral aromatase expression (both *cyp19a1a* and *cyp19a1b* genes). Similarly to BPS, BPAF exposure can also disrupt sex hormone levels and vitellogenin expression in zebrafish (Yang et al., 2014) and, in adult male rats, BPAF was associated with testosterone reduction by directly affecting testis function (Feng et al., 2012). In human fetal testis explants, low dose of BPS, or BPF is also sufficient to decrease basal testosterone secretion (Eladak et al., 2015). In the brain, it was recently shown that low-dose exposure to BPA and BPS might cause hyperactivity and brain changes in the developing zebrafish due to precocious hypothalamic neurogenesis (Kinch et al., 2015). Interestingly, such brain effects were paralleled with an increase of *cyp19a1b* expression. In *C. elegans*, BPA, and BPS exposure during early embryogenesis also affect neural functionality at adult stage (Mersha et al., 2015) and, in juvenile female rats, BPA, BPF, and BPS can affect 5α-reductase expression and dopamine-serotonin innervations in the prefrontal cortex (Castro et al., 2015).

The preoptic area and the hypothalamus are key integrative centers in the brain that play pivotal functions in the neuroendocrine regulation of homeostasis, reproduction, sexual behavior and stress response (Zohar et al., 2010 and references therein). The detailed analysis of the distribution of *cyp19a1b* transcripts on thin serial sections corresponding to the whole brain (7 dpf) provided evidence that exposure to xenoestrogenes, such as BPA or EE2, strongly induced expression of *cyp19a1b* transcripts in specific brain regions, including posterior telencephalon, preoptic area and caudal hypothalamus (**Figures 3, 4**). Increase in *cyp19a1b* promoter activity in these specific brain regions was also detected in transgenic larvae (EASZY assays; **Figure 2**). The different brain regions where *cyp19a1b* was upregulated following bisphenol exposure were

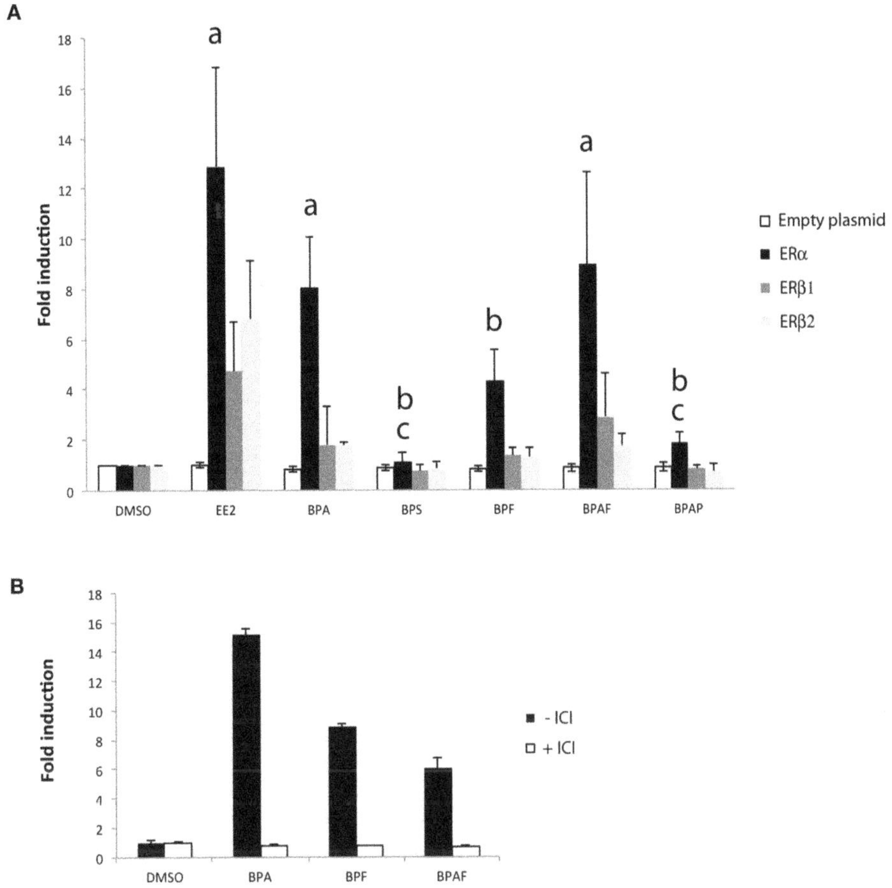

FIGURE 7 | (A) *Cyp19a1b*-luciferase assay in a glial cell context expressing either ERα, ERβ1, or ERβ2. Luciferase activity was measured in triplicate for each condition following treatment with EE2 or bisphenol analogs. Data are presented as mean ± SEM of five independent cellular treatment experiments. **a**: $p < 0.05$ vs. DMSO in ERα–containing cells; **b**: $p < 0.05$ vs. EE2 in ERα-containing cells; **c**: ERα vs. BPA. **(B)** *Cyp19a1b*-luciferase assay in a glial cell context expressing the ERα sub-type in presence or absence of ICI. Luciferase activity was measured in triplicate for each condition.

previously identified as sites of estrogen-induced *cyp19a1b* expression (Menuet et al., 2005; Lassiter and Linney, 2007; Tong et al., 2009; Mouriec et al., 2009a; Chung et al., 2011). In addition, we demonstrated that the caudal hypothalamus, and more precisely the lateral and posterior ventricular recesses (nrp), contains the highest amount of *cyp19a1b* transcripts after BPA or EE2 exposures. Importantly, BPS, BPF and BPAF were also able to strongly induce *cyp19a1b* expression in the nrp in the caudal hypothalamus, with a similar intensity compared to BPA and EE2 (**Figure 5**). Since various xenoestrogens can strongly stimulate *cyp19a1b* expression in similar and specific brain regions, this raise concern about the consequences of their combined actions on hypothalamic development and functioning.

Three distinct nuclear estrogen receptors (zfER) are characterized in zebrafish: ERα, ERβ1, and ERβ2, corresponding to *esr1*, *esr2b*, and *esr2a*, respectively. The three receptors can bind estradiol and are strongly expressed in the anterior and posterior preoptic area, and in the caudal hypothalamus (Menuet et al., 2002). As shown in this study, these two neuroendocrine regions are also the major sites of bisphenol-induced *cyp19a1b* expression (**Figures 3–6**). To define which estrogen receptors was implicated in the up-regulation of *cyp19a1b* gene, we used zebrafish *cyp19a1b* promoter luciferase reporter gene assay in a reconstituted glial cell context expressing one zebrafish ER subtype at a time (as previously reported (Menuet et al., 2005; Le Page et al., 2006). We showed here that BPA, used at a 10^{-6} M concentration, activates *cyp19a1b* promoter via its interaction with ER alpha, while the presence of either ER beta subtypes does not allow BPA to activate the promoter. BPF and BPAF are also able to stimulate *in vitro* the *cyp19a1b* promoter activity via the activation of ERα. This up-regulation was inhibited by the presence of the specific estrogen receptor antagonist ICI 182 780. (**Figure 7**). *In vitro* ligand competition assays confirmed that BPF and BPAF, in addition to BPA, physically bind zebrafish estrogen receptor alpha (**Figure 8**). Previous *in vitro* studies (reporter gene and ligand binding assays) performed in other cellular models also showed the ability of BPF and BPAF to act as an estrogen mimic that binds to estrogen receptors and subsequently exert *trans*-activation activities (Kitamura et al., 2005; Cabaton et al., 2009; Matsushima et al., 2010; Li et al.,

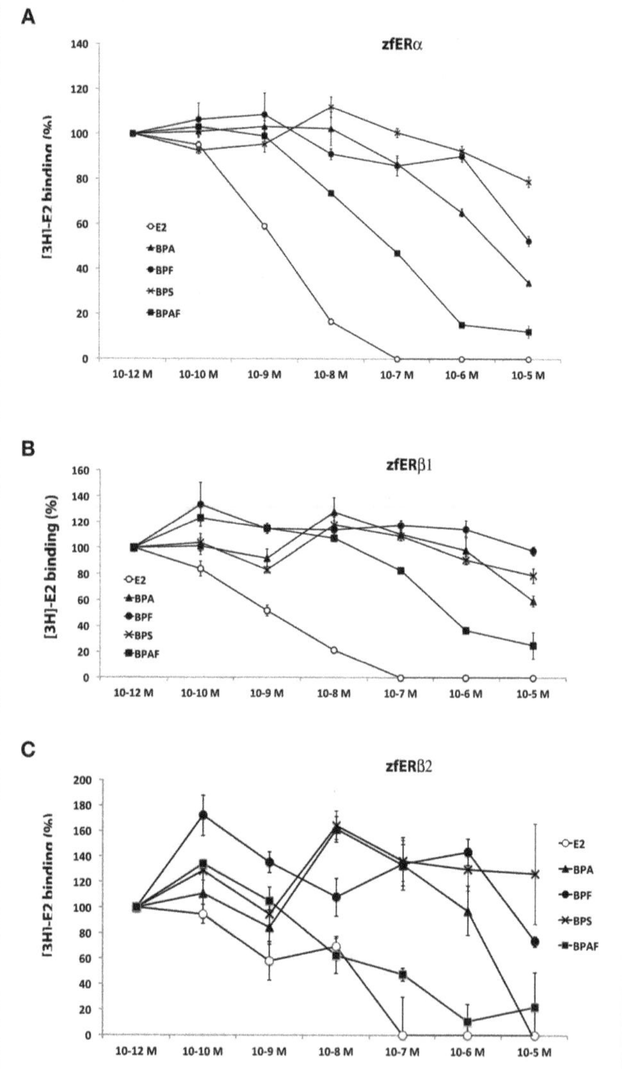

FIGURE 8 | *In vitro* bisphenols-and E2-binding activity to zebrafish estrogen receptors. (A–C) Competitive binding assays relative to [3H]17β-estradiol on ERα **(A)**, ERβ1 **(B)**, and ERβ2 **(C)**. Binding activity was measured in triplicate for each condition and data are presented as mean ± SEM of these 3 radioactivity countings. IC50 are provided in the Results section.

2012). In yeast assays, estrogenic activity for these BPA analogs was also reported (Hashimoto et al., 2001; Ruan et al., 2014).

As stated above, we showed that BPS significantly stimulated the expression of *cyp19a1b in vivo* but, interestingly, this effect did not involve the bisphenol-dependent activation of estrogen receptors in our *cyp19a1b*-luciferase reporter gene in the functional glial cell assay (**Figure 7**). This is in stark contrast with the data obtained with BPA, BPF, and BPAF, acting on *cyp19a1b* up-regulation via ERα subtype (**Figure 7**). It is possible that BPS has only a very weak affinity for the zebrafish estrogen receptors. This hypothesis was clearly reinforced by the ligand competition assays that showed almost no binding activity for BPS compared to other tested bisphenols (**Figure 8**). Previous *in vitro* studies have shown for BPS, lower (Chen et al., 2002; Kitamura et al., 2005; Rosenmai et al., 2014), similar (Hashimoto et al., 2001; Kitamura et al., 2005; Kuruto-Niwa et al., 2005; Grignard et al., 2012; Kang et al., 2014), or higher (Molina-Molina et al., 2013) estrogenic activity than BPA, depending on the experimental model. In the reporter gene assay, the lack of estrogenic activity for BPS could be linked to the absence of key transcriptional co-factors required for efficient estrogen receptor-dependent *trans*-activation. Alternatively, *in vivo* BPS-induced estrogenic activity could be mediated through a different pathway than estrogen receptors. BPS acts as an estrogen mimic in certain conditions, but can also antagonize androgen receptor (Hashimoto et al., 2001; Kitamura et al., 2005; Kuruto-Niwa et al., 2005; Grignard et al., 2012). Recent *in vitro* studies provide evidence that BPA analogs have a clear effect on androgen receptor activity as well as on steroid hormone synthesis (Rosenmai et al., 2014), suggesting that these compounds may interfere with the endocrine system through several modes of action. In addition, in the case of BPAF and in human breast cells, estrogenic activity has been proven to be mediated through both genomic (ERα) and nongenomic pathways (Li et al., 2014).

We did not observe a significant induction of the expression of *cyp19a1b* gene expression in the brain of larvae treated with BPAP, using RT-qPCR and EASZY strategies (**Figures 1, 2**). These data were confirmed in the glial cell context *cyp19a1b*-luciferase reporter gene assay (**Figure 7**). The detailed analysis of *cyp19a1b* transcripts distribution carried out in the whole brains of BPAP-treated larvae revealed that *cyp19a1b* transcripts were, indeed, not detected in telencephalon or preoptic area and very weakly in the caudal hypothalamus (**Figure 6**). Taken together, these data suggest that BPAP might have no or a very weak estrogenic activity in the brain *in vivo*, compared to other bisphenols tested here (BPA, BPS, BPF, and BPAF). To the best of our knowledge, there is only one study that reports low estrogenic activities for BPAP in a recombinant gene yeast assay (Zhang et al., 2009). Our data suggest that BPAP might be a safer alternative to BPA and to other BPA analogs currently used. Presently, BPAP use in industry is not (yet) a common BPA substitute as its environmental concentrations, as measured in food or in indoor dust, is very low compared to other bisphenols (Liao et al., 2012b; Liao and Kannan, 2013).

In conclusion, this work shows that BPA, BPF, BPAF, and BPS exhibit estrogenic activity on the *cyp19a1b* gene (aromatase B), a brain specific gene, which is considered as one of the most, if not the most, E2-sensitive gene in fish (Brion et al., 2012; Lee et al., 2012; Petersen et al., 2013). Thus, BPA analogs, because of their widespread use and their potential to persist in the environment, may be equally as harmul as BPA to developing brains. In contrast, BPAP appears to have no estrogenic activity in the brain of zebrafish. To confirm that BPAP could be a safer alternative to BPA, studies investigating its effects on other tissues and signaling pathways will be required. A replacemant of BPA by any of these coumpounds should be considered with caution and further studies are clearly required to clarify the precise *in vivo* effects of BPA analogs and their mechanisms of actions.

AUTHOR CONTRIBUTIONS

PC, designed the study, developed the methodology, conducted experiments and wrote the manuscript. JC, developed methodology and conducted experiments. CV, maintained embryo and larva development and helped with qPCR analysis. TC, helped with the statistics and editing the article. OK, EP, helped with the design of the study and editing the article.

ACKNOWLEDGMENTS

The authors are grateful to Master Students Athénais Méaude, Emeline Tanguy, and Kevin Dufeil for their precious help in this study. The valuable assistance of the staff of the zebrafish facilities (LPGP, SFR Biosit), in particular Amelie Patinote, is also greatly appreciated. This reseach was supported by funds from the European INTERREG project TC2N.

REFERENCES

Becerra, V., and Odermatt, J. (2012). Detection and quantification of traces of bisphenol A and bisphenol S in paper samples using analytical pyrolysis-GC/MS. *Analyst* 137, 2250–2259. doi: 10.1039/c2an15961a

Blair, R. M., Fang, H., Branham, W. S., Hass, B. S., Dial, S. L., Moland, C. L., et al. (2000). The estrogen receptor relative binding affinities of 188 natural and xenochemicals: structural diversity of ligands. *Toxicol. Sci.* 54, 138–153. doi: 10.1093/toxsci/54.1.138

Bondesson, M., Hao, R., Lin, C. Y., Williams, C., and Gustafsson, J. A. (2014). Estrogen receptor signaling during vertebrate development. *Biochim. Biophys. Acta* 1849, 142–151. doi: 10.1016/j.bbagrm.2014.06.005

Boon, W. C., Chow, J. D., and Simpson, E. R. (2010). The multiple roles of estrogens and the enzyme aromatase. *Prog. Brain Res.* 181, 209–232. doi: 10.1016/S0079-6123(08)81012-6

Briggs, J. P. (2002). The zebrafish: a new model organism for integrative physiology. *Am. J. Physiol. Regul. Integr. Comp. Physiol.* 282, R3–R9. doi: 10.1152/ajpregu.00589.2001

Brion, F., Le Page, Y., Piccini, B., Cardoso, O., Tong, S. K., Chung, B. C., et al. (2012). Screening estrogenic activities of chemicals or mixtures *in vivo* using transgenic (cyp19a1b-GFP) zebrafish embryos. *PLoS ONE* 7:e36069. doi: 10.1371/journal.pone.0036069

Cabaton, N., Dumont, C., Severin, I., Perdu, E., Zalko, D., Cherkaoui-Malki, M., et al. (2009). Genotoxic and endocrine activities of bis(hydroxyphenyl)methane (bisphenol F) and its derivatives in the HepG2 cell line. *Toxicology* 255, 15–24. doi: 10.1016/j.tox.2008.09.024

Calafat, A. M., Kuklenyik, Z., Reidy, J. A., Caudill, S. P., Ekong, J., and Needham, L. L. (2005). Urinary concentrations of bisphenol A and 4-nonylphenol in a human reference population. *Environ. Health Perspect.* 113, 391–395. doi: 10.1289/ehp.7534

Calafat, A. M., Weuve, J., Ye, X., Jia, L. T., Hu, H., Ringer, S., et al. (2009). Exposure to bisphenol A and other phenols in neonatal intensive care unit premature infants. *Environ. Health Perspect.* 117, 639–644. doi: 10.1289/ehp.0800265

Castro, B., Sanchez, P., Torres, J. M., and Ortega, E. (2015). Bisphenol A, bisphenol F and bisphenol S affect differently 5alpha-reductase expression and dopamine-serotonin systems in the prefrontal cortex of juvenile female rats. *Environ. Res.* 142, 281–287. doi: 10.1016/j.envres.2015.07.001

Chen, M. Y., Ike, M., and Fujita, M. (2002). Acute toxicity, mutagenicity, and estrogenicity of bisphenol-A and other bisphenols. *Environ. Toxicol.* 17, 80–86. doi: 10.1002/tox.10035

Chung, E., Genco, M. C., Megrelis, L., and Ruderman, J. V. (2011). Effects of bisphenol A and triclocarban on brain-specific expression of aromatase in early zebrafish embryos. *Proc. Natl. Acad. Sci. U.S.A.* 108, 17732–17737. doi: 10.1073/pnas.1115187108

Coumailleau, P., Pellegrini, E., Adrio, F., Diotel, N., Cano-Nicolau, J., Nasri, A., et al. (2015). Aromatase, estrogen receptors and brain development in fish and amphibians. *Biochim. Biophys. Acta* 1849, 152–162. doi: 10.1016/j.bbagrm.2014.07.002

D'Amico, L. A., Boujard, D., and Coumailleau, P. (2011). Proliferation, migration and differentiation in juvenile and adult Xenopus laevis brains. *Brain Res.* 1405, 31–48. doi: 10.1016/j.brainres.2011.06.032

D'Amico, L. A., Boujard, D., and Coumailleau, P. (2013). The neurogenic factor NeuroD1 is expressed in post-mitotic cells during juvenile and adult Xenopus neurogenesis and not in progenitor or radial glial cells. *PLoS ONE* 8:e66487. doi: 10.1371/journal.pone.0066487

Diotel, N., Le Page, Y., Mouriec, K., Tong, S. K., Pellegrini, E., Vaillant, C., et al. (2010). Aromatase in the brain of teleost fish: expression, regulation and putative functions. *Front. Neuroendocrinol.* 31, 172–192. doi: 10.1016/j.yfrne.2010.01.003

Eladak, S., Grisin, T., Moison, D., Guerquin, M. J., N'Tumba-Byn, T., Pozzi-Gaudin, S., et al. (2015). A new chapter in the bisphenol A story: bisphenol S and bisphenol F are not safe alternatives to this compound. *Fertil. Steril.* 103, 11–21. doi: 10.1016/j.fertnstert.2014.11.005

Farabollini, F., Porrini, S., Della Seta, D., Bianchi, F., and Dessi-Fulgheri, F. (2002). Effects of perinatal exposure to bisphenol A on sociosexual behavior of female and male rats. *Environ. Health Perspect.* 110(Suppl. 3), 409–414. doi: 10.1289/ehp.02110s3409

Feng, Y., Yin, J., Jiao, Z., Shi, J., Li, M., and Shao, B. (2012). Bisphenol AF may cause testosterone reduction by directly affecting testis function in adult male rats. *Toxicol. Lett.* 211, 201–209. doi: 10.1016/j.toxlet.2012.03.802

Fenichel, P., Dechaux, H., Harthe, C., Gal, J., Ferrari, P., Pacini, P., et al. (2012). Unconjugated bisphenol A cord blood levels in boys with descended or undescended testes. *Hum. Reprod.* 27, 983–990. doi: 10.1093/humrep/der451

Fetter, E., Krauss, M., Brion, F., Kah, O., Scholz, S., and Brack, W. (2014). Effect-directed analysis for estrogenic compounds in a fluvial sediment sample using transgenic cyp19a1b-GFP zebrafish embryos. *Aquat. Toxicol.* 154, 221–229. doi: 10.1016/j.aquatox.2014.05.016

Galea, L. A., and Barha, C. K. (2011). Maternal bisphenol A (BPA) decreases attractiveness of male offspring. *Proc. Natl. Acad. Sci. U.S.A.* 108, 11305–11306. doi: 10.1073/pnas.1108769108

Gallart-Ayala, H., Moyano, E., and Galceran, M. T. (2011). Analysis of bisphenols in soft drinks by on-line solid phase extraction fast liquid chromatography-tandem mass spectrometry. *Anal. Chim. Acta* 683, 227–233. doi: 10.1016/j.aca.2010.10.034

Gould, J. C., Leonard, L. S., Maness, S. C., Wagner, B. L., Conner, K., Zacharewski, T., et al. (1998). Bisphenol A interacts with the estrogen receptor alpha in a distinct manner from estradiol. *Mol. Cell. Endocrinol.* 142, 203–214. doi: 10.1016/S0303-7207(98)00084-7

Grignard, E., Lapenna, S., and Bremer, S. (2012). Weak estrogenic transcriptional activities of Bisphenol A and Bisphenol S. *Toxicol. In Vitro* 26, 727–731. doi: 10.1016/j.tiv.2012.03.013

Hao, R., Bondesson, M., Singh, A. V., Riu, A., McCollum, C. W., Knudsen, T. B., et al. (2013). Identification of estrogen target genes during zebrafish embryonic development through transcriptomic analysis. *PLoS ONE* 8:e79020. doi: 10.1371/journal.pone.0079020

Hashimoto, Y., Moriguchi, Y., Oshima, H., Kawaguchi, M., Miyazaki, K., and Nakamura, M. (2001). Measurement of estrogenic activity of chemicals for the development of new dental polymers. *Toxicol. In Vitro* 15, 421–425. doi: 10.1016/S0887-2333(01)00046-7

Hill, R. A., and Boon, W. C. (2009). Estrogens, brain, and behavior: lessons from knockout mouse models. *Semin. Reprod. Med.* 27, 218–228. doi: 10.1055/s-0029-1216275

Hojo, Y., Murakami, G., Mukai, H., Higo, S., Hatanaka, Y., Ogiue-Ikeda, M., et al. (2008). Estrogen synthesis in the brain-role in synaptic plasticity and memory. *Mol. Cell. Endocrinol.* 290, 31–43. doi: 10.1016/j.mce.2008.04.017

Huang, Y. Q., Wong, C. K., Zheng, J. S., Bouwman, H., Barra, R., Wahlstrom, B., et al. (2012). Bisphenol A (BPA) in China: a review of sources, environmental levels, and potential human health impacts. *Environ. Int.* 42, 91–99. doi: 10.1016/j.envint.2011.04.010

Ji, K., Hong, S., Kho, Y., and Choi, K. (2013). Effects of bisphenol s exposure on endocrine functions and reproduction of zebrafish. *Environ. Sci. Technol.* 47, 8793–8800. doi: 10.1021/es400329t

Kajta, M., and Wojtowicz, A. K. (2013). Impact of endocrine-disrupting chemicals on neural development and the onset of neurological disorders. *Pharmacol. Rep.* 65, 1632–1639. doi: 10.1016/S1734-1140(13)71524-X

Kang, J. S., Choi, J. S., Kim, W. K., Lee, Y. J., and Park, J. W. (2014). Estrogenic potency of bisphenol S, polyethersulfone and their metabolites generated by the rat liver S9 fractions on a MVLN cell using a luciferase reporter gene assay. *Reprod. Biol. Endocrinol.* 12:102. doi: 10.1186/1477-7827-12-102

Kausch, U., Alberti, M., Haindl, S., Budczies, J., and Hock, B. (2008). Biomarkers for exposure to estrogenic compounds: gene expression analysis in zebrafish (Danio rerio). *Environ. Toxicol.* 23, 15–24. doi: 10.1002/tox.20306

Kawai, K., Murakami, S., Senba, E., Yamanaka, T., Fujiwara, Y., Arimura, C., et al. (2007). Changes in estrogen receptors alpha and beta expression in the brain of mice exposed prenatally to bisphenol A. *Regul. Toxicol. Pharmacol.* 47, 166–170. doi: 10.1016/j.yrtph.2006.04.002

Keiter, S., Baumann, L., Farber, H., Holbech, H., Skutlarek, D., Engwall, M., et al. (2012). Long-term effects of a binary mixture of perfluorooctane sulfonate (PFOS) and bisphenol A (BPA) in zebrafish (Danio rerio). *Aquat. Toxicol.* 118–119, 116–129. doi: 10.1016/j.aquatox.2012.04.003

Kinch, C. D., Ibhazehiebo, K., Jeong, J. H., Habibi, H. R., and Kurrasch, D. M. (2015). Low-dose exposure to bisphenol A and replacement bisphenol S induces precocious hypothalamic neurogenesis in embryonic zebrafish. *Proc. Natl. Acad. Sci. U.S.A.* 112, 1475–1480. doi: 10.1073/pnas.1417731112

Kitamura, S., Suzuki, T., Sanoh, S., Kohta, R., Jinno, N., Sugihara, K., et al. (2005). Comparative study of the endocrine-disrupting activity of bisphenol A and 19 related compounds. *Toxicol. Sci.* 84, 249–259. doi: 10.1093/toxsci/kfi074

Krishnan, A. V., Stathis, P., Permuth, S. F., Tokes, L., and Feldman, D. (1993). Bisphenol-A: an estrogenic substance is released from polycarbonate flasks during autoclaving. *Endocrinology* 132, 2279–2286.

Kuruto-Niwa, R., Nozawa, R., Miyakoshi, T., Shiozawa, T., and Terao, Y. (2005). Estrogenic activity of alkylphenols, bisphenol S, and their chlorinated derivatives using a GFP expression system. *Environ. Toxicol. Pharmacol.* 19, 121–130. doi: 10.1016/j.etap.2004.05.009

Lam, S. H., Lee, S. G., Lin, C. Y., Thomsen, J. S., Fu, P. Y., Murthy, K. R., et al. (2011). Molecular conservation of estrogen-response associated with cell cycle regulation, hormonal carcinogenesis and cancer in zebrafish and human cancer cell lines. *BMC Med. Genomics* 4:41. doi: 10.1186/1755-8794-4-41

Lassiter, C. S., and Linney, E. (2007). Embryonic expression and steroid regulation of brain aromatase cyp19a1b in zebrafish (Danio rerio). *Zebrafish* 4, 49–57. doi: 10.1089/zeb.2006.9995

Lee, O., Tyler, C. R., and Kudoh, T. (2012). Development of a transient expression assay for detecting environmental oestrogens in zebrafish and medaka embryos. *BMC Biotechnol.* 12:32. doi: 10.1186/1472-6750-12-32

Leon-Olea, M., Martyniuk, C. J., Orlando, E. F., Ottinger, M. A., Rosenfeld, C. S., Wolstenholme, J. T., et al. (2014). Current concepts in neuroendocrine disruption. *Gen. Comp. Endocrinol.* 203, 158–173. doi: 10.1016/j.ygcen.2014.02.005

Le Page, Y., Diotel, N., Vaillant, C., Pellegrini, E., Anglade, I., Merot, Y., et al. (2010). Aromatase, brain sexualization and plasticity: the fish paradigm. *Eur. J. Neurosci.* 32, 2105–2115. doi: 10.1111/j.1460-9568.2010.07519.x

Le Page, Y., Scholze, M., Kah, O., and Pakdel, F. (2006). Assessment of xenoestrogens using three distinct estrogen receptors and the zebrafish brain aromatase gene in a highly responsive glial cell system. *Environ. Health Perspect.* 114, 752–758. doi: 10.1289/ehp.8141

Levi, L., Pekarski, I., Gutman, E., Fortina, P., Hyslop, T., Biran, J., et al. (2009). Revealing genes associated with vitellogenesis in the liver of the zebrafish (Danio rerio) by transcriptome profiling. *BMC Genomics* 10:141. doi: 10.1186/1471-2164-10-141

Li, M., Guo, J., Gao, W., Yu, J., Han, X., Zhang, J., et al. (2014). Bisphenol AF-induced endogenous transcription is mediated by ERalpha and ERK1/2 activation in human breast cancer cells. *PLoS ONE* 9:e94725. doi: 10.1371/journal.pone.0094725

Li, Y., Burns, K. A., Arao, Y., Luh, C. J., and Korach, K. S. (2012). Differential estrogenic actions of endocrine-disrupting chemicals bisphenol A, bisphenol AF, and zearalenone through estrogen receptor alpha and beta *in vitro*. *Environ. Health Perspect.* 120, 1029–1035. doi: 10.1289/ehp.1104689

Liao, C., and Kannan, K. (2011). Widespread occurrence of bisphenol A in paper and paper products: implications for human exposure. *Environ. Sci. Technol.* 45, 9372–9379. doi: 10.1021/es202507f

Liao, C., and Kannan, K. (2013). Concentrations and profiles of bisphenol A and other bisphenol analogues in foodstuffs from the United States and their implications for human exposure. *J. Agric. Food Chem.* 61, 4655–4662. doi: 10.1021/jf400445n

Liao, C., Liu, F., Alomirah, H., Loi, V. D., Mohd, M. A., Moon, H. B., et al. (2012a). Bisphenol S in urine from the United States and seven Asian countries: occurrence and human exposures. *Environ. Sci. Technol.* 46, 6860–6866. doi: 10.1021/es301334j

Liao, C., Liu, F., Guo, Y., Moon, H. B., Nakata, H., Wu, Q., et al. (2012b). Occurrence of eight bisphenol analogues in indoor dust from the United States and several Asian countries: implications for human exposure. *Environ. Sci. Technol.* 46, 9138–9145. doi: 10.1021/es302004w

Liao, C., Liu, F., and Kannan, K. (2012c). Bisphenol s, a new bisphenol analogue, in paper products and currency bills and its association with bisphenol a residues. *Environ. Sci. Technol.* 46, 6515–6522. doi: 10.1021/es300876n

Liu, X., Lee, J., Ji, K., Takeda, S., and Choi, K. (2012). Potentials and mechanisms of genotoxicity of six pharmaceuticals frequently detected in freshwater environment. *Toxicol. Lett.* 211, 70–76. doi: 10.1016/j.toxlet.2012.03.003

Matsushima, A., Liu, X., Okada, H., Shimohigashi, M., and Shimohigashi, Y. (2010). Bisphenol AF is a full agonist for the estrogen receptor ERalpha but a highly specific antagonist for ERbeta. *Environ. Health Perspect.* 118, 1267–1272. doi: 10.1289/ehp.0901819

Menuet, A., Pellegrini, E., Anglade, I., Blaise, O., Laudet, V., Kah, O., et al. (2002). Molecular characterization of three estrogen receptor forms in zebrafish: binding characteristics, transactivation properties, and tissue distributions. *Biol. Reprod.* 66, 1881–1892. doi: 10.1095/biolreprod66.6.1881

Menuet, A., Pellegrini, E., Brion, F., Gueguen, M. M., Anglade, I., Pakdel, F., et al. (2005). Expression and estrogen-dependent regulation of the zebrafish brain aromatase gene. *J. Comp. Neurol.* 485, 304–320. doi: 10.1002/cne.20497

Mersha, M. D., Patel, B. M., Patel, D., Richardson, B. N., and Dhillon, H. S. (2015). Effects of BPA and BPS exposure limited to early embryogenesis persist to impair non-associative learning in adults. *Behav. Brain Funct.* 11:27. doi: 10.1186/s12993-015-0071-y

Miyatake, M., Miyagawa, K., Mizuo, K., Narita, M., and Suzuki, T. (2006). Dynamic changes in dopaminergic neurotransmission induced by a low concentration of bisphenol-A in neurones and astrocytes. *J. Neuroendocrinol.* 18, 434–444. doi: 10.1111/j.1365-2826.2006.01434.x

Molina-Molina, J. M., Amaya, E., Grimaldi, M., Saenz, J. M., Real, M., Fernandez, M. F., et al. (2013). *In vitro* study on the agonistic and antagonistic activities of bisphenol-S and other bisphenol-A congeners and derivatives via nuclear receptors. *Toxicol. Appl. Pharmacol.* 272, 127–136. doi: 10.1016/j.taap.2013.05.015

Mouriec, K., Gueguen, M. M., Manuel, C., Percevault, F., Thieulant, M. L., Pakdel, F., et al. (2009a). Androgens upregulate cyp19a1b (aromatase B) gene expression in the brain of zebrafish (Danio rerio) through estrogen receptors. *Biol. Reprod.* 80, 889–896. doi: 10.1095/biolreprod.108.073643

Mouriec, K., Lareyre, J. J., Tong, S. K., Le Page, Y., Vaillant, C., Pellegrini, E., et al. (2009b). Early regulation of brain aromatase (cyp19a1b) by estrogen receptors during zebrafish development. *Dev. Dyn.* 238, 2641–2651. doi: 10.1002/dvdy.22069

Naderi, M., Wong, M. Y., and Gholami, F. (2014). Developmental exposure of zebrafish (Danio rerio) to bisphenol-S impairs subsequent reproduction potential and hormonal balance in adults. *Aquat. Toxicol.* 148, 195–203. doi: 10.1016/j.aquatox.2014.01.009

Negri-Cesi, P. (2015). Bisphenol a interaction with brain development and functions. *Dose Response* 13:1559325815590394. doi: 10.1177/155932581559 0394

Palanza, P., Gioiosa, L., vom Saal, F. S., and Parmigiani, S. (2008). Effects of developmental exposure to bisphenol A on brain and behavior in mice. *Environ. Res.* 108, 150–157. doi: 10.1016/j.envres.2008.07.023

Paris, F., Balaguer, P., Terouanne, B., Servant, N., Lacoste, C., Cravedi, J. P., et al. (2002). Phenylphenols, biphenols, bisphenol-A and 4-tert-octylphenol exhibit alpha and beta estrogen activities and antiandrogen activity in reporter cell lines. *Mol. Cell. Endocrinol.* 193, 43–49. doi: 10.1016/S0303-7207(02) 00094-1

Pellegrini, E., Diotel, N., Vaillant-Capitaine, C., Pérez Maria, R., Gueguen, M. M., Nasri, A., et al. (2015). Steroid modulation of neurogenesis: focus on radial glial cells in zebrafish. *J. Steroid Biochem. Mol. Biol.* doi: 10.1016/j.jsbmb.2015.06.011. [Epub ahead of print].

Petersen, K., Fetter, E., Kah, O., Brion, F., Scholz, S., and Tollefsen, K. E. (2013). Transgenic (cyp19a1b-GFP) zebrafish embryos as a tool for assessing combined effects of oestrogenic chemicals. *Aquat. Toxicol.* 138–139, 88–97. doi: 10.1016/j.aquatox.2013.05.001

Rezg, R., El-Fazaa, S., Gharbi, N., and Mornagui, B. (2014). Bisphenol A and human chronic diseases: current evidences, possible mechanisms, and future perspectives. *Environ. Int.* 64, 83–90. doi: 10.1016/j.envint.2013.12.007

Richter, C. A., Birnbaum, L. S., Farabollini, F., Newbold, R. R., Rubin, B. S., Talsness, C. E., et al. (2007). *In vivo* effects of bisphenol A in laboratory rodent studies. *Reprod. Toxicol.* 24, 199–224. doi: 10.1016/j.reprotox.2007.06.004

Rochester, J. R. (2013). Bisphenol A and human health: a review of the literature. *Reprod. Toxicol.* 42, 132–155. doi: 10.1016/j.reprotox.2013.08.008

Rosenmai, A. K., Dybdahl, M., Pedersen, M., Alice van Vugt-Lussenburg, B. M., Wedebye, E. B., Taxvig, C., et al. (2014). Are structural analogues to bisphenol a safe alternatives? *Toxicol. Sci.* 139, 35–47. doi: 10.1093/toxsci/kfu030

Ruan, T., Liang, D., Song, S., Song, M., Wang, H., and Jiang, G. (2014). Evaluation of the in vitro estrogenicity of emerging bisphenol analogs and their respective estrogenic contributions in municipal sewage sludge in China. *Chemosphere.* 124, 150–155. doi: 10.1016/j.chemosphere.2014.12.017

Rubin, B. S., Lenkowski, J. R., Schaeberle, C. M., Vandenberg, L. N., Ronsheim, P. M., and Soto, A. M. (2006). Evidence of altered brain sexual differentiation in mice exposed perinatally to low, environmentally relevant levels of bisphenol A. *Endocrinology* 147, 3681–3691. doi: 10.1210/en.2006-0189

Ruggeri, B., Ubaldi, M., Lourdusamy, A., Soverchia, L., Ciccocioppo, R., Hardiman, G., et al. (2008). Variation of the genetic expression pattern after exposure to estradiol-17beta and 4-nonylphenol in male zebrafish (Danio rerio). *Gen. Comp. Endocrinol.* 158, 138–144. doi: 10.1016/j.ygcen.2008.05.012

Saili, K. S., Tilton, S. C., Waters, K. M., and Tanguay, R. L. (2013). Global gene expression analysis reveals pathway differences between teratogenic and non-teratogenic exposure concentrations of bisphenol A and 17beta-estradiol in embryonic zebrafish. *Reprod. Toxicol.* 38, 89–101. doi: 10.1016/j.reprotox.2013.03.009

Sawyer, S. J., Gerstner, K. A., and Callard, G. V. (2006). Real-time PCR analysis of cytochrome P450 aromatase expression in zebrafish: gene specific tissue distribution, sex differences, developmental programming, and estrogen regulation. *Gen. Comp. Endocrinol.* 147, 108–117. doi: 10.1016/j.ygcen.2005.12.010

Schecter, A., Malik, N., Haffner, D., Smith, S., Harris, T. R., Paepke, O., et al. (2010). Bisphenol A (BPA) in U.S. food. *Environ. Sci. Technol.* 44, 9425–9430. doi: 10.1021/es102785d

Segner, H. (2009). Zebrafish (Danio rerio) as a model organism for investigating endocrine disruption. *Comp. Biochem. Physiol. Toxicol. Pharmacol.* 149, 187–195. doi: 10.1016/j.cbpc.2008.10.099

Staples, C. A., Tilghman Hall, A., Friederich, U., Caspers, N., and Klecka, G. M. (2011). Early life-stage and multigeneration toxicity study with bisphenol A and fathead minnows (Pimephales promelas). *Ecotoxicol. Environ. Saf.* 74, 1548–1557. doi: 10.1016/j.ecoenv.2011.05.010

Sun, L., Zha, J., and Wang, Z. (2009). Interactions between estrogenic chemicals in binary mixtures investigated using vitellogenin induction and factorial analysis. *Chemosphere* 75, 410–415. doi: 10.1016/j.chemosphere.2008.11.083

Sun, Y., Irie, M., Kishikawa, N., Wada, M., Kuroda, N., and Nakashima, K. (2004). Determination of bisphenol A in human breast milk by HPLC with column-switching and fluorescence detection. *Biomed. Chromatogr.* 18, 501–507. doi: 10.1002/bmc.345

Tian, Y. H., Baek, J. H., Lee, S. Y., and Jang, C. G. (2010). Prenatal and postnatal exposure to bisphenol a induces anxiolytic behaviors and cognitive deficits in mice. *Synapse* 64, 432–439. doi: 10.1002/syn.20746

Tong, S. K., Mouriec, K., Kuo, M. W., Pellegrini, E., Gueguen, M. M., Brion, F., et al. (2009). A cyp19a1b-gfp (aromatase B) transgenic zebrafish line that expresses GFP in radial glial cells. *Genesis* 47, 67–73. doi: 10.1002/dvg.20459

Tse, W. K., Yeung, B. H., Wan, H. T., and Wong, C. K. (2013). Early embryogenesis in zebrafish is affected by bisphenol A exposure. *Biol. Open* 2, 466–471. doi: 10.1242/bio.20134283

Vandenberg, L. N., Chahoud, I., Heindel, J. J., Padmanabhan, V., Paumgartten, F. J., and Schoenfelder, G. (2010). Urinary, circulating, and tissue biomonitoring studies indicate widespread exposure to bisphenol A. *Environ. Health Perspect.* 118, 1055–1070. doi: 10.1289/ehp.0901716

Vandenberg, L. N., Colborn, T., Hayes, T. B., Heindel, J. J., Jacobs, D. R. Jr., Lee, D. H., et al. (2012). Hormones and endocrine-disrupting chemicals: low-dose effects and nonmonotonic dose responses. *Endocr. Rev.* 33, 378–455. doi: 10.1210/er.2011-1050

Vinas, P., Campillo, N., Martinez-Castillo, N., and Hernandez-Cordoba, M. (2010). Comparison of two derivatization-based methods for solid-phase microextraction-gas chromatography-mass spectrometric determination of bisphenol A, bisphenol S and biphenol migrated from food cans. *Anal. Bioanal. Chem.* 397, 115–125. doi: 10.1007/s00216-010-3464-7

Vinggaard, A. M., Korner, W., Lund, K. H., Bolz, U., and Petersen, J. H. (2000). Identification and quantification of estrogenic compounds in recycled and virgin paper for household use as determined by an *in vitro* yeast estrogen screen and chemical analysis. *Chem. Res. Toxicol.* 13, 1214–1222. doi: 10.1021/tx000146b

Vogel, S. A. (2009). The politics of plastics: the making and unmaking of bisphenol a "safety". *Am. J. Public Health* 99(Suppl. 3), S559–S566. doi: 10.2105/AJPH.2008.159228

Wang, X., Dong, Q., Chen, Y., Jiang, H., Xiao, Q., Wang, Y., et al. (2013). Bisphenol A affects axonal growth, musculature and motor behavior in developing zebrafish. *Aquat. Toxicol.* 142–143, 104–113. doi: 10.1016/j.aquatox.2013.07.011

Wetherill, Y. B., Akingbemi, B. T., Kanno, J., McLachlan, J. A., Nadal, A., Sonnenschein, C., et al. (2007). *In vitro* molecular mechanisms of bisphenol A action. *Reprod. Toxicol.* 24, 178–198. doi: 10.1016/j.reprotox.2007.05.010

Wolstenholme, J. T., Taylor, J. A., Shetty, S. R., Edwards, M., Connelly, J. J., and Rissman, E. F. (2011). Gestational exposure to low dose bisphenol A alters social behavior in juvenile mice. *PLoS ONE* 6:e25448. doi: 10.1371/journal.pone.0025448

Wu, M., Xu, H., Shen, Y., Qiu, W., and Yang, M. (2011). Oxidative stress in zebrafish embryos induced by short-term exposure to bisphenol A, nonylphenol, and their mixture. *Environ. Toxicol. Chem.* 30, 2335–2341. doi: 10.1002/etc.634

Xu, X., Tian, D., Hong, X., Chen, L., and Xie, L. (2011). Sex-specific influence of exposure to bisphenol-A between adolescence and young adulthood on mouse behaviors. *Neuropharmacology* 61, 565–573. doi: 10.1016/j.neuropharm.2011.04.027

Yang, X., Liu, Y., Li, J., Chen, M., Peng, D., Liang, Y., et al. (2014). Exposure to Bisphenol AF disrupts sex hormone levels and vitellogenin expression in zebrafish. *Environ. Toxicol.* 31, 285–294. doi: 10.1002/tox.22043

Yang, Y., Yin, J., Yang, Y., Zhou, N., Zhang, J., Shao, B., et al. (2012). Determination of bisphenol AF (BPAF) in tissues, serum, urine and feces of orally dosed rats by ultra-high-pressure liquid chromatography-electrospray tandem mass spectrometry. *J. Chromatogr. B Analyt. Technol. Biomed. Life Sci.* 901, 93–97. doi: 10.1016/j.jchromb.2012.06.005

Zalko, D., Jacques, C., Duplan, H., Bruel, S., and Perdu, E. (2011). Viable skin efficiently absorbs and metabolizes bisphenol A. *Chemosphere* 82, 424–430. doi: 10.1016/j.chemosphere.2010.09.058

Zhang, H. C., Chen, L. Y., Liu, S. S., and Yin, D. Q. (2009). [Jointed estrogenic activities of bisphenol A and three of its analogs]. *Huan Jing Ke Xue= Huanjing kexue / [bian ji, Zhongguo ke xue yuan huan jing ke xue wei yuan hui "Huan jing ke xue" bian ji wei yuan hui.]*, 30, 260–265.

Zohar, Y., Munoz-Cueto, J. A., Elizur, A., and Kah, O. (2010). Neuroendocrinology of reproduction in teleost fish. *Gen. Comp. Endocrinol.* 165, 438–455. doi: 10.1016/j.ygcen.2009.04.017

17

Resveratrol Ameliorates the Anxiety- and Depression-Like Behavior of Subclinical Hypothyroidism Rat: Possible Involvement of the HPT Axis, HPA Axis, and Wnt/β-Catenin Pathway

Jin-Fang Ge†, Ya-Yun Xu†, Gan Qin, Jiang-Qun Cheng and Fei-Hu Chen**

Anhui Key Laboratory of Bioactivity of Natural Products, School of Pharmacy, Anhui Medical University, Hefei, Anhui, China

Edited by:
*Fumihiko Maekawa,
National Institute for Environmental Studies, Japan*

Reviewed by:
*Guillaume L. Poirier,
University of Massachusetts Medical School, USA
Jacques Epelbaum,
INSERM CNRS Université Paris Descartes, France*

***Correspondence:**
*Jin-Fang Ge
gejinfang@ahmu.edu.cn;
Fei-Hu Chen
cfhchina@sohu.com*

†Jin-Fang Ge and Ya-Yun Xu contributed equally to this work.

Metabolic disease subclinical hypothyroidism (SCH) is closely associated with depression-like behavior both in human and animal studies, and our previous studies have identified the antidepressant effect of resveratrol (RES) in stressed rat model. The aim of this study was to investigate whether RES would manifest an antidepressant effect in SCH rat model and explore the possible mechanism. A SCH rat model was induced by hemi-thyroid electrocauterization, after which the model rats in the RES and LT4 groups received a daily intragastric injection of RES at the dose of 15 mg/kg or LT4 at the dose of 60 μg/kg for 16 days. The rats' plasma concentrations of thyroid hormones were measured. Behavioral performance and hypothalamic–pituitary–adrenal (HPA) activity were evaluated. The protein expression levels of the Wnt/β-catenin in the hippocampus were detected by western blot. The results showed that RES treatment downregulated the elevated plasma thyroid-stimulating hormone concentration and the hypothalamic mRNA expression of thyrotropin-releasing hormone in the SCH rats. RES-treated rats showed increased rearing frequency and distance in the open-field test, increased sucrose preference in the sucrose preference test, and decreased immobility in the forced swimming test compared with SCH rats. The ratio of the adrenal gland weight to body weight, the plasma corticosterone levels, and the hypothalamic corticotrophin-releasing hormone mRNA expression were reduced in the RES-treated rats. Moreover, RES treatment upregulated the relative ratio of phosphorylated-GSK3β (p-GSK3β)/GSK3β and protein levels of p-GSK3β, cyclin D1, and c-myc, while downregulating the relative ratio of phosphorylated-β-catenin (p-β-catenin)/β-catenin and expression of GSK3β in the hippocampus. These findings suggest that RES exerts anxiolytic- and antidepressant-like effect in SCH rats by downregulating hyperactivity of the HPA axis and regulating both the HPT axis and the Wnt/β-catenin pathway.

Keywords: depression, hypothalamus–pituitary–adrenal axis, hypothalamic–pituitary–thyroid axis, resveratrol, subclinical hypothyroidism, Wnt/β-catenin pathway

INTRODUCTION

Imbalances in thyroid hormone homeostasis are associated with both functional and structural brain alterations, resulting in neurobehavioral alterations, including depression (1, 2). Subclinical hypothyroidism (SCH) is defined as an elevated plasma thyroid-stimulating hormone (TSH) level associated with normal total or free thyroxine (fT4) and triiodothyronine (T3) levels. Although the hypometabolism symptoms, including fatigue, weakness, and cold intolerance, are dormant and non-specific in SCH patients, increasing evidence suggests that SCH is associated with neuropsychiatric disorders such as cognitive dysfunction (2) and depression (3, 4). Depression is observed more frequently among individuals with SCH than those with overt hypothyroidism (3), and SCH patients exhibit a twofold higher prevalence of depressive-like symptoms than healthy individuals (5). In our previous study, SCH induced depression-like behavior in rats accompanied by subtle hyperactivity of the hypothalamus–pituitary–adrenal (HPA) axis (6). Clinical studies have demonstrated that treatment with levothyroxine (LT4) improves mood and normalizes the elevated relative cerebral glucose metabolism in several brain areas of depression patients (7, 8). However, the correct dosage of LT4 remains elusive. Moreover, the unpredictable clinical effects of the currently available antidepressants, including poor efficacy and adverse reactions, make the development of new drugs to alleviate depression in SCH patients an urgent clinical need.

Resveratrol (*trans*-3,5,4′-trihydroxy-*trans*-stilbene, RES), a polyphenol component found mainly in grape and *Polygonum cuspidatum*, possesses multiple biological and pharmacological activities, including metabolism regulation (9) and antioxidant effects (10). Recently, our results (11), together with findings from other studies (12–15), have demonstrated that RES alleviates depression-like behavior in a rat model of chronic unpredicted mild stress (CUMS) through its antioxidant effects and by ameliorating hyperactivity of the HPA axis. In addition, the monoaminergic system and the molecular markers related to depression were also altered by RES treatment (16). However, it remains unknown whether RES can alleviate the depression-like symptoms in SCH, which is complicated with the balance of both the hypothalamic–pituitary–thyroid (HPT) axis and the HPA axis. Clinic studies showed that RES was well tolerated with the dose ranging from 200 mg (17) to 1000 mg (18) daily. According to the formula for dose translation based on body surface area (BSA), the corresponding dose in rats should range from 18 to 90 mg/kg. With regard to animal research, it has been reported that RES (20, 40, and 80 mg/kg) could significantly decreased the immobility time of mice in the despair tests (19). Consistently, results of our previous study also demonstrated that RES (15 mg/kg/day × 7 day) could significantly alleviate the depression-like behavior of CUMS rat (11). Thus, the dose of 15 mg/kg/day was chosen in this study.

Multiple approaches have been adopted to evaluate the antidepressant potential of compounds in animal models, including behavioral tests and biochemical/neurochemical assays. In rodents, spontaneous motor activity and anxiety are often analyzed in terms of exploratory behavior, especially during exposure to an open field (20). And the clinical symptoms/signs of depression such as anhedonia (incapability to perform rewarded behaviors) and helplessness are usually measured using the sucrose preference test (SPT) and the forced swimming test (FST), respectively (13). In this study, these behavior tasks were used, and the activity of the HPA axis was also detected.

Several studies in recent years have implicated the canonical Wnt signaling pathway in mood disorders such as bipolar disorder (21) and major depression (22). Activation of the canonical Wnt pathway leads to the inhibition of GSK-3β, allowing β-catenin to be stabilized in the cytosol and translocated to the nucleus, where it activates the transcription of target genes (23). Mutant mice with a heterozygous GSK-3β deletion showed decreased evidence of depression in the FST (23), and infusion of L803-mts, a selective GSK-3 inhibitor, also decreased immobility in the same test (24). Additionally, upregulated β-catenin has been used as a marker for antidepressive-like effects (24). Furthermore, thyroid hormone exerts a negative effect on the canonical Wnt signaling pathway, as demonstrated in a previous study (25). Thyroid hormone stimulates cell proliferation, represses the expression of key members of the Wnt signaling pathway, and suppresses β-catenin levels (25). Therefore, the Wnt/β-catenin pathway may participate in SCH-associated depression.

In this study, in order to explore the potential antidepressant-like effect of RES in the SCH rats and the possible mechanisms, behavior performance were evaluated using a series of behavioral tasks [open-field test (OFT), SPT, and FST]. Moreover, the activities of the HPA axis, the HPT axis, and the canonical Wnt pathway were assessed biochemically.

EXPERIMENTAL PROCEDURES

Drugs

Resveratrol was purchased from Sigma Chemical Co. (St. Louis, MO, USA). LT4 was purchased from Berlin-Chemie AG (Berlin, Germany). Both drugs were dissolved in an aqueous solution of 0.5% sodium carboxymethyl cellulose to be a mixed suspension. Control and untreated model rats received a daily intragastric injection of 0.5% sodium carboxymethyl cellulose.

Animals

Male, 2-month-old Sprague-Dawley rats were purchased from the Anhui Experimental Animal Center of China. They were housed three to four per cage (43 cm length × 31 cm width × 19 cm height) with access to food and water *ad libitum* and were maintained under a 12:12-h light/dark cycle. The light onset is at 8 o'clock. The ambient temperature was maintained at 21–22°C with 50–60% relative humidity. The rats were handled for 5 min daily over 7 days before drug administration. All experimental procedures in this study were approved by the Animal Care and Use Committee at the University of Science and Technology of China, which complies with the National Institute of Health Guide for the Care and Use of Laboratory Animals (NIH publication No. 85-23, revised 1985).

Animal Model of SCH

The SCH rat model was established *via* hemi-electrocauterization, according to the procedures in our previous study (6). In brief, 33 rats underwent hemi-thyroid electrocauterization to establish the SCH model, and 8 sham rats underwent the same operation, but the thyroid tissues were exposed without electrocauterization. The SCH model was evaluated 2 weeks later, and the success rate of SCH modeling was 75.8% (25/33), according to the criterion that the plasma TSH concentration was higher than the 97.5 percentile of the sham group accompanied by a plasma fT4 level between the 2.5 and 97.5 percentile of the sham group. Consequently, 24 successful SCH rats were randomly divided into 3 groups with 8 rats in each group: an untreated model group, a RES treatment group (15 mg/kg/day + model) and an LT4 treatment group (60 μg/kg/day + model). The rats in the RES and LT4 groups received a daily intragastric injection of RES and LT4 at the corresponding dose for 16 days, respectively, and the rats in the sham and untreated model groups simultaneously received the same injection with 0.5% sodium carboxymethyl cellulose. To prevent hypocalcemia resulting from destruction of the parathyroid glands by electrocauterization, the rats were provided with 0.1% (w/v) calcium lactate in their drinking water after surgery.

Behavioral Tests

Behavioral tests were performed in a soundproof room with a neutral environment in the order listed in **Figure 1**. Briefly, SPT was carried out on day (D) 34, OFT on D 35, and FST on D 36 and D 37. All of the tests were carried out between 0900 and 1430 hours, with matching between the groups. The observers were blind to the treatment. The behavioral performance was monitored and recorded by a digital camera above the apparatus interfaced to a computer running the ANY-maze video imaging software (Stoelting Co., Wood Dale, IL, USA).

Sucrose Preference Test

After a 12-h period of food and water deprivation, the animals were individually housed in a cage (28 cm length × 17 cm width × 14.5 cm height) during the test and given two bottles (capacity: 250 ml) containing either water or a 2% sucrose solution. Six hours later, the volumes of water and sucrose consumed were measured. The percentage of the total liquid ingested was sucrose solution that was used as a measure of the sensitivity to reward.

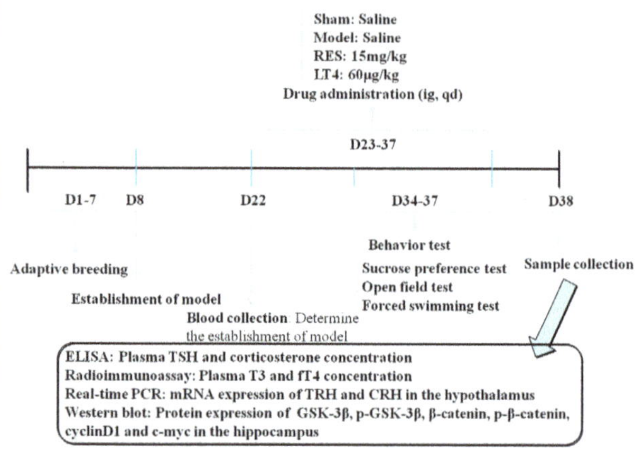

FIGURE 1 | Schedule of the experimental design. RES, resveratrol; LT4, levothyroxine; T3, triiodothyronine; fT4, free thyroxine; CRH, corticotrophin-releasing hormone; TRH, thyrotropin-releasing hormone.

Open-Field Test

The open-field apparatus consisted of a black square arena (100 cm × 100 cm), with a 30-cm-high wall. The floor was marked with a grid dividing it into 16 equally sized squares. During a 5-min observation period, the rat was placed at one corner of the apparatus facing the wall. After the 5-min test, rats were returned to their home cages, and the open field was cleaned with 75% ethyl alcohol and permitted to dry between tests. The total distance; average velocity; the distance, frequency, and duration in the center; and the frequencies of rearing, grooming, and defecation were recorded.

Forced Swimming Test

The behavioral cylinder was 60 cm high and 25 cm in diameter, maintained at 24–25°C, and filled with 30 cm of water, so that rats could not support themselves by touching the bottom with their paws. The FST paradigm includes two sections: an initial 15-min pretest followed by a 5-min test 24 h later. Rats were considered immobile when they did not make any active movements. Struggling was indicated when the rats made active movements with their forepaws in and out of the water along the side of the swim chamber. Swimming was indicated when the rats made active swimming or circular movements.

Measurement of Plasma Concentrations of Thyroid Hormones and Corticosterone

Two weeks after the operation, blood samples (approximately 1 ml) were collected from the angular vein to test whether the SCH rat model was successfully established. Twenty-four hours after the last behavioral test, the rats were deeply anesthetized with chloral hydrate, and blood was taken from the abdominal aorta. Plasma concentrations of TSH and corticosterone were measured using ELISA kits (TSH: Cusabio Biotech. Co., Ltd., Wuhan, Hubei, China; corticosterone: Enzo Life Sciences, Inc., USA), according to the manufacturer's instructions, and fT4 and T3 were measured with radioimmunoassay kits (North Institute of Biological Technology, Beijing, China), with the apparatus used in the assay that came from University of Science and Technology of China Zonkia (AnHui Ustc ZonKia Scientific Instruments Co., Ltd., Anhui China).

The Ratio of the Adrenal Gland Weight to Body Weight

The adrenal glands of each side were removed and weighed immediately postmortem. The ratio of the average of both glands weight to body weight was measured.

RNA Isolation and Real Time PCR

After blood collection, eight rats in each group were sacrificed by decapitation to collect the hypothalamus. The hypothalamus was rapidly dissected and frozen quickly in liquid nitrogen before storage at −80°C. Total RNA was extracted using the TRIzol (Invitrogen, Carlsbad, CA, USA) method. cDNA was synthesized using reverse transcriptase (Promega, WI, USA). Q-PCR was performed using the SYBR Green PCR Kit (Applied Biosystems, USA) and an ABI Prism 7000 Sequence Detector system in a 25-μl total reaction volume for 40 cycles (15 s at 95°C and 60 s at 62°C). The primers used in our study were as follows: rat β-actin 5′-TTGCTGACAGGATGCAGAA-3′ and 5′-ACCAATCCACACAGAGTACTT-3′; thyrotropin-releasing hormone (TRH) 5′-AGCTCAGCATCTTGGAAAGC-3′ and 5′-CCAGCAGCAACCAAGTC-3′; and corticotrophin-releasing hormone (CRH) 5′-CAGAACAACAGTGCGGGCTCA-3′ and 5′-AAGGCAGACAGGGCGACAGAG-3′. The relative amount of each target gene was calculated using the $2^{-\Delta\Delta Ct}$ method.

Western Blot Assays

The hippocampus was homogenized in radioimmunoprecipitation assay (RIPA) buffer (50 mM Tris–HCl at pH 7.4, 0.1% SDS, 1% NP-40, 0.25% sodium deoxycholate, 150 mM NaCl, 1 mM EDTA, 1 mM EGTA, and 1 mM Na_3VO_4). Before homogenization, a protease inhibitor cocktail (Roche, IN, USA) and the phosphatase inhibitor PhosSTOP (Roche, IN, USA) were added. Protein quantitation was conducted using a Lowry Protein Assay Kit (Meiji Biotech Co., Ltd., Shanghai, China). The same quantity (approximately 50 μg) of protein from each animal was loaded and separated by 15% SDS-PAGE and then transferred onto a polyvinylidene difluoride membrane (Amersham Biosciences, UK). The membrane was blocked with 5% skim milk for 1 h, incubated with antibodies targeting GSK3β, p-GSK3β (Ser9), β-catenin, p-β-catenin (1:1000; Cell Signaling Technology, USA), cyclin D1, c-myc (1:1000; ImmunoWay, Newark, DE, USA), or β-actin (1:1000; Bioworld Technology, Inc., USA) at 4°C overnight, and then incubated with a horseradish peroxidase-conjugated secondary antibody (1:10,000) at 37°C for 1 h. The blots were developed with the Easy Enhanced Chemiluminescence Western Blot Kit (Pierce Biotechnology, Rockford, IL, USA). The protein bands were scanned and analyzed using Image J software (NIH).

Statistical Analyses

All statistical analyses were performed using SPSS (Statistical Package for the Social Sciences) version 12.0.1 (SPSS Inc., Chicago, IL, USA). The data are expressed as the means ± SEM, and $P < 0.05$ was considered statistically significant. The distribution of the data was determined by the Kolmogorov–Smirnov test. Between-group effects on body weight, TSH, fT4, and T3 were analyzed by repeated measures ANOVA with group and days as the factors. Statistical analyses of the between-group effects of RES on behavioral performance, the ratio of the adrenal gland weight to body weight, plasma corticosterone, the hypothalamic mRNA expression of CRH and TRH, and the hippocampal protein expression of GSK3β, p-GSK3β (Ser9), β-catenin, p-β-catenin, cyclin D1, and c-myc were carried out using ANOVA followed by LSD *post hoc* tests. Correlation analysis was performed using a Pearson correlation test.

RESULTS

RES Administration Decreased the Elevated Plasma TSH and the Hypothalamic TRH mRNA in SCH Rats

The repeated measures ANOVA revealed that both the treatment [$F(5,140) = 11.975$, $P < 0.001$] and time [$F(3,28) = 76.925$, $P < 0.001$] had a significant effect on the TSH levels, with no significant interaction [$F(5,140) = 0.583$, $P = 0.614$]. When it comes to the T3 levels, the results showed that neither the time [$F(5,140) = 0.555$, $P = 0.461$] nor the treatment [$F(3,28) = 0.673$, $P = 0.574$] had a significant effect, with no significant interaction [$F(5,140) = 0.452$, $P = 0.718$]. Moreover, repeated measures ANOVA revealed a significant interaction between the treatments and weeks in body weight [$F(15,140) = 23.989$, $P < 0.001$]. The individual factor treatment also had a significant effect [$F(5,140) = 26.113$, $P < 0.001$], but the factor time did not [$F(3,28) = 2.509$, $P = 0.122$].

As shown in **Table 1**, before the treatment, SCH rats in the untreated model, RES and LT4 groups showed elevated plasma TSH level [$F(3,28) = 13.263$, $P < 0.01$; LSD: sham vs. untreated model: $P = 0.002$, sham vs. RES: $P < 0.001$, sham vs. LT4: $P < 0.001$] with normal plasma fT4 [$F(3,28) = 0.737$, $P = 0.539$; LSD: sham vs. untreated model: $P = 0.378$, sham vs. RES: $P = 0.689$, sham vs. LT4: $P = 0.876$] and T3 [$F(3,28) = 1.505$, $P = 0.235$; LSD: sham vs. untreated model: $P = 0.778$, sham vs. RES: $P = 0.701$, sham vs. LT4: $P = 0.423$] concentrations compared with the sham ones. After 16 days of treatment, both RES

TABLE 1 | Concentrations of plasma total triiodothyronine (T3), free thyroxine (fT4), thyroid-stimulating hormone (TSH) in sham ($n = 8$), model ($n = 8$), RES ($n = 8$), and LT4 ($n = 8$) before and after treatment.

Group	n	T3 (nmol/L)		fT4 (pmol/L)		TSH (mIU/L)	
		Before	After	Before	After	Before	After
Sham	8	0.78 ± 0.03	0.72 ± 0.04	9.45 ± 0.34	5.78 ± 0.51	0.45 ± 0.06	0.46 ± 0.05
Model	8	0.75 ± 0.04	0.74 ± 0.05	9.44 ± 0.41	6.36 ± 0.40	2.28 ± 0.34**	1.31 ± 0.03**
RES	8	0.78 ± 0.05	0.66 ± 0.16	9.36 ± 0.49	6.84 ± 0.53	2.58 ± 0.29**	0.55 ± 0.09#
LT4	8	0.79 ± 0.02	0.81 ± 0.05	8.91 ± 0.25	15.67 ± 0.85**,##	2.68 ± 0.28**	0.09 ± 0.01##

The data were presented as mean ± SEM.
***P < 0.01 compared with sham group.*
#P < 0.05 and ##P < 0.01 compared with model group.
RES, resveratrol; LT4, levothyroxine.

and LT4 decreased the elevated TSH level of untreated model rats [$F(3,28) = 11.269$, $P < 0.01$; LSD: RES vs. untreated model: $P = 0.028$, LT4 vs. untreated model: $P < 0.01$]. No significant difference was found between sham rats and RES- or LT4-treated rats (LSD: RES vs. sham: $P = 0.213$, LT4 vs. untreated model: $P = 0.711$). Consistent with this result, the hypothalamic mRNA expression of TRH was inhibited by treatment with RES or LT4 [**Figure 2**, $F(3,16) = 6.668$, $P < 0.001$; LSD: RES vs. untreated model: $P = 0.050$, LT4 vs. untreated model: $P = 0.01$, RES vs. sham: $P = 0.221$, LT4 vs. untreated model: $P = 0.611$]. No significant difference was observed between the plasma T3 concentrations of the groups [**Table 1**, $F(3,28) = 2.563$, $P = 0.458$]. LT4, but not RES, increased the plasma fT4 concentrations compared to sham or untreated model rats [**Table 1**, $F(3, 28) = 60.583$, $P < 0.01$; LSD: RES vs. sham: $P = 0.202$; LT4 vs. sham: $P < 0.001$; RES vs. untreated model: $P = 0.340$, LT4 vs. untreated model: $P < 0.001$].

RES Administration Did Not Reverse the Decreased Bodyweight in the SCH Rats

Figure 3A shows the effect of RES on the body weight and behaviors of the SCH rats. Repeated measures ANOVA revealed a significant interaction between the treatments and weeks in body weight [$F(15,140) = 3.707$, $P < 0.01$]. The individual factor weeks also had a significant effect [$F(5,140) = 165.550$, $P < 0.01$], but the factor treatments did not [$F(3,28) = 1.633$, $P = 0.198$]. A significant difference in body weight was noticed in week 5 in the sham rats compared to the untreated model rats [$F(3,28) = 3.179$, $P = 0.035$; LSD: sham vs. untreated model: $P = 0.027$, RES vs. untreated model: $P = 0.785$, LT4 vs. untreated model: $P = 0.745$, RES vs. sham: $P = 0.015$, LT4 vs. untreated model: $P = 0.052$]. However, no change in body weight was observed during the experimental period in the untreated model rats compared to the RES- or LT4-treated rats, indicating that neither drug had an effect on the body weights of untreated model rats.

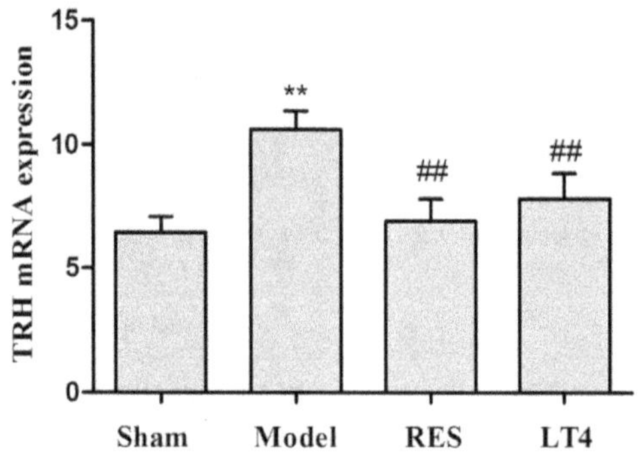

FIGURE 2 | Effect of RES on hypothalamic TRH mRNA expression in the SCH rats. The mRNA expression of TRH in the hypothalamus is illustrated. The data are presented as the means ± SEM, with $n = 8$ for each group. *$P < 0.05$ and **$P < 0.01$ compared to the sham group. #$P < 0.05$ and ##$P < 0.01$ compared to the untreated model group. RES, resveratrol; TRH, thyrotropin-releasing hormone; SCH, subclinical hypothyroidism.

RES Administration Alleviated the Anxiety- and Depressive-Like Behavior in the SCH Rats

The sucrose preference of the untreated model rats was remarkably lower than that of the sham group. Both the RES and LT4 groups showed an elevated sucrose preference index compared to the untreated model rats [**Figure 3B**, $F(3,28) = 6.387$, $P = 0.001$; LSD: RES vs. untreated model: $P = 0.002$, LT4 vs. untreated model: $P = 0.035$, RES vs. sham: $P = 0.849$, LT4 vs. untreated model: $P = 0.224$], indicating an anti-anhedonia effect of RES and LT4.

In the OFT (**Figures 3C–G**), the untreated model group traveled over a shorter total distance [$F(3,28) = 9.983$, $P < 0.01$; LSD: RES vs. untreated model: $P = 0.002$, LT4 vs. untreated model: $P = 0.018$, RES vs. sham: $P = 0.022$, LT4 vs. untreated model: $P = 0.004$] and at a lower velocity [$F(3,28) = 9.987$, $P < 0.01$; LSD: RES vs. untreated model: $P = 0.002$, LT4 vs. untreated model: $P = 0.017$, RES vs. sham: $P = 0.023$, LT4 vs. untreated model: $P = 0.004$] than the sham group, and these measures were ameliorated by the RES and LT4 treatments. These results indicate that both drug treatments improved the SCH rats' locomotor activity. Moreover, a decreased number of rearing was observed in the untreated model rats, and this behavior was increased in the SCH rats treated with RES or LT4 [$F(3,28) = 13.560$, $P < 0.01$; LSD: RES vs. untreated model: $P = 0.001$, LT4 vs. untreated model: $P = 0.008$, RES vs. sham: $P = 0.006$, LT4 vs. untreated model: $P = 0.001$], indicating that both drug treatments improved exploratory behavior. As the total distance and frequency of rearing are also used as measures of anxiety (26), these data revealed that the drug treatments may have decreased the high anxiety levels in the untreated model rats. However, no differences in the number of grooming behaviors and defecations were observed between the SCH rats with and without RES treatment.

In the FST (**Figures 3H–J**), the untreated model rats spent a longer time immobile [$F(3,28) = 4.792$, $P < 0.01$; LSD: RES vs. untreated model: $P = 0.014$, LT4 vs. untreated model: $P = 0.004$, RES vs. sham: $P = 0.351$, LT4 vs. untreated model: $P = 0.646$] and less time swimming [$F(3,28) = 3.557$, $P = 0.023$; LSD: RES vs. untreated model: $P = 0.014$, LT4 vs. untreated model: $P = 0.004$, RES vs. sham: $P = 0.351$, LT4 vs. untreated model: $P = 0.646$], and these changes were reversed by RES or LT4 treatment, indicating that RES alleviated the despairing behavior in the SCH rats.

RES Administration Decreased the Ratio of the Adrenal Gland Weight to Body Weight, Plasma Corticosterone, and Hypothalamic CRH mRNA in SCH Rats

Although the ratio of the adrenal gland weight to body weight was significantly increased in the untreated model rats (**Figure 4A**), both RES and LT4 significantly decreased the ratio compared to the sham group [$F(3,28) = 22.777$, $P < 0.001$; LSD: sham vs. untreated model: $P < 0.001$, RES vs. untreated model: $P < 0.001$, LT4 vs. untreated model: $P < 0.001$, RES vs. sham: $P = 0.011$, LT4 vs. untreated model: $P = 0.604$]. After the hemi-thyroid electrocauterization, plasma corticosterone in the

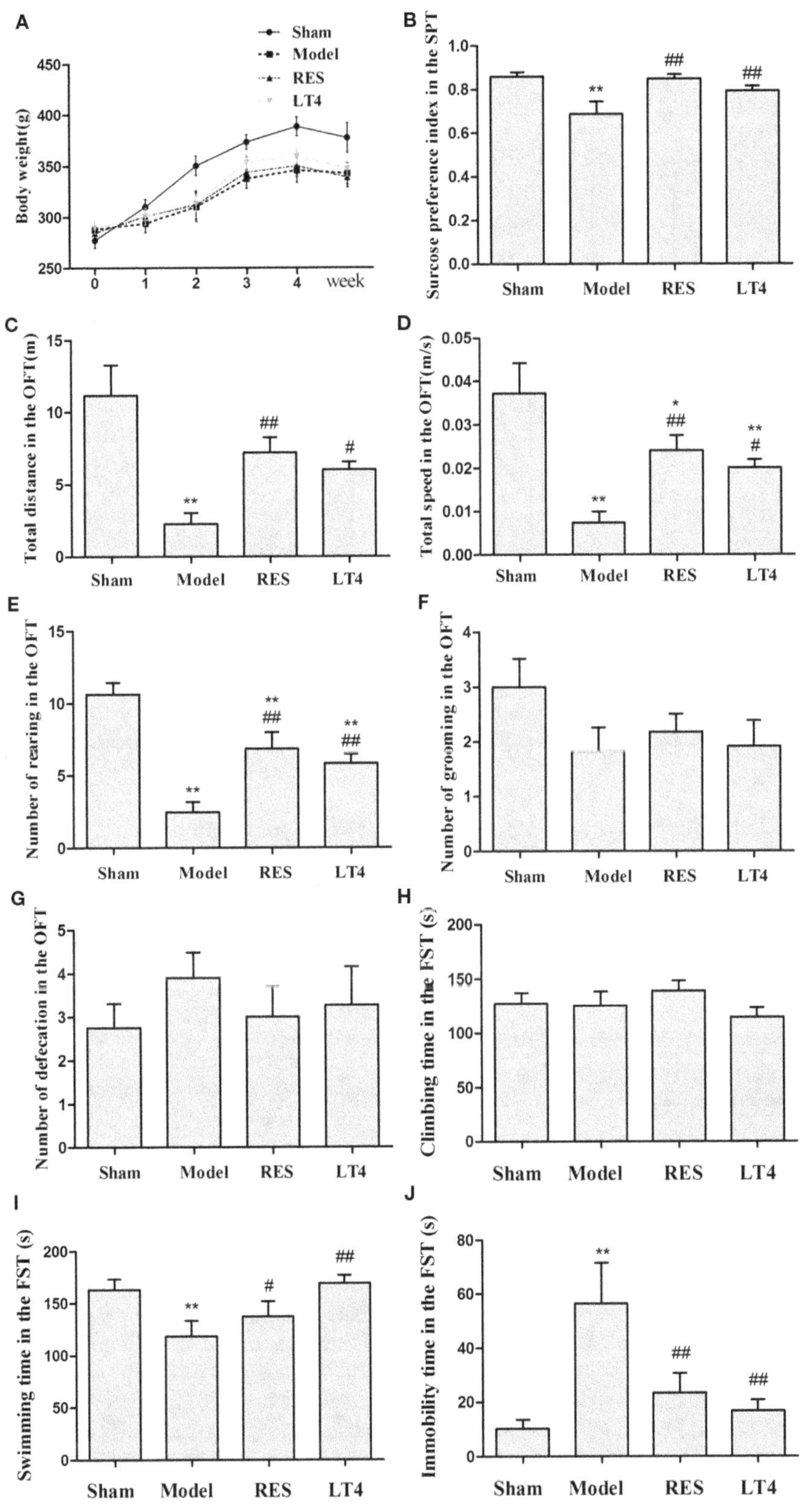

FIGURE 3 | Effect of RES on the body weight and behaviors of the SCH rats. The body weight **(A)**, sucrose preference **(B)**, and performance in the OFT **(C–G)** and FST **(H–J)** were observed. The data are presented as the means ± SEM, with $n = 8$ for each group. $^{*}P < 0.05$ and $^{**}P < 0.01$ compared to the sham group. $^{\#}P < 0.05$ and $^{\#\#}P < 0.01$ compared to the untreated model group. RES, resveratrol; SCH, subclinical hypothyroidism; OFT, open-field test; FST, forced swimming test.

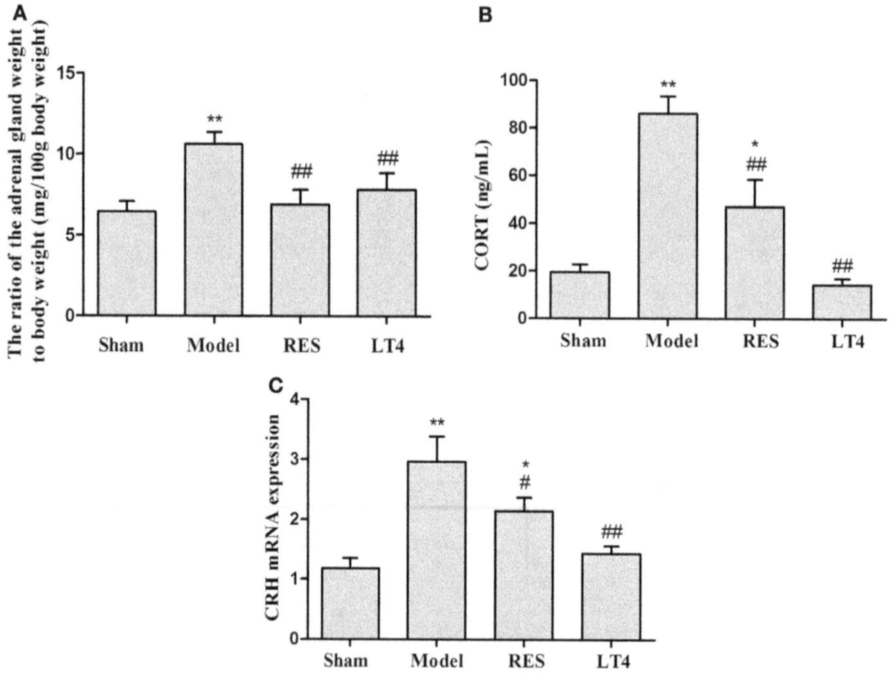

FIGURE 4 | Effects of RES on the ratio of the adrenal gland weight to body weight, the plasma corticosterone, and the expression of CRH mRNA in the hypothalamus in SCH rats. The ratio of the adrenal gland weight to body weight **(A)**, the plasma corticosterone **(B)**, and the expression of CRH mRNA in the hypothalamus **(C)** are shown. The data are presented as the means ± SEM, with $n = 8$ for each group. *$P < 0.05$ and **$P < 0.01$ compared to the sham group. #$P < 0.05$ and ##$P < 0.01$ compared to the untreated model group. RES = resveratrol, SCH = subclinical hypothyroidism, CRH = corticotrophin-releasing hormone.

untreated model rats increased significantly, while treatment with either RES or LT4 decreased the elevated corticosterone levels [**Figure 4B**, $F(3,28) = 19.066$, $P < 0.01$]. In line with this result, the elevated hypothalamic CRH mRNA expression noted in the untreated model rats was decreased by treatment with either RES or LT4 [**Figure 4C**, $F(3,28) = 9.468$, $P < 0.01$].

RES Administration Decreased Activation of the Canonical Wnt Pathway in the Hippocampus of SCH Rats

Figure 5 shows the protein expression levels of GSK-3β, p-GSK-3β (Ser9), β-catenin, p-β-catenin, cyclin D1, and c-myc in rat hippocampi. Compared with those of the sham group, a lower protein expression of p-GSK-3β [**Figure 5A**, $F(3,28) = 23.969$, $P < 0.01$] and relative ratio of p-GSK-3β/GSK-3β [$F(3,28) = 21.902$, $P < 0.01$] and a higher protein expression of GSK-3β [$F(3,28) = 23.673$, $P < 0.01$] were observed in the hippocampus of the untreated model rats, which was reversed by the RES or LT4 treatment.

As shown in **Figure 5B**, a higher protein expression of p-β-catenin [**Figure 5B**, $F(3,28) = 11.322$, $P < 0.01$] and relative ratio of p-β-catenin/β-catenin [**Figure 5B**, $F(3,28) = 11.641$, $P < 0.01$] were observed in the hippocampus of the untreated model rats. Conversely, the protein expression of β-catenin [**Figure 5B**, $F(3,28) = 7.44$, $P = 0.002$] was lower than that of the sham group. These changes were reversed by treatment with RES or LT4.

Consistently, hippocampal protein levels of cyclin D1 [**Figure 5C**, $F(3,28) = 7.457$, $P < 0.01$] and c-myc [$F(3,28) = 8.922$, $P < 0.01$] were lower in the untreated model rats than in the sham ones, but these changes were improved by treatment with RES or LT4. Altogether, these results indicate that the canonical Wnt pathway was activated in the hippocampus of the untreated model rats and that activation was ameliorated by the RES treatment.

Results of Pearson correlation analysis showed that the expressions of p-β-catenin/β-catenin were both negatively correlated to cyclin D1 ($r = -0.566$, $P = 0.004$) or c-myc ($r = -0.565$, $P = 0.004$).

DISCUSSION

In this study, we explored the antidepressant effects of RES in SCH rats. The results showed that RES treatment could alleviate anxiety- and depression-like behavior in SCH rats, as indicated by their increased rearing frequency and moving distance in the OFT, their elevated sucrose preference index, and their decreased immobility in the FST. Moreover, RES treatment improved the imbalance of HPA and HPT axes observed in the SCH rats. Furthermore, RES treatment downregulated activation of the canonical Wnt pathway in the hippocampus of SCH rats.

Subclinical hypothyroidism is a common thyroid dysfunction that occurs in 4–20% of the adult population. The risk of SCH progressing to overt hypothyroidism is approximately 7% (27), and both overt and SCH are associated with an increase in

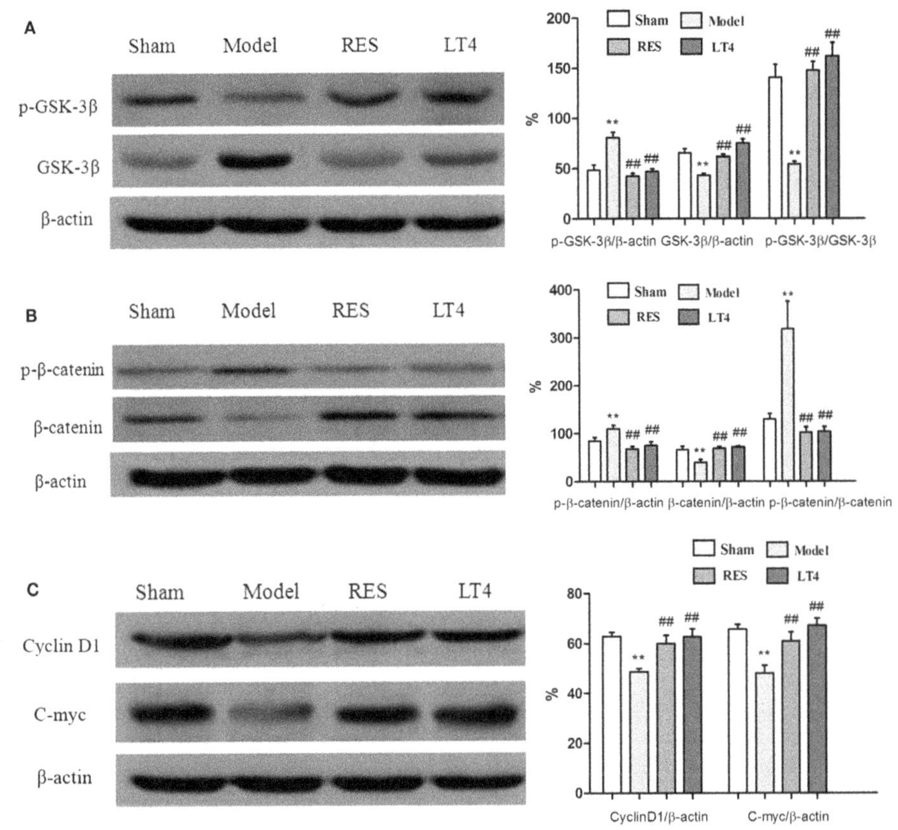

FIGURE 5 | Effects of RES on the activation of the canonical Wnt pathway in the hippocampi of SCH rats. Representative blots and the quantitative analysis of GSK3β and p-GSK3β **(A)**, β-catenin and p-β-catenin **(B)**, cyclin D1 and c-myc **(C)** are presented. The data are presented as the means ± SEM, with $n = 8$ for each group. $^{*}P < 0.05$ and $^{**}P < 0.01$ compared to the sham group. $^{\#}P < 0.05$ and $^{\#\#}P < 0.01$ compared to the untreated model group. RES, resveratrol; SCH, subclinical hypothyroidism.

the number and severity of depressive-like symptoms (28, 29). LT4 is the routine clinical treatment for SCH. In this study, our results show that the imbalance of the HPT axis in SCH rats was improved by the treatment of LT4, as indicated by the decrease of both the plasma TSH and the hypothalamic TRH mRNA expression. However, the possibility of overtreatment is one of the adverse effects of LT4 treatment, and the risk ranges from 14 to 21% (30). Consistently, with a dose parallel to the routine dose used clinically, LT4-treated SCH rats showed significantly higher plasma fT4 concentration than the sham rats in our study.

The adverse side effects of LT4, including the hyperthyroxinemia, make the development of new therapeutic drugs to treat SCH necessary. Recently, a new concept of antidepressant mechanisms of action has been proposed based on the findings that antidepressants showed immediate antioxidant effects in the treatment of major depressive disorder (31). Increasing evidence from animal studies suggests that treatment with antioxidants can reduce oxidative stress and alleviate depressive-like behaviors (32). RES is a polyphenol antioxidant that has versatile biological and pharmacological activities, including neuroprotective effects (19, 33). Our results reveal that treatment with RES decreases both the plasma TSH concentration and the hypothalamic TRH mRNA expression in SCH rats without increasing the plasma concentration of fT4. Although the specific mechanism remains unknown, this effect might be partly attributable to the capacity of RES to regulate TSH secretion by manipulating the levels of SIRT1 (34).

The OFT provides simultaneous measures of locomotion, exploration, and anxiety (26). In this study, the untreated model rats showed a decrease in the total distance traveled and the frequency of rearing in the OFT, which was increased in the SCH rats treated with RES, indicating that RES treatment improved the decreased locomotor activity and exploration in the untreated model rats. Moreover, the decreased total distance traveled and frequency of rearing indicated a higher level of anxiety in the untreated model rats, which may also have been reduced by the treatment with RES and LT4. The SPT is commonly used to assess anhedonia, which is a prominent symptom of depression in rodents. Immobility in the FST is taken as an index of despair behavior, which is another prominent symptom of depression. In this study, the SCH rats showed decreased sucrose preference index in the SPT and increased immobility in the FST, indicating a depression-like behavior in SCH rats, which was consistent with the findings in our previous study (6). Moreover, Detke et al. found that antidepressant drugs, which inhibit norepinephrine reuptake (desipramine or reboxetine) effectively, reduced immobility and selectively increased climbing behavior without affecting swimming, whereas the selective serotonin reuptake inhibitor (SSRI), which works through the serotonin system, reduced immobility and selectively increased swimming, without affecting climbing. In this study, our results showed that both RES and LT4 reduced immobility behaviors in the model rats (35). Thus, it is possible that RES might have an analogous therapeutic effect with the SSRIs in certain types of depression. Further studies are in need to verify the reliability of this hypothesis.

Treatment of thyroid dysfunction could reduce the psychiatric symptoms of depression in general (36), and clinical studies have shown an improvement in depressive-like symptoms after treatment with LT4 in SCH patients (37, 38). Thus, LT4 was selected as a positive control in this study. The results showed the expected antidepressant effect of LT4 on the SCH rats. Similarly, RES-treated rats showed an increased sucrose preference index and decreased immobility in the FST. These results indicate that treatment with RES also alleviated the depression-like behavior of the SCH rats.

Hyperactivity of the HPA axis is one of the most potent factors that trigger depression episodes (39), and abnormalities in HPA axis function are also well documented in rats with hypothyroidism (6). Similarly, the SCH rats displayed elevated adrenal mass, plasma corticosterone, and hypothalamic CRH mRNA expression. However, these changes were ameliorated by treatment with RES. Although RES reportedly stimulated cortisol biosynthesis and secretion in H295R adrenocortical cells *in vitro* (40), our results and other reports indicate that RES reduced the serum corticosterone concentration in stressed rats (11, 14) and unstressed mice (41). This discrepancy about the effect of RES on the HPA axis may be partly ascribed to the different experimental techniques and methods in the different studies.

Studies on human brains have evaluated the levels or activity of total GSK-3β protein in the prefrontal cortex in mood disorders, including depression (22, 42), and increasing evidence suggests that inhibition of GSK-3β might contribute to antidepressant activity (43). Consistent with the report that the enzymatic activity of GSK-3β was increased in depressed suicide victims (42), lower pGSK-3β and pGSK-3β/GSK-3β levels in the hippocampus were found in the SCH rats, which could induce depression-like behavior in this study (6). However, the increased GSK-3β levels were improved by the treatment with RES. L803-mts, a known GSK-3β inhibitor (24), induced an anti-immobility effect in the FST. Moreover, a lower GSK-3β level expressed in heterozygotic GSK-3β$^{+/-}$ mice was associated with reduced immobility time in the FST (44). These results suggest a role for GSK-3β in the antidepressive-like effects of RES and highlight GSK-3β as a potential target in the treatment of SCH-associated depression.

β-catenin, a substrate of GSK-3β (45), has been implicated in brain development, cognitive activity, and dendritic growth (46). Phosphorylation of β-catenin by GSK-3β enhances the degradation of the protein, whereas phosphorylation of GSK-3β stabilizes β-catenin and promotes its accumulation in the cell cytoplasm. The unphosphorylated β-catenin can then migrate into the nucleus, where it associates with transcription factors to stimulate gene expression (47). β-catenin protein levels were lower in the postmortem prefrontal cortices of depressed subjects compared to non-depressed controls (22), and β-catenin levels in the hippocampus can serve as a marker for antidepressant behavior (48). Consistent with these results, the protein levels of p-β-catenin and p-β-catenin/β-catenin were upregulated in the hippocampus of the SCH rats, indicating β-catenin degradation. Together with these reports, the findings from this study reinforce the clinical observation that depressed subjects display a high GSK-3β activation state and low β-catenin levels (22).

Recent studies have demonstrated that cyclin D1 and c-myc, critical genes involved in cell proliferation and differentiation, were important target genes of the Wnt signaling pathway. Overexpression of cyclin D1 and c-myc is highly associated with the accumulation of β-catenin and mutational defects of the Wnt signaling pathway (49). In this study, protein levels of cyclin D1 and c-myc were decreased due to the increased β-catenin protein levels in the SCH rats, which was improved by RES treatment, further confirming the therapeutic effect of RES. Several recent studies have focused on the relationship between β-catenin and cyclin D1 or c-myc. For instance, a strong correlation was reported between β-catenin deregulation and cyclin D1 expression in primary colorectal tumors (50). Brabletz et al. (51) also reported a tight correlation between nuclear β-catenin accumulation and c-myc expression in colorectal adenomas. In this study, the results of Pearson's correlation test suggested a significant positive association between the expression of p-β-catenin/β-catenin and cyclin D1 or c-myc. Based on our findings, the abnormal expression of β-catenin and its associated dysfunction of cyclin D1 and c-myc may play a key role in SCH-associated depression.

In this study, we first observed that RES alleviates depression-like behavior in SCH rats, which may be due to the regulation of HPA and HPT axes and the activity of the Wnt/β-catenin pathway in the hippocampus. Consistent with reports that RES does not cause adverse effects (15, 52), our results confirm that RES does not cause hyperthyroxinemia, which is a potential therapeutic advantage over LT4 treatment. However, this study presented several limitations. First, RES was administered only in a single dose. Thus, its dose relationship and long-term side-effects should be determined using different doses in future studies. Second, considering our previous finding that RES could alleviate the depression-like behavior of CUMS rats, together with the reports that RES treatment does not cause adverse effects (15, 52), we did not administer RES to the sham rats, which might make it subtly difficult to interpret many of the results. Third, although LT4 treatment was selected as a positive control in this study, the effect of RES on the depression-like behavior of the SCH rats was not compared with that of conventional antidepressant medications, such as fluoxetine.

In conclusion, our results demonstrate that RES improved anxiety- and depression-like behavior in SCH rats. This effect may be due, at least in part, to regulation of the HPA and HPT axes and the Wnt/β-catenin pathway in the hippocampus. Compared with the possible adverse effects of LT4 treatment, including cardiovascular events and symptoms associated with excess thyroid hormone, such as nervousness and palpitations (53), the credible efficacy with high safety margins (54, 55) of RES make it a promising candidate for the treatment of SCH-associated depression.

AUTHOR CONTRIBUTIONS

Associate Prof. Jin-Fang Ge and Prof. Fei-Hu Chen designed the study, and wrote the protocol and the first draft of the manuscript. Prof. Jin-Fang Ge and Dr. Ya-Yun Xu managed the literature searches and the statistical analyses. Ya-Yun Xu, Gan Qin, and Jiang-Qun Cheng performed animal model experiments. All authors contributed to and have approved the final manuscript.

REFERENCES

1. He XS, Ma N, Pan ZL, Wang ZX, Li N, Zhang XC, et al. Functional magnetic resource imaging assessment of altered brain function in hypothyroidism during working memory processing. *Eur J Endocrinol* (2011) **164**:951–9. doi:10.1530/EJE-11-0046
2. Zhu DF, Wang ZX, Zhang DR, Pan ZL, He S, Hu XP, et al. fMRI revealed neural substrate for reversible working memory dysfunction in subclinical hypothyroidism. *Brain* (2006) **129**:2923–30. doi:10.1093/brain/awl215
3. Chueire VB, Romaldini JH, Ward LS. Subclinical hypothyroidism increases the risk for depression in the elderly. *Arch Gerontol Geriatr* (2007) **44**:21–8. doi:10.1016/j.archger.2006.02.001
4. Davis JD, Stern RA, Flashman LA. Cognitive and neuropsychiatric aspects of subclinical hypothyroidism: significance in the elderly. *Curr Psychiatry Rep* (2003) **5**:384–90. doi:10.1007/s11920-003-0073-6
5. Almeida C, Brasil MA, Costa AJ, Reis FA, Reuters V, Teixeira P, et al. Subclinical hypothyroidism: psychiatric disorders and symptoms. *Rev Bras Psiquiatr* (2007) **29**:157–9. doi:10.1590/S1516-44462007000200013
6. Ge JF, Peng YY, Qi CC, Chen FH, Zhou JN. Depression-like behavior in subclinical hypothyroidism rat induced by hemi-thyroid electrocauterization. *Endocrine* (2014) **45**:430–8. doi:10.1007/s12020-013-0001-4
7. Bauer M, London ED, Rasgon N, Berman SM, Frye MA, Altshuler LL, et al. Supraphysiological doses of levothyroxine alter regional cerebral metabolism and improve mood in bipolar depression. *Mol Psychiatry* (2005) **10**:456–69. doi:10.1038/sj.mp.4001647
8. Uhl I, Bez JA, Stamm T, Pilhatsch M, Assion HJ, Norra C, et al. Influence of levothyroxine in augmentation therapy for bipolar depression on central serotonergic function. *Pharmacopsychiatry* (2014) **47**:180–3. doi:10.1055/s-0034-1383654
9. Cottart CH, Nivet-Antoine V, Beaudeux JL. Review of recent data on the metabolism, biological effects, and toxicity of resveratrol in humans. *Mol Nutr Food Res* (2014) **58**:7–21. doi:10.1002/mnfr.201200589
10. Shin SM, Cho IJ, Kim SG. Resveratrol protects mitochondria against oxidative stress through AMP-activated protein kinase-mediated glycogen synthase kinase-3beta inhibition downstream of poly(ADP-ribose)polymerase-LKB1 pathway. *Mol Pharmacol* (2009) **76**:884–95. doi:10.1124/mol.109.058479
11. Ge JF, Peng L, Cheng JQ, Pan CX, Tang J, Chen FH, et al. Antidepressant-like effect of resveratrol: involvement of antioxidant effect and peripheral regulation on HPA axis. *Pharmacol Biochem Behav* (2013) **11**(4–115):64–9. doi:10.1016/j.pbb.2013.10.028
12. Hurley LL, Akinfiresoye L, Kalejaiye O, Tizabi Y. Antidepressant effects of resveratrol in an animal model of depression. *Behav Brain Res* (2014) **268**:1–7. doi:10.1016/j.bbr.2014.03.052
13. Krishnan V, Nestler EJ. Animal models of depression: molecular perspectives. *Curr Top Behav Neurosci* (2011) **7**:121–47. doi:10.1007/7854_2010_108
14. Liu D, Zhang Q, Gu J, Wang X, Xie K, Xian X, et al. Resveratrol prevents impaired cognition induced by chronic unpredictable mild stress in rats. *Prog Neuropsychopharmacol Biol Psychiatry* (2014) **49**:21–9. doi:10.1016/j.pnpbp.2013.10.017
15. Poirier GL, Imamura N, Zanoletti O, Sandi C. Social deficits induced by peripubertal stress in rats are reversed by resveratrol. *J Psychiatr Res* (2014) **57**:157–64. doi:10.1016/j.jpsychires.2014.05.017
16. Yu Y, Wang R, Chen C, Du X, Ruan L, Sun J, et al. Antidepressant-like effect of trans-resveratrol in chronic stress model: behavioral and neurochemical evidences. *J Psychiatr Res* (2013) **47**:315–22. doi:10.1016/j.jpsychires.2012.10.018
17. Witte AV, Kerti L, Margulies DS, Floel A. Effects of resveratrol on memory performance, hippocampal functional connectivity, and glucose metabolism in healthy older adults. *J Neurosci* (2014) **34**:7862–70. doi:10.1523/JNEUROSCI.0385-14.2014
18. Chow HH, Garland LL, Heckman-Stoddard BM, Hsu CH, Butler VD, Cordova CA, et al. A pilot clinical study of resveratrol in postmenopausal women with high body mass index: effects on systemic sex steroid hormones. *J Transl Med* (2014) **12**:223. doi:10.1186/s12967-014-0223-0
19. Xu Y, Wang Z, You W, Zhang X, Li S, Barish PA, et al. Antidepressant-like effect of trans-resveratrol: involvement of serotonin and noradrenaline system. *Eur Neuropsychopharmacol* (2010) **20**:405–13. doi:10.1016/j.euroneuro.2010.02.013
20. Brenes Saenz JC, Villagra OR, Fornaguera Trias J. Factor analysis of forced swimming test, sucrose preference test and open field test on enriched, social and isolated reared rats. *Behav Brain Res* (2006) **169**:57–65. doi:10.1016/j.bbr.2005.12.001
21. de Sousa RT, Zanetti MV, Talib LL, Serpa MH, Chaim TM, Carvalho AF, et al. Lithium increases platelet serine-9 phosphorylated GSK-3beta levels in drug-free bipolar disorder during depressive episodes. *J Psychiatr Res* (2015) **62**:78–83. doi:10.1016/j.jpsychires.2015.01.016
22. Karege F, Perroud N, Burkhardt S, Fernandez R, Ballmann E, La Harpe R, et al. Protein levels of beta-catenin and activation state of glycogen synthase kinase-3beta in major depression. A study with postmortem prefrontal cortex. *J Affect Disord* (2012) **136**:185–8. doi:10.1016/j.jad.2011.09.024
23. Voleti B, Duman RS. The roles of neurotrophic factor and Wnt signaling in depression. *Clin Pharmacol Ther* (2012) **91**:333–8. doi:10.1038/clpt.2011.296
24. Kaidanovich-Beilin O, Milman A, Weizman A, Pick CG, Eldar-Finkelman H. Rapid antidepressive-like activity of specific glycogen synthase kinase-3 inhibitor and its effect on beta-catenin in mouse hippocampus. *Biol Psychiatry* (2004) **55**:781–4. doi:10.1016/j.biopsych.2004.01.008
25. Wang L, Shao YY, Ballock RT. Thyroid hormone interacts with the Wnt/beta-catenin signaling pathway in the terminal differentiation of growth plate chondrocytes. *J Bone Miner Res* (2007) **22**:1988–95. doi:10.1359/jbmr.070806
26. Walsh RN, Cummins RA. The open-field test: a critical review. *Psychol Bull* (1976) **83**:482–504. doi:10.1037/0033-2909.83.3.482
27. Cooper DS. Clinical practice. Subclinical hypothyroidism. *N Engl J Med* (2001) **345**:260–5. doi:10.1056/NEJM200107263450406
28. Farmer A, Korszun A, Owen MJ, Craddock N, Jones L, Jones I, et al. Medical disorders in people with recurrent depression. *Br J Psychiatry* (2008) **192**:351–5. doi:10.1192/bjp.bp.107.038380
29. Najafi L, Malek M, Hadian A, Ebrahim Valojerdi A, Khamseh ME, Aghili R. Depressive symptoms in patients with subclinical hypothyroidism – the effect of treatment with levothyroxine: a double-blind randomized clinical trial. *Endocr Res* (2015) **40**(3):121–6. doi:10.3109/07435800.2014.896924
30. Canaris GJ, Manowitz NR, Mayor G, Ridgway EC. The Colorado thyroid disease prevalence study. *Arch Intern Med* (2000) **160**:526–34. doi:10.1001/archinte.160.4.526
31. Behr GA, Moreira JC, Frey BN. Preclinical and clinical evidence of antioxidant effects of antidepressant agents: implications for the pathophysiology

of major depressive disorder. *Oxid Med Cell Longev* (2012) **2012**:609421. doi:10.1155/2012/609421
32. Reus GZ, Dos Santos MA, Abelaira HM, Titus SE, Carlessi AS, Matias BI, et al. Antioxidant treatment ameliorates experimental diabetes-induced depressive-like behavior and reduces oxidative stress in brain and pancreas. *Diabetes Metab Res Rev* (2016) **32**:278–88. doi:10.1002/dmrr.2732
33. Li H, Yan Z, Zhu J, Yang J, He J. Neuroprotective effects of resveratrol on ischemic injury mediated by improving brain energy metabolism and alleviating oxidative stress in rats. *Neuropharmacology* (2011) **60**:252–8. doi:10.1016/j.neuropharm.2010.09.005
34. Akieda-Asai S, Zaima N, Ikegami K, Kahyo T, Yao I, Hatanaka T, et al. SIRT1 regulates thyroid-stimulating hormone release by enhancing PIP5Kgamma activity through deacetylation of specific lysine residues in mammals. *PLoS One* (2010) **5**:e11755. doi:10.1371/journal.pone.0011755
35. Detke MJ, Rickels M, Lucki I. Active behaviors in the rat forced swimming test differentially produced by serotonergic and noradrenergic antidepressants. *Psychopharmacology* (1995) **121**:66–72. doi:10.1007/BF02245592
36. Geffken GR, Ward HE, Staab JP, Carmichael SL, Evans DL. Psychiatric morbidity in endocrine disorders. *Psychiatr Clin North Am* (1998) **21**:473–89. doi:10.1016/S0193-953X(05)70017-4
37. Miller KJ, Parsons TD, Whybrow PC, van Herle K, Rasgon N, van Herle A, et al. Memory improvement with treatment of hypothyroidism. *Int J Neurosci* (2006) **116**:895–906. doi:10.1080/00207450600550154
38. Samuels MH, Schuff KG, Carlson NE, Carello P, Janowsky JS. Health status, psychological symptoms, mood, and cognition in L-thyroxine-treated hypothyroid subjects. *Thyroid* (2007) **17**:249–58. doi:10.1089/thy.2006.0252
39. Swaab DF, Bao AM, Lucassen PJ. The stress system in the human brain in depression and neurodegeneration. *Ageing Res Rev* (2005) **4**:141–94. doi:10.1016/j.arr.2005.03.003
40. Li D, Dammer EB, Sewer MB. Resveratrol stimulates cortisol biosynthesis by activating SIRT-dependent deacetylation of P450scc. *Endocrinology* (2012) **153**:3258–68. doi:10.1210/en.2011-2088
41. Wang Z, Gu J, Wang X, Xie K, Luan Q, Wan N, et al. Antidepressant-like activity of resveratrol treatment in the forced swim test and tail suspension test in mice: the HPA axis, BDNF expression and phosphorylation of ERK. *Pharmacol Biochem Behav* (2013) **112**:104–10. doi:10.1016/j.pbb.2013.10.007
42. Karege F, Perroud N, Burkhardt S, Schwald M, Ballmann E, La Harpe R, et al. Alteration in kinase activity but not in protein levels of protein kinase B and glycogen synthase kinase-3beta in ventral prefrontal cortex of depressed suicide victims. *Biol Psychiatry* (2007) **61**:240–5. doi:10.1016/j.biopsych.2006.04.036
43. Jope RS, Roh MS. Glycogen synthase kinase-3 (GSK3) in psychiatric diseases and therapeutic interventions. *Curr Drug Targets* (2006) **7**:1421–34. doi:10.2174/138945010607011421
44. O'Brien WT, Harper AD, Jove F, Woodgett JR, Maretto S, Piccolo S, et al. Glycogen synthase kinase-3beta haploinsufficiency mimics the behavioral and molecular effects of lithium. *J Neurosci* (2004) **24**:6791–8. doi:10.1523/JNEUROSCI.4753-03.2004
45. Peifer M, Polakis P. Wnt signaling in oncogenesis and embryogenesis – a look outside the nucleus. *Science* (2000) **287**:1606–9. doi:10.1126/science.287.5458.1606
46. Yu X, Malenka RC. Beta-catenin is critical for dendritic morphogenesis. *Nat Neurosci* (2003) **6**:1169–77. doi:10.1038/nn1132
47. Dale TC. Signal transduction by the Wnt family of ligands. *Biochem J* (1998) **329**(Pt 2):209–23. doi:10.1042/bj3290209
48. Pilar-Cuellar F, Vidal R, Pazos A. Subchronic treatment with fluoxetine and ketanserin increases hippocampal brain-derived neurotrophic factor, beta-catenin and antidepressant-like effects. *Br J Pharmacol* (2012) **165**:1046–57. doi:10.1111/j.1476-5381.2011.01516.x
49. Li YJ, Wei ZM, Meng YX, Ji XR. Beta-catenin up-regulates the expression of cyclinD1, c-myc and MMP-7 in human pancreatic cancer: relationships with carcinogenesis and metastasis. *World J Gastroenterol* (2005) **11**:2117–23. doi:10.3748/wjg.v11.i14.2117
50. Yan W, Wu K, Herman JG, Brock MV, Fuks F, Yang L, et al. Epigenetic regulation of DACH1, a novel Wnt signaling component in colorectal cancer. *Epigenetics* (2013) **8**:1373–83. doi:10.4161/epi.26781
51. Brabletz T, Jung A, Dag S, Reu S, Kirchner T. [beta-Catenin induces invasive growth by activating matrix metalloproteinases in colorectal carcinoma]. *Verh Dtsch Ges Pathol* (2000) **84**:175–81.
52. Boocock DJ, Faust GE, Patel KR, Schinas AM, Brown VA, Ducharme MP, et al. Phase I dose escalation pharmacokinetic study in healthy volunteers of resveratrol, a potential cancer chemopreventive agent. *Cancer Epidemiol Biomarkers Prev* (2007) **16**:1246–52. doi:10.1158/1055-9965.EPI-07-0022
53. Helfand M; U.S. Preventive Services Task Force. Screening for subclinical thyroid dysfunction in nonpregnant adults: a summary of the evidence for the U.S. Preventive Services Task Force. *Ann Intern Med* (2004) **140**:128–41. doi:10.7326/0003-4819-140-2-200401200-00015
54. Kumar A, Negi G, Sharma SS. Neuroprotection by resveratrol in diabetic neuropathy: concepts & mechanisms. *Curr Med Chem* (2013) **20**:4640–5. doi:10.2174/09298673113209990151
55. Timmers S, Hesselink MK, Schrauwen P. Therapeutic potential of resveratrol in obesity and type 2 diabetes: new avenues for health benefits? *Ann N Y Acad Sci* (2013) **1290**:83–9. doi:10.1111/nyas.12185

18

In Utero Bisphenol A Exposure Induces Abnormal Neuronal Migration in the Cerebral Cortex of Mice

*Wenting Ling[1], Toshihiro Endo[1], Ken-ichiro Kubo[2], Kazunori Nakajima[2], Masaki Kakeyama[1,3] and Chiharu Tohyama[1,4]**

[1] *Laboratory of Environmental Health Sciences, Center for Disease Biology and Integrative Medicine, Graduate School of Medicine, The University of Tokyo, Tokyo, Japan,* [2] *Department of Anatomy, Keio University School of Medicine, Tokyo, Japan,* [3] *Laboratory for Systems Neuroscience and Preventive Medicine, Faculty of Human Sciences, Waseda University, Tokorozawa, Japan,* [4] *Environmental Biology Laboratory, Faculty of Medicine, University of Tsukuba, Tsukuba, Japan*

Edited by:
Fumihiko Maekawa, National Institute for Environmental Studies, Japan

Reviewed by:
Noriyuki Koibuchi, Gunma University Graduate School of Medicine, Japan
Jaeho Yang, Catholic University of Daegu, South Korea

***Correspondence:**
Chiharu Tohyama
tohyamac-tky@umin.org

Bisphenol A (BPA) has been known to have endocrine-disrupting activity to induce reproductive and behavioral abnormalities in offspring of laboratory animal species. However, morphological basis of this abnormality during brain development is largely unknown. Cerebral cortex plays a crucial role in higher brain function, and its precisely laminated structure is formed by neuronal migration. In the present study, transfecting a plasmid (pCAG-mCherry) by *in utero* electroporation (IUE), we visualized developing neurons and investigated the possible effects of *in utero* BPA exposure on neuronal migration. Pregnant mice were exposed to BPA by osmotic pump at estimated daily doses of 0, 40 (BPA-40), or 400 (BPA-400) µg/kg from embryonic day 14.5 (E14.5) to E18.5. IUE was performed at E14.5 and neuronal migration was analyzed at E18.5. Compared with the control group, neuronal migration in the cortical plate was significantly decreased in the BPA-40 group; however, there was no significant difference in the BPA-400 group. Among several neuronal migration-related genes and cortical layer-specific genes, TrkB in the BPA-400 group was found significantly upregulated. In conclusion, *in utero* exposure to low BPA dose was found to disrupt neuronal migration in the cerebral cortex in a dose-specific manner.

Keywords: bisphenol A, low dose, brain development, cerebral cortex, environmental chemicals, neuronal migration

INTRODUCTION

Bisphenol A (BPA, 4,4′-dihydroxy-2,2-diphenylpropane) is a monomer used worldwide for manufacturing plastics, such as polycarbonates and epoxy resins. Humans are widely exposed to BPA *via* leaching from plastic bottles, sealants for canned food, and other environmental sources. Low

---

Abbreviations: BDNF, brain-derived neurotrophic factor; BPA, bisphenol A; BrdU, 5-bromodeoxyuridine; Cdk5, cyclin-dependent kinase 5; Cux2, cut-like homeobox 2; DISC1, disrupted in schizophrenia 1; E, embryonic day; GAPDH, glyceraldehyde-3-phosphate dehydrogenase; IUE, *in utero* electroporation; Kitl, kit ligand; Lhx2, LIM homeobox protein 2; MAP2, microtubule-associated protein 2; PBS, phosphate-buffered saline; PBST, PBS containing 0.05% Triton X-100; PFA, paraformaldehyde; PND, postnatal day; Slitrk1, SLIT and NTRK-like family, member 1; Tle3, transducin-like enhancer of split 3, homolog of Drosophila E; TrkB, neurotrophic tyrosine kinase, receptor, type 2.

doses of BPA exposure during the perinatal period can result in numerous effects on health, ranging from reversible physiological responses to more long-term adverse effects. Exposure to BPA early in life has been reported to be associated with behavioral problems in children (1–3), presumably due to their limited capacity to metabolize BPA and to the fact that the blood–brain barrier is not fully developed. BPA has also been suggested to have adverse effects on neuronal development in human infants (4). Furthermore, animal studies have shown that offspring born to dams exposed to low doses of BPA during gestation and the early postnatal period had abnormal brain morphologies (5–9). However, the mechanisms by which maternal BPA exposure affects embryonic brain development are still largely unknown.

The laminated structure of the cerebral cortex is formed by highly tuned neuronal migration. Perturbations of this neuronal migration result in neurological and developmental abnormalities. Although neuronal migration has been suggested as a target of chemical exposure, it has not been widely studied in the context of developmental neurotoxicity. A few studies have reported that neuronal migration can be interrupted by environmental chemicals, such as methylmercury (10, 11) and toluene (12). The aim of the present study was to examine the possible effects of prenatal exposure to low doses of BPA on the process of neuronal migration. For this, we used *in utero* electroporation (IUE), a gene-transfer technique that enabled us to introduce fluorescent protein expression vectors into neuronal progenitor cells and visualize the process of migration (13, 14). We found that prenatal exposure to BPA interrupted neuronal migration in the cerebral cortex in a dose-specific manner.

MATERIALS AND METHODS

Pregnant ICR mice were purchased from CLEA Japan (Tokyo, Japan). The day of vaginal plug observation was designated as E0.5. Mice were housed in an animal room maintained at a temperature of 22–24°C, humidity at 40–60%, and under 12-h light/12-h dark cycles (lights on and off at 0800 and 2000 hours, respectively). Food (Labo MR Stock, Nosan, Yokohama, Japan) and water were provided *ad libitum*. Pregnant mice were exposed to BPA (Wako Pure Chemical Ind., Osaka, Japan) at a daily dose equivalent to 0, 40, or 400 μg/kg b.w. from E14.5 to E18.5 by implanting an osmotic pump (Alzet, Micro-Osmotic Pump, Model 1007D, Cupertino, CA, USA) into the peritoneal cavity. According to the doses given to the dams, the control and BPA exposed groups were named as Control, BPA-40, and BPA-400, respectively. The experimental protocols for the animal experiments were approved by the Animal Care and Use Committee of the University of Tokyo.

A plasmid (pCAG-mCherry, a kind gift from Dr. Masanori Matsuzaki at the National Institute for Basic Biology, Okazaki, Japan) was purified using the EndoFree Plasmid Kit (Qiagen K.K., Tokyo, Japan) according to the manufacturer's protocol. The purified plasmid was diluted with phosphate-buffered saline (PBS) to a final concentration of 3 μg/μl before use.

In utero electroporation was performed at E14.5, as described previously (13, 14). Briefly, time-pregnant mice were deeply anesthetized by an intraperitoneal injection of sodium pentobarbital solution (Dainippon Sumitomo Pharma, Osaka, Japan) at a dose of 50 mg/kg b.w. After the uterus was carefully pulled out from the abdominal cavity, an aliquot (approximately 1 μl) of plasmid solution colored by 0.01% fast green was injected into the lateral ventricle of the embryo and was transfected by electroporation (30–35 V, 50 ms, four pulses) using a square wave electroporator (CUY21SC, Nepa Gene Co., Chiba, Japan) with a forceps-type electrode (CUY650P5). The uterus was returned to the abdominal cavity, and an osmotic pump was implanted in the peritoneal cavity, followed by a closure of the abdomen with sutures. In this study, plasmids were successfully transfected into more than half of embryonic brains.

Mice were sacrificed at E18.5. Embryonic brains were collected, fixed with 4% paraformaldehyde (PFA) in PBS overnight at 4°C, and immersed consecutively in 20 and 30% sucrose in PBS at 4°C. Then, brains were embedded in O.C.T. compound (Sakura Finetek, Tokyo, Japan), and stored at −80°C until analysis. Frozen brains were cut into 20 μm thick coronal sections by cryostat (CM3050S, Leica Microsystems K.K., Tokyo, Japan).

To visualize the cortical plate (CP) boundary, microtubule-associated protein 2 (Map2) immunostaining was performed. Briefly, brain tissue sections were washed in PBS containing 0.05% Triton X-100 (PBST) and fixed in 4% PFA for 10 min. After blocking with 3% bovine serum albumins in PBST at room temperature for 1 h, the brain sections were incubated with anti-MAP2 antibodies that were conjugated to Alexa Fluor 488 (Merck Millipore Japan Headquarters, Tokyo, Japan) for 3 h. Following additional washing with PBST, the sections were mounted with 4′,6-diamidino-2-phenylindole (DAPI, Vector Laboratories, Burlingame, CA, USA). Images were acquired using a Leica microscope (DM6000 B, Leica Microsystems K.K.), processed with Neurolucida (MBF Bioscience) and Image-J (NIH) software.

Cell distribution in the CP was evaluated using a bin analysis, as described previously (15). The CP was equally divided into 10 bins in which the bin closest to the ventricle was numbered as Bin 1 and the bin closest to the pia mater was numbered as Bin 10. In each bin, the number of fluorescent cells (mCherry-positive cells) was estimated as a percentage of the total number in all 10 bins, using Image-J software (National Institute of Health, Bethesda, MD, USA). Embryonic brains that were successfully transfected with fluorescent protein vectors were selected for cell migration analysis. One to three brains from each litter were randomly selected, and total two to four litters in each dosed group were analyzed.

For body weight and mRNA analyses, another set of BPA-exposed pregnant mice was used. At PND 0, we checked the litter size and body weight and randomly selected one male from each litter, followed by the analysis of a total of six pups in each dosed group. Forebrains were dissected, snap frozen in liquid nitrogen, and stored at −80°C until analysis.

Total RNAs were extracted using the RNeasy Mini Kit (Qiagen) according to the manufacturer's instructions. cDNA synthesis was performed using the PrimeScript RT reagent Kit (Takara, Otsu, Japan). Quantitative real-time PCR was performed using the Thunderbird qPCR mix (Toyobo, Osaka, Japan) and LightCycler (Roche Diagnostic Co., Tokyo, Japan). Primer design and specificity check were performed by Primer-BLAST (NCBI, Bethesda, MD, USA). The mRNA expression of the target gene in each sample was normalized with glyceraldehyde-3-phosphate dehydrogenase (GAPDH).

For statistical analysis, one-way ANOVA (for litter size, body weight, and mRNA expression) and two-way ANOVA (for neuronal migration) followed by the Tukey–Kramer's *post hoc* test were used. All data are expressed as mean ± SEM. p-Values <0.05 were considered statistically significant.

RESULTS

There was no significant difference in litter size between control dams and BPA-exposed dams. In addition, no statistical differences in body weight were observed between groups for either sex at PND 0 (**Table 1**).

To investigate whether *in utero* BPA exposure affects neuronal migration, IUE was performed at E14.5 to introduce a fluorescent protein expression vector (pCAG-mCherry) into neural progenitor cells, and the distribution of mCherry-positive neurons was analyzed at E18.5 in the three groups (Control, BPA-40, and BPA-400) (**Figure 1A**). At E18.5, mCherry-positive cells were found in ventricular zone (VZ), subventricular zone (SVZ), intermediate zone (IZ), and CP (**Figures 1B,C**). Beneath the subplate (SP), not only mCherry-positive cells but also axons of projection neurons overlapped together exhibiting intense mCherry fluorescent signals, and it was very difficult to differentiate each single mCherry-positive cell from mCherry signals in IZ, so only the mCherry-positive cells migrated into the CP were subjected to a bin analysis to examine the cell distribution in CP (**Figure 1B**). In the control group, the majority of mCherry-positive neurons were located in layers II/III (corresponding to Bins 8 and 9) of the cerebral cortex. In the BPA-40 group, the percentage of mCherry-positive neurons in Bin 9 was significantly lower than that in the control group or the BPA-400 group. There were no significant differences in the distribution of mCherry-positive neurons in the CP between the BPA-400 group and the control group (**Figure 1D**). These data show that prenatal exposure to BPA suppresses neuronal migration in a dose-specific manner.

Neuronal migration is guided by various molecular cues. Thus, we examined the forebrain mRNA expression of genes that are known to be important for neuronal migration and layer formation, such as brain-derived neurotrophic factor (BDNF), neurotrophic tyrosine kinase receptor type 2 (TrkB), Reelin, cyclin-dependent kinase 5 (Cdk5), and disrupted in schizophrenia 1 (DISC1), and the neocortical layer II/III laminar-specific genes, such as transducin-like enhancer of split 3, homolog of Drosophila E (Tle3), kit ligand (Kitl), LIM homeobox protein 2 (Lhx2), cut-like homeobox 2 (Cux2), and SLIT and NTRK-like family, member 1 (Slitrk1) (**Figure 2**). TrkB, a receptor for neurotrophins, was significantly increased in the BPA-400 group

TABLE 1 | Litter size and pup body weight after *in utero* BPA exposure[a].

Group[b]	Litter size			Body weight (g)	
	All pups	Male	Female	Male	Female
Control	14.8 ± 0.8	6.67 ± 0.61	8.17 ± 0.79	1.67 ± 0.05	1.60 ± 0.04
BPA-40	13.7 ± 1.5	5.83 ± 1.10	7.83 ± 1.01	1.81 ± 0.05	1.71 ± 0.05
BPA-400	15.0 ± 0.7	8.50 ± 0.80	6.50 ± 1.09	1.77 ± 0.03	1.69 ± 0.03

[a]*Data are shown as mean ± SEM.*
[b]*n = 6 dams per treatment.*

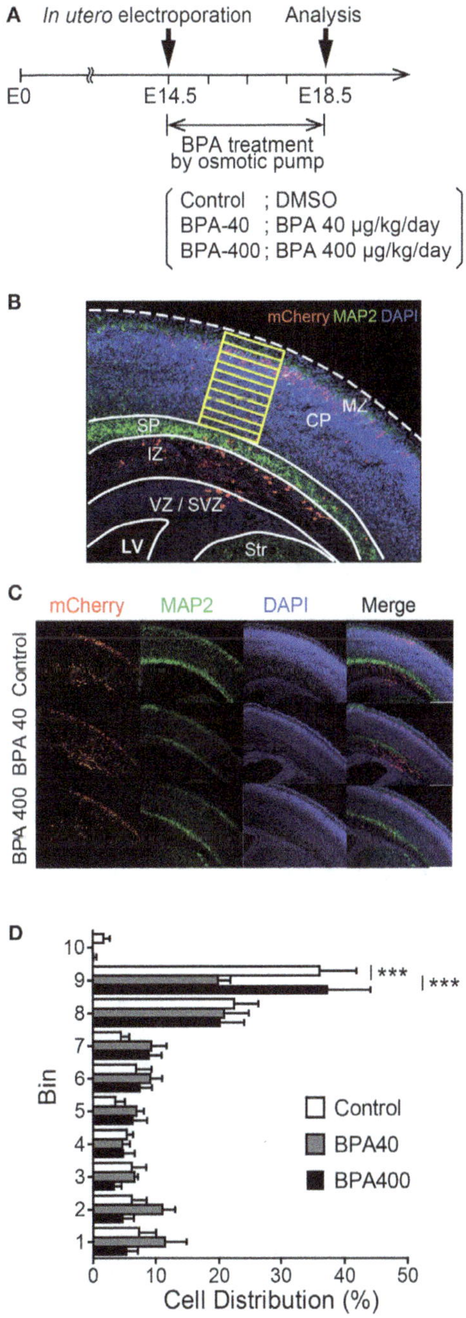

FIGURE 1 | Effects of prenatal BPA exposure on neuronal migration in the developing cerebral cortex. (A) Diagram of the experiment design. **(B)** Bin analysis was performed to evaluate differences in cell distribution. MZ, marginal zone; CP, cortical plate; SP, subplate; IZ, intermediate zone; SVZ, subventricular zone; VZ, ventricular zone; LV, lateral ventricle; Str, striatum. **(C)** Representative photographs of brain sections in the Control, BPA-40, and BPA-400 groups. **(D)** Distribution of mCherry-positive neurons in the CP at E18.5. Data are shown as mean ± SEM, $n = 4$ (control), $n = 5$ (BPA-40), $n = 5$ (BPA-400), $^{***}p < 0.01$.

compared with the control group. No significant difference in the mRNA expression of other genes was observed among the control, BPA-40, and BPA-400 groups.

DISCUSSION

In this study, we used IUE to transfect neural progenitor cells with plasmids that express fluorescent protein, and found that *in utero* low doses of BPA exposure significantly perturbed neuronal migration in the embryonic cerebral cortex in mice. The neurons born in VZ at E14.5 are mostly excitatory projection neurons that undergo radial migration in the cerebral cortex before reaching their final destination in layers II/III. Neurons located in layers II/III are commissural projection neurons extending axons to the opposite hemisphere across the corpus callosum. It has been reported that abnormalities in higher brain function observed in various neurological diseases are considered to be associated with the inappropriate positioning of neurons, which in turn leads to inaccurate projections and impairment of synaptogenesis (16, 17). Thus, it is possible that abnormal neuronal migration observed after low doses of BPA exposure could be a cause of abnormal brain function, but the direct link between delayed neuronal migration and high brain functions warrant future studies.

A previous study reported that BPA exposure from E0.5 at a daily dose of 20 μg/kg b.w. significantly decreased the number of 5-bromodeoxyuridine (BrdU)-positive cells in the VZ at E14.5 and E16.5 and increased the number of BrdU-positive cells in the CP at E14.5 compared with the control group, indicating that prenatal BPA exposure accelerates neuronal migration (18). However, the same research group also reported that when BrdU-positive cells were labeled at E14.5 in mice exposed to BPA *in utero*, there was subsequently a significant increase in labeled cells in cortical layers V and VI and a decrease in labeled cells in layer IV when the brains were examined at postnatal week 3 (19). Another *in vitro* study reported that BPA treatment increased the tangential migration of interneurons in cortical slices (20). In cerebral cortex, inhibitory neurons and excitatory neurons are born at different time periods and different places. Inhibitory neurons are born in the ganglionic eminence and migrate tangentially, whereas excitatory neurons are born in the VZ and migrate radially. The differences between results from previous studies and our study may be due to different exposure durations, doses, and neuronal types studied. The present study showed that the prenatal BPA exposure suppressed radial migration of excitatory neurons in the developing cerebral cortex.

The daily doses of 40 and 400 μg/kg used in this study are low doses compared with 5 mg/kg/day, which is regarded as the cutoff dose for low-dose effects regardless of the exposure route and duration (21). The observation of the present study, an abnormal neuronal migration in the mouse embryonic brain, can be added to the list of toxic phenotypes induced by low doses of BPA. Our study provides an example of a dose-specific response to BPA, as shown by the distinct disturbance of neural migration in the BPA-40 group that was absent in the BPA-400 group. A number of previous studies have investigated the effects of low doses of BPA and have shown that the dose–response curve has an inverted U-shape (22, 23). BPA can bind to the estrogen receptor and

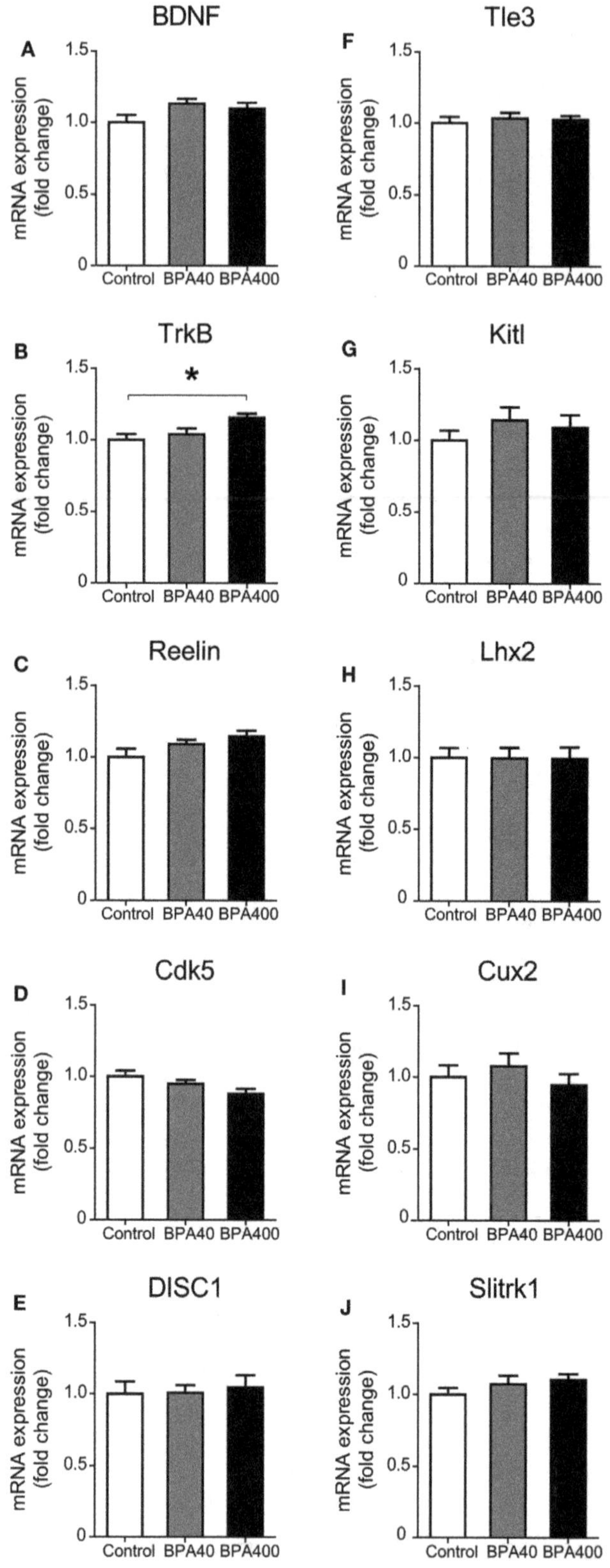

FIGURE 2 | mRNA expression of neuronal migration-related genes [BDNF (A), TrkB (B), Reelin (C), Cdk5 (D), and DISC1(E)] and cortical layer-specific genes [Tle3 (F), Kitl (G), Lhx2 (H), Cux2 (I), and Slitrk1 (J)] in mouse forebrain. Data are shown as mean ± SEM, $n = 6$ per treatment, $^{*}p < 0.05$.

has been shown to have estrogenic properties. As hormones are known to act in a non-monotonic dose–response manner, the low-dose-specific response to BPA may be regulated by interactions between BPA and hormone receptors (22, 23). For further study, the mode of action of BPA needs to be studied extending a dose range that includes multiple lower BPA doses.

In order to investigate the molecular basis of BPA-induced impairment of neuronal migration observed in the developing brain, we analyzed several migration guidance genes and neuron-specific markers for layer II/III. We identified a significantly enhanced gene expression of TrkB upon high dose BPA exposure. TrkB is a receptor for neurotrophins, which mediate neuronal migration, differentiation, and survival through beneficial trophic effects (24). Therefore, a plausible explanation for the dose-specific effects of BPA on neuronal migration would be that compensatory mechanisms may have been triggered in the BPA-400 group, such that higher TrkB expression minimized the effects of BPA exposure on neuronal migration. However, in order to elucidate mechanisms of BPA-induced abnormal neuronal migration, gene expressions of other neurotrophins (NGF, NT3, and NT4/5) and receptors (Trk A and Trk C) in specific brain regions, such as CP, need to be investigated in future studies. Migration guidance genes, such as Reelin, and several layer II/III-specific genes did not show any significant differences in expression between the control and BPA-40 groups. Because of the limited time point of the determination of mRNA levels on PND 0, it can be speculated that BPA may have disrupted expression of layer-specific genes in later time points. A recent study showed that perinatal exposure to BPA in mice at levels relevant to those exposed to humans transgenerationally altered behaviors and gene expression in brains, including expression of genes for several estrogen receptors, oxytocin, and vasopressin (25). Another recent study (9) showed reduction in overall length and branching number of basal dendrites of hippocampal CA1 pyramidal neurons in 3-week-old mouse pups, and spine densities in aged mice, both of which were born to dams administered BPA (40 or 400 μg/kg per day) during gestation. However, in the present study, we did not find any altered expression in genes, except TrkB as described above, that are relevant to neuronal migration or morphogenesis in BPA-exposed groups. The link of micromorphologically altered neuronal development with the molecular basis warrants prospective studies.

AUTHOR CONTRIBUTIONS

WL, TE, MK, and CT conceived this study. WL and TE performed experiments. WL analyzed experimental data. WL, TE, MK, and CT interpreted the data. K-iK and KN provided guidance and technical supports on IUE. WL and CT wrote the manuscript.

ACKNOWLEDGMENTS

This work was supported in part by grants from the Food Safety Commission Japan (No. 0902) and JSPS Kakenhi (No. 24221003) to CT and from the Strategic Research Program for Brain Sciences to KN. English language editing by Enago is greatly appreciated.

REFERENCES

1. Harley KG, Gunier RB, Kogut K, Johnson C, Bradman A, Calafat AM, et al. Prenatal and early childhood bisphenol A concentrations and behavior in school-aged children. *Environ Res* (2013) **126**:43–50. doi:10.1016/j.envres.2013.06.004
2. Hong SB, Hong YC, Kim JW, Park EJ, Shin MS, Kim BN, et al. Bisphenol A in relation to behavior and learning of school-age children. *J Child Psychol Psychiatry* (2013) **54**:890–9. doi:10.1111/jcpp.12050
3. Evans SF, Kobrosly RW, Barrett ES, Thurston SW, Calafat AM, Weiss B, et al. Prenatal bisphenol A exposure and maternally reported behavior in boys and girls. *Neurotoxicology* (2014) **45**:91–9. doi:10.1016/j.neuro.2014.10.003
4. Yang CW, Chou WC, Chen KH, Cheng AL, Mao IF, Chao HR, et al. Visualized gene network reveals the novel target transcripts Sox2 and Pax6 of neuronal development in trans-placental exposure to bisphenol A. *PLoS One* (2014) **9**:e100576. doi:10.1371/journal.pone.0100576
5. Elsworth JD, Jentsch JD, Vandevoort CA, Roth RH, Jr DE, Leranth C. Prenatal exposure to bisphenol A impacts midbrain dopamine neurons and hippocampal spine synapses in non-human primates. *Neurotoxicology* (2013) **35**:113–20. doi:10.1016/j.neuro.2013.01.001
6. Mathisen GH, Yazdani M, Rakkestad KE, Aden PK, Bodin J, Samuelsen M, et al. Prenatal exposure to bisphenol A interferes with the development of cerebellar granule neurons in mice and chicken. *Int J Dev Neurosci* (2013) **31**:762–9. doi:10.1016/j.ijdevneu.2013.09.009
7. Sadowski RN, Wise LM, Park PY, Schantz SL, Juraska JM. Early exposure to bisphenol A alters neuron and glia number in the rat prefrontal cortex of adult males, but not females. *Neuroscience* (2014) **279**:122–31. doi:10.1016/j.neuroscience.2014.08.038
8. Tiwari SK, Agarwal S, Chauhan LK, Mishra VN, Chaturvedi RK. Bisphenol-A impairs myelination potential during development in the hippocampus of the rat brain. *Mol Neurobiol* (2015) **51**:1395–416. doi:10.1007/s12035-014-8817-3
9. Kimura E, Matsuyoshi C, Miyazaki W, Benner S, Hosokawa M, Yokoyama K, et al. Prenatal exposure to bisphenol A impacts neuronal morphology in the hippocampal CA1 region in developing and aged mice. *Arch Toxicol* (2015). doi:10.1007/s00204-015-1485-x
10. Fahrion JK, Komuro Y, Li Y, Ohno N, Littner Y, Raoult E, et al. Rescue of neuronal migration deficits in a mouse model of fetal Minamata disease by increasing neuronal Ca2+ spike frequency. *Proc Natl Acad Sci U S A* (2012) **109**:5057–62. doi:10.1073/pnas.1120747109
11. Guo BQ, Yan CH, Cai SZ, Yuan XB, Shen XM. Low level prenatal exposure to methylmercury disrupts neuronal migration in the developing rat cerebral cortex. *Toxicology* (2013) **304**:57–68. doi:10.1016/j.tox.2012.11.019
12. Gospe SM Jr, Zhou SS. Prenatal exposure to toluene results in abnormal neurogenesis and migration in rat somatosensory cortex. *Pediatr Res* (2000) **47**:362–8. doi:10.1203/00006450-200003000-00013
13. Tabata H, Nakajima K. Efficient in utero gene transfer system to the developing mouse brain using electroporation: visualization of neuronal migration in the developing cortex. *Neuroscience* (2001) **103**:865–72. doi:10.1016/S0306-4522(01)00016-1
14. Tabata H, Nakajima K. Labeling embryonic mouse central nervous system cells by in utero electroporation. *Dev Growth Differ* (2008) **50**:507–11. doi:10.1111/j.1440-169X.2008.01043.x
15. Tomita K, Kubo K, Ishii K, Nakajima K. Disrupted-in-schizophrenia-1 (Disc1) is necessary for migration of the pyramidal neurons during mouse hippocampal development. *Hum Mol Genet* (2011) **20**:2834–45. doi:10.1093/hmg/ddr194
16. Tomasi D, Volkow ND. Abnormal functional connectivity in children with attention-deficit/hyperactivity disorder. *Biol Psychiatry* (2012) **71**:443–50. doi:10.1016/j.biopsych.2011.11.003
17. Maximo JO, Cadena EJ, Kana RK. The implications of brain connectivity in the neuropsychology of autism. *Neuropsychol Rev* (2014) **24**:16–31. doi:10.1007/s11065-014-9250-0

18. Nakamura K, Itoh K, Yaoi T, Fujiwara Y, Sugimoto T, Fushiki S. Murine neocortical histogenesis is perturbed by prenatal exposure to low doses of bisphenol A. *J Neurosci Res* (2006) **84**:1197–205. doi:10.1002/jnr.21020
19. Nakamura K, Itoh K, Sugimoto T, Fushiki S. Prenatal exposure to bisphenol A affects adult murine neocortical structure. *Neurosci Lett* (2007) **420**:100–5. doi:10.1016/j.neulet.2007.02.093
20. Yeo M, Berglund K, Hanna M, Guo JU, Kittur J, Torres MD, et al. Bisphenol A delays the perinatal chloride shift in cortical neurons by epigenetic effects on the Kcc2 promoter. *Proc Natl Acad Sci U S A* (2013) **110**:4315–20. doi:10.1073/pnas.1300959110
21. Melnick R, Lucier G, Wolfe M, Hall R, Stancel G, Prins G, et al. Summary of the national toxicology program's report of the endocrine disruptors low-dose peer review. *Environ Health Perspect* (2002) **110**:427–31. doi:10.1289/ehp.02110427
22. Welshons WV, Thayer KA, Judy BM, Taylor JA, Curran EM, vom Saal FS. Large effects from small exposures. I. Mechanisms for endocrine-disrupting chemicals with estrogenic activity. *Environ Health Perspect* (2003) **111**:994–1006. doi:10.1289/ehp.5494
23. Vandenberg LN. Non-monotonic dose responses in studies of endocrine disrupting chemicals: bisphenol A as a case study. *Dose Response* (2014) **12**:259–76. doi:10.2203/dose-response.13-020.Vandenberg
24. Medina DL, Sciarretta C, Calella AM, Von Bohlen Und Halbach O, Unsicker K, Minichiello L. TrkB regulates neocortex formation through the Shc/PLCgamma-mediated control of neuronal migration. *EMBO J* (2004) **23**:3803–14. doi:10.1038/sj.emboj.7600399
25. Wolstenholme JT, Edwards M, Shetty SR, Gatewood JD, Taylor JA, Rissman EF, et al. Gestational exposure to bisphenol A produces transgenerational changes in behaviors and gene expression. *Endocrinology* (2012) **153**:3828–38. doi:10.1210/en.2012-1195

19

Therapeutic Use of Non-invasive Brain Stimulation in Dystonia

Angelo Quartarone[1,2], Vincenzo Rizzo[3], Carmen Terranova[3], Alberto Cacciola[2], Demetrio Milardi[1,2], Alessandro Calamuneri[1], Gaetana Chillemi[3] and Paolo Girlanda[3]*

[1] Department of Biomedical, Dental Sciences and Morphological and Functional Images, University of Messina, Messina, Italy, [2] Centro Neurolesi Bonino Pulejo (IRCCS), Messina, Italy, [3] Department of Clinical and Experimental Medicine, University of Messina, Messina, Italy

Edited by:
Takashi Hanakawa,
National Center of Neurology and Psychiatry, Japan

Reviewed by:
Shinichi Furuya,
Sony Computer Science Laboratories, Japan
Christian K. E. Moll,
University Medical Center Hamburg-Eppendorf, Germany

***Correspondence:**
Angelo Quartarone
aquartar65@gmail.com

Repetitive transcranial magnetic stimulation (rTMS) and transcranial direct current stimulation (tDCS) are non-invasive methods for stimulating cortical neurons that have been increasingly used in the neurology realm and in the neurosciences applied to movement disorders. In addition, these tools have the potential to be delivered as clinically therapeutic approach. Despite several studies support this hypothesis, there are several limitations related to the extreme variability of the stimulation protocols, clinical enrolment and variability of rTMS and tDCS after effects that make clinical interpretation very difficult. Aim of the present study will be to critically discuss the state of art therapeutically applications of rTMS and tDCS in dystonia.

Keywords: dystonia, neuroplasticity, transcranial magnetic stimulation, basal ganglia, non-invasive brain stimulation

INTRODUCTION

Dystonia can be defined as a "movement disorder characterized by sustained or intermittent muscle contractions causing abnormal, often repetitive, movements, postures, or both" (Albanese et al., 2013).

Dystonia encompasses a heterogeneous group of syndromes that can be classified per the anatomical distribution in: focal, segmental, multifocal, hemidystonia, and generalized dystonia.

In addition, according to the etiology, dystonia can be categorized in inherited (i.e., autosomal dominant, recessive, X-linked, or mitochondrial), acquired (i.e., vascular, iatrogenic, neoplastic, traumatic, or psychogenic) and idiopathic (sporadic or familiar) (Albanese et al., 2013).

The pathophysiology of dystonia remains highly speculative although clinical heterogeneity suggests that it may be a multifactorial disease.

The paucity of symptomatic animal models is one of the reason why dystonia pathophysiology remains largely obscure (Raike et al., 2005).

Recent developed symptomatic animal models have also established the critical role of the cerebellum in dystonia, suggesting that basal ganglia and cerebellum are nodes in an integrated network that is dysfunctional in dystonia (Wilson and Hess, 2013; Richter and Richter, 2014; Pappas et al., 2015). Dystonia treatment can only partially alleviate symptoms and mainly relies on the injection of botulinum toxin in the hyperactive muscles, while the use of levodopa, anticholinergic and antiepileptic drugs has been proven to be largely ineffective (Albanese et al., 2015).

Deep brain stimulation (DBS) of the internal portion of globus pallidus (GPi) is the gold-standard of functional neurosurgical interventions for dystonia in the most severe patients and there are several evidences providing its efficacy and safety (Moro et al., 2017). On the other hand, it remains an invasive procedure so that alternative treatments are needed (Albanese et al., 2015).

In the last few years, gamma-knife and focused ultrasound lesions, which do not require surgical incision of the skull, have challenged the routine application of both the classic radiofrequency lesions and DBS. However, the application of dystonia is very limited (Higuchi et al., 2016).

Finally, transcranial magnetic stimulation (TMS) has been used in the last 20 years to explore non-invasively cortical excitability, shedding also important new insights into the pathophysiology of dystonia (Quartarone and Hallett, 2013).

In addition, TMS is a valuable technique that can be potentially used for diagnostic and therapeutic purposes in dystonia. However, the inter-subject variability in the TMS after-effects and the different pathophysiological mechanisms in the different form of dystonia, have limited diagnostic and therapeutic applications. Nevertheless, TMS can be used to differentiate between organic and psychogenic dystonia (Quartarone et al., 2009).

TMS has been proposed as noninvasive treatment in focal hand dystonia, where pharmacological options or injections of botulinum toxin are often ineffective. Finally, TMS can be considered as an adjuvant treatment in patients with cervical dystonia in conjunction with botulinum remaining the gold standard of treatment.

Hence in the present narrative review, we will describe how TMS can be used as therapeutic tool in dystonia in comparison with other noninvasive brain techniques such as transcranial direct current stimulation (tDCS).

NON-INVASIVE BRAIN STIMULATION TECHNIQUES

TMS and tDCS can stimulate the cerebral cortex painlessly through the intact skull and can produce long lasting changes in cortical excitability.

TMS was originally conceived as a non-invasive method to test the efficiency of motor pathways from the cortex to spinal cord (Rothwell, 1997).

Several experimental evidences suggest that TMS activates axons of the excitatory and inhibitory interneurons that synapse into pyramidal output neurons. In this way, the responsiveness to TMS may represent an indirect measure of the excitability of intrinsic cortical circuits. TMS can also produce long lasting changes in cortical excitability when the pulses are delivered in a repetitive fashion (Siebner and Rothwell, 2003).

Several protocols of non-invasive brain stimulation (NIBS) have been used in the last 20 years, the most common of whom are: repetitive TMS (rTMS), theta-burst stimulation (TBS) and tDCS. In all these cases, electromyography (EMG) amplitude of the motor evoked potentials (MEP) in response to single TMS stimulus is used as read out of the induced cortical plasticity.

The after effects of rTMS depend on the frequency of stimulation employed: if the pulses are given at frequency of 5 Hz or higher they facilitate excitability, whereas at frequency of 1 Hz, or lower, they depress excitability for at least 30–60 min (Quartarone et al., 2006). Thetaburst stimulation (TBS) is a protocol translated from animal studies characterized by repetitive sequences where short bursts are applied in the frequency range of EEG theta rhythms.

There are two main protocols i) the intermittent TBS (iTBS) which has facilitatory effects and ii) the continuous TBS (cTBS) which instead produces inhibitory effects. Their effect can be long lasting, up to 1 h, after the end of the conditioning protocol (Huang et al., 2005).

tDCS takes advantage of a weak polarizing direct current (1–2 mA) applied via small electrodes on the intact scalp. Several experimental evidences suggest that this small current is sufficient to polarize neurons changing their firing frequency. Anodal stimulation tends to increase cortical excitability while cathodal tends to decrease it (Nitsche and Paulus, 2001).

NIBS has been used to explore therapeutic opportunities in a bewildering variety of neurological conditions. It is now clear that, in order to get more tangible clinical effects, repeated rTMS sessions are needed (Khedr et al., 2005).

The mechanisms of action of TMS responsible for the long-lasting effects on cortical excitability are still sketchy. Changes in the effectiveness of synapses between cortical neurons such as long term depression (LTD) and long term potentiation (LTP) have been postulated based on pharmacological studies in humans. Indeed, the after effects of rTMS are abolished by a single dose of the NMDA antagonist dextromethorphan (Stefan et al., 2002). Similarly, another NMDA-antagonist, the memantine can block the after effects of some rTMS protocols (Huang et al., 2007). In addition the LTD-like depression produced by PAS10 is abolished by nimodipine, an L-type voltage-gated-Ca^{2+}-channel blocker (Weise et al., 2017). Finally, several evidences suggest that TMS modulation of BDNF-TrkB pathway could play a permissive role in determining the NMDA dependent after-effects on synaptic plasticity (Wang et al., 2011).

PATHOPHYSIOLOGY OF DYSTONIA AND THERAPEUTIC NIBS

Since dystonia etiology is very heterogeneous, dystonia pathophysiology can be a very complex puzzle (Marsden et al., 1985).

Despite the basal ganglia have been traditionally involved in dystonia, several evidences in animal models and in humans studies suggest that dystonia can be considered a network disorder (Quartarone and Hallett, 2013).

However, although it is tempting to locate the neuronal damage to a single node of the cortico-sub-cortical loop, there are now compelling evidences suggesting that, in a network perspective, it is also important to consider how remote healthy nodes of the brain may react and rearrange themselves in response to the primary damage. Such plastic reorganization may be either adaptive, compensatory, or maladaptive thus worsening the deficit (Quartarone and Hallett, 2013).

In keeping with this hypothesis, increased glucose metabolism over the striatum and anatomically related cortical motor regions such as supplementary motor area (SMA), lateral premotor cortex (PMC), anterior cingulate cortex (ACC) and dorsolateral prefrontal cortex (DLPCF) have been reported (Lerner et al., 2004; Asanuma et al., 2005).

However, several evidences suggest also an involvement of the cerebellar cortex and its direct connections with the basal ganglia and the motor cortex (Neumann et al., 2015; Cacciola et al., 2016, 2017; Milardi et al., 2016). This hypothesis is also supported by some neurophysiological data showing an abnormal cerebellar modulation over motor cortex in dystonic patients (Brighina et al., 2009).

Since dystonic patients have not overt cerebellar signs such as incoordination, loss of balance or falling, it has been postulated a compensative role of cerebellum thus pointing it out as a good candidate for therapeutic neuromodulation.

THERAPEUTIC APPROACHES IN DYSTONIA: STATE OF ART

In keeping with the pathophysiological considerations discussed above, NIBS has been applied over primary motor cortex (M1), PMC, ACC and the cerebellar cortex which are important relays of the cortico-striatal and cerebello-thalamic loops.

Since TMS affects the superficial layers of the cerebral cortex it is unlikely that it may stimulate directly basal ganglia structures. On the other hand, it has been demonstrated that rTMS over the human PFC may exert remote effects on the ipsilateral caudate nucleus via a cortico-striatal release of dopamine (Strafella et al., 2001). In addition rTMS over M1 induces a reduction in raclopride binding in the left putamen if compared with rTMS of the left occipital cortex (Strafella et al., 2003).

Therefore, it can be hypothesized that some of the potential therapeutic action in movement disorders are mediated by remote sub-cortical effects.

One possible strategy in dystonia is an increase of inhibitory mechanisms. In keeping with this hypothesis, it has been reported that 30 min of inhibitory low frequency stimulation over M1 may reduce writing pressure for at least 3 h in patients with focal hand dystonia (FHD) (Siebner et al., 1999).

Similarly, 1 Hz rTMS over PMC improved handwriting velocity and hand discomfort during writing (Tyvaert et al., 2006). In addition, the effect of rTMS was compared in three different motor areas including PMC in patients with FHD. This study revealed that rTMS (20 min 0.2 Hz rTMS) over PMC is more effective than M1 and SMA repetitive stimulation (Murase et al., 2005). The clinical effects were paralleled by increased cortical inhibition as indexed by a prolonged cortical silent period (Murase et al., 2005). In the same study the authors did not report any therapeutic effect of rTMS over M1 (Murase et al., 2005); the discrepancy with the study of Siebner could be due to the different parameters of stimulation (Siebner et al., 1999).

A similar beneficial effect was obtained in a subsequent study employing cTBS over the left PMC which however did not restore deficient inhibitory mechanisms (Veugen et al., 2013).

The beneficial effects of PMC stimulation are in keeping with an open trial of epidural PMC stimulation after at least 1 month of stimulation (Lalli et al., 2012).

Another study has used rTMS over PMC (Lefaucheur et al., 2004), however the lack of a placebo arm makes the interpretation of data very difficult. In this study the authors applied inhibitory rTMS over PMC for 5 consecutive days in patients with generalized secondary dystonia showing a significant clinical effect as indexed by the reduction of the Burke-Fahn-Marsden scale (Lefaucheur et al., 2004).

It is interesting to note that the parameters of cortical excitability, tested with TMS, can be used as prognostic markers of response to rTMS. For instance, it has been reported that only patients with a modulation of cortical inhibition do respond to rTMS treatment (Kimberley et al., 2015).

Altogether, these data suggest a potential therapeutic role of rTMS over PMC. The efficacy of PMC neuromodulation is not surprising considering that PMC is implicated in sensory-motor integration and motor learning.

Another potential target of stimulation is the somatosensory cortex (SCC). It has been indeed shown that 5 Hz rTMS may enhance tactile discrimination in healthy subjects (Ragert et al., 2003). In addition, it has been widely reported that patients with FHD have significant alterations of sensory-motor integration (Quartarone et al., 2003) as well as distortion of the fingers representation map in SCC (Butterworth et al., 2003).

High frequency stimulation over SCC is not beneficial in FHD, with no effect on tactile discrimination in comparison to controls (Schneider et al., 2010). In addition, it is interesting to note that the improvement of tactile discrimination in healthy controls after rTMS, was associated with an increased connectivity in the stimulated SCC, bilateral PMC and basal ganglia, which was not the case in FHD. Therefore, it can be postulated that a cortical-subcortical disconnection may be the basis of the ineffectiveness of rTMS (Schneider et al., 2010).

In another placebo controlled study, low frequency 1 Hz stimulation was delivered over SCC 30 min per day for 4 consecutive weeks in 15 patients affected by writer's cramp (Havrankova et al., 2010). The procedure was successful only in 4 out of 15 patients and was strictly related to the precise coil localization of a narrow strip over the post central sulcus (Havrankova et al., 2010).

ACC has been used as another potential target since this area has an increased activation with PET studies in patients with blepharospasm (Ceballos-Baumann and Brooks, 1998; Kerrison et al., 2003). Low frequency stimulation (0.2 Hz), delivered in a randomized controlled study, can significantly reduce eye blink rate, the number of sustained blinks and the time to eye closure (Kranz et al., 2009). This clinical effects was associated with a normalization of the blink recovery cycle (Kranz et al., 2010).

A new appealing target for NIBS is cerebellum since several evidences suggest that the cerebellum may play a compensatory role in dystonia (Jinnah and Hess, 2006; Quartarone and Hallett, 2013).

In a randomized controlled study, iTBS was delivered bilaterally over the cerebellum for 5 consecutive days for 2 weeks in 20 right handed patients affected by cervical dystonia.

This protocol induced a transient improvement of dystonia and was paralleled by a restoration of the topographic specificity of PAS with a disappearance of the facilitation on Fist Dorsal Interosseus (FDI) (Koch et al., 2014).

On the other hand, tDCS has brought conflicting results, in one study tDCS over the cerebellum was successful in FHD (Bradnam et al., 2015), while in other study it did not work (Sadnicka et al., 2014).

Similarly cathodal tDCS tested over M1 in a randomized double blind sham-controlled study was not successful in a population of writer's cramp patients and musicians cramp (Benninger et al., 2011; Buttkus et al., 2011).

Finally, since there is an enhanced sensory-motor integration, another feasible strategy is to provide independent inputs from dystonic muscles via an asynchronous afferent stimulation avoiding any temporal coupling of the evoked afferent inputs (Schabrun et al., 2009).

The idea is that a period of asynchronous afferent stimulation or non-associative stimulation (NAS) may reverse maladaptive cortical changes and alleviate symptoms.

By using a NAS protocol consisting of asynchronous electrical stimuli (never delivered together with a random inter-stimulus interval ranging from 0.15 to 2.85 as well as with stimulus intensity set to evoke a tiny muscle contraction) applied to the motor points of FDI and abductor pollicis brevis (APB) for 1 h, it has been demonstrated in FHD patients that NAS transiently normalizes the distorted motor map and can significantly reduce movement variability during cycling drawing (Schabrun et al., 2009).

LIMITATIONS AND FUTURE PERSPECTIVES

There are several factors that that strongly limit the interpretation of results after rTMS studies.

Perhaps the most important limitation is the lack of an optimal placebo condition, the so called sham condition. In theory, tilting the coil should dramatically reduce the biological effects of TMS, however several modeling studies in animals are now suggesting that tilting the coil over the skull does not exclude the possibility of a tiny cortical activation (Lisanby et al., 2001).

On the other hand, by using shield equipped coils and a tilt of 90 degrees it is possible to minimize the effective magnetic field (Duecker and Sack, 2013).

Another not risible issue is that active rTMS, besides its cortical effects, is associated with a characteristic click sound and a stimulation of trigeminal afferents. Therefore, to mimic click sound and trigeminal stimulation new dedicated sham shielded coils have been designed with a delivered magnetic field of only 10% compared to active coils.

Another limitation is that most of the studies have addressed primary dystonia while the therapeutic effect of NIBS in secondary dystonia is still unknown.

Despite therapeutic cerebellar stimulation is promising, the gold standard in dystonia is targeting the motor areas strictly connected with basal ganglia (Bharath et al., 2015).

The major limitation of all these studies are the small sample size, the presence of different phenotypes in the same cohort of patients, as well as the fact that several different parameters of stimulation have been adopted across studies.

Despite this extreme variability, it looks like that to be successful NIBS needs to be delivered in a multisession design. Some single session studies have shown positive results that however were not persistent (Murase et al., 2005; Furuya et al., 2014).

There are other possible confounding factors such as preliminary exercise, time of the day and concomitant medications (Ridding and Ziemann, 2010).

Finally, in most studies, stimulation was not performed under neuronavigation to maintain an adequate coil position during stimulation sessions.

Nevertheless, these preliminary results reinforce the idea that NIBS can represent a promising alternative therapeutic opportunity in dystonia.

Several recommendations could be considered in future therapeutic trials: first, it will be important in future studies to determine the best stimulation target, second to use multisession designs with neuronavigation and finally to increase the sample size with multicenter approaches. Another requirement is to design more efficient stimulation protocols to prolong the therapeutic effects. Last but not list, rTMS could be used, soon, to pre-select possible candidates to invasive surgical stimulation approaches.

AUTHOR CONTRIBUTIONS

AQ: work conception and design, drafting the work, work revision, final approval, and global agreement. VR: data interpretation, work revision, final approval, and global agreement. CT, AlbC, DM, AleC: work conception and design, work revision, final approval, GC: data interpretation, drafting the work. PG: work conception and design, guarantor of integrity of entire study, manuscript revision for important intellectual content, final approval.

REFERENCES

Albanese, A., Bhatia, K., Bressman, S. B., Delong, M. R., Fahn, S., Fung, V. S. C., et al. (2013). Phenomenology and classification of dystonia: a consensus update. *Mov. Disord.* 28, 863–873. doi: 10.1002/mds.25475

Albanese, A., Romito, L. M., and Calandrella, D. (2015). Therapeutic advances in dystonia. *Mov. Disord.* 30, 1547–1556. doi: 10.1002/mds.26384

Asanuma, K., Carbon-Correll, M., and Eidelberg, D. (2005). Neuroimaging in human dystonia. *J. Med. Invest.* 52 (Suppl.), 272–279. doi: 10.2152/jmi.52.272

Benninger, D. H., Lomarev, M., Lopez, G., Pal, N., Luckenbaugh, D. A., and Hallett, M. (2011). Transcranial direct current stimulation for the treatment of focal hand dystonia. *Mov. Disord.* 26, 1698–1702. doi: 10.1002/mds.23691

Bharath, R. D., Munivenkatappa, A., Gohel, S., Panda, R., Saini, J., Rajeswaran, J., et al. (2015). Recovery of resting brain connectivity ensuing mild traumatic brain injury. *Front. Hum. Neurosci.* 9:513. doi: 10.3389/fnhum.2015.00513

Bradnam, L. V., Graetz, L. J., McDonnell, M. N., and Ridding, M. C. (2015). Anodal transcranial direct current stimulation to the cerebellum improves handwriting and cyclic drawing kinematics in focal hand dystonia. *Front. Hum. Neurosci.* 9:286. doi: 10.3389/fnhum.2015.00286

Brighina, F., Romano, M., Giglia, G., Saia, V., Puma, A., Giglia, F., et al. (2009). Effects of cerebellar TMS on motor cortex of patients with focal dystonia: a preliminary report. *Exp. Brain Res.* 192, 651–656. doi: 10.1007/s00221-008-1572-9

Butterworth, S., Francis, S., Kelly, E., McGlone, F., Bowtell, R., and Sawle, G. V. (2003). Abnormal cortical sensory activation in dystonia: An fMRI study. *Mov. Disord.* 18, 673–682. doi: 10.1002/mds.10416

Buttkus, F., Baur, V., Jabusch, H. C., De La Cruz Gomez-Pellin, M., Paulus, W., Nitsche, M. A., et al. (2011). Single-session tDCS-supported retraining does not improve fine motor control in musician's dystonia. *Restor. Neurol. Neurosci.* 29, 85–90. doi: 10.3233/RNN-2011-0582

Cacciola, A., Milardi, D., Livrea, P., Flace, P., Anastasi, G., and Quartarone, A. (2017). The Known and Missing Links Between the Cerebellum, Basal Ganglia, and Cerebral Cortex. *Cerebellum* 16, 753–755. doi: 10.1007/s12311-017-0850-0

Cacciola, A., Milardi, D., and Quartarone, A. (2016). Role of cortico-pallidal connectivity in the pathophysiology of dystonia. *Brain* 139:e48. doi: 10.1093/brain/aww102

Ceballos-Baumann, A. O., and Brooks, D. J. (1998). Activation positron emission tomography scanning in dystonia. *Adv. Neurol.* 78, 135–152.

Duecker, F., and Sack, A. T. (2013). Pre-Stimulus Sham TMS Facilitates Target Detection. *PLoS ONE* 8:e57765. doi: 10.1371/journal.pone.0057765

Furuya, S., Nitsche, M. A., Paulus, W., and Altenmüller, E. (2014). Surmounting retraining limits in Musicians' dystonia by transcranial stimulation. *Ann. Neurol.* 75, 700–707. doi: 10.1002/ana.24151

Havrankova, P., Jech, R., Walker, N. D., Operto, G., Tauchmanova, J., Vymazal, J., et al. (2010). Repetitive TMS of the somatosensory cortex improves writer's cramp and enhances cortical activity. *Neuroendocrinol. Lett.* 31, 73–86.

Higuchi, Y., Matsuda, S., and Serizawa, T. (2016). Gamma knife radiosurgery in movement disorders: indications and limitations. *Mov. Disord.* 32, 28–35. doi: 10.1002/mds.26625

Huang, Y.-Z., Chen, R.-S., Rothwell, J. C., and Wen, H.-Y. (2007). The after-effect of human theta burst stimulation is NMDA receptor dependent. *Clin. Neurophysiol.* 118, 1028–1032. doi: 10.1016/j.clinph.2007.01.021

Huang, Y. Z., Edwards, M. J., Rounis, E., Bhatia, K. P., and Rothwell, J. C. (2005). Theta burst stimulation of the human motor cortex. *Neuron* 45, 201–206. doi: 10.1016/j.neuron.2004.12.033

Jinnah, H. A., and Hess, E. J. (2006). A new twist on the anatomy of dystonia: the basal ganglia and the cerebellum? *Neurology* 67, 1740–1741. doi: 10.1212/01.wnl.0000246112.19504.61

Kerrison, J. B., Lancaster, J. L., Zamarripa, F. E., Richardson, L. A., Morrison, J. C., Holck, D. E. E., et al. (2003). Positron emission tomography scanning in essential blepharospasm. *Am. J. Ophthalmol.* 136, 846–852. doi: 10.1016/S0002-9394(03)00895-X

Khedr, E. M., Ahmed, M. A., Fathy, N., and Rothwell, J. C. (2005). Therapeutic trial of repetitive transcranial magnetic stimulation after acute ischemic stroke. *Neurology* 65, 466–468. doi: 10.1212/01.wnl.0000173067.84247.36

Kimberley, T. J., Borich, M. R., Schmidt, R. L., Carey, J. R., and Gillick, B. (2015). Focal hand dystonia: individualized intervention with repeated application of repetitive transcranial magnetic stimulation. *Arch. Phys. Med. Rehabil.* 96, S122–S128. doi: 10.1016/j.apmr.2014.07.426

Koch, G., Porcacchia, P., Ponzo, V., Carrillo, F., Cáceres-Redondo, M. T., Brusa, L., et al. (2014). Effects of two weeks of cerebellar theta burst stimulation in cervical dystonia patients. *Brain Stimul.* 7, 564–572. doi: 10.1016/j.brs.2014.05.002

Kranz, G., Shamim, E. A., Lin, P. T., Kranz, G. S., and Hallett, M. (2010). Transcranial magnetic brain stimulation modulates blepharospasm: a randomized controlled study. *Neurology* 75, 1465–1471. doi: 10.1212/WNL.0b013e3181f8814d

Kranz, G., Shamim, E. A., Lin, P. T., Kranz, G. S., Voller, B., and Hallett, M. (2009). Blepharospasm and the modulation of cortical excitability in primary and secondary motor areas. *Neurology* 73, 2031–2036. doi: 10.1212/WNL.0b013e3181c5b42d

Lalli, S., Piacentini, S., Franzini, A., Panzacchi, A., Cerami, C., Messina, G., et al. (2012). Epidural premotor cortical stimulation in primary focal dystonia: clinical and 18F-fluoro deoxyglucose positron emission tomography open study. *Mov. Disord.* 27, 533–538. doi: 10.1002/mds.24949

Lefaucheur, J. P., Fnelon, G., Mnard-Lefaucheur, I., Wendling, S., and Nguyen, J. P. (2004). Low-frequency repetitive TMS of premotor cortex can reduce painful axial spasms in generalized secondary dystonia: A pilot study of three patients. *Neurophysiol. Clin.* 34, 141–145. doi: 10.1016/j.neucli.2004.07.003

Lerner, A., Shill, H., Hanakawa, T., Bushara, K., Goldfine, A., and Hallett, M. (2004). Regional cerebral blood flow correlates of the severity of writer's cramp symptoms. *Neuroimage* 21, 904–913. doi: 10.1016/j.neuroimage.2003.10.019

Lisanby, S. H., Gutman, D., Luber, B., Schroeder, C., and Sackeim, H. A. (2001). Sham TMS: Intracerebral measurement of the induced electrical field and the induction of motor-evoked potentials. *Biol. Psychiatry* 49, 460–463. doi: 10.1016/S0006-3223(00)01110-0

Marsden, C. D., Obeso, J. A., Zarranz, J. J., and Lang, A. E. (1985). The anatomical basis of symptomatic hemidystonia. *Brain* 108, 463–483. doi: 10.1093/brain/108.2.463

Milardi, D., Arrigo, A., Anastasi, G., Cacciola, A., Marino, S., Mormina, E., et al. (2016). Extensive direct subcortical cerebellum-basal ganglia connections in human brain as revealed by constrained spherical deconvolution tractography. *Front. Neuroanat.* 10:29. doi: 10.3389/fnana.2016.00029

Moro, E., LeReun, C., Krauss, J. K., Albanese, A., Lin, J. P., Walleser Autiero, S., et al. (2017). Efficacy of pallidal stimulation in isolated dystonia: a systematic review and meta-analysis. *Eur. J. Neurol.* 24, 552–560. doi: 10.1111/ene.13255

Murase, N., Rothwell, J. C., Kaji, R., Urushihara, R., Nakamura, K., Murayama, N., et al. (2005). Subthreshold low-frequency repetitive transcranial magnetic stimulation over the premotor cortex modulates writer's cramp. *Brain* 128, 104–115. doi: 10.1093/brain/awh315

Neumann, W. J., Jha, A., Bock, A., Huebl, J., Horn, A., Schneider, G. H., et al. (2015). Cortico-pallidal oscillatory connectivity in patients with dystonia. *Brain* 138, 1894–1906. doi: 10.1093/brain/awv109

Nitsche, M. A., and Paulus, W. (2001). Sustained excitability elevations induced by transcranial DC motor cortex stimulation in humans. *Neurology* 57, 1899–1901. doi: 10.1212/WNL.57.10.1899

Pappas, S. S., Darr, K., Holley, S. M., Cepeda, C., Mabrouk, O. S., Wong, J. M. T., et al. (2015). Forebrain deletion of the dystonia protein torsinA causes dystonic-like movements and loss of striatal cholinergic neurons. *Elife* 4:e08352. doi: 10.7554/eLife.08352

Quartarone, A., Bagnato, S., Rizzo, V., Siebner, H. R., Dattola, V., Scalfari, A., et al. (2003). Abnormal associative plasticity of the human motor cortex in writer's cramp. *Brain* 126, 2586–2596. doi: 10.1093/brain/awg273

Quartarone, A., and Hallett, M. (2013). Emerging concepts in the physiological basis of dystonia. *Mov. Disord.* 28, 958–967. doi: 10.1002/mds.25532

Quartarone, A., Rizzo, V., Terranova, C., Morgante, F., Schneider, S., Ibrahim, N., et al. (2009). Abnormal sensorimotor plasticity in organic but not in psychogenic dystonia. *Brain* 132, 2871–2877. doi: 10.1093/brain/awp213

Quartarone, A., Siebner, H. R., and Rothwell, J. C. (2006). Task-specific hand dystonia: can too much plasticity be bad for you? *Trends Neurosci.* 29, 192–199. doi: 10.1016/j.tins.2006.02.007

Ragert, P., Dinse, H. R., Pleger, B., Wilimzig, C., Frombach, E., Schwenkreis, P., et al. (2003). Combination of 5 Hz repetitive transcranial magnetic stimulation (rTMS) and tactile coactivation boosts tactile discrimination in humans. *Neurosci. Lett.* 348, 105–108. doi: 10.1016/S0304-3940(03)00745-6

Raike, R. S., Jinnah, H. A., and Hess, E. J. (2005). Animal models of generalized dystonia. *NeuroRx* 2, 504–512. doi: 10.1602/neurorx.2.3.504

Richter, F., and Richter, A. (2014). Genetic animal models of dystonia: common features and diversities. *Prog. Neurobiol.* 121, 91–113. doi: 10.1016/j.pneurobio.2014.07.002

Ridding, M. C., and Ziemann, U. (2010). Determinants of the induction of cortical plasticity by non-invasive brain stimulation in healthy subjects. *J. Physiol.* 588, 2291–2304. doi: 10.1113/jphysiol.2010.190314

Rothwell, J. C. (1997). Techniques and mechanisms of action of transcranial stimulation of the human motor cortex. *J. Neurosci. Methods* 74, 113–122. doi: 10.1016/S0165-0270(97)02242-5

Sadnicka, A., Hamada, M., Bhatia, K. P., Rothwell, J. C., and Edwards, M. J. (2014). Cerebellar stimulation fails to modulate motor cortex plasticity in writing dystonia. *Mov. Disord.* 29, 1304–1307. doi: 10.1002/mds.25881

Schabrun, S. M., Stinear, C. M., Byblow, W. D., and Ridding, M. C. (2009). Normalizing motor cortex representations in focal hand dystonia. *Cereb. Cortex* 19, 1968–1977. doi: 10.1093/cercor/bhn224

Schneider, S. A., Pleger, B., Draganski, B., Cordivari, C., Rothwell, J. C., Bhatia, K. P., et al. (2010). Modulatory effects of 5Hz rTMS over the primary somatosensory cortex in focal dystonia - An fMRI-TMS Study. *Mov. Disord.* 25, 76–83. doi: 10.1002/mds.22825

Siebner, H. R., and Rothwell, J. (2003). Transcranial magnetic stimulation: new insights into representational cortical plasticity. *Exp. Brain Res.* 148, 1–16. doi: 10.1007/s00221-002-1234-2

Siebner, H. R., Tormos, J. M., Ceballos-Baumann, A. O., Auer, C., Catala, M. D., Conrad, B., et al. (1999). Low-frequency repetitive transcranial magnetic stimulation of the motor cortex in writer's cramp. *Neurology* 52, 529–537.

Stefan, K., Kunesch, E., Benecke, R., Cohen, L. G., and Classen, J. (2002). Mechanisms of enhancement of human motor cortex excitability induced by interventional paired associative stimulation. *J. Physiol.* 543, 699–708. doi: 10.1113/jphysiol.2002.023317

Strafella, A. P., Paus, T., Barrett, J., and Dagher, A. (2001). Repetitive transcranial magnetic stimulation of the human prefrontal cortex induces dopamine release in the caudate nucleus. *J. Neurosci.* 21, 1–4.

Strafella, A. P., Paus, T., Fraraccio, M., and Dagher, A. (2003). Striatal dopamine release induced by repetitive transcranial magnetic stimulation of the human motor cortex. *Brain* 126, 2609–2615. doi: 10.1093/brain/awg268

Tyvaert, L., Houdayer, E., Devanne, H., Monaca, C., Cassim, F., and Derambure, P. (2006). The effect of repetitive transcranial magnetic stimulation on dystonia: a clinical and pathophysiological approach. *Neurophysiol. Clin.* 36, 135–143. doi: 10.1016/j.neucli.2006.08.007

Veugen, L. C., Hoffland, B. S., Stegeman, D. F., and Van De Warrenburg, B. P. (2013). Inhibition of the dorsal premotor cortex does not repair surround inhibition in writer's cramp patients. *Exp. Brain Res.* 225, 85–92. doi: 10.1007/s00221-012-3350-y

Wang, H.-Y., Crupi, D., Liu, J., Stucky, A., Cruciata, G., Di Rocco, A., et al. (2011). Repetitive transcranial magnetic stimulation enhances BDNF–TrkB signaling in both brain and lymphocyte. *J. Neurosci.* 31, 11044–11054. doi: 10.1523/JNEUROSCI.2125-11.2011

Weise, D., Mann, J., Rumpf, J.-J., Hallermann, S., and Classen, J. (2017). Differential regulation of human paired associative stimulation-induced and theta-burst stimulation-induced plasticity by L-type and T-type Ca^{2+} channels. *Cereb. Cortex* 27, 4010–4021. doi: 10.1093/cercor/bhw212

Wilson, B. K., and Hess, E. J. (2013). Animal models for dystonia. *Mov. Disord.* 28, 982–989. doi: 10.1002/mds.25526

20

Avian Test Battery for the Evaluation of Developmental Abnormalities of Neuro- and Reproductive Systems

Takaharu Kawashima[1*], *Walaa M. S. Ahmed*[2,3], *Koki Nagino*[1,4], *Takayoshi Ubuka*[4,5] *and Kazuyoshi Tsutsui*[4]

[1] Center for Environmental Biology and Ecosystem Studies, National Institute for Environmental Studies, Tsukuba, Japan, [2] Center for Environmental Health Sciences, National Institute for Environmental Studies, Tsukuba, Japan, [3] Department of Clinical Pathology, Faculty of Veterinary Medicine, Beni-Suef University, Beni-Suef, Egypt, [4] Laboratory of Integrative Brain Sciences, Department of Biology and Center for Medical Life Science, Waseda University, Tokyo, Japan, [5] Jeffrey Cheah School of Medicine and Health Sciences, Brain Research Institute Monash Sunway, Monash University Malaysia, Bandar Sunway, Malaysia

Edited by:
Kazuaki Nakamura,
National Research Institute for Child Health and Development, Japan

Reviewed by:
Ei-Ichi Izawa,
Keio University, Japan
Takashi Bungo,
Hiroshima University, Japan

***Correspondence:**
Takaharu Kawashima
kawataka@nies.go.jp

Most of the currently used toxicity assays for environmental chemicals use acute or chronic systemic or reproductive toxicity endpoints rather than neurobehavioral endpoints. In addition, the current standard approaches to assess reproductive toxicity are time-consuming. Therefore, with increasing numbers of chemicals being developed with potentially harmful neurobehavioral effects in higher vertebrates, including humans, more efficient means of assessing neuro- and reproductive toxicity are required. Here we discuss the use of a Galliformes-based avian test battery in which developmental toxicity is assessed by means of a combination of chemical exposure during early embryonic development using an embryo culture system followed by analyses after hatching of sociosexual behaviors such as aggression and mating and of visual memory via filial imprinting. This Galliformes-based avian test battery shows promise as a sophisticated means not only of assessing chemical toxicity in avian species but also of assessing the risks posed to higher vertebrates, including humans, which are markedly sensitive to nervous or neuroendocrine system dysfunction.

Keywords: embryo culture system, sociosexual behavior, imprinting behavior, developmental neurotoxicity, Galliformes

INTRODUCTION

Avian experimental models are an important tool for elucidating fundamental principles in research fields such as embryology, endocrinology, genetics, neurology, and ethology (Le Douarin, 2004; Stern, 2005; Emery, 2006; Nakamori et al., 2013). Since the embryos of common Galliformes such as the chicken *(Gallus gallus domesticus)* and Japanese quail (*Coturnix japonica*) can easily be observed and directly manipulated during embryogenesis, they have become the model organisms most widely used in developmental biology (Le Douarin and Dieterlen-Lièvre, 2013; Nakamura and Funahashi, 2013; Sato, 2013; Suzuki, 2013). Recently, Japanese quail has also been used as a model organism in neurophysiological and neuroendocrine studies of sociosexual behavior (Ubuka et al., 2013; Ubuka and Tsutsui, 2014).

Recently, it has been suggested that similarities exist between mammals and birds in the sex differentiation of core sexual behaviors that is induced by gonadal hormones during embryonic development (Maekawa et al., 2014). Furthermore, Clayton and Emery (2015) have proposed that avian experimental models for human cognition could be adapted for studying the neural basis of complex cognition; reasoning, e.g., mean flexibility, problem solving, prospection, and declarative knowledge, and understanding the evolution and neurobiology of cognition, e.g. specific cognitive functions and critical roles of the avian and mammalian brain. Thus, avian experimental models represent a potentially powerful platform for elucidating the developmental mechanisms of the nervous and reproductive systems in higher vertebrates, including humans.

The negative effects of endocrine-disrupting chemicals, such as pesticides and herbicides, on neurodevelopmental processes and reproductive functions in wildlife and humans have been known for over a quarter of a century (Colborn et al., 1993; Lewis and Ford, 2012). Recently, house dust and flame retardants have also been identified as endocrine-disrupting chemicals (Suzuki et al., 2013). It has been proposed that endocrine-disrupting chemicals exert greater toxic effects during periods when organisms are more sensitive to hormonal disruption, such as during the intrauterine, perinatal, and juvenile periods and during puberty (Frye et al., 2012).

The existing developmental neurotoxicity tests have been carried out for some chemicals such as pesticides and their effects have been studied. However, there are problems to correspond to the large number of new chemicals because of high costs, long test period and high numbers of pregnant laboratory mammals used. Moreover, for inspection of embryonic development, the mothers have to be sacrificed which are of ethical concern (Lu et al., 2014). Therefore, simpler and alternative methods are desired. Avian culture techniques using embryonic tissues may offer certain advantages over *in vivo* experiments especially when developmental toxicity is anticipated (Neubert, 1982). The avian models are advantageous at three points in comparison to the conventional mammalian model for the assessment of the developmental toxicity: (1) direct manipulation, (2) continuous observation, and (3) reduction of unnecessary sacrifices of the pregnant individuals. In conventional developmental toxicity studies, the toxic effects of test compounds are examined in fetuses by using pregnant model organisms, such as rats and mice. However, avian embryos may be a better platform than mammalian embryos because the former can be observed and manipulated directly. Moreover, innovative avian embryo culture systems (ECSs) now allow continuous quantitative observations after administration of the test compound (Perry, 1988; Kawashima et al., 2005). Avian models also have ethical advantages because mammalian toxicity tests usually require sacrifice of the pregnant animals prior to examination of embryonic development, whereas avian models do not.

To allow more detailed evaluation of the neuro- and reproductive toxicities of environmental chemicals, new neurobehavioral endpoints in avian test models, such as sex differentiation in the gonads and brain, need to be established. Here we discuss the usefulness of an avian test battery with Galliformes for the assessment of developmental toxicity by using a combination of chemical exposure during early embryonic development by using an ECS followed by analyses after hatching of sociosexual behaviors such as aggression and mating and of visual memory via filial imprinting. Although, avian model systems are already commonly used in basic research (Le Douarin and Dieterlen-Lièvre, 2013; Nakamura and Funahashi, 2013), this article presents one of most alternative solutions as the evaluation of developmental abnormalities of neuro- and reproductive systems.

AVIAN BIORESOURCES

Genetically homogeneous inbred strains of rats or mice are often used in toxicity studies to ensure reproducibility of the experimental results. However, no fully genetically inbred avian strains are currently available. It has now been more than half a century since the Japanese quail was evaluated and recommended as a laboratory animal by Padgett and Ivey (1959), and since then the Japanese quail has become of high value to researchers, especially those in the fields of embryology and physiology, because of its hardiness, ease of handling, precocity, and high egg productivity. In 1980, our group at the National Institute for Environmental Studies (NIES), Japan, began developing a closed colony of Japanese quail with the goal of establishing a new experimental model organism. This Japanese quail is maintained by means of rotational crossbreeding (**Figure 1A**) and is fixed with a yellow-brown plumage color mutation (**Figures 1B,C**). This strain is named NIES-L as mentioned below.

Recently, a draft genome sequence of the NIES-L quail was produced by means of next-generation sequencing, and 100 microsatellite markers have been developed as useful tools

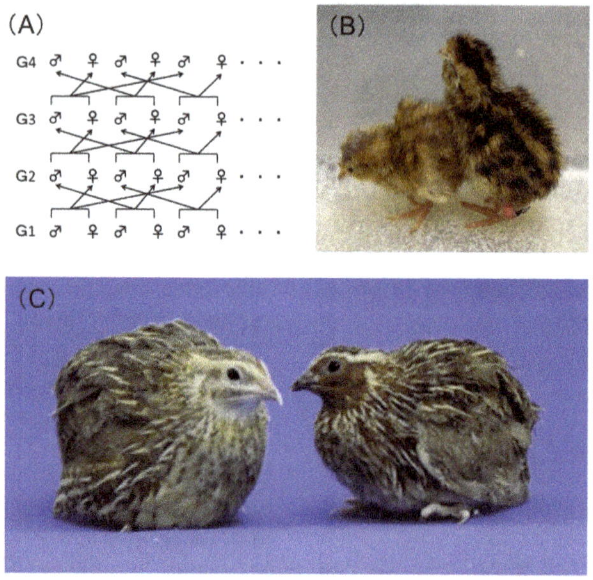

FIGURE 1 | Closed colony of Japanese quail at the National Institute for Environmental Studies, Japan. (A) Overview of the rotational crossbreeding of the NIES-L quail strain from generations 1 (G1)–4 (G4). **(B)** Newly hatched NIES-L quail chicks with the yellow-brown plumage color phenotype (left) and the wild-type phenotype (right). **(C)** Male (right) and female (left) adult NIES-L quails.

for evaluating the genetic variation within and between quail populations (Kawahara-Miki et al., 2013). Tadano et al. (2014) compared the estimated level of inbreeding within the NIES-L colony with that of a commercial random-bred colony by using polymorphic microsatellite marker analyses and confirmed that the heterozygosity in the NIES-L colony is gradually being lost over time. Our group is also using specific alleles of the microsatellite loci to monitor for genetic contamination in the colony by genetic markers developed. The Japanese quail is a potentially useful experimental organism not only for studies in the field of poultry science but also in the field of basic research and/or environmental studies, which are more necessary to analyze genetically.

About 35 years ago, we started to select and breed Japanese quails for high (H) and low (i.e., NIES-L) serum antibody titers against inactivated Newcastle disease virus (Takahashi et al., 1984), but the H quails have been extinct. It is clear that heterozygosity in the NIES-L closed colony is being gradually lost over time. However, it is difficult to establish mutant quail strains and maintain inbred strains because they are particularly susceptible to inbreeding depression (Sittmann et al., 1966). Indeed, no inbred strain of Japanese quail surviving more than 20 consecutive generations of full-sib mating has ever been developed, unlike in mouse and rat. Therefore, if we could fully establish an inbred strain of Japanese quail by continuing our breeding of NIES-L, this model organism would be useful for toxicity testing and would provide a simple and reproducible platform for the assessment of nervous and reproductive system developmental toxicity in birds and mammals.

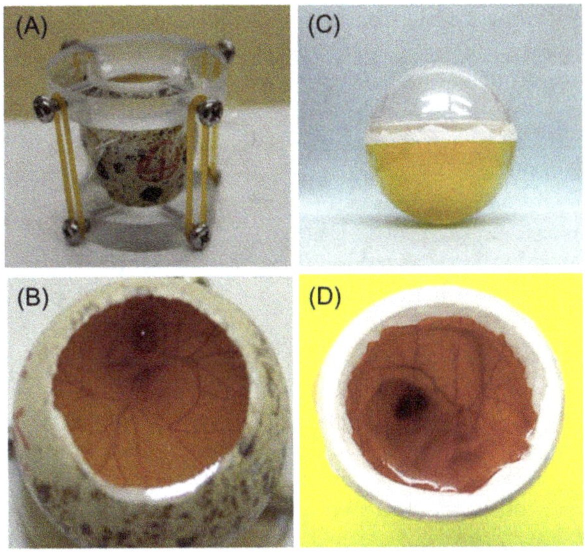

FIGURE 2 | Photographs of two quail embryo culture systems (ECSs). **(A)** Perry's ECS (System II) uses a surrogate eggshell for the period from blastoderm to embryogenesis. **(B)** Perry's ECS (System III) uses a surrogate eggshell during embryonic growth until hatching. **(C)** Alternative ECS using an artificial culture vessel for the period from blastoderm to embryogenesis. Developing quail embryos can be observed by tipping the vessel slightly, allowing easy determination of the developmental stage. The volumes of the lower halves of the plastic cases (diameter across the equatorial plane, 26 mm) were comparable with those of quail eggs. **(D)** Alternative ECS using an artificial culture vessel during embryonic growth until hatching.

AVIAN EMBRYO CULTURE SYSTEM

The first avian whole ECS was established in chicken by Perry (1988) and developed further by Naito et al. (1990). An ECS has also been developed for Japanese quail (Ono et al., 1994). Perry's ECS (1988) covers the period from fertilization of the ovum to hatching and comprises three culture systems (Perry, 1988). System I is used to culture embryos obtained from the oviduct in the early cleavage stages, that is, to culture embryos from fertilization to blastoderm formation (Phase I). Systems II (**Figure 2A**) and III (**Figure 2B**) use a surrogate eggshell to culture embryos obtained from newly laid eggs through the period of embryogenesis (Phase II) and from embryonic growth to hatching (Phase III).

Our group has also succeeded in cultivating newly laid chicken or quail eggs through the period of embryogenesis (Phase II) by using a clear, egg-shaped artificial culture vessel (**Figure 2C**), which allowed direct observation of the developmental stage at any time throughout the cultivation period simply by tipping the vessel (Kawashima et al., 2005). In a comparison of our ECS, which uses an artificial culture vessel, and Perry's System II culture system, which uses a surrogate eggshell culture vessel, no obvious detrimental effects were found in Phase II embryos cultured by using our shell-less culture method (Kawashima et al., 2005).

Attempts to culture avian embryos *in vitro* from embryonic growth to hatching (i.e., Phase III) have also been made. Auerbach et al. (1974) cultured 3- to 4-day-old chicken embryos in Petri dishes and obtained approximately 40% viability at 14 days of total incubation with a maximum development period of 18 days. Dunn and Boone (1976) cultured 3-day-old chicken embryos in egg-shaped plastic wrap and reported that the maximum developmental stage reached was almost before hatching. Ono and Wakasugi (1983) cultured quail embryos, preincubated for 2.5 days, by using a plastic wrap technique, but the embryos did not survive beyond 14 days. Finally, Kamihira et al. (1998) succeeded in culturing 2-day-old quail embryos to hatching by using a gas-permeable Teflon membrane (Milliwrap; Nihon Millipore Co., Tokyo, Japan) with calcium supplementation and oxygen aeration (**Figure 2D**). Therefore, it is now possible to cultivate avian embryos in an artificial vessel throughout the whole embryonic growth phase.

Avian-based toxicity screening tests that are simple to conduct, rapid, and cost-effective are urgently required to obtain preliminary information on the effects of exposure to endocrine-disrupting chemicals in vertebrates (Flint et al., 2012; Oshima et al., 2012). An avian *in ovo* model called the sex reversal test has been established that uses Japanese quail embryos (Shibuya et al., 2004). Histologically, intact male Japanese quail embryos in the later embryonic stages just before hatching develop both left and right testes, whereas intact female embryos develop only a left-side ovary. Exposure of the embryo to estrogen or to an estrogen-like chemical such as an endocrine-disrupting chemical during an early embryonic developmental stage causes transformation of the left testis into an ovotestis and persistence of the left oviduct in genetic males (Shibuya et al., 2005). Therefore, the sex reversal test using an avian ECS represents a high-throughput, quantitative approach for the evaluation of the estrogenic effects of endocrine-disrupting or other chemicals.

Avian ECSs offer ethical advantages over other *in vivo* means of toxicity screening, especially when developmental toxicity of a chemical is anticipated. Furthermore, avian ECSs offer the additional advantage of allowing direct quantitative determination of the effects of test chemicals on the fetus without any maternal influence through placental transmission. Furthermore, because avian ECSs facilitate direct observation and manipulation, it is now possible to investigate the time-specific influences of chemicals with embryonic toxicity on the embryo. Suitable ECSs should be developed depending on the research or testing goal.

FEATURES OF AVIAN NEUROBEHAVIOR

Avian experimental models may also be useful for assessing aspects of neurobehavior such as the sociosexual behaviors of aggression and mating using Japanese quail (Ubuka et al., 2013). Indeed, some avian species have already been used as models of learning and memory in studies examining the neural basis of cognition (Emery, 2006). Corvids, songbirds, and domestic fowl are currently considered the best models available to examine specific aspects of the neurobiology underlying learning and cognition (Clayton and Emery, 2015). To apply the usefulness of avian models for learning and cognition to the developmental toxicity research, we need to establish new endpoints appropriate for the evaluation of neurotoxic and neurobehavioral effects.

Japanese quails have been used as a model organism in studies of the neurophysiological and neuroendocrine bases of aggression and reproductive behavior for a long period (Selinger and Bermant, 1967; Mills et al., 1997; Ubuka et al., 2013; Ubuka and Tsutsui, 2014). Sexually mature male quail frequently fight with intense aggression and display a series of stereotypical actions. They often approach, chase, and peck their opponent (peck), grab the back of their opponent's head or neck with their beak (grab), attempt to ride on the back of their opponent (mount), or ride on the back of their opponent and lower their cloaca close to their opponent's cloaca (cloacal contact-like action). Since the behavior of each quail can be recorded and analyzed by using a digital video camera, the numbers of pecks, grabs, mounts, and cloacal contact-like actions attempted by each animal can be quantified (see in **Supplementary Movie 1**). Since the frequency of these actions represents the degree of the sociosexual behavior of individual male quails (Ubuka et al., 2013), these actions represent novel endpoints that could be used to assess developmental toxicity.

Imprinting, which occurs limitedly during the initial stage of avian chicks, may be useful to establish a behavioral index for investigating the neural plasticity involved in juvenile learning (Yamaguchi et al., 2012; Nakamori et al., 2013). Imprinting is characterized by a high learning efficiency and robust memory retention, which are features that distinguish it from general learning and memory. Maekawa et al. (2006) established an experimental procedure for imprinting to visual stimuli presented on a liquid crystal display. After training, the chicks are placed on a running wheel, and an angle sensor is used to record the number of forward and backward rotations of the wheel as the chick is shown either images they had been shown since hatching or new, previously unseen images. The effects of imprinting on neural activity in the visual wulst can also be investigated by using *in vivo* intrinsic optical imaging techniques (Maekawa et al., 2007). It may also be possible to apply a measurement system of juvenile learning and memory that utilizes avian imprinting behavior as a novel means of rapidly assessing developmental neurotoxicity in early childhood.

Imprinting in Japanese quail has also been reported. It has been found that Japanese quail will imprint on achromatic stimuli, flashing lights, and models of quail hens (Mills et al., 1997). Imprinting in chicks may be a good model of learning in human infants because human infants and chicks share a critical period during which they are sensitive to specific experiences. Therefore, uncovering the molecular mechanisms underlying the imprinting process will help clarify the juvenile learning, which has an obvious critical period (Suzuki et al., 2012). Since future studies are expected to reveal the molecular mechanisms underlying learning and memory in higher vertebrates, new developmental neurotoxicity endpoints are also likely to be established in the future.

CAN AVIAN TEST BATTERY BE ALTERNATIVE TO DEVELOPMENTAL NEUROTOXICITY TESTS FOR HUMAN?

The combination of an avian ECS followed by neurobehavioral assessment is also a promising means of assessing developmental neurotoxicity. For many chemicals, it is high prenatal exposure that induces postnatal neurobehavioral disorders (Grandjean and Landrigan, 2006; Huizink and Mulder, 2006). However, even if exposure to a certain chemical is not found to induce apparently morphological abnormalities in the fetal and infantile brain, the chemical may still cause functional disorders and affect learning and memory. By using brain functions such as behavior, memory, and learning as advanced endpoints, it may be possible to use avian-based assay systems in place of the currently used tests of developmental neurotoxicity. However, given that the morphological development of the brain may differ between humans and birds, further studies are needed to determine how best to extrapolate test results.

Most of the currently used toxicity studies for environmental chemicals use acute or chronic systemic or reproductive toxicity endpoints and use mammalian or avian laboratory animals. However, since exposure in mammalian models is usually based on how much chemical is administered to the mother, it is difficult to determine exactly how much the fetus receives through the placenta. The Organization for Economic Cooperation and Development has established a series of standardized ecological risk assessments for chemicals such as endocrine disruptors (Buschmann, 2013). Although, these tests are accepted internationally as standard methods for evaluating the risk to human health and wildlife posed by persistent and degradable chemicals in the environment, neurobehavioral endpoints of toxicity are rarely examined. In addition, given the increasing number of new chemicals that potentially have neurotoxic effects in vertebrates, including humans, a rapid means of assessing the neurotoxic effects of these chemicals in humans is required.

Recently, it has been suggested that neonicotinoid pesticides have caused a decline in wild bird populations (Hallmann et al., 2014; Gibbons et al., 2015). Since the use of neonicotinoid pesticides is rapidly increasing throughout the world, the effects of these pesticides on human health are now a concern. Even if neonicotinoid pesticides were found not to adversely affect the morphological development of the embryonic human brain, the question of whether or not they cause postnatal neurobehavioral disorders would remain. Therefore, there is an urgent need to establish animal-based evaluation systems that can be used to assess neurotoxic effects of neonicotinoid pesticides. The avian test battery represents a potentially rapid and cost-effective way of conducting these assays.

CONCLUSION

Avian test batteries represent a potentially rapid, cost-effective, ethical alternative to the currently available means of assessing developmental toxicity using higher vertebrates. Here we have discussed using a Galliformes-based avian test battery in which developmental toxicity is assessed by means of a combination of chemical exposure during early embryonic development by using an ECS followed by analyses in later life of sociosexual behaviors such as aggression and mating and of visual memory via filial imprinting. However, to fully harness the potential of this novel means of chemical toxicity screening, it will be necessary to establish a variety of evaluation systems and experimental models before we can extrapolate the test results to humans.

AUTHOR CONTRIBUTIONS

All authors contributed to substantial contributions to the conception or design of the work. TK, WA, and KN designed this work. TK, TU, and KT revised the important intellectual content critically. TK wrote the article and all authors contributed to the editing.

ACKNOWLEDGMENTS

We thank Dr. Shinji Takahashi for his helpful insights. This work was supported by JSPS KAKENHI Grant Number 26660262 and by the National Institute for Environmental Studies [1416AT001].

REFERENCES

Auerbach, R., Kubai, L., Knighton, D., and Folkman, J. (1974). A simple procedure for the long-term cultivation of chicken embryos. *Dev. Biol.* 41, 391–394. doi: 10.1016/0012-1606(74)90316-9

Buschmann, J. (2013). The OECD guidelines for the testing of chemicals and pesticides. *Methods Mol. Boil.* 947, 37–56. doi: 10.1007/978-1-62703-131-8_4

Clayton, N. S., and Emery, N. J. (2015). Avian models for human cognitive neuroscience: a proposal. *Neuron* 86, 1330–1342. doi: 10.1016/j.neuron.2015.04.024

Colborn, T., vom Saal, F. S., and Soto, A. M. (1993). Developmental effects of endocrine-disrupting chemicals in wildlife and humans. *Environ. Health Perspect.* 101, 378–384. doi: 10.1289/ehp.93101378

Dunn, B. E., and Boone, M. A. (1976). Growth of the chick embryo *in vitro*. *Poult. Sci.* 55, 1067–1071. doi: 10.3382/ps.0551067

Emery, N. J. (2006). Cognitive ornithology: the evolution of avian intelligence. *Philos. Trans. R. Soc. Lond. B. Biol. Sci.* 361, 23–43. doi: 10.1098/rstb.2005.1736

Flint, S., Markle, T., Thompson, S., and Wallace, E. (2012). Bisphenol a exposure, effects, and policy: a wildlife perspective. *J. Environ. Manage.* 104, 19–34. doi: 10.1016/j.jenvman.2012.03.021

Frye, C. A., Bo, E., Calamandrei, G., Calzà, L., Dessì-Fulgheri, F., Fernández, M., et al. (2012). Endocrine disrupters: a review of some sources, effects, and mechanisms of actions on behaviour and neuroendocrine systems. *J. Neuroendocrinol.* 24, 144–159. doi: 10.1111/j.1365-2826.2011.02229.x

Gibbons, D., Morrissey, C., and Mineau, P. (2015). A review of the direct and indirect effects of neonicotinoids and fipronil on vertebrate wildlife. *Environ. Sci. Pollut. Res.* 22, 103–118. doi: 10.1007/s11356-014-3180-5

Grandjean, P., and Landrigan, P. J. (2006). Developmental neurotoxicity of industrial chemicals. *Lancet* 368, 2167–2178. doi: 10.1016/S0140-6736(06)69665-7

Hallmann, C. A., Foppen, R. P. B., van Turnhout, C. A. M., de Kroon, H., and Jongejans, E. (2014). Declines in insectivorous birds are associated with high neonicotinoid concentrations. *Nature* 511, 341–343. doi: 10.1038/nature13531

Huizink, A. C., and Mulder, E. J. H. (2006). Maternal smoking, drinking or cannabis use during pregnancy and neurobehavioral and cognitive functioning in human offspring. *Neurosci. Biobehav. Rev.* 30, 24–41. doi: 10.1016/j.neubiorev.2005.04.005

Kamihira, M., Oguchi, S., Tachibana, A., Kitagawa, Y., and Iijima, S. (1998). Improved hatching for *in vitro* quail embryo culture using surrogate eggshell and artificial vessel. *Dev. Growth Differ.* 40, 449–455. doi: 10.1046/j.1440-169X.1998.t01-2-00010.x

Kawahara-Miki, R., Sano, S., Nunome, M., Shimmura, T., Kuwayama, T., Takahashi, S., et al. (2013). Next-generation sequencing reveals genomic features in the Japanese quail. *Genomics* 101, 345–353. doi: 10.1016/j.ygeno.2013.03.006

Kawashima, T., Kumata, K., Tamaki, Y., Kuwana, T., and Hashimoto, K. (2005). An avian embryo culture system for embryogenesis using an artificial vessel: possible conservation benefits in the rescue and management of endangered avian species. *Zoo Biol.* 24, 519–529. doi: 10.1002/zoo.20068

Le Douarin, N. M. (2004). The avian embryo as a model to study the development of the neural crest: a long and still ongoing story. *Mech. Dev.* 121, 1089–1102. doi: 10.1016/j.mod.2004.06.003

Le Douarin, N. M., and Dieterlen-Lièvre, F. (2013). How studies on the avian embryo have opened new avenues in the understanding of development: a view about the neural and hematopoietic systems. *Dev. Growth Differ.* 55, 1–14. doi: 10.1111/dgd.12015

Lewis, C., and Ford, A. T. (2012). Infertility in male aquatic invertebrates: a review. *Aquat. Toxicol.* 120–121, 79–89. doi: 10.1016/j.aquatox.2012.05.002

Lu, Z. G., Li, M. H., Wang, J. S., Wei, D. D., and Liu, Q. W. (2014). Developmental toxicity and neurotoxicity of two matrine-type alkaloids, matrine and sophocarpine, in zebrafish (*Danio rerio*) embryos/larvae. *Reprod. Toxicol.* 47, 33–41. doi: 10.1016/j.reprotox.2014.05.015

Maekawa, F., Komine, O., Sato, K., Kanamatsu, T., Uchimura, M., Tanaka, K., et al. (2006). Imprinting modulates processing of visual information in the visual wulst of chicks. *BMC Neurosci.* 7:75. doi: 10.1186/1471-2202-7-75

Maekawa, F., Nakamori, T., Uchimura, M., Fujiwara, K., Yada, T., Tsukahara, S., et al. (2007). Activation of cholecystokinin neurons in the dorsal pallium of the telencephalon is indispensable for the acquisition of chick imprinting behavior. *J. Neurochem.* 102, 1645–1657. doi: 10.1111/j.1471-4159.2007.04733.x

Maekawa, F., Tsukahara, S., Kawashima, T., Nohara, K., and Ohki-Hamazaki. (2014). The mechanisms underlying sexual differentiation of behavior and physiology in mammals and birds: relative contributions of sex steroids and sex chromosomes. *Front. Neurosci.* 8:242. doi: 10.3389/fnins.2014.00242

Mills, A. D., Crawford, L. L., Domjan, M., and Faure, J. M. (1997). The behavior of the Japanese or domestic quail *Coturnix japonica*. *Neurosci. Biobehav. Rev.* 21, 261–281. doi: 10.1016/S0149-7634(96)00028-0

Naito, M., Nirasawa, K., and Oishi, T. (1990). Development in culture of the chick embryo from fertilized ovum to hatching. *J. Exp. Zool.* 254, 322–326. doi: 10.1002/jez.1402540311

Nakamori, T., Maekawa, F., Sato, K., Tanaka, K., and Ohki-Hamazaki, H. (2013). Neural basis of imprinting behavior in chicks. *Dev. Growth Differ.* 55, 198–206. doi: 10.1111/dgd.12028

Nakamura, H., and Funahashi, J. (2013). Electroporation: past, present and future. *Dev. Growth Differ.* 55, 1–14. doi: 10.1111/dgd.12012

Neubert, D. (1982). The use of culture techniques in studies on prenatal toxicity. *Pharmacol. Ther.* 18, 397–434. doi: 10.1016/0163-7258(82)90039-0

Ono, T., Murakami, T., Mochii, M., Agata, K., Kino, K., Otsuka, K., et al. (1994). A complete culture system for avian transgenesis, supporting quail embryos from the single-cell stage to hatching. *Dev. Biol.* 161, 126–130. doi: 10.1006/dbio.1994.1014

Ono, T., and Wakasugi, N. (1983). Development of cultured quail embryos. *Poult. Sci.* 62, 532–536. doi: 10.3382/ps.0620532

Oshima, A., Yamashita, R., Nakamura, K., Wada, M., and Shibuya, K. (2012). *In ovo* exposure to nonylphenol and bisphenol A resulted in dose-independent feminization of male gonads in Japanese quail (*Coturnix japonica*) embryos. *Environ. Toxicol. Chem.* 31, 1091–1097. doi: 10.1002/etc.1787

Padgett, C. A., and Ivey, W. D. (1959). Coturnix quail as a laboratory research animal. *Science* 129, 267–268. doi: 10.1126/science.129.3344.267

Perry, M. M. (1988). A complete culture system for the chick embryo. *Nature* 331, 70–72. doi: 10.1038/331070a0

Sato, Y. (2013). Dorsal aorta formation: separate origins, lateral-to-medial migration, and remodeling. *Dev. Growth Differ.* 55, 113–129. doi: 10.1111/dgd.12010

Selinger, H. E., and Bermant, G. (1967). Hormonal control of aggressive behavior in Japanese quail (Coturnix *Coturnix japonica*). *Behaviour.* 28, 255–268. doi: 10.1163/156853967X00037

Shibuya, K., Mizitani, M., Sato, K., Itabashi, M., and Nunoya, T. (2005). Comparative evaluation of sex reversal effects of natural and synthetic estrogens in sex reversal test using F1(AWE × WE). Japanese quail embryos. *J. Poult. Sci.* 42, 119–129. doi: 10.2141/jpsa.42.119

Shibuya, K., Mizutani, M., Wada, M., Sato, K., and Nunoya, T. (2004). A new screening model using F1(AWE × WE) Japanese quail embryo for evaluating sex reversal effects. *J. Toxicol. Pathol.* 17, 245–252. doi: 10.1293/tox.17.245

Sittmann, K., Abplanalp, H., and Fraser, R. A. (1966). Inbreeding depression in Japanese quail. *Genetics* 54, 371–379.

Stern, C. D. (2005). The chick: a great model system becomes even greater. *Dev. Cell* 8, 9–17. doi: 10.1016/j.devcel.2004.11.018

Suzuki, G., Tue, N. M., Malarvannan, G., Sudaryanto, A., Takahashi, S., Tanabe, S., et al. (2013). Similarities in the endocrine-disrupting potencies of indoor dust and flame retardants by using human osteosarcoma (U2OS) cell-based reporter gene assays. *Environ. Sci. Technol.* 47, 2898–2908. doi: 10.1021/es304691a

Suzuki, K., Maekawa, F., Suzuki, S., Nakamori, T., Sugiyama, H., Kanamatsu, T., et al. (2012). Elevated expression of brain-derived neurotrophic factor facilitates visual imprinting in chicks. *J. Neurochem.* 123, 800–810. doi: 10.1111/jnc.12039

Suzuki, T. (2013). How is digit identity determined during limb development? *Dev. Growth Differ.* 55, 130–138. doi: 10.1111/dgd.12022

Tadano, R., Nunome, M., Mizutani, M., Kawahara-Miki, R., Fujiwara, A., Takahashi, S., et al. (2014). Cost-effective development of highly polymorphic microsatellite in Japanese quail facilitated by next-generation sequencing. *Anim. Genet.* 45, 881–884. doi: 10.1111/age.12227

Takahashi, S., Inooka, S., and Mizuma, Y. (1984). Selective breeding for high and low antibody responses to inactivated Newcastle disease virus in Japanese quails. *Poult. Sci.* 63, 595–599. doi: 10.3382/ps.0630595

Ubuka, T., Haraguchi, S., Tobari, Y., Narihiro, M., Ishikawa, K., Hayashi, T., et al. (2013). Hypothalamic inhibition of socio-sexual behaviour by increasing neuroestrogen synthesis. *Nat. Commun.* 5, 3061. doi: 10.1038/ncomms4061

Ubuka, T., and Tsutsui, K. (2014). Review: neuroestrogen regulation of socio-sexual behavior of males. *Front. Neurosci.* 8:323. doi: 10.3389/fnins.2014.00323

Yamaguchi, S., Aoki, N., Kitajima, T., Iikubo, E., Katagiri, S., Matsushima, T., et al. (2012). Thyroid hormone determines the start of the sensitive period of imprinting and primes later learning. *Nat. Commun.* 3, 1081. doi: 10.1038/ncomms2088

21

Learning and Memory Deficits in Male Adult Mice Treated with a Benzodiazepine Sleep-Inducing Drug during the Juvenile Period

Yusuke Furukawa[1,2], Kentaro Tanemura[3], Katsuhide Igarashi[4], Maky Ideta-Otsuka[4], Ken-Ichi Aisaki[1], Satoshi Kitajima[1], Masanobu Kitagawa[2] and Jun Kanno[1,5]*

[1] Division of Cellular and Molecular Toxicology, Biological Safety Research Center, National Institute of Health Sciences, Tokyo, Japan, [2] Department of Comprehensive Pathology, Graduate School, Tokyo Medical and Dental University, Tokyo, Japan, [3] Laboratory of Animal Reproduction and Development, Graduate School of Agricultural Science, Tohoku University, Sendai, Japan, [4] Life Science Tokyo Advanced Research Center, Hoshi University School of Pharmacy and Pharmaceutical Sciences, Tokyo, Japan, [5] Japan Bioassay Research Center, Japan Organization of Occupational Health and Safety, Hadano, Japan

Edited by:
Fumihiko Maekawa,
National Institute for Environmental Studies, Japan

Reviewed by:
Mauro Ceccanti,
Sapienza University of Rome, Italy
Masaki Kakeyama,
Waseda University, Japan

***Correspondence:**
Kentaro Tanemura
kentaro@m.tohoku.ac.jp

Gamma-aminobutyric acid (GABA), the major inhibitory neurotransmitter in the mammalian central nervous system, is also known to be important for brain development. Therefore, disturbances of GABA receptor (GABA-R) mediated signaling (GABA-R signal) during brain development may influence normal brain maturation and cause late-onset brain malfunctions. In this study, we examined whether the stimulation of the GABA-R signal during brain development induces late-onset adverse effects on the brain in adult male mice. To stimulate the GABA-R signal, we used either the benzodiazepine sleep-inducing drug triazolam (TZ) or the non-benzodiazepine drug zolpidem (ZP). We detected learning and memory deficits in mice treated with TZ during the juvenile period, as seen in the fear conditioning test. On the other hand, ZP administration during the juvenile period had little effect. In addition, decreased protein expression of GluR1 and GluR4, which are excitatory neurotransmitter receptors, was detected in the hippocampi of mice treated with TZ during the juvenile period. We measured mRNA expression of the immediate early genes (IEGs), which are neuronal activity markers, in the hippocampus shortly after the administration of TZ or ZP to juvenile mice. Decreased IEG expression was detected in mice with juvenile TZ administration, but not in mice with juvenile ZP administration. Our findings demonstrate that TZ administration during the juvenile period can induce irreversible learning and memory deficits in adult mice. It may need to take an extra care for the prescription of benzodiazepine sleep-inducing drugs to juveniles because it might cause learning and memory deficits.

Keywords: sleep-inducing drug, triazolam, zolpidem, GABA receptor signal, behavioral battery test

INTRODUCTION

Normal brain development requires various neuronal signals must be activated at the appropriate timing and with the proper extent in the developmental brain (Rice and Barone, 2000). Excitatory glutamate receptor (Glu-R) signals and inhibitory gamma-aminobutyric acid (GABA) receptor (GABA-R) signals are the most important neuronal signals in the adult brain. These neuronal signals are also known to be important for brain development. These signals have roles in neuronal cellular proliferation and differentiation, neuronal migration, the construction of neuronal circuits, and the reorganization of neuronal circuits (Luján et al., 2005). Therefore, the stimulation of these neuronal signals with external factors, such as chemical compounds, may interfere with normal brain development and result in late-onset functional deficits during adulthood. We have previously reported that the transient activation of Glu-R signals in the prenatal mouse brain with domoic acid results in aberrant emotional behavior, as well as learning and memory deficits, as revealed by a mouse behavioral battery tests (BBT) (Tanemura et al., 2009). On the other hand, Haas et al. have shown that prenatal GABA-R signal activation with the anxiolytic drug Diazepam (DZP) leads to the inhibition of neuronal migration and the disruption of cerebral cortex neuronal circuits (Haas et al., 2013). In addition, Shen et al. have shown that neonatal activation of GABA-R signals by DZP results in increased anxiety-like behavior (Shen et al., 2012). However, the behavioral tests applied in these studies were limited, and their results were not analyzed in an integrated manner. We therefore believe that analyses of several behavioral tests during the adult stage following the activation of GABA-R signals during brain development are critically needed.

In this study, we report the results of the BBT that we conducted. These include the open field test, the light/dark transition test, the elevated plus maze test, the contextual/cued fear conditioning test, and the pre-pulse inhibition test. The results of these tests will help us to understand the effects of GABA-R signal activation during brain development with the benzodiazepine (BZD) sleep-inducing drug triazolam (TZ: original brand name "Halcion") or the non-BZD drug zolpidem (ZP: originally marketed as "Ambien" and available worldwide under many brand names) on behavior during the adult stage (Pakes et al., 1981; Holm and Goa, 2000). These sleep-inducing drugs have similar pharmacokinetic and pharmacodynamic effects in humans (Lobo and Greene, 1997). They are preferentially used as drugs for the treatment of insomnia owing to their lack of carryover effects on the next day (Neubauer, 2007). Their reported side effects include drug-dependence, withdrawal symptoms, psychiatric symptoms (excitement stimulation, confusion, aggression, noctambulation, hallucinations, delusions, and agitation), transient anterograde amnesia before and after sleeping, or arousal during sleep (Pakes et al., 1981; Jonas et al., 1992; Toner et al., 2000; Greenblatt and Roth, 2012). Treatment of sleep disorders in children using hypnotic drugs is common (Kahn et al., 1989; Stores, 1996; Owens et al., 2003; Weiss and Garbutt, 2010; Felt and Chervin, 2014), although their safety in children has not been established (FDA, 2008, 2013). These chemicals act by suppressing excitatory neuronal activity by inducing hyperpolarization following the cellular influx of chloride ions when they bind to GABA (A)-R alpha and gamma receptors. GABA (A)-R is found as pentamers of a combination of 19 subunits (α1–6, β1–3, γ1–3, δ, ϵ, θ, π, and ρ1–3). The BZD chemical TZ binds to GABA (A)–R α1, 2, 3, 5, and 6 subtypes in any combination, along with the γ2 subtype. The non-BZD chemical ZP binds only to combinations of GABA (A)–R α1 and γ2 subtypes (Rudolph and Knoflach, 2011).

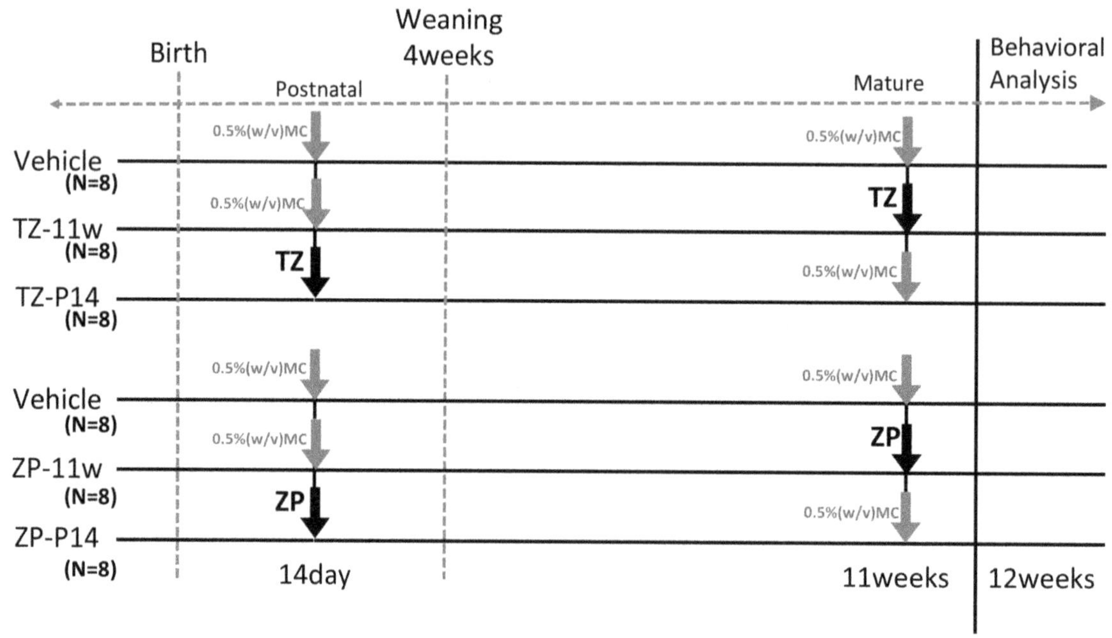

FIGURE 1 | Experimental schedule. This figure describes the experimental schedules for triazolam (TZ) and zolpidem (ZP) treatment. The gray arrow indicates vehicle and the black arrows indicate TZ 1 mg/kg or ZP 50 mg/kg. All mice received the drug three times by gavage. The two ages of 2 weeks (2 w) and 11 weeks (11 w) were selected. TZ and ZP were administered to the mice at one of the two time points and vehicle was administered at the other two time points. The mice were weaned at 4 weeks. Male mice were selected and were housed in new cages (4 mice per cage). A behavioral battery tests (BBT) was carried out starting at 12 weeks of age. Each group consisted of eight mice (6 group, 48 mice total).

MATERIALS AND METHODS

Animal Experiment

All animal experiments were conducted with permission from the Animal Ethics Committee at the National Institute of Health Sciences. Pregnant female C57BL/6NCrSlc mice at embryonic day 11 were purchased from Japan SLC Inc. (Shizuoka, Japan). The mice were housed in plastic cages and maintained under a 12-h light/12-h dark cycle with water and chow (CRF-1, Oriental Yeast Co. Ltd., Tokyo, Japan) provided *ad libitum*. Triazolam (TZ: 8-chloro-6-(2-chlorophhenyl)-1-methyl-4H-1, 2, 4 -triazolo[4,3-a]-1, 4-benzodiazepine; Sigma Aldrich Co. Steinheim, Germany), and Zolpidem (ZP: N,N,6-Trimethyl-2-(4-methylphenyl)-imidazo[1,2-a]pyridine-3-acetamide; Sigma Aldrich Co., Steinheim, Germany) were dissolved in 0.5% (w/v) methyl cellulose solution (Wako Pure Chemical Industries, Ltd. Osaka, Japan) and administered by gavage at the doses of 1 and 50 mg/kg. In the vehicle group, 0.5% (w/v) methyl cellulose solution (MC) was administered by gavage. Administration and experimental schedules are shown in **Figure 1**. Mice in the Vehicle group (8 mice per experimental group, 16 mice total) were treated with 0.5% (w/v) MC at 2 weeks and 11 weeks of age. The TZ-2w group (8 mice) was treated with TZ at 2 weeks of age and with 0.5% (w/v) MC at 11 weeks of age. The ZP-2w group (8 mice) was treated with ZP at 2 weeks of age and with 0.5% (w/v) MC at 11 weeks of age. The TZ-11w group (8 mice) was treated with 0.5% (w/v) MC at 2 weeks of age and with TZ at 11 weeks of age. The ZP-11w group (8 mice) was treated with 0.5% (w/v) MC at 2 weeks of age and with ZP at 11 weeks of age. Subsequently, a series of BBT were conducted at 12 weeks of age. After the BBT, the brains of the mice were dissected, and the hippocampus was removed for biochemical analysis at 13 weeks of age.

Mouse Behavioral Battery Test

We conducted a behavioral battery test (BBT), including the open field test (OF), the light/dark transition test (LD), the elevated plus maze test (EP), the contextual/cued fear conditioning test (FZ), and the additional pre-pulse inhibition test (PPI). For the OF, LD, EP, and FZ methods details, refer to the Tanemura et al. (2009). In the present study, we added the PPI further for information processing analysis. Experimental apparatuses and image analysis software was obtained from O'Hara & Co., Ltd., Japan. Image analysis software (Image OF4, Image LD2,

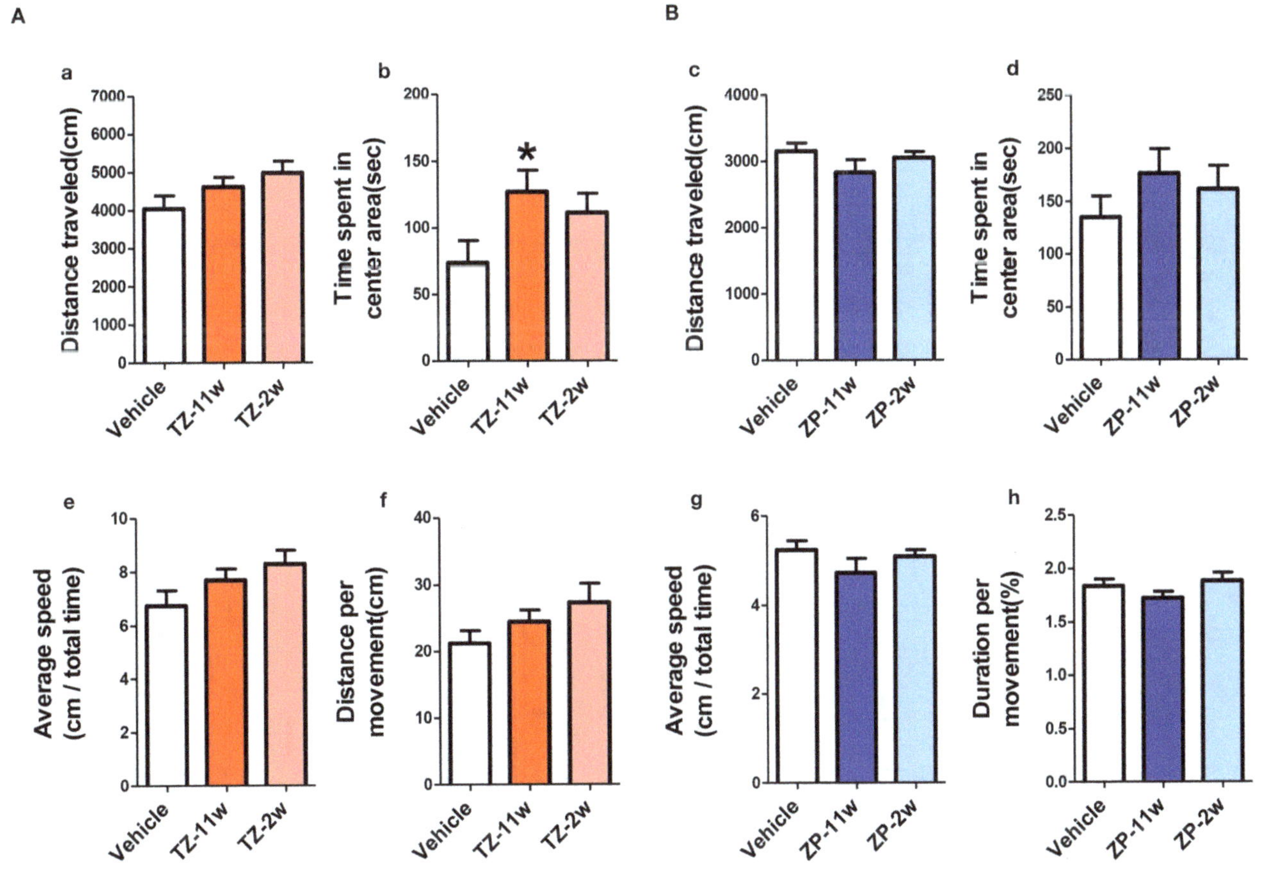

FIGURE 2 | Results of the open field (OF) test. (A,B) The scores of the OF test (total test time, 600 s) are shown. **(Aa,Bc)** Distance traveled (cm) during the test period (600 s) is shown. **(Ab,Bd)** Time spent in the center area (seconds) is shown. **(Ab)** Statistically significant increases were detected in the TZ-11w group. **(Ae,Bg)** Average speed (cm/total time) is shown. **(Af,Bh)** Distance per movement (cm) is shown. $n = 8$, mean ± SEM. Asterisk (*) indicates a statistically significant difference (*$p < 0.05$, Student's t-test) compared to the Vehicle group.

Image EP2, and Image FZ2) were developed using the public domain ImageJ program. All experiments were performed with 8 mice per group (TZ experimental: 3 groups, ZP experimental: 3 groups). We thus had 6 groups for a total of 48 mice. The experimental tests were conducted between 13:30 and 16:30. The level of background noise during BBT was about 50 dB. After each trial, the apparatus was wiped and cleaned. The pre-pulse inhibition test apparatus consists of a light source and a sound system, and a startle measurement load cell. These are set into a soundproof box. The software for the operation of the apparatus and the data analysis is the SR-9040 (O'Hara & Co., Ltd., Tokyo, Japan). The white background noise level is set to 70 dB in the soundproof box. The mouse is put into a plastic cylinder and kept there for 90 s before the test. The test schedule consists of three blocks, and the total trial time is 30 min. Breakdown of each block is as follows: 80, 85, 95, 100, 105, and 110 dB pulse × 3 (acclimation block), 120 dB pulse × 10 (acoustic startle response block). The combinations of pre-pulse are 80–120, 85–120, 95–120, 100–120, 105–120 dB, with a delay of 100 ms × 6 (pre-pulse inhibition measurement block). These combinations were presented in a pseudorandom order, such that each trial type was presented once within a block. The inhibition ratio (%) of the startle response is calculated as follows: (1–pre-pulse [80, 85, 95, 100, or 105 dB] startle response value / acoustic startle response value) × 100.

Western Blotting

Hippocampal extracts were dissolved in Tris-buffered saline (pH 7.4) containing protease inhibitors (Nacalai Tesque, Inc., Kyoto, Japan) and phosphatase inhibitors (Nacalai Tesque, Inc., Kyoto, Japan). Equal volume of the total protein solutions were added to 2 × sample buffer solution (Nacalai Tesque, Inc., Kyoto, Japan). The amount of protein was quantified using Qubit protein assay kits (Life Technologies Co., California, USA). The protein samples (30 μg/well) were subjected to SDS-PAGE (7.5% polyacrylamide), and transferred to a nitrocellulose membrane. The membranes were blocked in Blocking-one (Nacalai Tesque, Inc., Kyoto, Japan) at room temperature for 90 min and incubated with primary antibodies, such as those against acetyl-tubulin (sc-23950, Santa Cruz Biotechnology, Inc., California, USA), MAP2 (sc-20172), GluR1 (T9026, Sigma Aldrich Co., Steinheim, Germany), and GluR4 (SAB450126) overnight at room temperature. The membranes were then washed with phosphate buffered saline (pH 7.4) with 0.05% Tween-20 (PBS-T). The membranes were then incubated with peroxidase-conjugated secondary antibodies for 2 h at room temperature. After several PBS-T washes, the membranes were incubated with chemi-lumi one L (Nacalai Tesque, Inc., Kyoto, Japan) for signal production. The signal was photographed using an LAS-3000 (Fujifilm Co., Ltd., Tokyo, Japan). The intensity of each protein band was measured

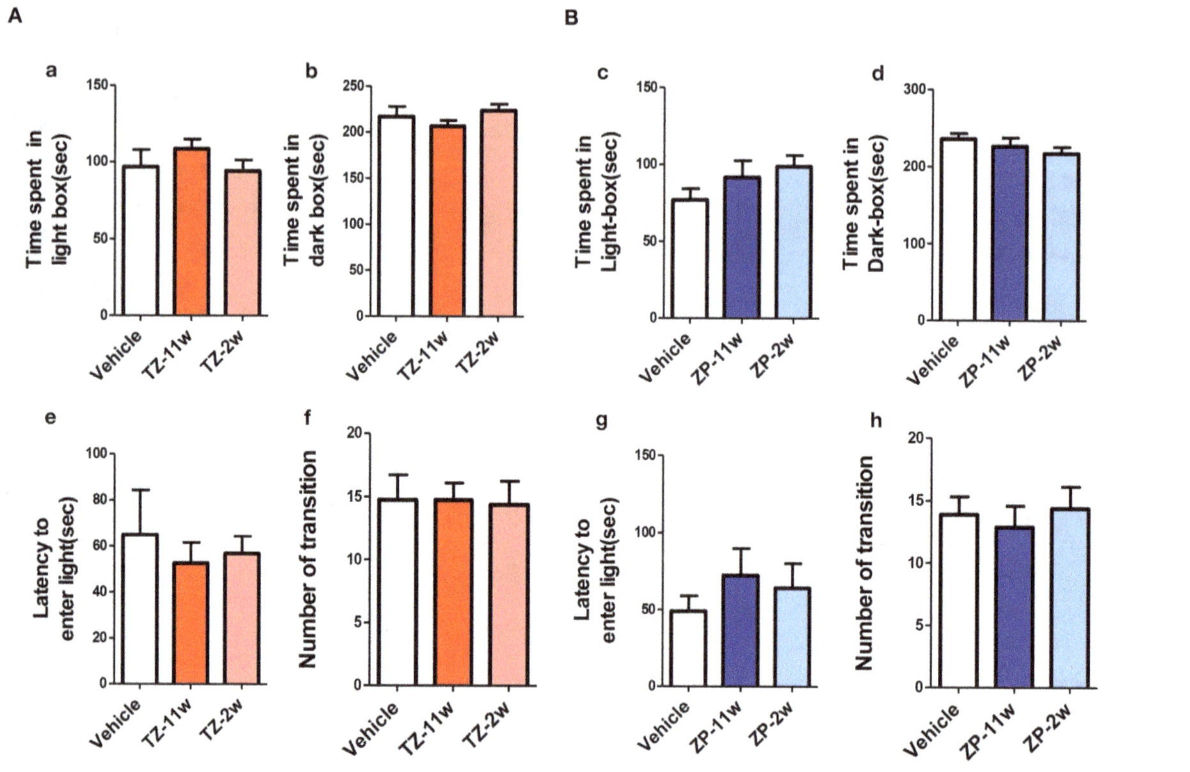

FIGURE 3 | Results of the light/dark transition (LD) test. (A,B) The scores for the LD test (total test time, 360 s) are shown. **(Aa,Bc)** Time spent in the light box (seconds). **(Ab,Bd)** Light box distance traveled (seconds) is shown. **(Ae,Bg)** The number of transitions between the dark box and the light box. **(Af,Bh)** Latency (seconds) to enter the light box for the first time. No significant differences compared with the Vehicle group were detected in the LD. The number of mice per group was eight and the scores are shown as the mean ± SEM.

using the Gel Analyzer program in ImageJ, and normalized to the intensity of the acetyl-tubulin band using the following formula: (intensity of each protein band/acetyl-tubulin band intensity) $\times$ 100. We present each normalized band intensity as a percentage of its intensity in the Vehicle group. The changes in protein expression associated with TZ and ZP treatment were calculated as follows: Ratio (%) = (Vehicle, TZ and ZP group individual value/Vehicle group average value) $\times$ 100.

Quantitative RT-PCR

Duplicate homogenate hippocampal samples were treated with DNaseI (amplification grade, Invitrogen Corp., Carlsbad, CA, USA) for 15 min at room temperature. They were then incubated with Super-Script II (Invitrogen) for 50 min at 42°C for reverse transcription. Quantitative real time PCR was performed using an ABI PRISM 7900 HT sequence detection system (Applied Biosystems, Foster City, CA, USA) using SYBR Premix Ex Taq (Takara Bio Inc., Japan) with initial denaturation at 95°C for 10 s followed by 45 cycles of 5 s at 95°C and 60 s at 60°C. Ct values were obtained. The primers were synthesized by FASMAC Co., Ltd., Japan. Expression of genes of interest was normalized to that of *Actb* and presented as fold change over baseline using the delta-delta CT method. Fold changes of relative gene expression levels compared to those of Vehicle animals were calculated (Livak and Schmittgen, 2001).

Primers

Arc: forward 5′-TACCGTTAGCCCCTATGCCATC-3′, reverse 5′-TGATATTGCTGAGCCTCAACTG-3′

c-Fos: forward 5′-ATGGGCTCTCCTGTCAACACAC-3′, reverse 5′-ATGGCTGTCACCGTGGGGATAAAG-3′

Nr4a1: forward 5′- TTAAGAGGTGGGTCGGGTTC -3′, reverse 5′- GCAATCCTTCTCGCACACTA -3′

ActB: forward 5′-GGACTCATCGTACTCCTGCTT-3′, reverse 5′-GAGATTACTGCTCTGGCTCCT-3′.

Statistical Analysis

Statistical analysis was conducted using Prism 5.01 (SAS Institute, California, USA). Data was analyzed using Student's unpaired *t*-tests. Values in graphs are expressed as the mean ± standard error of the mean (SEM).

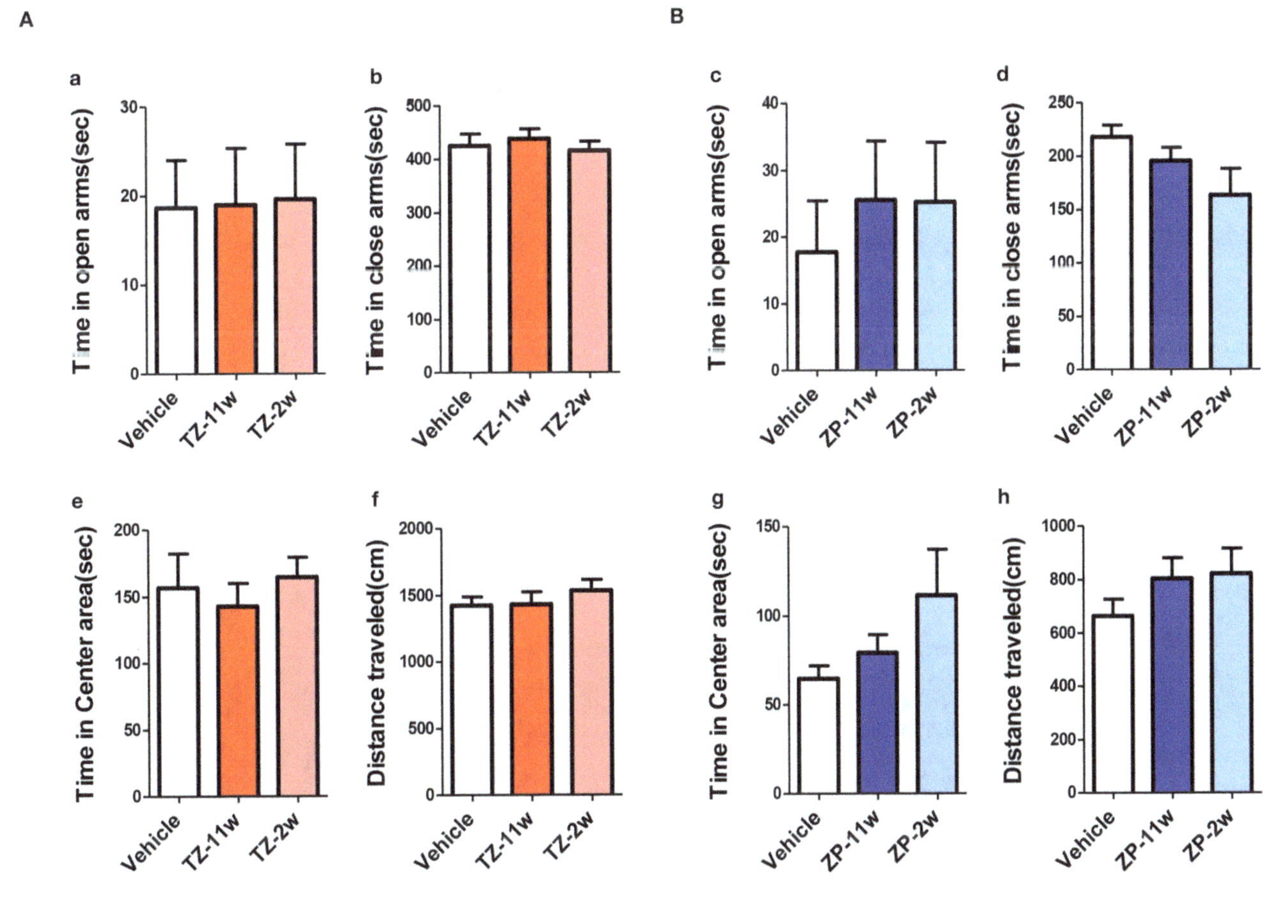

FIGURE 4 | Results of the elevated plus maze (EP) test. EP tests were conducted to analyze emotional behavioral changes in TZ- and ZP-treated mice. **(A,B)** The scores of the EP test (total test time, 600 s) are shown. **(Aa,Bc)** Time spent in the open arm (seconds). **(Ab,Bd)** Time spent in the closed arm (seconds). **(Ae,Bg)** Time spent in the center area (seconds). **(Af,Bh)** Total distance moved (cm). No significant differences with the Vehicle group were detected in the EP. The number of mice per group was eight and the scores are shown as the mean ± SEM.

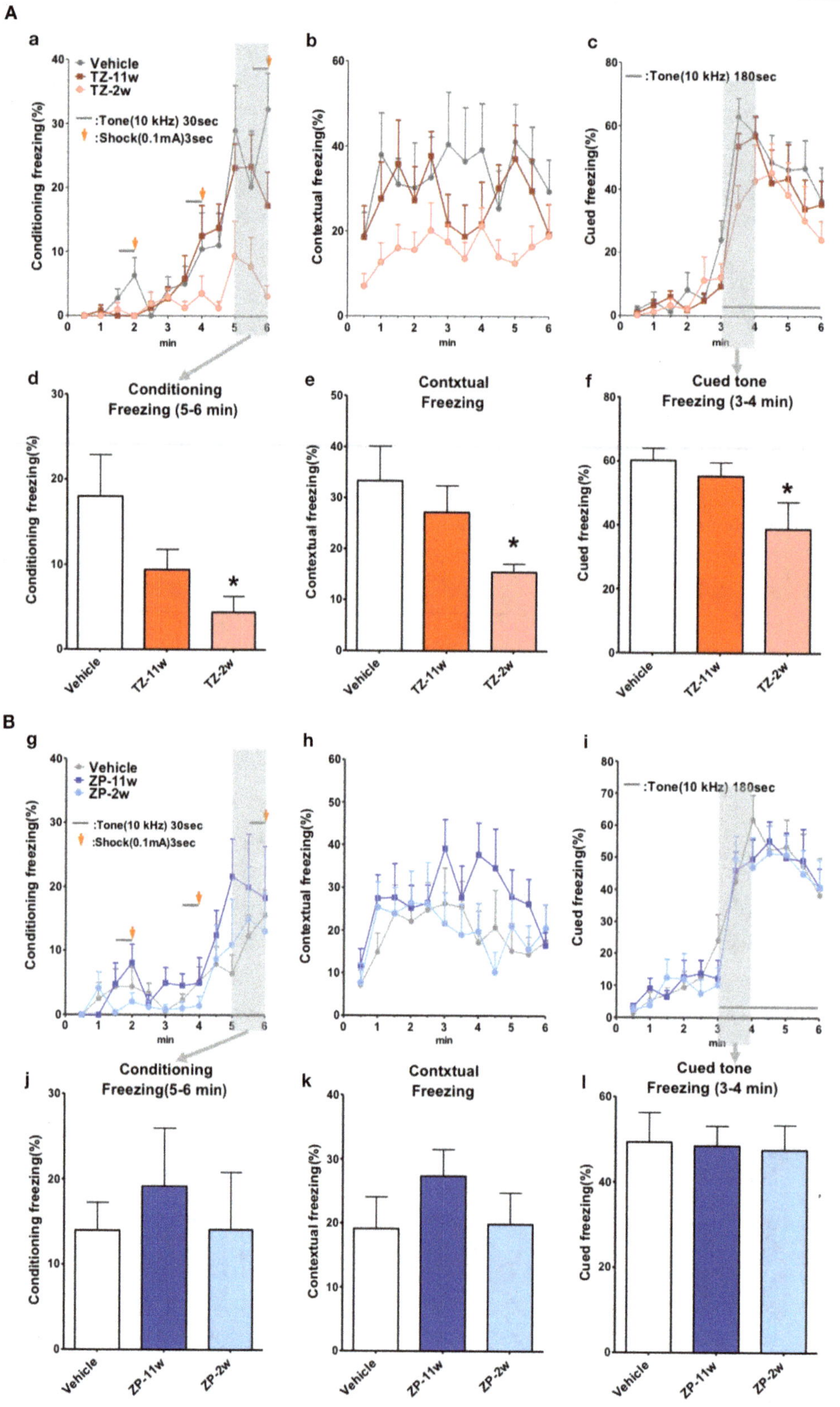

FIGURE 5 | Results of the fear conditioning test. (A,B) Fear conditioning test was conducted to analyze the effects of TZ and ZP on learning and contextual memory, i.e., place (test-box) and sound (cued tone). **(Aa,d,Bg,j)** The total conditioning time was 360 s. Three cycles consisting of a tone (30 s) and a mild foot shock

(Continued)

FIGURE 5 | Continued
(arrows: 0.1 mA, 3 s) were carried out for each mouse after it was allowed to explore the box freely for 90 s. **(Aa,Bg)** The time course of the freezing % scores is plotted for the conditioning test. As the cycles of the conditioning were repeated, the freezing percentages increased in the Vehicle group and in all groups other than the TZ-2w group. This indicates successful conditioning. On the other hand, the freezing % remained low in the TZ-2w group. **(Ad,Bj)** The average freezing % scores during the later period (180–360 s) of the conditioning test are shown. A significant decrease in freezing % was observed in the TZ-2w group. **(Ab,e,Bh,k)** Contextual tests were conducted 24 h after the conditioning test to analyze the effects of triazolam on place memory function. **(Ab,Bh)** The time course of the freezing % scores is plotted for the contextual test. The total time of the test is 360 s. **(Ae,Bk)** The average freezing % scores in the contextual test are shown. A significant decrease in freezing % was detected in the TZ-2w group. **(Ac,f,Bi,l)** The cued test was conducted 24 h after the contextual test to analyze the effects of triazolam on cued memory function. The total time of the test is 360 s. **(Ac,Bi)** The time course of the freezing % scores was plotted for the cued test. The tone was presented to the mice during the later period of the test (180–360 s). **(Af,Bl)** The average freezing % scores for the first one minute period after the tone are presented. The freezing % scores of the TZ-2w group were significantly lower than those of the Vehicle group. The number of mice per group was eight and the scores are shown as the mean ± SEM. Asterisk (*) indicate statistically significant differences (*$p < 0.05$, Student's *t*-test) compared to the Vehicle group.

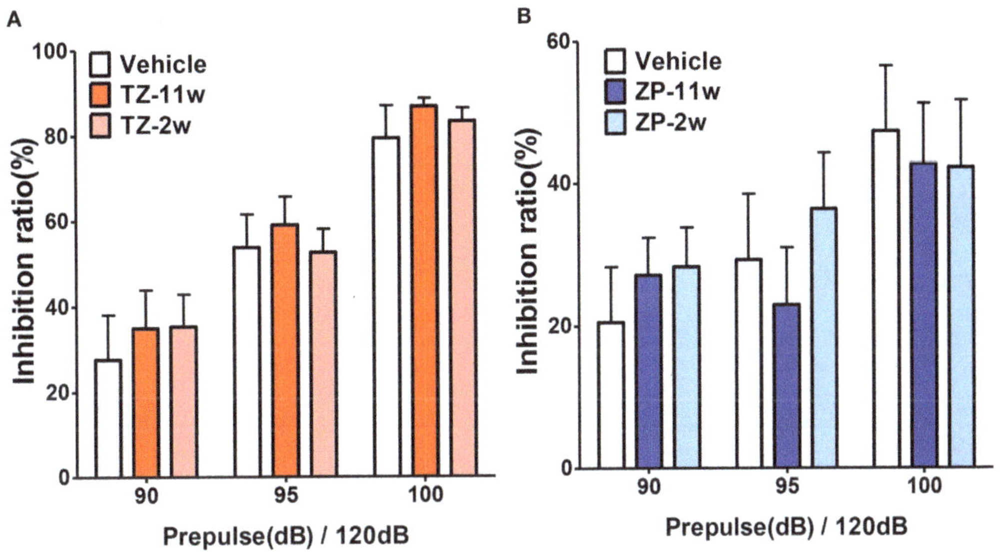

FIGURE 6 | Results of the pre-pulse inhibition (PPI) test. (A,B) The pre-pulse inhibition test was conducted to analyze the effects of sleep-inducing drugs on sensory information processing. The scores indicated the inhibition (%) of the startle response to a 120-dB sound with pre-pulse sounds of 90, 95, 100, and 105 dB when compared to the response to a 120-dB sound without a pre-pulse sound. No significant differences were found in the PPI test. The number of mice per group was eight and the scores are shown as the mean ± SEM.

RESULT

Results of Behavioral Battery Tests in the TZ-11w, TZ-2w, ZP-11w, and ZP-2w Groups

In the open field test (**Figure 2**), the total distance traveled and the time spent in the center region were significantly longer in the TZ-11w group (**Figure 2Ab**). Exposure to either chemical did not lead to any changes in the results of the light/dark transition test (**Figure 3**) or the elevated plus maze test (**Figure 4**). In the fear conditioning test, only the TZ-2w group did not show an increase in freezing % during the later period of the conditioning trial (**Figures 5Aa,d, Bg,j**, $p < 0.05$). In addition, in the contextual test, only the TZ-2w group had significantly lower freezing percentages (**Figures 5Ab,e, Bh,k**, $p < 0.05$). All other groups responded quickly to the tone and showed high freezing responses, while mice in the TZ-2w group had slower responses to the tone, which resulted in lower freezing responses (**Figures 5Ac,f, Bi,l**, $p < 0.05$). These results indicate that the administration of TZ during the juvenile period induces deficits in learning and memory. Exposure to either chemical did not lead to any changes in the results of the pre-pulse inhibition test (**Figure 6**). Significant differences were not observed in any of the tests in our BBT in the ZP-11w and ZP-2w groups. The results of the series of BBT performed on the TZ-11w, TZ-2w, ZP-11w, and ZP-2w groups during the adult stage are summarized in **Table 1**.

Protein Expression in the Adult Hippocampus in the TZ-11w, TZ-2w, ZP-11w, and ZP-2w Groups

We analyzed expression of several proteins in the adult mice hippocampus following juvenile or adult stage exposure to triazolam or zolpidem using western blotting (**Figure 7**). Although, no differences were detected in the TZ-11w, ZP-2w, and ZP-11w groups, MAP2 (**Figures 7A,Bb**, $p < 0.05$) was increased and GluR1 and GluR4 (**Figures 7A,Ba,b**, $p <$

TABLE 1 | A summary for the behavioral change at adult stage with different developmental exposure of triazolam 1 mg/kg B.W. and zolpidem 50 mg/kg B.W.

Test name	Behavioral tasks	Triazolam 1 mg/kg		Zolpidem 50 mg/kg	
		TZ-11w	TZ-2w	ZP-11w	ZP-2w
Open field	Distance traveled	1.14	1.23	0.90	0.97
	Center region time	1.72*	1.51	1.31	1.20
	Average speed	1.14	1.23	0.90	0.97
	Moving speed	1.03	1.09	0.96	0.97
	Moving episode number	0.99	0.98	1.00	0.97
	Total movement duration	1.12*	1.14*	0.93	1.00
	Distance per movement	1.15	1.29	0.91	1.00
	Duration per movement	1.14	1.19	0.94	1.03
Light/Dark transition	Dark distance	0.95	0.96	0.86	0.89
	Light distance	1.08	0.92	1.06	1.18
	Dark time	0.95	1.03	0.96	0.92
	Light time	1.12	0.97	1.19	1.28
	Number of transitions	1.00	0.97	0.93	1.04
	Latency to enter light	0.81	0.87	1.47	1.31
Elevated plus maze	Total distance	1.01	1.08	1.21	1.24
	Total center time	0.91	1.05	1.22	1.73
	Total open area	1.02	1.05	1.45	1.43
	Total close area	1.03	0.98	0.90	0.75
	Total arm select number	0.90	0.97	1.41	1.47
Fear conditioning	Total conditioning freezing %	0.83	0.27	1.57	0.91
	Conditioning 5–6 min freezing %	0.52	0.24*	1.39	1.02
	Total contextual freezing %	0.82	0.47*	1.43	0.72
	Cued tone 3–6 min freezing %	0.89	0.72	0.98	0.96
	Cued tone 3–4 min freezing %	0.92	0.64*	0.92	0.93
Pre-pulse inhibition	Pre-pulse 90 dB	1.07	1.28	1.32	1.38
	Pre-pulse 95 dB	1.19	0.98	0.78	1.24
	Pre-pulse 100 dB	1.07	1.05	0.90	0.89

The number indicates the fold change to vehicle and the asterisk indicates for the tests with the statistically significant difference to vehicle group [$p < 0.05$ (Student's t -test)].*

0.05) were decreased in the TZ-2w group. Both GluR1 and GluR4 belong to the AMPA-type glutamate receptor family and are known to be necessary for long-term potentiation in the hippocampus (Sanderson et al., 2008; Lee and Kirkwood, 2011). Therefore, decreases in the levels of GluR1 and GluR4 may be important mechanisms underlying the learning and memory deficits in mice exposed during the juvenile period.

mRNA Expression of Immediate Early Response Genes (IEGs) in the TZ-2w and ZP-2w Groups

We analyzed mRNA expression levels of IEGs (*Arc*, *c-fos*, and *Nr4a1*) in the hippocampus shortly (8 h) after TZ and ZP administration during the juvenile period. We observed decreased mRNA expression of IEGs in the TZ-2w group, but not in the ZP-2w group (**Figure 8**).

DISCUSSION

In this study, we analyzed the late-onset effects of the stimulation of the GABA-R signal using a behavioral battery tests (BBT) and several biochemical assays. We stimulated the GABA-R signal of mice by the oral administration of the sleep-inducing drugs TZ (1 mg/kg body weight [B.W.]) or ZP (50 mg/kg B.W.) during juvenile (TZ-2w, ZP-2w) and adult stages (TZ-11w, ZP-11w).

The results of the BBT indicate that spontaneous activity, as measured in the open field test, was significantly increased in the TZ-11w group. Reactivity to a novel environment may be changed in mice exposed to TZ during adulthood. On the other hand, deficits in learning and memory were detected by the fear conditioning test only in the TZ-2w group. The freezing response was decreased in all three stages (conditioning test, contextual test, and cued test) of the fear conditioning test. Although, the TZ-11w, ZP-11w, and ZP-2w groups had increases in freezing % as the cycles of tone and mild foot-shock were repeated, the

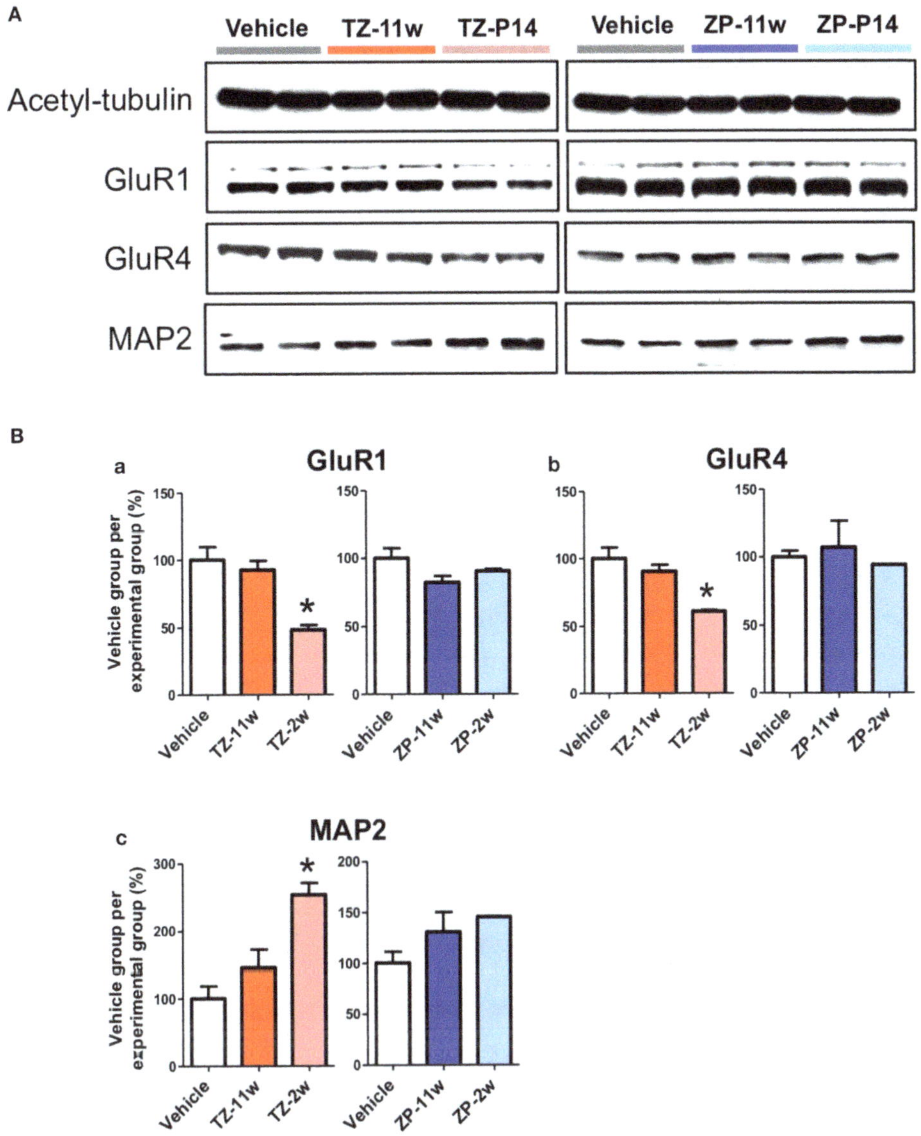

FIGURE 7 | Protein expression in the hippocampus during the adult stage following exposure to TZ and ZP during development. The expression levels of several proteins were analyzed by western blotting to explore the effects of triazolam on the hippocampus during adulthood. **(A)** Acetyl-tubulin and AMPA-type glutamate receptors GluR1 and GluR4, as well as the neuronal cytoskeletal marker MAP2. **(Ba–c)** The expression of each protein was normalized to that of acetyl-tubulin expression and its ratio (%) to the expression in the Vehicle group is shown. The number of samples was two and the value is shown as the mean ± SEM. Asterisk (*) indicate statistically significant differences (*$p < 0.05$, Student's t-test) compared to the Vehicle group.

TZ-2w group did not have an increase in freezing %, even during the later period of the test. These results may indicate that TZ-2w mice lose their ability to make short-term memories, which are needed for quick responses in this situation. In addition, TZ-2w mice had significantly lower scores in the contextual test. This may indicate deficits in spatial memory (Clark and Squire, 1998). In the cued test, a delay of the freezing response to the tone was detected in the TZ-2w group, which may indicate mild deficits in cued memory. We believe that these learning and memory deficits are the most serious effects of TZ treatment in the TZ-2w group.

To identify the molecular mechanisms underlying the late-onset learning and memory deficits, we first analyzed the expressions of several proteins in the hippocampus. We observed late-onset protein expression changes in the TZ-2w group. For example, MAP2 expression was increased in TZ-2w mice. MAP2 is a protein specifically expressed in the dendrites of neurons and plays an important role in the stabilization of tubulin structure in neuronal filaments (Caceres et al., 1983). There are also several reports of decreases in MAP2 levels in Alzheimer's disease and Parkinson's disease (Li et al., 2008; Liu et al., 2011). However, no increases in MAP2 levels have been reported thus

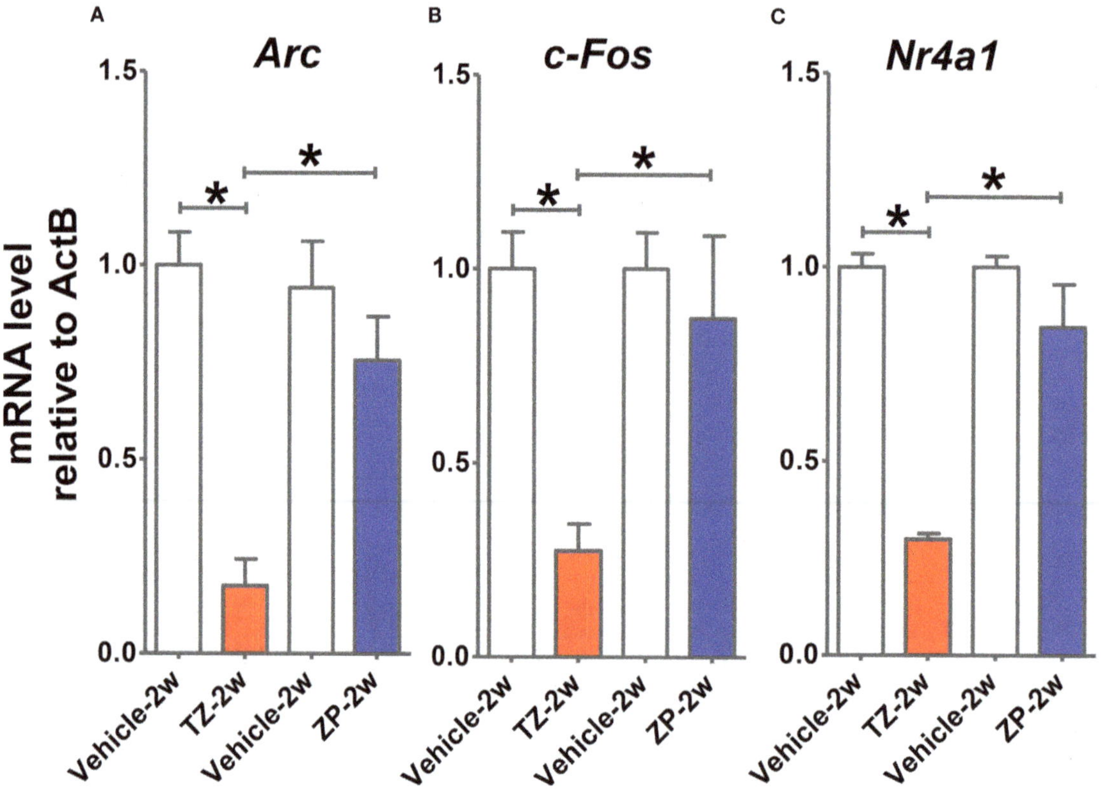

FIGURE 8 | Comparisons of immediate early response gene (IEG) mRNA expression levels in the hippocampus shortly after TZ or ZP exposure. Eight hours after TZ or ZP administration to juvenile (2-week-old) mice, we examined the mRNA expression levels of multiple IEGs in the hippocampus. Significant decreases in the expressions of **(A)** *Arc*, **(B)** *c-Fos*, and **(C)** *Nr4a1* were observed in the TZ-2w group. The number of the samples in each group was three and the values are shown as mean ± SEM. Asterisk (*) indicate statistically significant differences (*$p < 0.05$, Student's *t*-test) compared to the Vehicle group.

far. It is therefore still unclear how this increase in MAP2 levels relates to the deficits induced by triazolam. In addition, the expression levels of GluR1 and GluR4 were decreased in the TZ-2w group. GluR1 and GluR4 are AMPA-type glutamate receptors and are known to be important for learning and memory, as they induce long-term potentiation and synaptic plasticity (Sanderson et al., 2008; Lee and Kirkwood, 2011). Therefore, the deficits of learning and memory in the adult stage in neonatally exposed mice may be related to decreases in GluR1 and GluR4 levels. None of the ZP-treated groups and TZ-11w groups had changes in MAP2, GluR1, or GluR4 protein expression.

We hypothesize that TZ may have greater inhibitory effects on the hippocampus during the juvenile period and that may be a trigger of learning and memory deficits. Therefore, we measured changes in IEG mRNA expression in the hippocampi of juvenile mice shortly after TZ or ZP exposure (8 h). As expected, TZ had a greater inhibitory effect on the juvenile hippocampus than ZP. Indeed, the expression levels of all three IEGs (*Arc*, *c-fos*, and *Nr4a1*) were decreased in response to TZ treatment. IEGs are known to be induced rapidly following neuronal activation and are considered as markers of activated neurons (Sheng and Greenberg, 1990). The TZ-specific suppression of neuronal activity during the juvenile period may thus be responsible for the TZ-specific learning and memory deficits.

In summary, our findings demonstrate that the BZD sleep-inducing drug TZ can lead to learning and memory deficits with juvenile exposure. In contrast, ZP, which is a non-BZD, did not induce deficits in brain functional development. Decreased IEG expression was detected in mice treated with TZ during the juvenile period, but not in mice treated with ZP during the juvenile period. Therefore, we suggest that decreased IEG expression may be one of the triggers for the long-lasting adverse effects of TZ on the brain. The learning and memory deficits induced by TZ may be dependent on the timing of the exposure, as GABA-R signal has different functions in different brain developmental stages and in different brain regions containing GABA-Rs (Rice and Barone, 2000). GABA-R signal is reported to have a critical role in the reconstruction of synapses during the juvenile period (Steward and Falk, 1986; Herschkowitz et al., 1997). Therefore, juvenile exposure to TZ may interfere with synapse reconstruction and affect the proper development of learning and memory.

We have previously reported the aberration of emotional behavior associated with deficits in learning and memory in adult male mice treated with domoic acid (the chemical compound for the excessive activation of glutamate receptor mediated signal; Glu-R signal) at prenatal period by the administration to pregnant female mice (Tanemura et al., 2009). Nevertheless, we could not find the correlativity with this study using TZ. The following points can be given as that reasons. In previous study, we used mice in prenatal period does not correspond in the degree of maturation of hippocampus from juvenile period (Rice and Barone, 2000; Luján et al., 2005). Moreover, the domoic acid and TZ are completely different mechanism of action. We demonstrated that TZ administration cause the IEGs expression inhibitory in the juvenile period hippocampus. However, the domoic acid administration is known to increase IEG expression in hippocampus (Scallet et al., 2004). For these reasons, current study cannot be directly compared with previous one. We guessed that there might be several differences between the effects induced by disturbances of GABA-R and Glu-R signals, as each neuronal signal has the particular function to construct the neuronal circuits and reorganization depending on brain development (Steward and Falk, 1986; Rice and Barone, 2000; Luján et al., 2005). In addition, we guessed that the various aberrations of behavioral manners might be induced by the various disturbances of neural signals by the neuroactive chemical compounds.

In conclusion, our study indicates that juvenile TZ exposure may lead to learning and memory deficits. GABA-R agonists, such as BZD, are used for the treatment of both sleep disorders and anxiety disorders in both adults and children (Chevreuil et al., 2010; Weiss and Garbutt, 2010; Pelayo and Yuen, 2012). Therefore, considering the possible influence of GABA-R agonists on brain development, their careful prescription to children is warranted.

AUTHOR CONTRIBUTIONS

YF designed and performed experiments, analyzed data, and wrote the paper. KT designed the study, developed the methodology, conducted experiments, and editing the manuscript. KI helped with designed and editing the manuscript. MI helped with behavioral test and western blotting. KA, SK helped with the design of the study. MK, JK for the supervisor and design of the study.

ACKNOWLEDGMENTS

This study was supported in part by the Health Sciences Research Grants from the Ministry of Health, Labor, and Welfare, Japan (H23-KAGAKU-IPPAN-004, H27-KAGAKU-IPPAN-007).

REFERENCES

Caceres, A., Payne, M. R., Binder, L. I., and Steward, O. (1983). Immunocytochemical localization of actin and microtubule-associated protein MAP2 in dendritic spines. *Proc. Natl. Acad. Sci. U.S.A.* 80, 1738–1742. doi: 10.1073/pnas.80.6.1738

Chevreuil, C., Polard, E., Gicquel, G., Frémaux, T., and Bentué-Ferrer, D. (2010). [Pharmacologic treatment of insomnia in children and adolescent psychiatric patients]. *Therapie* 65, 1–12. doi: 10.2515/therapie/2010001

Clark, R. E., and Squire, L. R. (1998). Classical conditioning and brain systems: the role of awareness. *Science* 280, 77–81. doi: 10.1126/science.280.5360.77

FDA (2008). *Medication Guide Halcion Tablets/C-IV*. Silver Spring: US Food and Drug Administration (FDA).

FDA (2013). *Medication Guide Ambien (zolpidem tartrate) Tablets C-IV*. Silver Spring: US Food and Drug Administration (FDA).

Felt, B. T., and Chervin, R. D. (2014). Medications for sleep disturbances in children. *Neurol. Clin. Pract.* 4, 82–87. doi: 10.1212/01.CPJ.0000442521.30233.ef

Greenblatt, D. J., and Roth, T. (2012). Zolpidem for insomnia. *Expert Opin. Pharmacother.* 13, 879–893. doi: 10.1517/14656566.2012.667074

Haas, M., Qu, Z., Kim, T. H., Vargas, E., Campbell, K., Petrou, S., et al. (2013). Perturbations in cortical development and neuronal network excitability arising from prenatal exposure to benzodiazepines in mice. *Eur. J. Neurosci.* 37, 1584–1593. doi: 10.1111/ejn.12167

Herschkowitz, N., Kagan, J., and Zilles, K. (1997). Neurobiological bases of behavioral development in the first year. *Neuropediatrics* 28, 296–306. doi: 10.1055/s-2007-973720

Holm, K. J., and Goa, K. L. (2000). Zolpidem: an update of its pharmacology, therapeutic efficacy and tolerability in the treatment of insomnia. *Drugs* 59, 865–889. doi: 10.2165/00003495-200059040-00014

Jonas, J. M., Coleman, B. S., Sheridan, A. Q., and Kalinske, R. W. (1992). Comparative clinical profiles of triazolam versus other shorter-acting hypnotics. *J. Clin. Psychiatry* 53(Suppl.), 19–31. discussion; 32–33.

Kahn, A., Van de Merckt, C., Rebuffat, E., Mozin, M. J., Sottiaux, M., Blum, D., et al. (1989). Sleep problems in healthy preadolescents. *Pediatrics* 84, 542–546.

Lee, H. K., and Kirkwood, A. (2011). AMPA receptor regulation during synaptic plasticity in hippocampus and neocortex. *Semin. Cell Dev. Biol.* 22, 514–520. doi: 10.1016/j.semcdb.2011.06.007

Li, B., Yamamori, H., Tatebayashi, Y., Shafit-Zagardo, B., Tanimukai, H., Chen, S., et al. (2008). Failure of neuronal maturation in Alzheimer disease dentate gyrus. *J. Neuropathol. Exp. Neurol.* 67, 78–84. doi: 10.1097/nen.0b013e318160c5db

Liu, Q., Xie, F., Alvarado-Diaz, A., Smith, M. A., Moreira, P. I., Zhu, X., et al. (2011). Neurofilamentopathy in neurodegenerative diseases. *Open Neurol. J.* 5, 58–62. doi: 10.2174/1874205X01105010058

Livak, K. J., and Schmittgen, T. D. (2001). Analysis of relative gene expression data using real-time quantitative PCR and the 2(-Delta Delta C(T)) Method. *Methods* 25, 402–408. doi: 10.1006/meth.2001.1262

Lobo, B. L., and Greene, W. L. (1997). Zolpidem: distinct from triazolam? *Ann. Pharmacother.* 31, 625–632.

Luján, R., Shigemoto, R., and López-Bendito, G. (2005). Glutamate and GABA receptor signalling in the developing brain. *Neuroscience* 130, 567–580. doi: 10.1016/j.neuroscience.2004.09.042

Neubauer, D. N. (2007). The evolution and development of insomnia pharmacotherapies. *J. Clin. Sleep Med.* 3, S11–S15.

Owens, J. A., Rosen, C. L., and Mindell, J. A. (2003). Medication use in the treatment of pediatric insomnia: results of a survey of community-based pediatricians. *Pediatrics* 111, e628–e635. doi: 10.1542/peds.111.5.e628

Pakes, G. E., Brogden, R. N., Heel, R. C., Speight, T. M., and Avery, G. S. (1981). Triazolam: a review of its pharmacological properties and therapeutic efficacy in patients with insomnia. *Drugs* 22, 81–110. doi: 10.2165/00003495-198122020-00001

Pelayo, R., and Yuen, K. (2012). Pediatric sleep pharmacology. *Child Adolesc. Psychiatr. Clin. N. Am.* 21, 861–883. doi: 10.1016/j.chc.2012.08.001

Rice, D., and Barone, S. (2000). Critical periods of vulnerability for the developing nervous system: evidence from humans and animal models. *Environ. Health Perspect.* 108(Suppl. 3), 511–533. doi: 10.1289/ehp.00108s3511

Rudolph, U., and Knoflach, F. (2011). Beyond classical benzodiazepines: novel therapeutic potential of GABAA receptor subtypes. *Nat. Rev. Drug Discov.* 10, 685–697. doi: 10.1038/nrd3502

Sanderson, D. J., Good, M. A., Seeburg, P. H., Sprengel, R., Rawlins, J. N., and Bannerman, D. M. (2008). The role of the GluR-A (GluR1) AMPA receptor subunit in learning and memory. *Prog. Brain Res.* 169, 159–178. doi: 10.1016/S0079-6123(07)00009-X

Scallet, A. C., Kowalke, P. K., Rountree, R. L., Thorn, B. T., and Binienda, Z. K. (2004). Electroencephalographic, behavioral, and c-fos responses to acute domoic acid exposure. *Neurotoxicol. Teratol.* 26, 331–342. doi: 10.1016/j.ntt.2003.10.004

Shen, Q., Fuchs, T., Sahir, N., and Luscher, B. (2012). GABAergic control of critical developmental periods for anxiety- and depression-related behavior in mice. *PLoS ONE* 7:e47441. doi: 10.1371/journal.pone.0047441

Sheng, M., and Greenberg, M. E. (1990). The regulation and function of c-fos and other immediate early genes in the nervous system. *Neuron* 4, 477–4485. doi: 10.1016/0896-6273(90)90106-P

Steward, O., and Falk, P. M. (1986). Protein-synthetic machinery at postsynaptic sites during synaptogenesis: a quantitative study of the association between polyribosomes and developing synapses. *J. Neurosci.* 6, 412–4423.

Stores, G. (1996). Practitioner review: assessment and treatment of sleep disorders in children and adolescents. *J. Child Psychol. Psychiatry* 37, 907–925. doi: 10.1111/j.1469-7610.1996.tb01489.x

Tanemura, K., Igarashi, K., Matsugami, T. R., Aisaki, K., Kitajima, S., and Kanno, J. (2009). Intrauterine environment-genome interaction and children's development (2): brain structure impairment and behavioral disturbance induced in male mice offspring by a single intraperitoneal administration of domoic acid (DA) to their dams. *J. Toxicol. Sci.* 34(Suppl. 2), Sp279–Sp86. doi: 10.2131/jts.34.sp279

Toner, L. C., Tsambiras, B. M., Catalano, G., Catalano, M. C., and Cooper, D. S. (2000). Central nervous system side effects associated with zolpidem treatment. *Clin. Neuropharmacol.* 23, 54–58. doi: 10.1097/00002826-200001000-00011

Weiss, S. K., and Garbutt, A. (2010). Pharmacotherapy in pediatric sleep disorders. *Adolesc. Med. State Art Rev.* 21, 508–521.

22

Neuroendocrinal, Neurodevelopmental, and Embryotoxic Effects of Recombinant Tissue Plasminogen Activator Treatment for Pregnant Women with Acute Ischemic Stroke

Anna Steinberg[1,2]* *and Tiago P. Moreira*[1,2]

[1] *Department of Neurology, Karolinska University Hospital, Stockholm, Sweden,* [2] *Stroke Research Unit, Department of Clinical Neuroscience, Karolinska Institutet, Stockholm, Sweden*

Edited by:
Fumihiko Maekawa,
National Institute for Environmental Studies, Japan

Reviewed by:
Tin-Tin Win-Shwe,
National Institute for Environmental Studies, Japan
Masaki Kakeyama,
Waseda University, Japan

***Correspondence:**
Anna Steinberg
anna.steinberg@karolinska.se

Thrombolysis with recombinant tissue plasminogen activator (rTPA) was the first evidence-based treatment approved for acute stroke. Ischemic stroke is relatively uncommon in fertile women but treatment is often delayed or not given. In randomized trials, pregnancy has been an exclusion criterion for thrombolysis. Physiologic TPA has been shown to have neuroendocrine effects namely in vasopressin secretion. Important TPA effects in brain function and development include neurite outgrowth, migration of cerebellar granular neurons and promotion of long-term potentiation, among others. Until now, no neuroendocrine side-effects have been reported in pregnant women treated with rTPA. The effects of rTPA exposure in the fetus following intravenous thrombolysis in pregnant women are still poorly understood. This depends on low case frequency, short-duration of exposure and the fact that rTPA molecule is too large to pass the placenta. rTPA has a short half-life of 4–5 min, with only 10% of its concentration remaining in circulation after 20 min, which may explain its safety at therapeutically doses. Ischemic stroke during pregnancy occurs most often in the third trimester. Complication rates of rTPA in pregnant women treated for thromboembolic conditions and ischemic stroke were found to be similar when compared to non-pregnant women (7–9% mortality). In embryos of animal models so far, no indications of a teratogenic or mutagenic potential were found. Pregnancy is still considered a relative contraindication when treating acute ischemic stroke with rTPA, however, treatment risk must be balanced against the potential of maternal disability and/or death.

Keywords: rTPA, alteplase, brain development, toxicity, haemorrhagic, intravenous, teratogenic, uterine

NEUROENDOCRINE EFFECTS OF TISSUE PLASMINOGEN ACTIVATOR

Tissue plasminogen activator (TPA) is a serine protease that converts plasminogen into the fibrinolytic enzyme plasmin thus promoting fibrin dissolution in blood clots (Carmeliet et al., 1994). Endothelial cells are the major source of circulating TPA, which is released upon stimulation by factor X-a, bradykinin, fibrin, platelet activating factor, and thrombin (Booyse et al., 1986; Emeis, 1992). Other triggers of TPA released into the bloodstream include among others, anxiety, exercise, surgery, and electroconvulsive therapy, however, these conditions are also coupled to catecholamine release, which may thus be the shared trigger mechanism for both direct TPA release and TPA release from endothelial cells in these conditions. In support of this notion, TPA was demonstrated to be co-expressed and trafficked simultaneously with noradrenaline in the chromaffin cells of the adrenal glands (Parmer et al., 1993). Chromogranin A is one soluble protein that is co-released with TPA and catecholamines. It works as prohormone which, when cleaved into active peptides, inhibits the further release of catecholamines (Parmer et al., 1993). Experiments with knockout mice lacking TPA provided further evidence for a role of TPA in behavioral stress responses and catecholamine release. These mice exhibit deficient stress-induced anxiety behavior (Pawlak et al., 2003, 2005) and show anxiety-like behavior after intracerebroventricular injection of corticotrophin releasing factor (Matys et al., 2004).

TPA-cleaved plasmin regulates proteolysis of among other, laminin, collagen IV, proteoglycans, pro-brain-derived neurotrophic factor (pro-BDNF), and protease activated receptor-1 (Dityatev and Schachner, 2003; Pang et al., 2004). TPA has been shown to directly interact with low-density lipoprotein receptor-related protein (LRP) leading to phosphorylation of mitogen-activated protein kinase (MAPK) 1 and extracellular signal-regulated kinases-1 and 2 (Zhuo et al., 2000; Hu et al., 2006). In turn, serpins (including the CNS variant neuroserpin) and plasminogen activator inhibitor PAI-1 and -2 are the main inhibitors of the serine protease family including TPA, urokinase-type plasminogen activator (uPA), plasmin, and thrombin (Yepes and Lawrence, 2004).

Endogenous TPA is widely distributed in the neuroendocrine system. In the neuroendocrine cells of the hypophysis, the magnocellular neurons of the hypothalamic supra-optic nucleus, the chromaffin cells of the adrenal medulla, thyroid and parathyroid glands, endogenous TPA first enters the endoplasmic reticulum where it binds to a signal peptide and is transported through the Golgi complex. It is then released either via the regulated secretory pathway (vesicular) or the constitutive secretory pathway (direct release) (Kelly, 1985). Although there is one regulated secretory pathway, TPA gets rapidly released from storage vesicles originated from the Golgi complex and appears to be mediated by calcium ion influx (Gualandris et al., 1996). A similar mechanism of TPA co-release with parathyroid hormone has been described in parathyroid cells (Bansal and MacGregor, 1992).

In the brain, wide expression of neuronal TPA and the plasmin inhibitor neuroserpin are found in the developing and adult nervous system and have been shown to play a role in neuronal plasticity (Lee et al., 2015). TPA expression predominate in the lobar hemispheres, thalamus, medulla oblongata, and mesencephalon whereas neuroserpin, although also overlapping with TPA in the lobar hemispheres and mesencephalon, is more abundant in the spinal cord, substantia nigra and Purkinje cells (Teesalu et al., 2004). Moreover, TPA mRNA expression is seen in ventricular ependymal cells and meningeal blood vessel cells (Hashimoto et al., 1998).

In particular, a role of TPA in the neurohypophysis has been proposed for the osmotic regulation of body fluids. The antidiuretic hormone vasopressin (arginine-vasopressin or AVP) is synthesized in the magnocellular neurons of the hypothalamic supra-optic nucleus and paraventricular nucleus, and packed into neurosecretory granules, which are transported through their axons over to the neurohypophysary terminals (Miyata and Hatton, 2002). TPA immunoreactivity was observed at neurosecretory granules of vasopressin-positive magnocellular terminals and that of plasminogen was seen at astrocytes. With electron microscopy, Imamura et al. were able to show a specific localization of TPA at neurosecretory granules containing vasopressin, indicating that TPA is co-released along with the exocytosis of vasopressin and might be an early regulator of vasopressin release (Imamura et al., 2010).

TPA has been implicated in neurite outgrowth of neuronal cultures (Pittman et al., 1989), neuronal regeneration, migration of cerebellar granule neurons (Seeds et al., 1995), and prohormone synthesis (Sappino et al., 1993). TPA is capable of potentiating N-methyl-D-aspartate (NMDA) receptor activation by cleaving the NMDA receptor 1 (NMDAR1) subunit (Nicole et al., 2001). The significance TPA-induced cleavage of NMDAR1, as well as cleavage of pro-BDNF by plasmin is particularly relevant for learning and memory. On the one hand, TPA knockout (KO) mice show reduced maintenance of the long-term potential in the hippocampal CA1 area and exhibit less open-field exploration and poor performance in a context-conditioning task (Calabresi et al., 2000). On the other hand, mice overexpressing TPA show an enhancement of the long-term potential in the hippocampus with improved performance in spatial navigation learning tasks (Baranes et al., 1998; Madani et al., 1999). Long-term depression is absent in the striatum of TPA KO mice and has been coupled with decreased rearing activity and object exploration, as well as with poorer performance in a two-way active avoidance task (Calabresi et al., 2000). In 3 month-old Fischer rats, increased TPA mRNA expression is detected in Purkinje cerebellar neurons following 1 h of complex motor task learning in rats (Seeds et al., 1995). Ocular dominance plasticity in the visual cortex was also shown to be related to TPA and plasmin activities (Müller and Griesinger, 1998; Mataga et al., 2004). The authors have also suggested that a cascade of plasmin generated by TPA may selectively mediate cortical plasticity, perhaps via structural remodeling of axons (Müller and Griesinger, 1998; Mataga et al., 2004). Evidence for a function of TPA and the brain-specific protease inhibitor neuroserpin in regulating axonal growth has come from studies of cultured cells (for a recent review see Lee et al., 2015). Hashimoto and colleagues found evidence supporting TPA involvement in long-lasting cortical plasticity following psychotomimetic administration in the rat by observing increased mRNA expression in prefrontal cortex neurons projecting to the medial striatum (Hashimoto et al., 1998).

Finally, ischemic damage is suggested to lead to excess endogenous TPA activity in the brain and contribute to neurodegeneration via extracellular matrix degradation, microglia activation, and blood brain barrier leakage (Lee et al., 2015). Neuroserpin-knockout mice have worse ischemic damage and neurological outcomes than controls, with the effects attributed to TPA-mediated activation of microglia (Gelderblom et al., 2013). Experimental intravenous (exogenous) TPA administration was shown to increase cerebrovascular permeability and decrease cerebrovascular resistance (Tsirka et al., 1995; Yepes et al., 2003; Nassar et al., 2004).

TREATMENT WITH RECOMBINANT TPA IN PREGNANT WOMEN

About 85% of all strokes are ischemic and the remaining are hemorrhagic. Spontaneous reperfusion may occur through endogenous release of plasminogen activator, which stimulates plasmin formation from plasminogen. For larger occlusions this release seems insufficient to induce reperfusion in time to avoid a cerebral lesion. Administration of alteplase, a recombinant tissue plasminogen activator (rTPA) as an injectable drug, which is commonly used to treat myocardial infarction, stroke and thrombosis, is thus one method to enhance this endogenous procedure (for a recent review see Prabhakaran et al., 2015). Acute ischemic stroke in pregnant women occurs most commonly in the third trimester and is potentiated by an increased pro-coagulant state during pregnancy, higher risk for cervical and intracranial artery dissection peri-partum, as well as by persistent foramen ovale and other underlying cardiac conditions.

The thrombolytic effect of rTPA varies among species. Humans are proposed to have a more sensitive fibrinolytic system to the effects of rTPA (Korninger and Collen, 1981). Thus, in humans the effective and safe dose for acute stroke treatment is 0.9 mg/kg. In rats, a dose of 1.8 mg/kg up to 10 mg/kg induced recanalization of carotid artery occlusion in 17–71%, whereas in humans this is only achieved in 10–30% of cases. The 1.8 mg/kg dose in the rat is proposed to be equivalent to the human dose of 0.9 mg/kg in terms of efficacy (Tomkins et al., 2015). In rabbits, a dose of 5 mg/kg—but not of 3 or 10 mg/kg—is capable of dissolving an intracerebral clot embolized from the carotid artery (Bednar et al., 1993). Until now, randomized controlled trials have excluded pregnant women and patients with increased hemorrhage risk from participation in studies regarding thrombolysis treatment. In animals rTPA does not cross the placenta and there has been no evidence of teratogenicity (Chan et al., 2000; Leonhardt et al., 2006; De Keyser et al., 2007). To date there are no reports on rTPA being able to cross the human placenta. In 2006, Leonhardt et al. had reviewed 18 cases of pregnant women treated with rTPA for other thromboembolic conditions, mainly pulmonary embolism, deep vein thrombosis and thrombosed cardiac valve prosthesis and 10 cases of pregnant women treated with rTPA for acute stroke, including an own stroke case (Leonhardt et al., 2006). Good maternal neurological outcome was reported for all but two mothers who died (one with stroke, the other with mitral valve thrombosis) and one who developed cerebral infarction. Ineffective thrombolysis or partial arterial recanalization was reported in four mothers. Twenty children were born with good outcome, however, there were two spontaneous abortions, three pregnancy interruptions owing to maternal cause and one infant died at 2 weeks' post-partum. Thus, there was a similar rate of complications in pregnant women compared to non-pregnant women, with mortality at about 7% for the mother and about 23% for the child (half of the child losses occurred in three stroke cases; the other half in two pulmonary embolisms and one valve thrombosis). Possible explanations for child loss not addressed by this review may include the severity of the underlying maternal medical condition rather than a direct effect of rTPA treatment alone. Interruptions of pregnancy may also have been carried following medical decision. Later in 2006, Wiese et al. reported use of intravenous rTPA thrombolysis in a pregnant woman with acute cardioembolic stroke. The patient improved clinically, did not develop complications after receiving rTPA, and at 37 weeks' gestation, delivered a healthy infant (Wiese et al., 2006). Yamaguchi et al. reported a 36 year-old woman, who was 18 weeks pregnant and developed a sudden onset of motor aphasia and hemiparesis on the right side. The NIH stroke scale was 6, and the brain MRI indicated occlusion of the left middle cerebral artery branches. She was treated with intravenous rTPA with subsequent recanalization of the occluded left middle cerebral artery branches. The symptoms disappeared within a few hours after treatment. She delivered a healthy infant without any apparent complications (Yamaguchi et al., 2010). There are further cases of successful use of rTPA in pregnant women with acute stroke, the majority in the third trimester of pregnancy (Dapprich and Boessenecker, 2002; Elford et al., 2002; Johnson et al., 2005; Murugappan et al., 2006). In 2012, Li et al. reported one own stroke case and reviewed 10 previously published stroke cases. They reported good to complete recovery in 10 mothers and one death during endovascular treatment, resulting in the delivery of eight healthy infants, two medical terminations of pregnancy, and one fetus death (Li et al., 2012). In 2013 and 2014, two additional stroke cases with good outcome for the mothers and the fetuses were reported by Tassi and Ritter, respectively (Tassi et al., 2013; Mantoan Ritter et al., 2014). The most recent case of successful rTPA treatment in a pregnant woman at 39 weeks of gestation with normal delivery was reported in 2015 (Ritchie et al., 2015). So far, only one mother treated with rTPA for acute stroke suffered a significant uterine bleeding complication (Demchuk, 2013), however, caution about bias publication should be taken into account when reviewing case reports. Intravenously administered rTPA has a high affinity for fibrin strands and a short half-life of 4–5 min via liver metabolism, with only 10% of its concentration remaining in circulation after 20 min, which may explain its safety at therapeutic doses.

In menstruating women, Wein et al. described five subjects in the active arm of the National Institute of Neurological Disorders and Stroke (NINDS) intravenous thrombolysis trial, who were coded as actively menstruating. One subject who had a 1-year history of dysfunctional uterine bleeding required urgent uterine artery ligation. The authors also reported a case of a woman requiring transfusion after intravenous thrombolysis for acute ischaemic stroke (Wein et al., 2002).

So far, no neuroendocrine side-effects have been reported in pregnant women treated with alteplase.

EFFECTS OF EXPOSURE TO rTPA IN BRAIN DEVELOPMENT

As stated above, intravenous rTPA is too large a molecule (7200 KDa) to be able to pass the placental blood barrier. From clinical reports of IVT-treated pregnant women with stroke, there have been no signs of brain development issues on the surviving fetuses. The European Medicines Agency license for alteplase includes information on embryotoxicity (in the form of embryolethality and growth retardation) in pregnant rabbits given 3 mg/kg alteplase, which is over 3 times the therapeutical dose (0.9 mg/kg). However, no teratogenic effects were observed in animals treated with i.v. therapeutical doses and no effects on peri- or post-natal development or fertility were observed in rats treated with doses up to 10 mg/kg (Kojima et al., 1988) In subchronic toxicity studies in rats and marmosets no unexpected adverse effects were observed. No indicative signs of mutagenesis were found (preclinical safety data included in the European license documentation) (EMEA, 2002).

ONGOING STUDIES

Uncertainty whether fertile women with potential or known pregnancy should be treated may delay or halt thrombolysis and worsen stroke outcome. Maternal hemorrhagic complications have been reported in 8% with systemic thrombolysis across the spectrum of clinical thromboembolic indications (Cronin et al., 2008). More specifically, mortality in 172 pregnant women treated with a potent thrombolytic agent, streptokinase, was reported at 1.2% (Turrentine et al., 1995), which is far lower than the 9.5% mortality owed to stroke alone in pregnant women (Ritchie et al., 2015). Thus, considering this limited risk, pregnancy should not be considered an absolute contraindication. The risk during pregnancy must be balanced against the potential of a disabled outcome without treatment (Demchuk, 2013). To explore the safety of thrombolysis in pregnant women with acute stroke, and indeed within the whole group of fertile women, the Safe Implementation of Treatments in Stroke International Stroke Thrombolysis Register (SITS-ISTR), a prospective, international, observational registry for medical centers documenting stroke treatments (Wahlgren et al., 2007) has been expanded to include specific questions for women in the age group 13–50. The aim is to systematically collect data, to contribute to knowledge about treatment safety for these women, and to explore whether treatment in pregnant women, or indeed all women in fertile age is safe and not delayed. We estimate that a number of women will be treated despite pregnancy, partly because the condition was not considered when treatment was initiated, or because the potential benefit was judged higher than the risk. The overall aim of the study, Safe Implementation of Treatments in Stroke-Fertile Women Stroke Thrombolysis Study (SITS-FW), is to determine if pregnancy and even menstruation constitutes any safety issue when treated with thrombolysis, or if these patients can be given the same opportunity for treatment as other patients.

CONCLUSIONS

Pregnancy is still considered a relative contraindication for intravenous thrombolysis with rTPA for acute ischemic stroke within 4.5 h of symptom onset. However, the present and previous reviews indicate a similar maternal safety profile compared with non-pregnant women. This should be further analyzed in future prospective studies. It is reasonable to weigh in the benefit of rTPA vs. the risk for the fetus in this patient group and offer treatment for moderate to severe disabling stroke, particularly if there is no access to endovascular treatment. With the current ongoing implementation of mechanical thrombectomy for acute ischemic stroke in routine practice (Wahlgren et al., 2016), we expect more pregnant women to benefit from acute reperfusion strategies that may or not include intravenous thrombolysis in addition to mechanical thrombectomy for large vessel occlusions.

AUTHOR CONTRIBUTIONS

AS, Planned litterature review, wrote first draft with references. TM, Planned litterature review, wrote abstract, edited first draft, and wrote final version.

REFERENCES

Bansal, D. D., and MacGregor, R. R. (1992). Calcium-regulated secretion of tissue plasminogen activator and parathyroid hormone from human parathyroid cells. *J. Clin. Endocrinol. Metab.* 74, 266–271. doi: 10.1210/jcem.74.2.1730806

Baranes, D., Lederfein, D., Huang, Y. Y., Chen, M., Bailey, C. H., and Kandel, E. R. (1998). Tissue plasminogen activator contributes to the late phase of LTP and to synaptic growth in the hippocampal mossy fiber pathway. *Neuron* 21, 813–825. doi: 10.1016/S0896-6273(00)80597-8

Bednar, M. M., Raymond, S. J., and Gross, C. E. (1993). Tissue plasminogen activator: comparison of dose and route of administration in a rabbit model of thromboembolic stroke. *Neurol. Res.* 15, 405–408.

Booyse, F. M., Bruce, R., Dolenak, D., Grover, M., and Casey, L. C. (1986). Rapid release and deactivation of plasminogen activators in human endothelial cell cultures in the presence of thrombin and ionophore A23187. *Semin. Thromb. Hemost.* 12, 228–230. doi: 10.1055/s-2007-1003558

Calabresi, P., Napolitano, M., Centonze, D., Marfia, G. A., Gubellini, P., Teule, M. A., et al. (2000). Tissue plasminogen activator controls multiple forms of synaptic plasticity and memory. *Eur. J. Neurosci.* 12, 1002–1012. doi: 10.1046/j.1460-9568.2000.00991.x

Carmeliet, P., Schoonjans, L., Kieckens, L., Ream, B., Degen, J., Bronson, R., et al. (1994). Physiological consequences of loss of plasminogen activator gene function in mice. *Nature* 368, 419–424. doi: 10.1038/368419a0

Chan, W. S., Anand, S., and Ginsberg, J. S. (2000). Anticoagulation of pregnant women with mechanical heart valves: a systematic review of the literature. *Arch. Intern. Med.* 160, 191–196. doi: 10.1001/archinte.160.2.191

Cronin, C. A., Weisman, C. J., and Llinas, R. H. (2008). Stroke treatment: beyond the three-hour window and in the pregnant patient. *Ann. N.Y. Acad. Sci.* 1142, 159–178. doi: 10.1196/annals.1444.013

Dapprich, M., and Boessenecker, W. (2002). Fibrinolysis with alteplase in a pregnant woman with stroke. *Cerebrovasc. Dis.* 13, 290. doi: 10.1159/000057859

De Keyser, J., Gdovinová, Z., Uyttenboogaart, M., Vroomen, P. C., and Luijckx, G. J. (2007). Intravenous alteplase for stroke: beyond the guidelines and in particular clinical situations. *Stroke* 38, 2612–2618. doi: 10.1161/STROKEAHA.106.480566

Demchuk, A. M. (2013). Yes, intravenous thrombolysis should be administered in pregnancy when other clinical and imaging factors are favorable. *Stroke* 44, 864–865. doi: 10.1161/STROKEAHA.111.000134

Dityatev, A., and Schachner, M. (2003). Extracellular matrix molecules and synaptic plasticity. *Nat. Rev. Neurosci.* 4, 456–468. doi: 10.1038/nrn1115

Elford, K., Leader, A., Wee, R., and Stys, P. K. (2002). Stroke in ovarian hyperstimulation syndrome in early pregnancy treated with intra-arterial rt-PA. *Neurology* 59, 1270–1272. doi: 10.1212/01.WNL.0000032492.77156.35

EMEA (2002). *European Medicines Agency. Summary Information on a Referral Opinion following an Arbitration Pursuant to Article 29 of Directive 2001/83/EC, for Actilyse. CPMP/3346/02-EN.* London.

Emeis, J. J. (1992). Regulation of the acute release of tissue-type plasminogen activator from the endothelium by coagulation activation products. *Ann. N.Y. Acad. Sci.* 667, 249–258. doi: 10.1111/j.1749-6632.1992.tb51622.x

Gelderblom, M., Neumann, M., Ludewig, P., Bernreuther, C., Krasemann, S., Arunachalam, P., et al. (2013). Deficiency in serine protease inhibitor neuroserpin exacerbates ischemic brain injury by increased postischemic inflammation. *PLoS ONE* 8:e63118. doi: 10.1371/journal.pone.0063118

Gualandris, A., Jones, T. E., Strickland, S., and Tsirka, S. E. (1996). Membrane depolarization induces calcium-dependent secretion of tissue plasminogen activator. *J. Neurosci.* 16, 2220–2225.

Hashimoto, T., Kajii, Y., and Nishikawa, T. (1998). Psychotomimetic-induction of tissue plasminogen activator mRNA in corticostriatal neurons in rat brain. *Eur. J. Neurosci.* 10, 3387–3399. doi: 10.1046/j.1460-9568.1998.00343.x

Hu, K., Yang, J., Tanaka, S., Gonias, S. L., Mars, W. M., and Liu, Y. (2006). Tissue-type plasminogen activator acts as a cytokine that triggers intracellular signal transduction and induces matrix metalloproteinase-9 gene expression. *J. Biol. Chem.* 281, 2120–2127. doi: 10.1074/jbc.M504988200

Imamura, Y., Morita, S., Nakatani, Y., Okada, K., Ueshima, S., Matsuo, O., et al. (2010). Tissue plasminogen activator and plasminogen are critical for osmotic homeostasis by regulating vasopressin secretion. *J. Neurosci. Res.* 88, 1995–2006. doi: 10.1002/jnr.22370

Johnson, D. M., Kramer, D. C., Cohen, E., Rochon, M., Rosner, M., and Weinberger, J. (2005). Thrombolytic therapy for acute stroke in late pregnancy with intra-arterial recombinant tissue plasminogen activator. *Stroke* 36, e53–e55. doi: 10.1161/01.STR.0000166203.27135.27

Kelly, R. B. (1985). Pathways of protein secretion in eukaryotes. *Science* 230, 25–32. doi: 10.1126/science.2994224

Kojima, N., Tanaka, M., Naya, M., Imoto, H., Hara, T., Deguchi, T., et al. (1988). Teratogenic, peri and postnatal studies of GMK-527 (rt-PA) parts II, III and IV. *Jpn. Pharmacol. Ther.* 16, 93–142.

Korninger, C., and Collen, D. (1981). Studies on the specific fibrinolytic effect of human extrinsic (tissue-type) plasminogen activator in human blood and in various animal species *in vitro*. *Thromb. Haemost.* 46, 561–565.

Lee, T. W., Tsang, V. W., and Birch, N. P. (2015). Physiological and pathological roles of tissue plasminogen activator and its inhibitor neuroserpin in the nervous system. *Front. Cell Neurosci.* 9:396. doi: 10.3389/fncel.2015.00396

Leonhardt, G., Gaul, C., Nietsch, H. H., Buerke, M., and Schleussner, E. (2006). Thrombolytic therapy in pregnancy. *J. Thromb. Thrombolysis* 21, 271–276. doi: 10.1007/s11239-006-5709-z

Li, Y., Margraf, J., Kluck, B., Jenny, D., and Castaldo, J. (2012). Thrombolytic therapy for ischemic stroke secondary to paradoxical embolism in pregnancy: a case report and literature review. *Neurologist* 18, 44–48. doi: 10.1097/NRL.0b013e31823d7af0

Madani, R., Hulo, S., Toni, N., Madani, H., Steimer, T., Muller, D., et al. (1999). Enhanced hippocampal long-term potentiation and learning by increased neuronal expression of tissue-type plasminogen activator in transgenic mice. *EMBO J.* 18, 3007–3012. doi: 10.1093/emboj/18.11.3007

Mantoan Ritter, L., Schüler, A., Gangopadhyay, R., Mordecai, L., Arowele, O., Losseff, N., et al. (2014). Successful thrombolysis of stroke with intravenous alteplase in the third trimester of pregnancy. *J. Neurol.* 261, 632–634. doi: 10.1007/s00415-014-7286-y

Mataga, N., Mizuguchi, Y., and Hensch, T. K. (2004). Experience-dependent pruning of dendritic spines in visual cortex by tissue plasminogen activator. *Neuron* 44, 1031–1041. doi: 10.1016/j.neuron.2004.11.028

Matys, T., Pawlak, R., Matys, E., Pavlides, C., McEwen, B. S., and Strickland, S. (2004). Tissue plasminogen activator promotes the effects of corticotropin-releasing factor on the amygdala and anxiety-like behavior. *Proc. Natl. Acad. Sci. U.S.A.* 101, 16345–16350. doi: 10.1073/pnas.0407355101

Miyata, S., and Hatton, G. I. (2002). Activity-related, dynamic neuron-glial interactions in the hypothalamo-neurohypophysial system. *Microsc. Res. Tech.* 56, 143–157. doi: 10.1002/jemt.10012

Müller, C. M., and Griesinger, C. B. (1998). Tissue plasminogen activator mediates reverse occlusion plasticity in visual cortex. *Nat. Neurosci.* 1, 47–53. doi: 10.1038/248

Murugappan, A., Coplin, W. M., Al-Sadat, A. N., McAllen, K. J., Schwamm, L. H., Wechsler, L. R., et al. (2006). Thrombolytic therapy of acute ischemic stroke during pregnancy. *Neurology* 66, 768–770. doi: 10.1212/01.wnl.0000201272.90216.15

Nassar, T., Akkawi, S., Shina, A., Haj-Yehia, A., Bdeir, K., Tarshis, M., et al. (2004). *Front* and *in vivo* effects of tPA and PAI-1 on blood vessel tone. *Blood* 103, 897–902. doi: 10.1182/blood-2003-05-1685

Nicole, O., Docagne, F., Ali, C., Margaill, I., Carmeliet, P., Mackenzie, E. T., et al. (2001). The proteolytic activity of tissue-plasminogen activator enhances NMDA receptor-mediated signaling. *Nat. Med.* 7, 59–64. doi: 10.1038/83358

Pang, P. T., Teng, H. K., Zaitsev, E., Woo, N. T., Sakata, K., Zhen, S., et al. (2004). Cleavage of proBDNF by tPA/plasmin is essential for long-term hippocampal plasticity. *Science* 306, 487–491. doi: 10.1126/science.1100135

Parmer, R. J., Xi, X. P., Wu, H. J., Helman, L. J., and Petz, L. N. (1993). Secretory protein traffic. Chromogranin A contains a dominant targeting signal for the regulated pathway. *J. Clin. Invest.* 92, 1042–1054. doi: 10.1172/JCI116609

Pawlak, R., Magarinos, A. M., Melchor, J., McEwen, B., and Strickland, S. (2003). Tissue plasminogen activator in the amygdala is critical for stress-induced anxiety-like behavior. *Nat. Neurosci.* 6, 168–174. doi: 10.1038/nn998

Pawlak, R., Rao, B. S., Melchor, J. P., Chattarji, S., McEwen, B., and Strickland, S. (2005). Tissue plasminogen activator and plasminogen mediate stress-induced decline of neuronal and cognitive functions in the mouse hippocampus. *Proc. Natl. Acad. Sci. U.S.A.* 102, 18201–18206. doi: 10.1073/pnas.0509232102

Pittman, R. N., Ivins, J. K., and Buettner, H. M. (1989). Neuronal plasminogen activators: cell surface binding sites and involvement in neurite outgrowth. *J. Neurosci.* 9, 4269–4286.

Prabhakaran, S., Ruff, I., and Bernstein, R. A. (2015). Acute stroke intervention: a systematic review. *JAMA* 313, 1451–1462. doi: 10.1001/jama.2015.3058

Ritchie, J., Lokman, M., and Panikkar, J. (2015). Thrombolysis for stroke in pregnancy at 39 weeks gestation with a subsequent normal delivery. *BMJ Case Rep.* 2015:bcr2015209563. doi: 10.1136/bcr-2015-209563

Sappino, A. P., Madani, R., Huarte, J., Belin, D., Kiss, J. Z., Wohlwend, A., et al. (1993). Extracellular proteolysis in the adult murine brain. *J. Clin. Invest.* 92, 679–685. doi: 10.1172/JCI116637

Seeds, N. W., Williams, B. L., and Bickford, P. C. (1995). Tissue plasminogen activator induction in Purkinje neurons after cerebellar motor learning. *Science* 270, 1992–1994. doi: 10.1126/science.270.5244.1992

Tassi, R., Acampa, M., Marotta, G., Cioni, S., Guideri, F., Rossi, S., et al. (2013). Systemic thrombolysis for stroke in pregnancy. *Am. J. Emerg. Med.* 31, 448.e1–e3. doi: 10.1016/j.ajem.2012.05.040

Teesalu, T., Kulla, A., Simisker, A., Siren, V., Lawrence, D. A., Asser, T., et al. (2004). Tissue plasminogen activator and neuroserpin are widely expressed in the human central nervous system. *Thromb. Haemost.* 92, 358–368. doi: 10.1160/th02-12-0310

Tomkins, A. J., Hood, R. J., Levi, C. R., and Spratt, N. J. (2015). Tissue Plasminogen Activator for preclinical stroke research: neither "rat" nor "human" dose mimics clinical recanalization in a carotid occlusion model. *Sci. Rep.* 5, 16026. doi: 10.1038/srep16026

Tsirka, S. E., Gualandris, A., Amaral, D. G., and Strickland, S. (1995). Excitotoxin-induced neuronal degeneration and seizure are mediated by tissue plasminogen activator. *Nature* 377, 340–344. doi: 10.1038/377340a0

Turrentine, M. A., Braems, G., and Ramirez, M. M. (1995). Use of thrombolytics for the treatment of thromboembolic disease during pregnancy. *Obstet. Gynecol. Surv.* 50, 534–541. doi: 10.1097/00006254-199507000-00020

Wahlgren, N., Ahmed, N., Dávalos, A., Ford, G. A., Grond, M., Hacke, W., et al. (2007). Thrombolysis with alteplase for acute ischaemic stroke in the Safe Implementation of Thrombolysis in Stroke-Monitoring Study (SITS-MOST): an observational study. *Lancet* 369, 275–282. doi: 10.1016/S0140-6736(07)60149-4

Wahlgren, N., Moreira, T., Michel, P., Steiner, T., Jansen, O., Cognard, C., et al. (2016). Mechanical thrombectomy in acute ischemic stroke: consensus statement by ESO-Karolinska stroke update 2014/2015, supported by ESO, ESMINT, ESNR and EAN. *Int. J. Stroke* 11, 134–147. doi: 10.1177/1747493015609778

Wein, T. H., Hickenbottom, S. L., Morgenstern, L. B., Demchuk, A. M., and Grotta, J. C. (2002). Safety of tissue plasminogen activator for acute stroke in menstruating women. *Stroke* 33, 2506–2508. doi: 10.1161/01.STR.0000030108.47462.4F

Wiese, K. M., Talkad, A., Mathews, M., and Wang, D. (2006). Intravenous recombinant tissue plasminogen activator in a pregnant woman with cardioembolic stroke. *Stroke* 37, 2168–2169. doi: 10.1161/01.STR.0000230286.95513.c2

Yamaguchi, Y., Kondo, T., Ihara, M., Kawamata, J., Fukuyama, H., and Takahashi, R. (2010). [Intravenous recombinant tissue plasminogen activator in an 18-week pregnant woman with embolic stroke]. *Rinsho Shinkeigaku* 50, 315–319. doi: 10.5692/clinicalneurol.50.315

Yepes, M., and Lawrence, D. A. (2004). New functions for an old enzyme: nonhemostatic roles for tissue-type plasminogen activator in the central nervous system. *Exp. Biol. Med. (Maywood)* 229, 1097–1104.

Yepes, M., Sandkvist, M., Moore, E. G., Bugge, T. H., Strickland, D. K., and Lawrence, D. A. (2003). Tissue-type plasminogen activator induces opening of the blood-brain barrier via the LDL receptor-related protein. *J. Clin. Invest.* 112, 1533–1540. doi: 10.1172/JCI200319212

Zhuo, M., Holtzman, D. M., Li, Y., Osaka, H., Demaro, J., Jacquin, M., et al. (2000). Role of tissue plasminogen activator receptor LRP in hippocampal long-term potentiation. *J. Neurosci.* 20, 542–549.

23

SSRI and Motor Recovery in Stroke: Reestablishment of Inhibitory Neural Network Tonus

Camila B. Pinto[1,2], Faddi G. Saleh Velez[1], Fernanda Lopes[1], Polyana V. de Toledo Piza[1,3], Laura Dipietro[4], Qing M. Wang[5], Nicole L. Mazwi[6], Erica C. Camargo[7], Randie Black-Schaffer[6] and Felipe Fregni[1]*

[1] Laboratory of Neuromodulation and Center for Clinical Research Learning, Department of Physical Medicine and Rehabilitation, Harvard Medical School, Spaulding Rehabilitation Hospital, Harvard University, Boston, MA, United States, [2] Department of Neuroscience and Behavior, Psychology Institute, University of São Paulo, São Paulo, Brazil, [3] Department of Severe Patients, Hospital Israelita Albert Einstein, São Paulo, Brazil, [4] Highland Instruments, Cambridge, MA, United States, [5] Stroke Biological Recovery Laboratory, Department of Physical Medicine and Rehabilitation, Harvard Medical School, Spaulding Rehabilitation Hospital, Harvard University, Boston, MA, United States, [6] Department of Physical Medicine and Rehabilitation, Harvard Medical School, Spaulding Rehabilitation Hospital, Harvard University, Boston, MA, United States, [7] Department of Neurology, Harvard Medical School, Massachusetts General Hospital, Harvard University, Boston, MA, United States

Edited by:
Giancarlo Zito, Ospedale San Giovanni Calibita Fatebenefratelli, Italy

Reviewed by:
Leif Hertz, Institute of Metabolic Disease Research and Drug Development, China Medical University, China
Giovanni Assenza, Università Campus Bio-Medico, Italy
Filippo Zappasodi, Università degli Studi "G. d'Annunzio" Chieti - Pescara, Italy

***Correspondence:**
Felipe Fregni
fregni.felipe@mgh.harvard.edu

Selective serotonin reuptake inhibitors (SSRIs) are currently widely used in the field of the neuromodulation not only because of their anti-depressive effects but also due to their ability to promote plasticity and enhance motor recovery in patients with stroke. Recent studies showed that fluoxetine promotes motor recovery after stroke through its effects on the serotonergic system enhancing motor outputs and facilitating long term potentiation, key factors in motor neural plasticity. However, little is known in regards of the exact mechanisms underlying these effects and several aspects of it remain poorly understood. In this manuscript, we discuss evidence supporting the hypothesis that SSRIs, and in particular fluoxetine, modulate inhibitory pathways, and that this modulation enhances reorganization and reestablishment of excitatory-inhibitory control; these effects play a key role in learning induced plasticity in neural circuits involved in the promotion of motor recovery after stroke. This discussion aims to provide important insights and rationale for the development of novel strategies for stroke motor rehabilitation.

Keywords: stroke, motor rehabilitation, SSRIs, cortical excitability, inhibitory tonus, neuroplasticity

INTRODUCTION

Stroke is the second cause of death worldwide and the leading cause of death in upper-middle income countries; about 6.7 million people died from stroke in 2013 in the US (Mozaffarian et al., 2016). Among stroke survivors, recovery of motor function is frequently incomplete, with the majority of stroke patients unable to perform professional duties or activities of daily living 6 months after the event (Hummel and Cohen, 2005, 2006).

Current conventional therapies rely on behavioral treatments such as physiotherapy and occupational therapy (Winstein et al., 2016); however, these treatments only induce limited plastic and cortical reorganization changes (Veerbeek et al., 2014). Thus, considerable research efforts have been devoted to developing methods for enhancing neuroplasticity in stroke and increasing the efficacy of rehabilitation techniques.

To this end, the use of pharmacological agents such as selective serotonin reuptake inhibitors (SSRIs), in particular fluoxetine, is increasingly being explored by several research groups. It has been shown that SSRIs can modulate neural excitability, promote plastic changes and improve motor rehabilitation after stroke (Chollet et al., 2011; Siepmann et al., 2015). Chollet et al. reported positive results of the Flame (fluoxetine for motor recovery after acute ischemic stroke) trial. They hypothesized that fluoxetine enhances motor recovery after stroke through a coupling of its neuroprotective effect with the serotonergic system capability to enhance motor outputs and facilitate long term potentiation (LTP) (Chollet et al., 2011). The encouraging results of the Flame trial were further supported by the positive results of a Cochrane review of SSRIs for stroke recovery including 52 trials and 4,059 patients (Mead et al., 2013).

The similarity between the processes of stroke recovery and learning has also recently gained increasing attention, and it is being explored by several research groups with the goal of improving the therapeutic efficacy of technologies for stroke rehabilitation (Hogan et al., 2006; Krakauer, 2006). Neural repair and recovery after stroke involve mechanisms of neuronal excitability modulation that are very similar to those involved in memory and learning processes (Krakauer, 2006).

Although their exact function during these processes is still unclear (Clarkson et al., 2010), the important role of inhibitory networks has begun to be acknowledged. These networks are thought to play a key role in both early and late stages of learning-induced plastic circuits. In fact, a strong neural system to promote learning is a system that can rapidly shift between inhibition and excitation (Trevelyan, 2016).

While the exact mechanisms of action of SSRIs on the neural system after stroke are far from being understood, this review aims to discuss the potential role of SSRIs on inhibitory neural circuits as a possible mechanism underlying motor rehabilitation after stroke through cortical reorganization and enhancement of motor learning. We critically analyze evidence regarding: (i) The relationship between inhibitory neural activity and motor learning; (ii) Disruption of inhibitory activity after stroke; (iii) Evidence of SSRIs-induced enhancement of inhibitory tone; and (iv) Evidence of SSRIs-induced enhancement of motor learning through an increase of inhibitory tone in stroke.

Relationship between Inhibitory Neural Activity and Motor Learning

Motor learning leads to alteration in the cortical motor mapping, promoting changes in the motor and somatosensory representations. Motor learning involves neuronal excitability and inhibitory modulatory mechanisms that are very similar to the mechanisms involved in memory and non-motor learning processes (Krakauer, 2006).

Learning a new motor skill shares similar physiological traits with motor recovery from stroke. The similarities between these processes provide us with a model that can be applied to certain processes of functional recovery after stroke (Krakauer, 2006; Rossi et al., 2009; Krakauer and Mazzoni, 2011; Kitago and Krakauer, 2013; Costanzo, 2017). For instance, the modifications of motor behavior after exposure to stimuli or experiences (learning) are similar to those occurring during physical therapy; however, in the latter case the modifications underlie a process of re-learning of behaviors lost due to the structural alteration caused by the cerebrovascular accident (Krakauer, 2006; Krakauer and Mazzoni, 2011).

Additionally, memory plays an important role in the consolidation of newly learned behaviors, therefore the enhancement of mechanisms underlying both learning and memory is crucial for therapies aimed at promoting stroke motor recovery (Krakauer, 2006).

The neurophysiological mechanism underlying learning and memory is synaptic plasticity. Enhanced and more effective synaptic functions largely depend on facilitating the likelihood of neuronal inputs to happen; repeated stimuli generate a pattern of repeated activation on a determined pathway leading to an enhanced responsiveness of the post synaptic neuron (potentiation) (Feldman, 2009; Costanzo, 2017). On a cellular level these processes depend on changes in network excitability as regulated by long-term potentiation (LTP) and long-term depression (LTD) (Hagemann et al., 1998). LTP and LTD can induce changes in synaptic strengthening, thereby shaping learning and memory processing (Bliss and Collingridge, 1993; Lynch, 2004).

Although little is known about the spatiotemporal aspects of motor learning (Berger et al., 2017), the modulation of inhibitory activity is an important mechanism underlying motor cortex plasticity. In fact, inhibitory activity can change during early and late stages of the learning process (See **Figure 1**; Engel et al., 2001; Hensch and Stryker, 2004; Stagg et al., 2011).

The early stage of learning is characterized by reduction in inhibition, facilitating LTP process in the motor cortex (Nudo et al., 1996; Floyer-Lea et al., 2006). Local changes in inhibitory circuits (GABA concentrations) can unmask existent neural pathways within the cortex leading to rapid changes in the sensory and motor representations (Castro-Alamancos et al., 1995; Castro-Alamancos and Connors et al., 1996). It has been shown that during early learning a transient GABA decrease in the motor cortex correlates with the degree of motor learning (Floyer-Lea et al., 2006; Stagg, 2013). Despite the transient impact of lower inhibitory activity in acute phases of learning, this correlation may be inverted in late phases of learning consolidation.

In later stages of motor learning, a partial recovery in inhibitory tonus (restoration of the inhibitory tonus) can be associated with longer-term consolidation of learning (Shadmehr and Holcomb, 1997; Floyer-Lea et al., 2006).

An interesting study using TMS, tDCS and neuroimaging showed that the degree of learning is associated with a decrease in GABA activity induced by tDCS (Johnstone et al., 2016), thus supporting the notion that during early learning stages a decreased and transient inhibitory tone is desirable. However, subsequent inhibition seems necessary for consolidation of learning (Brosh and Barkai, 2009).

Taken all together, these studies suggest that understanding the balance between excitation and inhibition activity during motor learning is key to better understanding the process

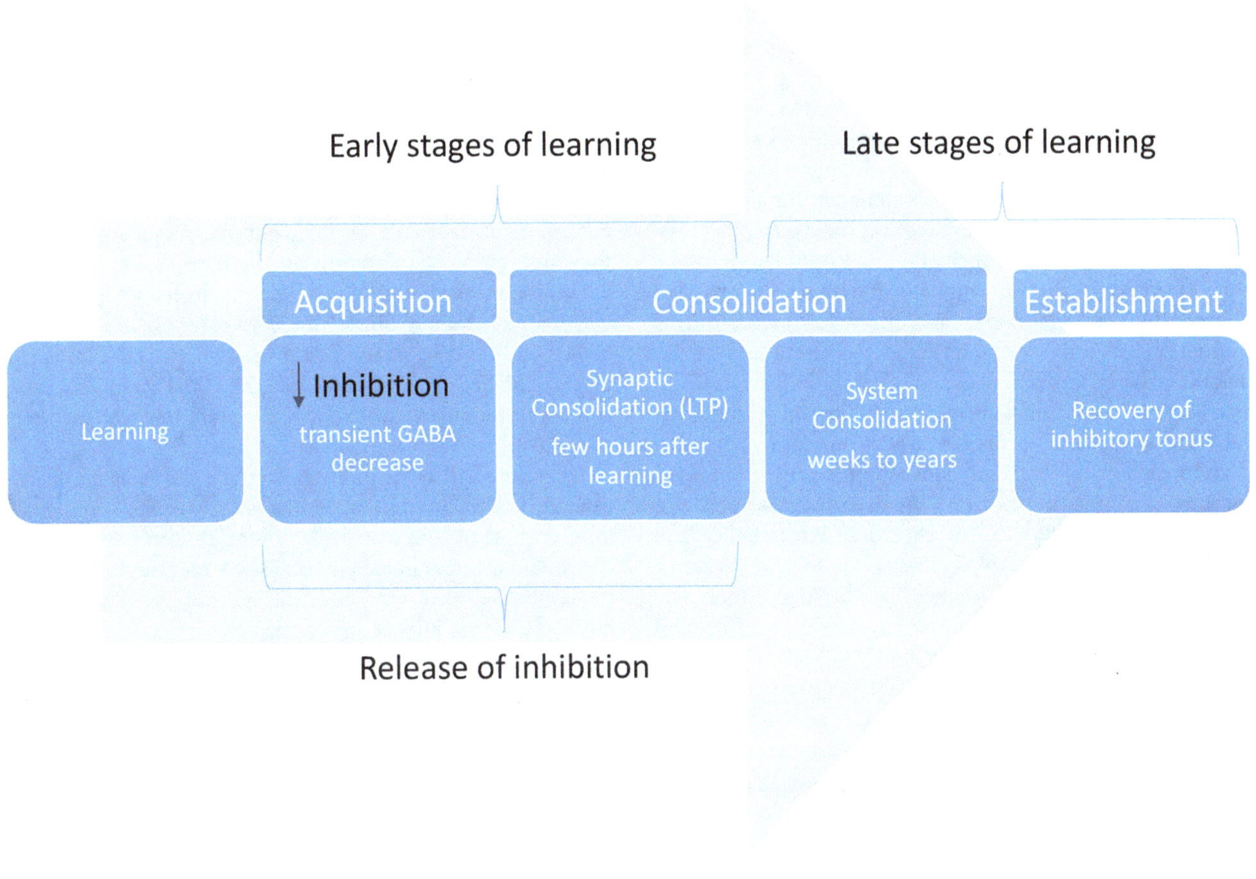

FIGURE 1 | Neurobiology of learning phases.

of motor learning. Assuming that stroke recovery and motor learning are somewhat similar processes (Hogan et al., 2006; Krakauer, 2006), this knowledge may help understand how to improve rehabilitation in stroke patients.

Disruption of Inhibitory Activity after Stroke

Following stroke, several structural and biological changes take place and the interactions between excitatory and inhibitory activity in learning-related circuits are crucial to drive motor cortex plasticity and recovery (Jones, 2017). In the very acute phase of stroke (hours after the event), inhibition of activity of cortical areas surrounding the injured site is a neuroprotective mechanism since increased excitability can result in glutamatergic toxicity and increase apoptosis (Schiene et al., 1996; Floyer-Lea et al., 2006).

After this initial phase, and similarly to early stages of learning, the excitation/inhibition ratio increases (Schiene et al., 1996). Two main neurophysiological changes have been associated with brain remodeling and recovery after stroke: (i) an initial increase in excitability in cortical regions and perilesional areas not affected by the stroke, and (ii) increased activity/excitability in the contralesional hemisphere. In this context, several studies showed that in stroke patients the inhibitory function is globally reduced in both hemispheres suggesting that the modulation of inhibitory circuits might result from a strategy that aims at compensating for motor impairment (Talelli et al., 2006; Di Lazzaro et al., 2012; Takeuchi and Izumi, 2012). Even though this enhanced excitability pattern is related to the enhanced plasticity and functional reorganization, both changes are required to be time dependent.

In the peri-lesional and distant cortical regions the down-regulation of the inhibitory tonus is important for altering cortical maps and promoting neuronal connectivity (*re-hardwiring*) (Schiene et al., 1996). Moreover, manipulation of the inhibitory tone promotes axonal and dendritic growth and guidance, cytoskeletal organization and the expression of genes related with adult brain remodeling (Urban et al., 2012; Nudo, 2013).

Widespread areas of enhanced cortical excitability appear after stroke, and are important for some of the compensatory re-organization (Collins, 2016). For example, Frost et al. (2003) showed that in adult squirrel monkeys an increased hand representation in ventral pre-motor areas (PMv) is observed after an experimental ischemic lesion of 50% of the M1 hand area. Additionally, the amount of reorganization was correlated with the size of the hand area lesion, suggesting that bigger lesions induce greater compensatory reorganization (Frost et al., 2003). Although the development of compensatory reorganization results in initial gain of function, it may inhibit further gain of function in later phases of stroke rehabilitation (Meintzschel and Ziemann, 2006; Carmichael, 2012).

In this regard, increased disinhibition of the widespread cortical areas increases the risk of competitive interaction between the areas (pre motor cortex and M1), thereby resulting in incomplete motor recovery (Takeuchi et al., 2007). On the other hand, the localized and transient disinhibition of the affected M1 in stroke patients may promote the motor recovery of normal patterns by facilitating M1 plasticity (Takeuchi and Izumi, 2012).

One example is the surrounding inhibitory theory that highlights the importance of inhibitory networks during the initiation of active voluntary tasks. During movement preparation, there is a local decrease of inhibition (decrease in GABAa) and a concomitant increase of inhibition in the brain neighboring areas; these processes avoid competition between local and neighboring areas and allow specific activation of the motor area in charge of generating the desired motor behavior (Pfurtscheller et al., 2005; Klimesch, 2012; Pfurtscheller and Lopes da Silva, 2017). In stroke patients, the local decrease of inhibitory activity prior to movement is reduced and there is a widespread disinhibition in the neighboring areas of the lesion (Reynolds and Ashby, 1999; Zaaroor et al., 2003; Hummel et al., 2009).

Therefore, stronger functional recovery is associated with a time-dependent increase of inhibition. In fact, an important aspect that has not been fully explored in human studies is the modulation of the inhibitory states; varying from disinhibition to inhibition in cortico-subcortical circuits according to the phase of learning. A shift in one direction only (i.e., disinhibitory state) has a low learning efficiency. In fact, that shift may be an index of cortical disorganization.

A Network Example of Disrupted Excitation-Inhibition Balance: Transcallosal Imbalance and Motor Recovery in Stroke

An example of imbalance in the excitation-inhibition ratio can be seen in the transcallosal interaction between motor cortices in stroke (Julkunen et al., 2016). Functional imaging and non-invasive brain stimulation have indicated that ipsilateral motor projections are enhanced early after stroke and that a pattern of hyper-excitation is commonly observed in the unaffected hemisphere (Turton et al., 1996; Netz et al., 1997; Werhahn et al., 2003; Murase et al., 2004; Oh et al., 2010). Although the underlying mechanism remains unclear, it is believed that latent ipsilateral motor projections are activated by disruption of the contralateral corticospinal projections in stroke patients (Feydy et al., 2002; Johansen-Berg et al., 2002). This results in the reconfiguration of motor networks through the establishment of alternative inputs for the cortico-spinal tracts. Then, parallel motor circuits are activated and begin to transfer the impaired functions to unaffected areas of the brain (Feydy et al., 2002; Lindenberg et al., 2010).

In later stages of stroke recovery, better motor recovery and outcome of functional rehabilitation are associated with a shift of activation back to the affected hemisphere by the reestablishment of the inhibitory tonus in the unaffected hemisphere as well as with recovery of connectivity and cessation of imbalance between the two hemispheres (Jaillard et al., 2005; Carter et al., 2010; Park et al., 2011).

A persistent increased activity of the unaffected hemisphere can result in alterations of transcallosal structure and function and it is associated with upper limb motor impairment and greater levels of arm motor dysfunction (Sato et al., 2015) in chronic stroke patients. In this context, several studies showed the importance of inhibition after stroke and the association between increased inhibition of the unaffected hemisphere with better functional outcomes (Conforto et al., 2008; Swayne et al., 2008). Additionally, patients with severe upper limb impairment display higher disinhibition of the unaffected hemisphere compared to patients with mild-moderate impairment (Liepert et al., 2000).

Therefore, it is hypothesized that the balance between excitatory and inhibitory inputs after stroke is crucial for long term stroke recovery and motor re-learning. These time dependent changes in balance between excitatory and inhibitory networks are also seen in healthy subjects (Guerra et al., 2016). However, after a stroke this process can be altered and jeopardize motor recovery. Consequently, longitudinal changes in the regulation of inhibitory functions seem to play a major role in this balance, since the lack of inhibition in later phases of stroke recovery is associated with worse motor function outcomes (see **Figure 2**; Crichton et al., 2016).

Can SSRIs Enhance Inhibitory Tone?

SSRIs are the most common treatment for major depressive disorder (MDD). Clinical and preclinical data of MDD patients indicate imbalanced activity in the right dorsolateral prefrontal cortex (DLPC) compared to the left cortex/counterpart (Grimm et al., 2008). It has been shown that impaired inhibition of the right hemisphere, as indexed by TMS measures such as intracortical inhibition (ICI), intracortical facilitation (ICF) and cortical silent period, is correlated with treatment responsiveness and recovery after depression (Mantovani et al., 2012). Several authors have also demonstrated that adults with MDD present deficits in GABAergic mediated transmission related with the severity of MDD (Robinson et al., 2003; Ye et al., 2008; Croarkin et al., 2014). Moreover, it has been shown that acute (intravenous infusion) (Bhagwagar, 2004) or chronic (2 months) (Sanacora et al., 2002) administration of SSRIs can increase cortical levels of GABA in depressed adults, leading to the normalization of GABA levels and possibly contributing to an antidepressant mechanism.

Besides that, in mouse models of social isolation, fluoxetine treatment can induce stress recovery independently of its serotonergic pathways. In these models, fluoxetine acts by increasing the neurosteroids levels in the brain allowing a normal allosteric increase of GABA-A synapses and therefore restoring inhibition (Matsumoto et al., 2007).

Several neurological conditions seem to depend on a balance between excitatory and inhibitory activity in the brain, and the inhibitory control of excitation may have a key role in this balance. Dysfunction in GABA-controlled inhibition is pathophysiologically correlated with several diseases and

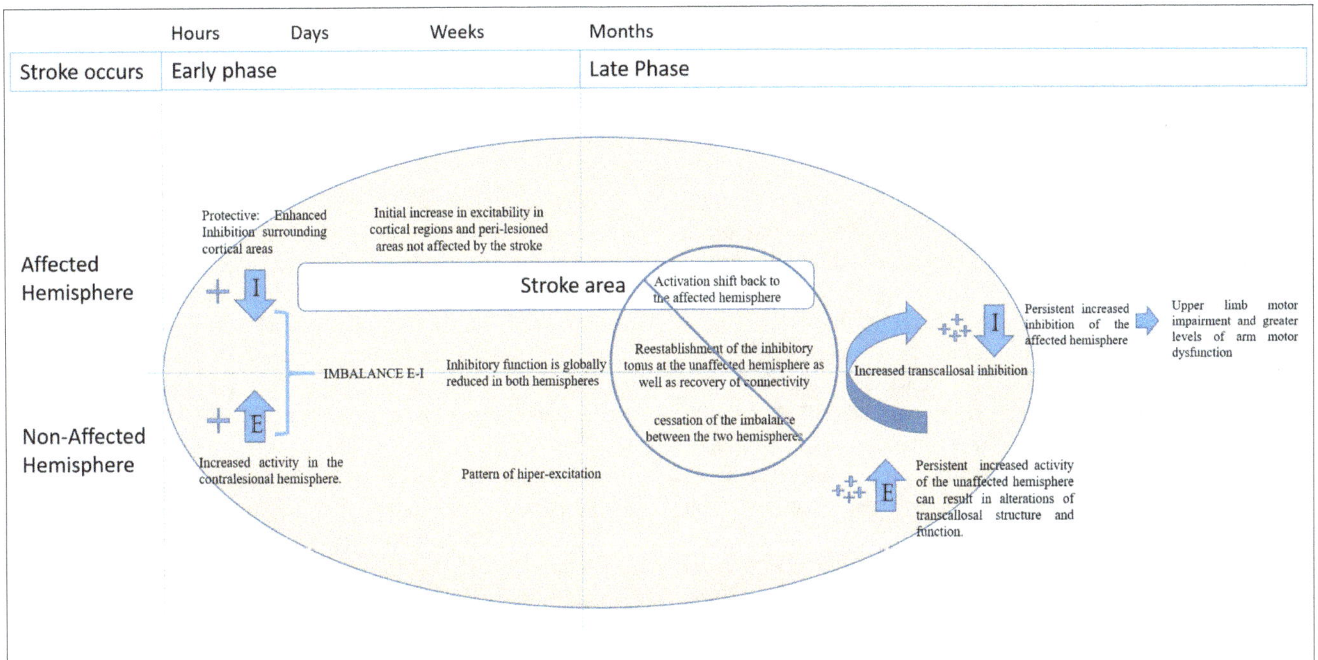

FIGURE 2 | Disruption of balance between excitation (E) and inhibition (I) of the affected and non-lesioned hemispheres throughout the time post stroke.

restoration of functional inhibition leads to better treatment outcomes. In particular, fluoxetine was shown to have positive effects on motor rehabilitation after stroke and preclinical data demonstrated that fluoxetine can directly up regulate GABA, increasing inhibitory activity (Tunnicliff et al., 1999; Robinson et al., 2003). In fact it is possible that one of the mechanisms of SSRIs in improving depression is through a reestablishment of normal learning patterns of prefrontal circuits.

SSRIs and Changes in Inhibitory Activity in Stroke

Inhibitory circuits play an essential role in post-stroke motor learning. SSRIs seem to exert an effect on excitation/inhibition pathways, leading to enhancement of motor function after a stroke. Although this mechanism is still underexplored in stroke, other disease models are clearer; some insights from these conditions can be extrapolated to better understand the potential role of this class of drugs in stroke patients.

Recent studies have shown the effects of drugs that are capable of modulating excitatory and inhibitory pathways and this may be how they facilitate functional recovery after brain lesions. Some of these pharmacological candidates are SSRIs (Pariente et al., 2001; Chollet et al., 2011), dopamine agonist (Scheidtmann et al., 2001), amphetamines (Bütefisch et al., 2002; Sawaki et al., 2002b) and cholinergic substances (ACR) (Sawaki et al., 2002a; Meintzschel and Ziemann, 2006).

Among these drugs, SSRIs have been shown to be able to produce different effects (inhibitory or excitatory) on motor cortex plasticity (Robol et al., 2004). The neuroplastic changes triggered by SSRIs can be responsible for the compensation of some of the neurophysiologic damage caused by the stroke. Several early studies suggested that serotonergic agents such as fluoxetine and citalopram have a positive effect on motor function in hemiplegic patients after stroke (Dam et al., 1996; Pariente et al., 2001; Zittel et al., 2008). The Flame trial, a large randomized placebo-controlled clinical trial, showed that the administration of fluoxetine during the acute stroke phase has a moderate effect size, resulting in improvement of a clinical motor function scale for upper and lower limbs outcome (Fugl-Meyer) (Chollet et al., 2011).

To date, the mechanism by which fluoxetine enhances rehabilitation after stroke remain unclear; however, some insights from animal-based models suggested that SSRIs may enhance overall brain excitability. Additionally, it has been shown that SSRIs can promote neuronal sprouting (Kokoeva et al., 2005; Hourai and Miyata, 2013; Ohira et al., 2013b) and cortical reorganization (26), restore blood flow (Rosenstein et al., 1998; Sun et al., 2003), and enhance neuroprotective mechanism (Lim et al., 2009); thereby improving neuronal survival and protecting cerebral tissue from hypoxia since it regulates the expression of hypoxia-inducible factor-1α (HIF-1α) and of heme oxygense-1 (HO-1) (Shin et al., 2009; Siepmann et al., 2015). Therefore, one hypothesis for the motor rehabilitation induced by fluoxetine is that the blockage of serotonin (5-HT) reuptake due to SSRI administration increases the availability of this neurotransmitter in the synaptic cleft thus enhancing signal transmission (Ganzer et al., 2013; Rief et al., 2016; Stahl, 2017) and consequently, increasing the excitatory input of glutamate and activating the NMDA receptors leading to a cascade of intracellular events. These events might generate synaptic modifications that culminate in a LTP leading synapse reprogramming and strengthening (Stahl, 2017).

Nevertheless, we also believe that this acute effect on enhancement of excitatory activity is followed by an increase in inhibitory activity. Studies exploring the effects exerted by SSRIs over motor cortex plasticity showed that SSRIs can also enhance inhibitory activity (Etherton et al., 2016). Studies have shown that serotonergic drugs induce changes in inhibitory activity. Indeed inhibition in the motor cortex was observed in healthy subjects 2.5 h after citalopram intake. A single dose of citalopram produced a transient enhanced GABAergic interneuronal control over corticospinal neurons, resulting in increases in the ICI, motor threshold and cortico-silent period (CSP) as well as mild decrease in the ICF (Robol et al., 2004). Therefore, citalopram was able to acutely decrease motor cortex excitability in healthy subjects.

In addition, pre-clinical data suggest that citalopram, fluoxetine and sertraline have anticonvulsive effects in the hippocampus inhibiting seizure like events. The effects of these SSRIs were likely due to regulation of pyramidal cell's excitability leading to vigorous inhibition of repetitive firing (Igelström and Heyward, 2012). However, in clinical studies an increase in seizures after administration of SSRIs was also described (Hill et al., 2015).

Recently, authors have been exploring the role of long term administration of fluoxetine treatment administration (Chen et al., 2011) inducing structural plasticity by promoting neuron "dematuration" (Kobayashi et al., 2010; Ohira et al., 2013a,b). This mechanism consists in a reverse effect on the normal maturate state of cells that can be induced by changes in GABAergic transmission; therefore, culminating in a juvenile-like state of fast-spiking inhibitory interneurons. In several studies, neuronal "dematuration" induced by fluoxetine was identified in different brain regions such as adult dentate granule cells, adult amygdala cells (Karpova et al., 2011), hippocampus, medial pre-frontal cortex (mPFC) (Guirado et al., 2014) and a subset of GABAergic interneurons, generated from Layer 1 inhibitory neuron progenitor cells (L1-INP cells) (Ohira et al., 2013a).

In this context, it is important to acknowledge that the same antidepressant can exert different regulatory effects in different brain regions and these effects vary depending on dose, regimen of use (single dose or prolonged use) and time of administration (in acute or chronic diseases phase). For example, a single dose of paroxetine can improve motor performance and induce hyper activation of the primary sensorimotor cortex (S1M1) (Loubinoux et al., 2005). However, prolonged paroxetine treatment (30 days 20 mg per day) induced hypo activation of S1M1 cells, but still resulted in improvement in finger tapping motor task (Gerdelat-Mas et al., 2005). These results indicate that SSRIs may have an acute effect on excitatory circuits that is led by enhancement of inhibitory activity.

Even though the exact mechanism by which this effect occurs is unknown, prior studies showed that some SSRIs can potentiate GABA-mediated inhibitory neurotransmission. Among SSRIs, fluoxetine's mechanism of action includes its 5-HT2C antagonism. Furthermore, 5-HT2C receptors are expressed on GABAergic neurons (Serrats et al., 2005; Invernizzi et al., 2007).

Furthermore, SSRIs can activate other receptors such as the 5-HT2B receptor that have been identified in multiple brain cells such as neurons, astrocytes, and Purkinje cells (Chen et al., 1995; Peng et al., 2014). However, animal studies have shown that its expression can be twice as much in astrocytes than in neurons (Lovatt et al., 2007; Dong et al., 2015). Astrocytes have a main role in the neuronal metabolic process in the brain and recent evidence shows that fluoxetine can alter this metabolic process through 5-HT2B receptor activity (Peng et al., 2014; Hertz et al., 2015a).

The activation of 5-HT2B leads to a cascade of effects that have been associated with the enhancement of learning and memory. Among those processes, animal studies showed that its activation can lead to raise of intracellular calcium levels in astrocytes and consequent increase of glycogenolysis and glycolysis, causing subsequent increase of lactate release that can either act as extra metabolic fuel for neurons or act in further signaling pathways (Li et al., 2011; Hertz et al., 2015a; Steinman et al., 2016). Other processes such as potassium homeostasis are also enhanced by this activation (Du et al., 2014). In this regard, it is known that lactate has a neuroprotective effects during brain ischemia and that glycogen metabolism have many implications for the brain activities. In addition, it is suggested that the 5-HT2B receptor plays an important role in neurogenesis driven by SSRI treatments since studies in animals lacking this receptor revealed a deficient response to the enhanced effects of fluoxetine in neurogenesis (Diaz et al., 2012, 2016).

Moreover, the effects exert by fluoxetine differ depending on its dose as different responses are seen in glycogen concentration in astrocytes with different doses of fluoxetine. Whereas lower concentration of fluoxetine causes an increase of glycogen in astrocytes the opposite effects are seen with an increased concentration of the drug. It is believe that this dual effect can be associated with aspects of either the therapeutic effect or adverse event of the medication (Bai et al., 2017). The effects of fluoxetine in the 5-HT2B receptor need to be further explored in human studies since its role in plasticity can be used to better explain the mechanism underling this drug effects in neuroplasticity and motor rehabilitation after stroke.

In this context, the astrocytic metabolism could have a role in regulation excitatory and inhibitory mechanism after stroke. The activation of GABA-A receptors in astrocytes can stimulate a similar mechanism enhancing regulation of calcium concentrations and further enhancement of glycogenolysis, a process that has already been associated with learning and memory tasks; therefore relevant in the setting of motor recovery (Hertz et al., 2015b). Finally, the effects of fluoxetine in the 5-HT2B receptor need to be further explored in human studies since its role in plasticity can be used to better explain the mechanism underlying this drug effects in neuroplasticity and motor rehabilitation after stroke.

SSRIs and Safety Considerations

Most studies to date have reported little or no side effects in relation of SSRI use in the stroke population; however, known potential adverse effects on mood disorders should be discussed. Due to their selective action, SSRIs present a more tolerable profile of adverse actions and there are differences between the main side effects of the different selective serotonin reuptake inhibitors. Overall, the most frequently reported adverse events are nausea, vomiting, abdominal pain, diarrhea, agitation, anxiety, insomnia, cycling for mania, headache, dizziness, fatigue, tremors, extrapyramidal effects, xerostomia, perspiration, loss or weight gain, sexual dysfunction, and dermatological reactions.

Moreover, SSRIs effects on patient with pre-existent cardiac disease or acute coronary syndrome are controversial as they may improve cardiac disease prognosis by inhibiting platelet aggregation but could potentially worsen prognosis by increasing risk of bleeding or of arrhythmias (Rieckmann and Kronish, 2013).

Another important aspect associated with increased serotonergic activity in the central nervous system is the Serotonergic syndrome, a potentially fatal condition (Peng et al., 2014). The most common symptoms include: hyperthermia, agitation, ocular clone, tremor, akathisia, deep tendon hyperreflexia, inducible or spontaneous clonus, muscular rigidity, dilated pupils, dry mucous membranes, increased intestinal sounds, spotted skin and diaphoresis (Boyer and Shannon, 2005). Although, serotonergic syndrome is commonly the result of the combination of SSRIs with drugs or dietary supplements that have a similar effect of increasing serotonin, it may occur after the initiation of a higher doses of single serotonergic drugs or increase of the dose of a serotonergic drug in particularly sensitive individuals. Selective serotonin reuptake inhibitors, such as fluoxetine, are perhaps the most implicitly associated drug group associated with serotonergic syndrome. They may contribute to the development of serotonin syndrome up to several weeks after drug discontinuation (Birmes et al., 2003).

Even though uncommon, the FLAME trial reported that among the 118 participants two in the active fluoxetine group have severe adverse events (hyponatremia and partial seizure). The most frequent adverse events in the active group were transient digestive disorders. To avoid serotonin syndrome, treatment was stopped in patients in the active group who developed depression and required the use of another antidepressant during the study (Chollet et al., 2011). Therefore, if this hypothesis that SSRIs improve motor function by modulating the excitatory-inhibitory balance is confirmed, other interventions that are safer may be best better first alternatives to SSRIs in this context.

SUMMARY

The mechanisms underlying the enhancement of motor learning via SSRIs are still unclear, and the exact effects of fluoxetine in motor recovery after stroke are yet to be proven. We discussed how this class of drugs might help reestablish the excitation-inhibitory balance by initially enhancing excitation that is followed by a compensatory inhibition. Different techniques such as functional magnetic resonance, magnetic resonance spectroscopy, transcranial magnetic stimulation, transcranial direct current stimulation and EEG have been used to show the role of neurochemical and neurophysiological markers as well as to quantify modifications of inhibitory and excitatory responses to several interventions. However, further work needs to be done to develop better methods to assess specific alterations in inhibitory pathways.

Ultimately SSRIs can have a broader action on promoting reorganization of neural activity following brain lesion. With the current evidence it is not possible to conclude whether the increased neural inhibition that follows use of SSRIs is indeed the result of its usage. However further studies can explore further this mechanism as to understand better how to use SSRIs and the potential limitations of this class of drugs that may also be detrimental in some cases.

AUTHOR CONTRIBUTIONS

CP: conception and design of the manuscript, acquisition of data, analysis and interpretation of data reviewed, drafting revising and important intellectual contribution, critical revision and final approval of the version; FS: conception and design of the manuscript, interpretation of data reviewed, drafting revising and important intellectual contribution, and critical revision; FL and PdTP: acquisition of data, analysis, and final review; LdP, NM, RB-S, QW, and EC: critical revision, review, and final approval of the version; FF: conception and design of the manuscript, analysis, critical revision, and final approval of the version.

REFERENCES

Bai, Q., Song, D., Gu, L., Verkhratsky, A., and Peng, L. (2017). Bi-phasic regulation of glycogen content in astrocytes via Cav-1/PTEN/PI3K/AKT/GSK-3β pathway by fluoxetine. *Psychopharmacology* 234, 1069–1077. doi: 10.1007/s00213-017-4547-3

Berger, D. J., Ferrari, F., Esposito, A., Masciullo, M., Molinari, M., Lacquaniti, F., et al. (2017). "Changes in muscle synergy organization after neurological lesions," in *Converging Clinical and Engineering Research on Neurorehabilitation II. Biosystems and Biorobotics*, Vol. 15, eds J. Ibáñez, J. González-Vargas, J. Azorín, M. Akay, and J. Pons (Cham: Springer International Publishing), 939–943.

Bhagwagar, Z. (2004). Increased brain GABA concentrations following acute administration of a selective serotonin reuptake Inhibitor. *Am. J. Psychiatry* 161, 368–370. doi: 10.1176/appi.ajp.161.2.368

Birmes, P., Coppin, D., Schmitt, L., and Lauque, D. (2003). Serotonin syndrome: a brief review. *Can. Med. Assoc. J.* 168, 1439–1442.

Bliss, T. V., and Collingridge, G. L. (1993). A synaptic model of memory: long-term potentiation in the hippocampus. *Nature* 361, 31–39. doi: 10.1038/361031a0

Boyer, E. W., and Shannon, M. (2005). The serotonin syndrome. *N. Engl. J. Med.* 352, 1112–1120. doi: 10.1056/NEJMra041867

Brosh, I., and Barkai, E. (2009). Learning-induced enhancement of feedback inhibitory synaptic transmission. *Learn. Mem.* 16, 413–416. doi: 10.1101/lm.1430809

Bütefisch, C. M., Davis, B. C., Sawaki, L., Waldvogel, D., Classen, J., Kopylev, L., et al. (2002). Modulation of use-dependent plasticity by d-amphetamine. *Ann. Neurol.* 51, 59–68. doi: 10.1002/ana.10056

Carmichael, S. T. (2012). Brain excitability in stroke: the Yin and Yang of stroke progression. *Arch. Neurol.* 69, 161–167. doi: 10.1001/archneurol.2011.1175

Carter, A. R., Astafiev, S. V., Lang, C. E., Connor, L. T., Rengachary, J., Strube, M. J., et al. (2010). Resting interhemispheric functional magnetic resonance imaging connectivity predicts performance after stroke. *Ann. Neurol.* 67, 365–375. doi: 10.1002/ana.21905

Castro-Alamancos, M., A., and Connors, B. W. (1996). Short-term plasticity of a thalamocortical pathway dynamically modulated by behavioral state. *Science* 272, 274–277. doi: 10.1126/science.272.5259.274

Castro-Alamancos, M., A, Donoghue, J. P., and Connors, B. W. (1995). Different forms of synaptic plasticity in somatosensory and motor areas of the neocortex. *J. Neurosci.* 15, 5324–5333.

Chen, J. L., Lin, W. C., Cha, J. W., So, P. T., Kubota, Y., and Nedivi, E. (2011). Structural basis for the role of inhibition in facilitating adult brain plasticity. *Nat. Neurosci.* 14, 587–594. doi: 10.1038/nn.2799

Chen, Y., Peng, L., Zhang, X., Stolzenburg, J. U., and Hertz, L. (1995). Further evidence that fluoxetine interacts with a 5-HT2C receptor in glial cells. *Brain Res. Bull.* 38, 153–159. doi: 10.1016/0361-9230(95)00082-P

Chollet, F., Tardy, J., Albucher, J.-F., Thalamas, C., Berard, E., Lamy, C., et al. (2011). Fluoxetine for motor recovery after acute ischaemic stroke (FLAME): a randomised placebo-controlled trial. *Lancet Neurol.* 10, 123–130. doi: 10.1016/S1474-4422(10)70314-8

Clarkson, A. N., Huang, B. S., Macisaac, S. E., Mody, I., and Carmichael, S. T. (2010). Reducing excessive GABA-mediated tonic inhibition promotes functional recovery after stroke. *Nature* 468, 305–309. doi: 10.1038/nature09511

Collins, K. (2016). *Investigation of Upper Limb Kinematics and Corticospinal Pathway Activity Early after Stroke.* East Angle, CA: Norwich University.

Conforto, A. B., dos Santos, R. L., Farias, S. N., Marie, S. K. N., Mangini, N., and Cohen, L. G. (2008). Effects of somatosensory stimulation on the excitability of the unaffected hemisphere in chronic stroke patients. *Clinics* 63, 735–740. doi: 10.1590/S1807-59322008000600005

Costanzo, L. S. (2017). *Physiology E-Book.* Elsevier Health Sciences. Available online at: https://books.google.com/books?id=H6BcDgAAQBAJ

Crichton, S. L., Bray, B. D., McKevitt, C., Rudd, A. G., and Wolfe, C. D. A. (2016). Patient outcomes up to 15 years after stroke: survival, disability, quality of life, cognition and mental health. *J. Neurol. Neurosurg. Psychiatr.* 87, 1091–1098. doi: 10.1136/jnnp-2016-313361

Croarkin, P. E., Nakonezny, P. A., Husain, M. M., Port, J. D., Melton, T., Kennard, B. D., et al. (2014). Evidence for pretreatment LICI deficits among depressed children and adolescents with nonresponse to fluoxetine. *Brain Stimul.* 7, 243–251. doi: 10.1016/j.brs.2013.11.006

Dam, M., Tonin, P., De Boni, A., Pizzolato, G., Casson, S., Ermani, M., et al. (1996). Effects of fluoxetine and maprotiline on functional recovery in poststroke hemiplegic patients undergoing rehabilitation therapy. *Stroke* 27, 1211–1214. doi: 10.1161/01.STR.27.7.1211

Diaz, S. L., Doly, S., Narboux-Nême, N., Fernández, S., Mazot, P., Banas, S. M., et al. (2012). 5-HT2B receptors are required for serotonin-selective antidepressant actions. *Mol. Psychiatry* 17, 154–163. doi: 10.1038/mp.2011.159

Diaz, S. L., Narboux-Nême, N., Boutourlinsky, K., Doly, S., and Maroteaux, L. (2016). Mice lacking the serotonin 5-HT2B receptor as an animal model of resistance to selective serotonin reuptake inhibitors antidepressants. *Eur. Neuropsychopharmacol.* 26, 265–279. doi: 10.1016/j.euroneuro.2015.12.012

Di Lazzaro, V., Profice, P., Pilato, F., Capone, F., Ranieri, F., Florio, L., et al. (2012). The level of cortical afferent inhibition in acute stroke correlates with long-term functional recovery in humans. *Stroke* 43, 250–252. doi: 10.1161/STROKEAHA.111.631085

Dong, L., Li, B., Verkhratsky, A., and Peng, L. (2015). Cell type-specific *in vivo* expression of genes encoding signalling molecules in the brain in response to chronic mild stress and chronic treatment with fluoxetine. *Psychopharmacology* 232, 2827–2835. doi: 10.1007/s00213-015-3921-2

Du, T., Liang, C., Li, B., Hertz, L., and Peng, L. (2014). Chronic fluoxetine administration increases expression of the L-channel gene Cav1.2 in astrocytes from the brain of treated mice and in culture and augments K+-induced increase in [Ca2+]i. *Cell Calc.* 55, 166–174. doi: 10.1016/j.ceca.2014.01.002

Engel, D., Pahner, I., Schulze, K., Frahm, C., Jarry, H., Ahnert-Hilger, G., et al. (2001). Plasticity of rat central inhibitory synapses through GABA metabolism. *J. Physiol.* 535, 473–482. doi: 10.1111/j.1469-7793.2001.00473.x

Etherton, M., Siddiqui, K. A., Ayres, A., and Schwamm, L. H. (2016). *Abstract WP174: Prestroke Selective Serotonin Reuptake Inhibitor Use and Functional Outcomes in Ischemic Stroke. Stroke 47, AWP174–AWP174.* Available online at: http://stroke.ahajournals.org/content/47/Suppl_1/AWP174

Feldman, D. E. (2009). Synaptic mechanisms for plasticity in neocortex. *Annu. Rev. Neurosci.* 32, 33–55. doi: 10.1146/annurev.neuro.051508.135516

Feydy, A., Carlier, R., Roby-Brami, A., Bussel, B., Cazalis, F., Pierot, L., et al. (2002). Longitudinal study of motor recovery after stroke: recruitment and focusing of brain activation. *Stroke* 33, 1610–1617. doi: 10.1161/01.STR.0000017100.68294.52

Floyer-Lea, A., Wylezinska, M., Kincses, T., and Matthews, P. M. (2006). Rapid modulation of GABA concentration in human sensorimotor cortex during motor learning. *J. Neurophysiol.* 95, 1639–1644. doi: 10.1152/jn.00346.2005

Frost, S. B., Barbay, S., Friel, K. M., Plautz, E. J., and Nudo, R. J. (2003). Reorganization of remote cortical regions after ischemic brain injury: a potential substrate for stroke recovery. *J. Neurophysiol.* 89, 3205–3214. doi: 10.1152/jn.01143.2002

Ganzer, P. D., Moxon, K. A., Knudsen, E. B., and Shumsky, J. S. (2013). Serotonergic pharmacotherapy promotes cortical reorganization after spinal cord injury. *Exp. Neurol.* 241, 84–94. doi: 10.1016/j.expneurol.2012.12.004

Gerdelat-Mas, A., Loubinoux, I., Tombaria, D., Rascolb, O., Cholleta, F., and Simonetta-Moreaua, M. (2005). Chronic administration of selective serotonin reuptake inhibitor (SSRI) paroxetine modulates human motor cortex excitability in healthy subjects. *Neuroimage* 27, 314–322. doi: 10.1016/j.neuroimage.2005.05.009

Grimm, S., Beck, J., Schuepbach, D., Hell, D., Boesiger, P., Bermpohl, F., et al. (2008). Imbalance between left and right dorsolateral prefrontal cortex in major depression is linked to negative emotional judgment: an fMRI study in severe major depressive disorder. *Biol. Psychiatry* 63, 369–376. doi: 10.1016/j.biopsych.2007.05.033

Guerra, A., Pogosyan, A., Nowak, M., Tan, H., Ferreri, F., Di Lazzaro, V., et al. (2016). Phase dependency of the human primary motor cortex and cholinergic inhibition cancelation during beta tACS. *Cereb. Cortex* 26, 3977–3990. doi: 10.1093/cercor/bhw245

Guirado, R., Perez-Rando, M., Sanchez-Matarredona, D., Castrén, E., and Nacher, J. (2014). Chronic fluoxetine treatment alters the structure, connectivity and plasticity of cortical interneurons. *Int. J. Neuropsychopharmacol.* 17, 1635–1646. doi: 10.1017/S1461145714000406

Hagemann, G., Redecker, C., Neumann-Haefelin, T., Freund, H. J., and Witte, O. W. (1998). Increased long-term potentiation in the surround of experimentally induced focal cortical infarction. *Ann. Neurol.* 44, 255–258. doi: 10.1002/ana.410440217

Hensch, T. K., and Stryker, M. P. (2004). Columnar architecture sculpted by GABA circuits in developing cat visual cortex. *Science* 303, 1678–1681. doi: 10.1126/science.1091031

Hertz, L., Rothman, D. L., Li, B., and Peng, L. (2015a). Chronic SSRI stimulation of astrocytic 5-HT2B receptors change multiple gene expressions/editings and metabolism of glutamate, glucose and glycogen: a potential paradigm shift. *Front. Behav. Neurosci.* 9:25. doi: 10.3389/fnbeh.2015.00025

Hertz, L., Xu, J., Song, D., Du, T., Li, B., Yan, E., et al. (2015b). Astrocytic glycogenolysis: mechanisms and functions. *Metab. Brain Dis.* 30, 317–333. doi: 10.1007/s11011-014-9536-1

Hill, T., Coupland, C., Morriss, R., Arthur, A., Moore, M., and Hippisley-Cox, J. (2015). Antidepressant use and risk of epilepsy and seizures in people aged 20 to 64 years: cohort study using a primary care database. *BMC Psychiatry* 15:315. doi: 10.1186/s12888-015-0701-9

Hogan, N., Krebs, H. I., Rohrer, B., Palazzolo, J. J., Dipietro, L., Fasoli, S. E., et al. (2006). Motions or muscles? Some behavioral factors underlying robotic assistance of motor recovery. *J. Rehabil. Res. Dev.* 43, 605–618. doi: 10.1682/JRRD.2005.06.0103

Hourai, A., and Miyata, S. (2013). Neurogenesis in the circumventricular organs of adult mouse brains. *J. Neurosci. Res.* 91, 757–770. doi: 10.1002/jnr.23206

Hummel, F. C., and Cohen, L. G. (2006). Non-invasive brain stimulation: a new strategy to improve neurorehabilitation after stroke? *Lancet Neurol.* 5, 708–712. doi: 10.1016/S1474-4422(06)70525-7

Hummel, F., and Cohen, L. G. (2005). Improvement of motor function with noninvasive cortical stimulation in a patient with chronic stroke. *Neurorehabil. Neural Repair* 19, 14–19. doi: 10.1177/1545968304272698

Hummel, F. C., Steven, B., Hoppe, J., Heise, K., Thomalla, G., Cohen, L. G., et al. (2009). Deficient intracortical inhibition (SICI) during movement preparation after chronic stroke. *Neurology* 72, 1766–1772. doi: 10.1212/WNL.0b013e3181a609c5

Igelström, K. M., and Heyward, P. M. (2012). Inhibition of hippocampal excitability by citalopram. *Epilepsia* 53, 2034–2042. doi: 10.1111/j.1528-1167.2012.03660.x

Invernizzi, R. W., Pierucci, M., Calcagno, E., Di Giovanni, G., Di Matteo, V., Benigno, A., et al. (2007). Selective activation of 5-HT2C receptors stimulates GABA-ergic function in the rat substantia nigra pars reticulata: a combined *in vivo* electrophysiological and neurochemical study. *Neuroscience* 144, 1523–1535. doi: 10.1016/j.neuroscience.2006.11.004

Jaillard, A., Martin, C. D., Garambois, K., Lebas, J. F., and Hommel, M. (2005). Vicarious function within the human primary motor cortex? a longitudinal fMRI stroke study. *Brain* 128, 1122–1138. doi: 10.1093/brain/awh456

Johansen-Berg, H., Rushworth, M. F., Bogdanovic, M. D., Kischka, U., Wimalaratna, S., and Matthews, P. M. (2002). The role of ipsilateral premotor cortex in hand movement after stroke. *Proc. Natl. Acad. Sci. U.S.A.* 99, 14518–14523. doi: 10.1073/pnas.222536799

Johnstone, A., Hinson, E., and Stagg, C. J. (2016). "tDCS and magnetic resonance imaging," in *Transcranial Direct Current Stimulation in Neuropsychiatric Disorders: Clinical Principles and Management*, eds A. Brunoni, M. Nitsche, and C. Loo (Cham: Springer International Publishing), 169–195.

Jones, T. A. (2017). Motor compensation and its effects on neural reorganization after stroke. *Nat. Rev. Neurosci.* 18, 267–280. doi: 10.1038/nrn.2017.26

Julkunen, P., Määttä, S., Säisänen, L., Kallioniemi, E., Könönen, M., Jäkälä, P., et al. (2016). Functional and structural cortical characteristics after restricted focal motor cortical infarction evaluated at chronic stage - indications from a preliminary study. *Clin. Neurophysiol.* 127, 2775–2784. doi: 10.1016/j.clinph.2016.05.013

Karpova, N. N., Pickenhagen, A., Lindholm, J., Tiraboschi, E., Kulesskaya, N., Agústsdóttir, A., et al. (2011). Fear erasure in mice requires synergy between antidepressant drugs and extinction training. *Science* 334, 1731–1734. doi: 10.1126/science.1214592

Kitago, T., and Krakauer, J. W. (2013). "Chapter 8 - Motor learning principles for neurorehabilitation," in *Neurological Rehabilitation, Handbook of Clinical Neurology*, Vol. 110, eds M. P. Barnes and D. C. Good (New York, NY: Elsevier), 93–103. doi: 10.1016/B978-0-444-52901-5.00008-3

Klimesch, W. (2012). Alpha-band oscillations, attention, and controlled access to stored information. *Trends Cogn. Sci.* 16, 606–617. doi: 10.1016/j.tics.2012.10.007

Kobayashi, K., Ikeda, Y., Sakai, A., Yamasaki, N., Haneda, E., Miyakawa, T., et al. (2010). Reversal of hippocampal neuronal maturation by serotonergic antidepressants. *Proc. Natl. Acad. Sci. U.S.A.* 107, 8434–8439. doi: 10.1073/pnas.0912690107

Kokoeva, M. V., Yin, H., and Flier, J. S. (2005). Neurogenesis in the hypothalamus of adult mice: potential role in energy balance. *Science* 310, 679–683. doi: 10.1126/science.1115360

Krakauer, J. W. (2006). Motor learning: its relevance to stroke recovery and neurorehabilitation. *Curr. Opin. Neurol.* 19, 84–90. doi: 10.1097/01.wco.0000200544.29915.cc

Krakauer, J. W., and Mazzoni, P. (2011). Human sensorimotor learning: adaptation, skill, and beyond. *Curr. Opin. Neurobiol.* 21, 636–644. doi: 10.1016/j.conb.2011.06.012

Li, B., Zhang, S., Zhang, H., Hertz, L., and Peng, L. (2011). Fluoxetine affects GluK2 editing, glutamate-evoked Ca^{2+} influx and extracellular signal-regulated kinase phosphorylation in mouse astrocytes. *J. Psychiatry Neurosci.* 36, 322–338. doi: 10.1503/jpn.100094

Liepert, J., Hamzei, F., and Weiller, C. (2000). Motor cortex disinhibition of the unaffected hemisphere after acute stroke. *Muscle Nerve* 23, 1761–1763. doi: 10.1002/1097-4598(200011)23:11<1761::AID-MUS14>3.0.CO;2-M

Lim, C.-M., Kim, S.-W., Park, J.-Y., Kim, C., Yoon, S. H., and Lee, J.-K. (2009). Fluoxetine affords robust neuroprotection in the postischemic brain via its anti-inflammatory effect. *J. Neurosci. Res.* 87, 1037–1045. doi: 10.1002/jnr.21899

Lindenberg, R., Renga, V., Zhu, L. L., Nair, D., and Schlaug, G. (2010). Bihemispheric brain stimulation facilitates motor recovery in chronic stroke patients. *Neurology* 75, 2176–2184. doi: 10.1212/WNL.0b013e318202013a

Loubinoux, I., Tombari, D., Pariente, J., Gerdelat-Mas, A., Franceries, X., Cassol, E., et al. (2005). Modulation of behavior and cortical motor activity in healthy subjects by a chronic administration of a serotonin enhancer. *Neuroimage* 27, 299–313. doi: 10.1016/j.neuroimage.2004.12.023

Lovatt, D., Sonnewald, U., Waagepetersen, H. S., Schousboe, A., He, W., Lin, J. H.-C., et al. (2007). The transcriptome and metabolic gene signature of protoplasmic astrocytes in the adult murine cortex. *J. Neurosci.* 27, 12255–12266. doi: 10.1523/JNEUROSCI.3404-07.2007

Lynch, M. A. (2004). Long-term potentiation and memory. *Physiol. Rev.* 84, 87–136. doi: 10.1152/physrev.00014.2003

Mantovani, A., Pavlicova, M., Avery, D., Nahas, Z., McDonald, W. M., Wajdik, C. D., et al. (2012). Long-term efficacy of repeated daily prefrontal transcranial magnetic stimulation (TMS) in treatment-resistant depression. *Depress. Anxiety* 29, 883–890. doi: 10.1002/da.21967

Matsumoto, K., Puia, G., Dong, E., and Pinna, G. (2007). GABA(A) receptor neurotransmission dysfunction in a mouse model of social isolation-induced stress: possible insights into a non-serotonergic mechanism of action of SSRIs in mood and anxiety disorders. *Stress* 10, 3–12. doi: 10.1080/10253890701200997

Mead, G. E., Hsieh, C.-F., Lee, R., Kutlubaev, M., Claxton, A., Hankey, G. J., et al. (2013). Selective serotonin reuptake inhibitors for stroke recovery: a systematic review and meta-analysis. *Stroke* 44, 844–850. doi: 10.1161/STROKEAHA.112.673947

Meintzschel, F., and Ziemann, U. (2006). Modification of practice-dependent plasticity in human motor cortex by neuromodulators. *Cereb. Cortex* 16, 1106–1115. doi: 10.1093/cercor/bhj052

Mozaffarian, D., Benjamin, E. J., Go, A. S., Arnett, D. K., Blaha, M. J., Cushman, M., et al. (2016). Heart disease and stroke statistics-2016 update a report from the American heart association. *Circulation* 133, e38–e48. doi: 10.1161/CIR.0000000000000366

Murase, N., Duque, J., Mazzocchio, R., and Cohen, L. G. (2004). Influence of interhemispheric interactions on motor function in chronic stroke. *Ann. Neurol.* 55, 400–409. doi: 10.1002/ana.10848

Netz, J., Lammers, T., and Hömberg, V. (1997). Reorganization of motor output in the non-affected hemisphere after stroke. *Brain* 120, 1579–1586. doi: 10.1093/brain/120.9.1579

Nudo, R. J. (2013). Recovery after brain injury: mechanisms and principles. *Front. Hum. Neurosci.* 7:887. doi: 10.3389/fnhum.2013.00887

Nudo, R. J., Milliken, G. W., Jenkins, W. M., and Merzenich, M. M. (1996). Use-dependent alterations of movement representations in primary motor cortex of adult squirrel monkeys. *J. Neurosci.* 16, 785–807.

Oh, B.-M., Kim, D.-Y., and Paik, N.-J. (2010). Disinhibition in the unaffected hemisphere is related with the cortical involvement of the affected hemisphere. *Int. J. Neurosci.* 120, 512–515. doi: 10.3109/00207451003760114

Ohira, K., Takeuchi, R., Iwanaga, T., and Miyakawa, T. (2013a). Chronic fluoxetine treatment reduces parvalbumin expression and perineuronal nets in gamma-aminobutyric acidergic interneurons of the frontal cortex in adult mice. *Mol. Brain* 6:43. doi: 10.1186/1756-6606-6-43

Ohira, K., Takeuchi, R., Shoji, H., and Miyakawa, T. (2013b). Fluoxetine-induced cortical adult neurogenesis. *Neuropsychopharmacology* 38, 909–920. doi: 10.1038/npp.2013.2

Pariente, J., Loubinoux, I., Carel, C., Albucher, J. F., Leger, A., Manelfe, C., et al. (2001). Fluoxetine modulates motor performance and cerebral activation of patients recovering from stroke. *Ann. Neurol.* 50, 718–729. doi: 10.1002/ana.1257

Park, C. H., Chang, W. H., Ohn, S. H., Kim, S. T., Bang, O. Y., Pascual-Leone, A., et al. (2011). Longitudinal changes of resting-state functional connectivity during motor recovery after stroke. *Stroke* 42, 1357–1362. doi: 10.1161/STROKEAHA.110.596155

Peng, L., Gu, L., Li, B., and Hertz, L. (2014). Fluoxetine and all other SSRIs are 5-HT2B agonists - importance for their therapeutic effects. *Curr. Neuropharmacol.* 12, 365–379. doi: 10.2174/1570159X12666140828221720

Pfurtscheller, G., and Lopes da Silva, F. H. (2017). Event-related EEG/MEG synchronization and desynchronization: basic principles. *Clin. Neurophysiol.* 110, 1842–1857. doi: 10.1016/S1388-2457(99)00141-8

Pfurtscheller, G., Neuper, C., Brunner, C., and Lopes Da Silva, F. (2005). Beta rebound after different types of motor imagery in man. *Neurosci. Lett.* 378, 156–159. doi: 10.1016/j.neulet.2004.12.034

Reynolds, C., and Ashby, P. (1999). Inhibition in the human motor cortex is reduced just before a voluntary contraction. *Neurology* 53, 730–735. doi: 10.1212/WNL.53.4.730

Rieckmann, N., and Kronish, I. (2013). Serotonin reuptake inhibitor use, depression, and long-term outcomes after an acute coronary syndrome: a prospective cohort study. *JAMA Intern. Med.* 173, 1150–1151. doi: 10.1001/jamainternmed.2013.910

Rief, W., Barsky, A. J., Bingel, U., Doering, B. K., Schwarting, R., Wöhr, M., et al. (2016). Rethinking psychopharmacotherapy: the role of treatment context and brain plasticity in antidepressant and antipsychotic interventions. *Neurosci. Biobehav. Rev.* 60, 51–64. doi: 10.1016/j.neubiorev.2015.11.008

Robinson, R. T., Drafts, B. C., and Fisher, J. L. (2003). Fluoxetine increases GABAA receptor activity through a novel modulatory site. *J. Pharmacol. Exp. Ther.* 304, 978–984. doi: 10.1124/jpet.102.044834

Robol, E., Fiaschi, A., and Manganotti, P. (2004). Effects of citalopram on the excitability of the human motor cortex: a paired magnetic stimulation study. *J. Neurol. Sci.* 221, 41–46. doi: 10.1016/j.jns.2004.03.007

Rosenstein, J. M., Mani, N., Silverman, W. F., and Krum, J. M. (1998). Patterns of brain angiogenesis after vascular endothelial growth factor administration *in vitro* and *in vivo*. *Proc. Natl. Acad. Sci. U.S.A.* 95, 7086–7091.

Rossi, S., Hallett, M., Rossini, P. M., and Pascual-Leone, A. (2009). Safety, ethical considerations, and application guidelines for the use of transcranial magnetic stimulation in clinical practice and research. *Clin. Neurophysiol.* 120, 2008–2039. doi: 10.1016/j.clinph.2009.08.016

Sanacora, G., Mason, G. F., Rothman, D. L., and Krystal, J. H. (2002). Increased occipital cortex GABA concentrations in depressed patients after therapy with selective serotonin reuptake inhibitors. *Am. J. Psychiatry* 159, 663–665. doi: 10.1176/appi.ajp.159.4.663

Sato, S., Bergmann, T. O., and Borich, M. R. (2015). Opportunities for concurrent transcranial magnetic stimulation and electroencephalography to characterize cortical activity in stroke. *Front. Hum. Neurosci.* 9:250. doi: 10.3389/fnhum.2015.00250

Sawaki, L., Boroojerdi, B., Kaelin-Lang, A., Burstein, A. H., Bütefisch, C. M., Kopylev, L., et al. (2002a). Cholinergic influences on use-dependent plasticity. *J. Neurophysiol.* 87, 166–171. doi: 10.1152/jn.00279.2001

Sawaki, L., Cohen, L. G., Classen, J., Davis, B. C., and Butefisch, C. M. (2002b). Enhancement of use-dependent plasticity by D-amphetamine 7446. *Neurology* 59, 1262–1264. doi: 10.1212/WNL.59.8.1262

Scheidtmann, K., Fries, W., Müller, F., and Koenig, E. (2001). Effect of levodopa in combination with physiotherapy on functional motor recovery after stroke: a prospective, randomised, double-blind study. *Lancet* 358, 787–790. doi: 10.1016/S0140-6736(01)05966-9

Schiene, K., Bruehl, C., Zilles, K., Qü, M., Hagemann, G., Kraemer, M., et al. (1996). Neuronal hyperexcitability and reduction of GABAA-receptor expression in the surround of cerebral photothrombosis. *J. Cereb. Blood Flow Metab.* 16, 906–914. doi: 10.1097/00004647-199609000-00014

Serrats, J., Mengod, G., and Cortés, R. (2005). Expression of serotonin 5-HT2C receptors in GABAergic cells of the anterior raphe nuclei. *J. Chem. Neuroanat.* 29, 83–91. doi: 10.1016/j.jchemneu.2004.03.010

Shadmehr, R., and Holcomb, H. H. (1997). Neural correlates of motor memory consolidation. *Science* 277, 821–825. doi: 10.1126/science.277.5327.821

Shin, T. K., Kang, M. S., Lee, H. Y., Seo, M. S., Kim, S. G., Kim, C. D., et al. (2009). Fluoxetine and sertraline attenuate postischemic brain injury in mice. *Korean J. Physiol. Pharmacol.* 13, 257–263. doi: 10.4196/kjpp.2009.13.3.257

Siepmann, T., Penzlin, A. I., Kepplinger, J., Illigens, B. M., Weidner, K., Reichmann, H., et al. (2015). Selective serotonin reuptake inhibitors to improve outcome in acute ischemic stroke: possible mechanisms and clinical evidence. *Brain Behav.* 5:e00373. doi: 10.1002/brb3.373

Stagg, C. J. (2013). Magnetic Resonance Spectroscopy as a tool to study the role of GABA in motor-cortical plasticity. *Neuroimage* 86, 19–27. doi: 10.1016/j.neuroimage.2013.01.009

Stagg, C. J., Bachtiar, V., and Johansen-Berg, H. (2011). The role of GABA in human motor learning. *Curr. Biol.* 21, 480–484. doi: 10.1016/j.cub.2011.01.069

Stahl, S. M. (2017). Mechanism of action of serotonin selective reuptake inhibitors. *J. Affect. Disord.* 51, 215–235. doi: 10.1016/S0165-0327(98)00221-3

Steinman, M. Q., Gao, V., and Alberini, C. M. (2016). The role of lactate-mediated metabolic coupling between astrocytes and neurons in long-term memory formation. *Front. Integr. Neurosci.* 10:10. doi: 10.3389/fnint.2016.00010

Sun, Y., Jin, K., Xie, L., Childs, J., Mao, X. O., Logvinova, A., et al. (2003). VEGF-induced neuroprotection, neurogenesis, and angiogenesis after focal cerebral ischemia. *J. Clin. Invest.* 111, 1843–1851. doi: 10.1172/JCI200317977

Swayne, O. B., Rothwell, J. C., Ward, N. S., and Greenwood, R. J. (2008). Stages of motor output reorganization after hemispheric stroke suggested by longitudinal studies of cortical physiology. *Cereb. Cortex* 18, 1909–1922. doi: 10.1093/cercor/bhm218

Takeuchi, N., and Izumi, S.-I. (2012). Maladaptive plasticity for motor recovery after stroke: mechanisms and approaches. *Neural Plast.* 2012:359728. doi: 10.1155/2012/359728

Takeuchi, N., Tada, T., Chuma, T., Matsuo, Y., and Ikoma, K. (2007). Disinhibition of the premotor cortex contributes to a maladaptive change in the affected hand after stroke. *Stroke* 38, 1551–1556. doi: 10.1161/STROKEAHA.106.470187

Talelli, P., Greenwood, R. J., and Rothwell, J. C. (2006). Arm function after stroke: neurophysiological correlates and recovery mechanisms assessed by transcranial magnetic stimulation. *Clin. Neurophysiol.* 117, 1641–1659. doi: 10.1016/j.clinph.2006.01.016

Trevelyan, A. J. (2016). Do cortical circuits need protecting from themselves? *Trends Neurosci.* 39, 502–511. doi: 10.1016/j.tins.2016.06.002

Tunnicliff, G., Schindler, N. L., Crites, G. J., Goldenberg, R., Yochum, A., and Malatynska, E. (1999). The GABA(A) receptor complex as a target for fluoxetine action. *Neurochem. Res.* 24, 1271–1276. doi: 10.1023/A:1020977123968

Turton, A., Wroe, S., Trepte, N., Fraser, C., and Lemon, R. N. (1996). Contralateral and ipsilateral EMG responses to transcranial magnetic stimulation during recovery of arm and hand function after stroke. *Electroencephalogr. Clin. Neurophysiol. Electromyogr. Mot. Control* 101, 316–328. doi: 10.1016/0924-980X(96)95560-5

Urban, E. T., Bury, S. D., Barbay, H. S., Guggenmos, D. J., Dong, Y., and Nudo, R. J. (2012). Gene expression changes of interconnected spared cortical neurons 7 days after ischemic infarct of the primary motor cortex in the rat. *Mol. Cell. Biochem.* 369, 267–286. doi: 10.1007/s11010-012-1390-z

Veerbeek, J. M., van Wegen, E., van Peppen, R., van der Wees, P. J., Hendriks, E., Rietberg, M., et al. (2014). What is the evidence for physical therapy poststroke? a systematic review and meta-analysis. *PLoS ONE* 9:e87987. doi: 10.1371/journal.pone.0087987

Werhahn, K. J., Conforto, A. B., Kadom, N., Hallett, M., and Cohen, L. G. (2003). Contribution of the ipsilateral motor cortex to recovery after chronic stroke. *Ann. Neurol.* 54, 464–472. doi: 10.1002/ana.10686

Winstein, C. J., Stein, J., Arena, R., Bates, B., Cherney, L. R., Cramer, S. C., et al. (2016). Guidelines for adult stroke rehabilitation and recovery: a guideline for healthcare professionals from the american heart association/american stroke association. *Stroke* 47, e98–e169. doi: 10.1161/STR.0000000000000098

Ye, Z. Y., Zhou, K. Q., Xu, T., Le, and Zhou, J. N. (2008). Fluoxetine potentiates GABAergic IPSCs in rat hippocampal neurons. *Neurosci. Lett.* 442, 24–29. doi: 10.1016/j.neulet.2008.06.072

Zaaroor, M., Pratt, H., and Starr, A. (2003). Time course of motor excitability before and after a task-related movement. *Neurophysiol. Clin. Neurophysiol.* 33, 130–137. doi: 10.1016/S0987-7053(03)00029-7

Zittel, S., Weiller, C., and Liepert, J. (2008). Citalopram improves dexterity in chronic stroke patients. *Neurorehabil. Neural Repair* 22, 311–314. doi: 10.1177/1545968307312173

24

Murine Depression Model and its Potential Applications for Discovering Foods and Farm Products with Antidepressant-Like Effects

*Tatsuhiko Goto [1,2], Shozo Tomonaga [3], Tsuyoshi Okayama [1,2,4] and Atsushi Toyoda [1,2,4]**

[1] Department of Biological Production Science, College of Agriculture, Ibaraki University, Ami, Ibaraki, Japan, [2] Department of Biological Production Science, Ibaraki University Cooperation between Agriculture and Medical Science, Ami, Ibaraki, Japan, [3] Graduate School of Agriculture, Kyoto University, Kyoto, Japan, [4] Department of Biological Production Science, United Graduate School of Agricultural Science, Tokyo University of Agriculture and Technology, Fuchu, Japan

Edited by:
Fumihiko Maekawa, National Institute for Environmental Studies, Japan

Reviewed by:
Bruno Bonaz, Grenoble Faculty of Medicine and Hospital, France
Keizo Takao, University of Toyama, Japan
Adriana Ximenes-da-Silva, Universidade Federal de Alagoas, Brazil

***Correspondence:**
Atsushi Toyoda
atsushi.toyoda.0516@vc.ibaraki.ac.jp

Advanced societies face increased health problems related to various stresses. Chronic psychological stress is a major risk factor for psychiatric disorders such as depression. Although therapeutic agents reduce several symptoms of depression, most have side effects in a broad range of the population. Furthermore, some victims of depression do not show significant improvement with any drugs, so alternative approaches are needed. Good dietary habits may potentially reduce depressive symptoms, but there is little scientific evidence thus far. Murine depression models are useful to test nutritional approaches *in vivo*. Our model mice subjected to a subchronic mild social defeat stress (sCSDS) paradigm show several alterations in physiological parameters and social behavior. These stress-induced symptoms in sCSDS mice can be used as cues to identify antidepressant-like natural resources including foods and farm products. We previously discovered that sCSDS mice show more vulnerability to social stress by changing dietary condition. In addition, we developed a more objective system for analyzing mouse behavior using a 3D depth-sensing camera to understand relationships between diet and behavior. The combination of sCSDS mice with 3D behavioral analysis is a powerful method for screening ingredients in foods and farm products for antidepressant-like effects.

Keywords: depression, food, behavior, metabolomics, social defeat stress, depth camera

INTRODUCTION

Advanced societies face increased health problems related to various stresses; chronic psychological stress in particular is a major risk factor for precipitating psychiatric disorders such as depression. A Global Burden of Disease study showed depression is the most disabling disorder worldwide (Whiteford et al., 2013). Since this issue will face the next generation of developing countries, it is imperative to find some solution. Therapeutic agents reduce several symptoms of depression, but most have several side effects in a broad population (Stevens et al., 2014; Galling et al., 2015). Moreover, some victims of depression do not show significant improvement with any drugs (treatment-resistant depression), so alternative approaches are needed (El-Hage et al., 2013). For prevention, it is more important to change dietary habits rather than resort to conventional treatments. Recently, interest has increased in Kampo (Watanabe et al., 2011) and functional foods (Arai, 1996). In fact, some reports indicate that Kampo (Ito et al., 2012; Hori et al., 2015) and functional ingredients (Tomonaga et al., 2008; Iio et al., 2012a) have antidepressant effects in animal models. This study further explores functional ingredients from natural sources for prevention and attenuation of symptoms of depression.

Chronic social defeat stress (CSDS) models of rats and mice are recognized as good animal models of depression. CSDS models establish social stress using male territorial aggression (Kudryavtseva et al., 1991; Miczek et al., 2008; Hammels et al., 2015). We previously studied CSDS rats and found that social stress induces alterations in the MAP kinase cascade, hypothalamic malonyl-CoA, peripheral leptin, digestive system, and behaviors (Iio et al., 2011, 2012b, 2014; Toyoda et al., 2015). Others have analyzed both central nervous system and peripheral tissues in relation to stress resilience using CSDS mice (Russo and Nestler, 2013; Hodes et al., 2014; Pfau and Russo, 2015). In addition, we have established a milder model of depression, subchronic mild social defeat stress (sCSDS; Goto et al., 2014, Goto and Toyoda, 2015) than CSDS (Krishnan et al., 2007). Since several models are required (Bartolomucci and Leopardi, 2009), sCSDS mice may provide insights about pathogenic mechanisms and preventive measures for depression.

The 3D behavioral analysis allows evaluation of more natural, realistic animal behavior. Although animals behave in 3D space and show several postures sterically, conventional animal monitoring systems have been primarily 2D video cameras. Recently, commercially available 3D depth-sensing cameras have been developed in the computer game industry, and can thus be affordably obtained (~$200/camera). Using 3D cameras, rats and mice have been monitored (Ou-Yang et al., 2011). Since behavioral scientists can derive depth information from animal behavior, the 3D camera enables discrimination of slight differences in 3D behavioral characteristics that have not been previously well detected.

In this article, we introduce features of our murine stress model and novel 3D monitoring system. We discuss the use of both for discovering foods and farm products providing antidepressant-like effects.

SUBCHRONIC MILD SOCIAL DEFEAT STRESS (SCSDS) MODEL MOUSE

Phenotypes of sCSDS (Figure 1A)

sCSDS mice are established by the method (Goto and Toyoda, 2015). Subject C57BL/6J mice are exposed to psychosocial stress from aggressive ICR mice for 10 consecutive days. During establishment, body weight gain, food intake, and water intake in sCSDS mice are significantly higher than those of non-stressed control mice (Goto et al., 2014). The sCSDS mice show increased body water content and social avoidance behavior after the stress. Moreover, nest-building behavior in sCSDS mice is significantly delayed compared to control mice (Otabi et al., 2016). In CSDS mice, social avoidance behavior has been widely reported (Tanaka et al., 2012; Russo and Nestler, 2013). Increased body weight gain has been reported in defeated mice (Goto et al., 2014) and lower ranking mice (Kim et al., 2015). Stress-induced polydipsia has been reported in both CSDS (Krishnan et al., 2007) and chronic mild stress (CMS) conditions (Gross and Pinhasov, 2016). Although, these features are supported by several studies, social stress-induced increases in body water content (Goto et al., 2014) and delays in nest-building behavior (Otabi et al., 2016) are, to our knowledge, unique findings.

Metabolomic Analyses of sCSDS (Figure 1A)

To find key metabolites altered by social defeat stress, we tested the blood plasma/serum, urine, and liver. Biochemical assays for blood serum components revealed that sCSDS mice showed low levels of albumin (ALB) and blood urea nitrogen (BUN) just after stress (Goto et al., 2014). Low levels of sodium were found in the urine of sCSDS mice. Metabolomics revealed that four liver metabolites, taurocyamine (GES), phosphorylcholine, D-alanyl-D-alanine (D-ala-D-ala), and 1-methylnicotinamide (MNA), were significantly upregulated in sCSDS mice vs. control mice (Goto et al., 2015a).

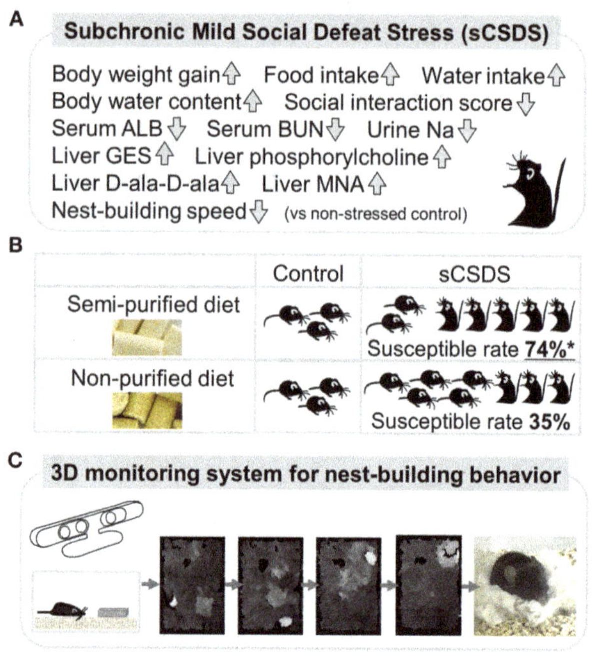

FIGURE 1 | Summary of a mouse model and 3D behavioral analysis. (A) Social stress-induced symptoms in sCSDS mice. **(B)** Dietary quality influence stress-vulnerability behavior in sCSDS mice. sCSDS mice fed semi-purified diet indicate significantly higher susceptible rate than sCSDS mice fed non-purified diet. $^{*}P < 0.05$ (Goto et al., in press). **(C)** 3D monitoring system of nest-building behavior. Temporal changes of nesting behavior are clearly identified by depth images (higher regions are indicated by whiter color).

Food Habits Attenuate Stress-Induced Symptoms in sCSDS (Figure 1B)

We established sCSDS mice under feeding conditions with two kinds of pellet food, a semi-purified and a non-purified diet. We confirmed that the increased body weight gain, food intake, and water intake of sCSDS mice during stress were common to both diets (Goto et al., in press). Interestingly, we found that the vulnerability of mice to social defeat stress was affected by diet quality. sCSDS mice fed a semi-purified diet were more susceptible than sCSDS mice fed a non-purified diet (Goto et al., in press). This may be due to changing gut environments, as gut microbiota and their metabolic products can affect animal brain function and behavior (Cryan and Dinan, 2012). Especially, commensal microbiota can influence the hypothalamus-pituitary-adrenal reaction to stress in mice (Sudo et al., 2004). And, gut microbiota can modulate brain development and modulation of the serotonergic system, which is directly related to mood, in the limbic system (Heijtz et al., 2011). Although the microflora of sCSDS mice have not been fully studied, intestinal flora will be influenced by both stress and food. Metabolomics with the sCSDS mice fed both diets hope to find some solutions to attenuate stress-induced behavior by changing the metabolic environments of peripheral tissues.

A NOVEL 3D BEHAVIORAL TESTING METHOD FOR INNATE BEHAVIOR (FIGURE 1C)

Infrared 3D depth-sensing cameras have been developed intensely in the computer game industry. Both Microsoft Kinect (Microsoft Corp., USA) and Xtion PRO LIVE (ASUSTek Computer Inc., Taiwan) have become commercially available and affordable. The 3D depth-sensing camera has thus recently become available for use in rodent behavioral tests. The first reported behavioral analyses using a 3D camera focused on locomotion and pose in rats and mice (Ou-Yang et al., 2011). Matsumoto et al. constructed skeleton models of rats using four 3D cameras simultaneously and analyzed social and sexual interactions and novel object recognition behavior (Matsumoto et al., 2013, 2014). We monitored nest-building behavior in mice using a 3D camera (Okayama et al., 2015), and confirmed its effective utilization in a genetic study (Goto et al., 2015b). Nakamura et al. have developed a gait analysis system for mice using a 3D camera (Nakamura et al., 2015). Hong et al. succeeded in automating measurement of mouse social behaviors with machine learning algorithms from images captured simultaneously by a 3D camera and two 2D video cameras (Hong et al., 2015). Although conventional testing has been performed with 2D video cameras, future animal behavioral testing will evolve dramatically through use of 3D cameras.

Our 3D monitoring system focused on nesting behavior in mice, because the steric nest can be evaluated as a visible behavior. Deacon codified a standard method of nest-building behavior in mice using pressed cotton and rated nest quality on a scale of 1–5 (Deacon, 2006). By utilizing 3D depth-sensing cameras, we are able to conduct objective 3D evaluation of the final nest in one point evaluation (Okayama et al., 2015). In addition, we have analyzed an untapped behavioral characteristic, the construction process of the nest. Our 3D monitoring system could discriminate slight differences in temporal nesting behavior using 3D depth images and Deacon score 1-5 (Goto et al., 2015b). Since nest-building behavior is altered by social stress (Otabi et al., 2016), several stress models such as CSDS, CMS, and restraint stress should also be analyzed while nest-building in future.

STRATEGY FOR FINDING ANTIDEPRESSANTS FROM NATURAL INGREDIENTS (FIGURE 2)

Using sCSDS mice, we will investigate functional ingredients from natural sources that should attenuate stress-induced symptoms. Since sCSDS mice fed a semi-purified diet show more vulnerable behavior than mice fed a non-purified diet (Goto et al., in press), a change to a semi-purified diet as a base diet would be a good approach to identify functional ingredients enhancing stress resilience behavior. A semi-purified diet is preferred for nutritional research because the non-purified diet contains unknown raw materials and ingredients. Since the non-purified diet potentially improves stress vulnerability, it would be worthwhile to note differences between semi-purified and non-purified diets. Components including dietary fiber, resistant starch, and unavailable carbohydrates will be targets in future studies. These components are available to gut microbiota, resulting in a variety of species living in the gut. The brain-gut axis (Kelly et al., 2015) should be a main target for food-mediated approaches to finding antidepressants and preventing stress-related diseases by shifting food habits. In addition, sCSDS mice show stress-induced symptoms described above. By checking these indicators, the depression model can be useful for screening antidepressant effects of functional food and farm products.

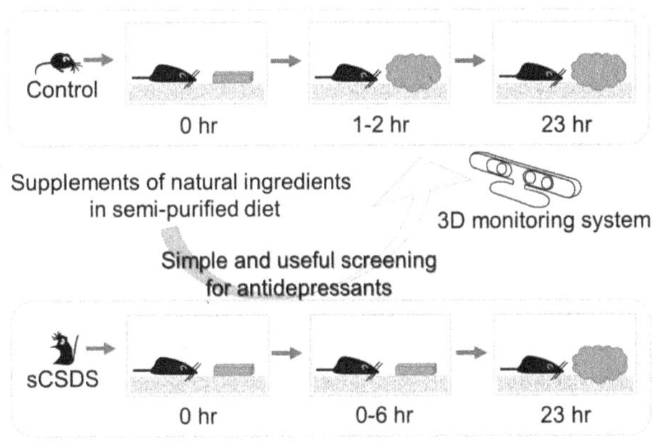

FIGURE 2 | Strategy for finding antidepressants from natural sources. The combination of sCSDS mice with 3D monitoring system is a powerful method for screening antidepressants from natural ingredients. Natural ingredients which rescue retarded nest-building can be screened.

Our novel 3D monitoring system for nest-building enabled us to detect small differences among groups in different treatments and strains (Okayama et al., 2015; Goto et al., 2015b). Furthermore, we found simple and useful nesting behavioral test (Otabi et al., 2016). By using this combined method with sCSDS mice and 3D monitoring systems, we can discern slight differences in innate behavior and screen candidate supplements quickly. In future, automated behavioral analysis for nesting behavior will make this method easy for many researchers.

Toyoda and colleagues conducted research in the interdisciplinary field of agricultural-medical science (http://iucam-ibaraki.wix.com/iucam), exploring functional food and farm products for prevention and attenuation of psychiatric symptoms. Establishing animal models of depression, searching and screening supplemental resources, and applying engineering techniques will be essential in the big data era. Now that the fundamental platform has been established, we can screen ingredients from natural sources such as dairy products, fruits, and vegetables.

CONCLUSIONS

In this article, we introduced our mouse model of depression and novel 3D evaluation system for nesting behavior. Good dietary habits should provide potential effects for reducing depressive symptoms and extending healthy life. The importance of food habits in overcoming stress can be shown by identifying antidepressant-like natural resources using sCSDS mice. The combination of sCSDS mice with 3D behavioral assays is a powerful method for screening the ingredients showing antidepressant-like effects in foods and farm products.

AUTHOR CONTRIBUTIONS

TG and AT wrote overall manuscript. ST and TO wrote a part of the manuscript about metabolome and 3D sensor, respectively. TG, ST, TO, and AT have checked the manuscript entirely and agree with submission.

REFERENCES

Arai, S. (1996). Studies on functional foods in Japan–state of the art. *Biosci. Biotechnol. Biochem.* 60, 9–15. doi: 10.1271/bbb.60.9

Bartolomucci, A., and Leopardi, R. (2009). Stress and depression: preclinical research and clinical implications. *PLoS ONE* 4:e4265. doi: 10.1371/journal.pone.0004265

Cryan, J. F., and Dinan, T. G. (2012). Mind-altering microorganisms: the impact of the gut microbiota on brain and behaviour. *Nat. Rev. Neurosci.* 13, 701–712. doi: 10.1038/nrn3346

Deacon, R. M. J. (2006). Assessing nest building in mice. *Nat. Protoc.* 1, 1117–1119. doi: 10.1038/nprot.2006.170

El-Hage, W., Leman, S., Camus, V., and Belzung, C. (2013). Mechanisms of antidepressant resistance. *Front. Pharmacol.* 4:146. doi: 10.3389/fphar.2013.00146

Galling, B., Calsina Ferrer, A., Abi Zeid Daou, M., Sangroula, D., Hagi, K., and Correll, C. U. (2015). Safety and tolerability of antidepressant co-treatment in acute major depressive disorder: results from a systematic review and exploratory meta-analysis. *Expert Opin. Drug Saf.* 14, 1587–1608. doi: 10.1517/14740338.2015.1085970

Goto, T., Kubota, Y., Tanaka, Y., Iio, W., Moriya, N., and Toyoda, A. (2014). Subchronic and mild social defeat stress accelerates food intake and body weight gain with polydipsia-like features in mice. *Behav. Brain Res.* 270, 339–348. doi: 10.1016/j.bbr.2014.05.040

Goto, T., Kubota, Y., and Toyoda, A. (2015a). Plasma and liver metabolic profiles in mice subjected to subchronic and mild social defeat stress. *J. Proteome Res.* 14, 1025–1032. doi: 10.1021/pr501044k

Goto, T., Kubota, Y., and Toyoda, A. (in press). Effects of diet quality on vulnerability to mild subchronic social defeat stress in mice. *Nutr. Neurosci.* doi: 10.1179/1476830515y.0000000017

Goto, T., Okayama, T., and Toyoda, A. (2015b). Strain differences in temporal changes of nesting behaviors in C57BL/6N, DBA/2N, and their F1 hybrid mice assessed by a three-dimensional monitoring system. *Behav. Processes* 119, 86–92. doi: 10.1016/j.beproc.2015.07.007

Goto, T., and Toyoda, A. (2015). A mouse model of subchronic and mild social defeat stress for understanding stress-induced behavioral and physiological deficits. *J. Vis. Exp.* 105:e52973. doi: 10.3791/52973

Gross, M., and Pinhasov, A. (2016). Chronic mild stress in submissive mice: marked polydipsia and social avoidance without hedonic deficit in the sucrose preference test. *Behav. Brain Res.* 298, 25–34. doi: 10.1016/j.bbr.2015.10.049

Hammels, C., Pishva, E., De Vry, J., van den Hove, D. L. A., Prickaerts, J., van Winkel, R., et al. (2015). Defeat stress in rodents: From behavior to molecules. *Neurosci. Biobehav. Rev.* 59, 111–140. doi: 10.1016/j.neubiorev.2015.10.006

Heijtz, R. D., Wang, S., Anuar, F., Qian, Y., Bjorkholm, B., Samuelsson, A., et al. (2011). Normal gut microbiota modulates brain development and behavior. *Proc. Natl. Acad. Sci. U.S.A.* 108, 3047–3052. doi: 10.1073/pnas.1010529108

Hodes, G. E., Pfau, M. L., Leboeuf, M., Golden, S. A., Christoffel, D. J., Bregman, D., et al. (2014). Individual differences in the peripheral immune system promote resilience versus susceptibility to social stress. *Proc. Natl. Acad. Sci. U.S.A.* 111, 16136–16141. doi: 10.1073/pnas.1415191111

Hong, W., Kennedy, A., Burgos-Artizzu, X. P., Zelikowsky, M., Navonne, S. G., Perona, P., et al. (2015). Automated measurement of mouse social behaviors using depth sensing, video tracking, and machine learning. *Proc. Natl. Acad. Sci. U.S.A.* 112, E5351–E5360. doi: 10.1073/pnas.1515982112

Hori, A., Ito, N., Oikawa, T., and Hanawa, T. (2015). Kososan, but not milnacipran, elicits antidepressant-like effects in a novel psychological stress-induced mouse model of depression. *Tradit. Kampo Med.* 2, 1–7. doi: 10.1002/tkm2.1013

Iio, W., Matsukawa, N., Tsukahara, T., Kohari, D., and Toyoda, A. (2011). Effects of chronic social defeat stress on MAP kinase cascade. *Neurosci. Lett.* 504, 281–284. doi: 10.1016/j.neulet.2011.09.047

Iio, W., Matsukawa, N., Tsukahara, T., and Toyoda, A. (2012a). The effects of oral taurine administration on behavior and hippocampal signal transduction in rats. *Amino Acids* 43, 2037–2046. doi: 10.1007/s00726-012-1282-2

Iio, W., Takagi, H., Ogawa, Y., Tsukahara, T., Chohnan, S., and Toyoda, A. (2014). Effects of chronic social defeat stress on peripheral leptin and its hypothalamic actions. *BMC Neurosci.* 15:72. doi: 10.1186/1471-2202-15-72

Iio, W., Tokutake, Y., Matsukawa, N., Tsukahara, T., Chohnan, S., and Toyoda, A. (2012b). Anorexic behavior and elevation of hypothalamic malonyl-CoA in socially defeated rats. *Biochem. Biophys. Res. Commun.* 421, 301–304. doi: 10.1016/j.bbrc.2012.04.004

Ito, N., Hori, A., Yabe, T., Nagai, T., Oikawa, T., Yamada, H., et al. (2012). Involvement of neuropeptide Y signaling in the antidepressant-like effect and hippocampal cell proliferation induced by kososan, a Kampo medicine, in the stress-induced depression-like model mice. *Biol. Pharm. Bull.* 35, 1775–1783. doi: 10.1248/bpb.b12-00466

Kelly, J. R., Kennedy, P. J., Cryan, J. F., Dinan, T. G., Clarke, G., and Hyland, N. P. (2015). Breaking down the barriers: the gut microbiome, intestinal permeability and stress-related psychiatric disorders. *Front. Cell. Neurosci.* 9:392. doi: 10.3389/fncel.2015.00392

Kim, B., Colon, E., Chawla, S., Vandenberg, L. N., and Suvorov, A. (2015). Endocrine disruptors alter social behaviors and indirectly influence social hierarchies via changes in body weight. *Environ. Health* 14:64. doi: 10.1186/s12940-015-0051-6

Krishnan, V., Han, M.-H., Graham, D. L., Berton, O., Renthal, W., Russo, S. J., et al. (2007). Molecular adaptations underlying susceptibility and resistance to social defeat in brain reward regions. *Cell* 131, 391–404. doi: 10.1016/j.cell.2007.09.018

Kudryavtseva, N. N., Bakshtanovskaya, I. V., and Koryakina, L. A. (1991). Social model of depression in mice of C57BL/6J strain. *Pharmacol. Biochem. Behav.* 38, 315–320. doi: 10.1016/0091-3057(91)90284-9

Matsumoto, J., Uehara, T., Urakawa, S., Takamura, Y., Sumiyoshi, T., Suzuki, M., et al. (2014). 3D video analysis of the novel object recognition test in rats. *Behav. Brain Res.* 272, 16–24. doi: 10.1016/j.bbr.2014.06.047

Matsumoto, J., Urakawa, S., Takamura, Y., Malcher-Lopes, R., Hori, E., Tomaz, C., et al. (2013). A 3D-video-based computerized analysis of social and sexual interactions in rats. *PLoS ONE* 8:e78460. doi: 10.1371/journal.pone.0078460

Miczek, K. A., Yap, J. J., and Covington, H. E. (2008). Social stress, therapeutics and drug abuse: preclinical models of escalated and depressed intake. *Pharmacol. Ther.* 120, 102–128. doi: 10.1016/j.pharmthera.2008.07.006

Nakamura, A., Funaya, H., Uezono, N., Nakashima, K., Ishida, Y., Suzuki, T., et al. (2015). Low-cost three-dimensional gait analysis system for mice with an infrared depth sensor. *Neurosci. Res.* 100, 55–62. doi: 10.1016/j.neures.2015.06.006

Okayama, T., Goto, T., and Toyoda, A. (2015). Assessing nest-building behavior of mice using a 3D depth camera. *J. Neurosci. Methods* 251, 151–157. doi: 10.1016/j.jneumeth.2015.05.019

Otabi, H., Goto, T., Okayama, T., Kohari, D., and Toyoda, A. (2016). Subchronic and mild social defeat stress alter mouse nest building behavior. *Behav. Processes* 122, 21–25. doi: 10.1016/j.beproc.2015.10.018

Ou-Yang, T.-H., Tsai, M.-L., Yen, C.-T., and Lin, T.-T. (2011). An infrared range camera-based approach for three-dimensional locomotion tracking and pose reconstruction in a rodent. *J. Neurosci. Methods* 201, 116–123. doi: 10.1016/j.jneumeth.2011.07.019

Pfau, M. L., and Russo, S. J. (2015). Peripheral and central mechanisms of stress resilience. *Neurobiol. Stress* 1, 66–79. doi: 10.1016/j.ynstr.2014.09.004

Russo, S. J., and Nestler, E. J. (2013). The brain reward circuitry in mood disorders. *Nat. Rev. Neurosci.* 14, 609–625. doi: 10.1038/nrn3381

Stevens, J. R., Jarrahzadeh, T., Brendel, R. W., and Stern, T. A. (2014). Strategies for the prescription of psychotropic drugs with black box warnings. *Psychosomatics* 55, 123–133. doi: 10.1016/j.psym.2013.08.009

Sudo, N., Chida, Y., Aiba, Y., Sonoda, J., Oyama, N., Yu, X.-N., et al. (2004). Postnatal microbial colonization programs the hpothalamic-pituitary-adrenal system for stress response in mice. *J. Physiol.* 558, 263–275. doi: 10.1113/jphysiol.2004.063388

Tanaka, K., Furuyashiki, T., Kitaoka, S., Senzai, Y., Imoto, Y., Segi-Nishida, E., et al. (2012). Prostaglandin E2-mediated attenuation of mesocortical dopaminergic pathway is critical for susceptibility to repeated social defeat stress in mice. *J. Neurosci.* 32, 4319–4329. doi: 10.1523/JNEUROSCI.5952-11.2012

Tomonaga, S., Yamane, H., Onitsuka, E., Yamada, S., Sato, M., Takahata, Y., et al. (2008). Carnosine-induced antidepressant-like activity in rats. *Pharmacol. Biochem. Behav.* 89, 627–632. doi: 10.1016/j.pbb.2008.02.021

Toyoda, A., Iio, W., Matsukawa, N., and Tsukahara, T. (2015). Influence of chronic social defeat stress on digestive system functioning in rats. *J. Nutr. Sci. Vitaminol.* 61, 280–284. doi: 10.3177/jnsv.61.280

Watanabe, K., Matsuura, K., Gao, P., Hottenbacher, L., Tokunaga, H., Nishimura, K., et al. (2011). Traditional Japanese Kampo Medicine: clinical research between modernity and traditional medicine-the state of research and methodological suggestions for the future. *Evid. Based Complement. Alternat. Med.* 2011:513842. doi: 10.1093/ecam/neq067

Whiteford, H. A., Degenhardt, L., Rehm, J., Baxter, A. J., Ferrari, A. J., Erskine, H. E., et al. (2013). Global burden of disease attributable to mental and substance use disorders: findings from the Global Burden of Disease Study 2010. *Lancet* 382, 1575–1586. doi: 10.1016/S0140-6736(13)61611-6

Permissions

All chapters in this book were first published in CFCDNDNTPTNINCET, by Frontiers; hereby published with permission under the Creative Commons Attribution License or equivalent. Every chapter published in this book has been scrutinized by our experts. Their significance has been extensively debated. The topics covered herein carry significant findings which will fuel the growth of the discipline. They may even be implemented as practical applications or may be referred to as a beginning point for another development.

The contributors of this book come from diverse backgrounds, making this book a truly international effort. This book will bring forth new frontiers with its revolutionizing research information and detailed analysis of the nascent developments around the world.

We would like to thank all the contributing authors for lending their expertise to make the book truly unique. They have played a crucial role in the development of this book. Without their invaluable contributions this book wouldn't have been possible. They have made vital efforts to compile up to date information on the varied aspects of this subject to make this book a valuable addition to the collection of many professionals and students.

This book was conceptualized with the vision of imparting up-to-date information and advanced data in this field. To ensure the same, a matchless editorial board was set up. Every individual on the board went through rigorous rounds of assessment to prove their worth. After which they invested a large part of their time researching and compiling the most relevant data for our readers.

The editorial board has been involved in producing this book since its inception. They have spent rigorous hours researching and exploring the diverse topics which have resulted in the successful publishing of this book. They have passed on their knowledge of decades through this book. To expedite this challenging task, the publisher supported the team at every step. A small team of assistant editors was also appointed to further simplify the editing procedure and attain best results for the readers.

Apart from the editorial board, the designing team has also invested a significant amount of their time in understanding the subject and creating the most relevant covers. They scrutinized every image to scout for the most suitable representation of the subject and create an appropriate cover for the book.

The publishing team has been an ardent support to the editorial, designing and production team. Their endless efforts to recruit the best for this project, has resulted in the accomplishment of this book. They are a veteran in the field of academics and their pool of knowledge is as vast as their experience in printing. Their expertise and guidance has proved useful at every step. Their uncompromising quality standards have made this book an exceptional effort. Their encouragement from time to time has been an inspiration for everyone.

The publisher and the editorial board hope that this book will prove to be a valuable piece of knowledge for researchers, students, practitioners and scholars across the globe.

List of Contributors

Suman Das
Department of Biomedical Engineering and Zlotowski Center for Neuroscience, Ben Gurion University of the Negev, Be'er Sheva, Israel
Department of Neuroscience, Erasmus Medical Center, Rotterdam, Netherlands
Department of Integrative Neurophysiology, Center for Neurogenomics and Cognitive Research, Vrije Universiteit Amsterdam, Amsterdam, Netherlands

Marcella Spoor, Tafadzwa M. Sibindi and Martijn Schonewille
Department of Neuroscience, Erasmus Medical Center, Rotterdam, Netherlands

Peter Holland and Opher Donchin
Department of Biomedical Engineering and Zlotowski Center for Neuroscience, Ben Gurion University of the Negev, Be'er Sheva, Israel
Department of Neuroscience, Erasmus Medical Center, Rotterdam, Netherlands

Chris I. De Zeeuw
Department of Neuroscience, Erasmus Medical Center, Rotterdam, Netherlands
Netherlands Institute for Neuroscience, Amsterdam, Netherlands

Maarten A. Frens
Department of Neuroscience, Erasmus Medical Center, Rotterdam, Netherlands
Faculty of Social and Behavioral Sciences

Keiko Nohara and Fumihiko Maekawa
Molecular Toxicology Section, National Institute for Environmental Studies, Tsukuba, Japan

Kazuaki Nakamura and Akito Tanoue
Department of Pharmacology, National Research Institute for Child Health and Development, Setagaya, Japan

Masaki Kakeyama
Faculty of Human Sciences, Waseda University, Tokorozawa, Japan

Chiharu Tohyama
Faculty of Medicine, University of Tsukuba, Tsukuba, Japan

Adriana Ximenes-da-Silva
Setor de Fisiologia, Instituto de Ciências Biológicas e da Saúde, Universidade Federal de Alagoas, Maceió, Brazil

Yousuke Ogata
Department of Advanced Neuroimaging, Integrative Brain Imaging Center, National Center of Neurology and Psychiatry, Kodaira, Japan
Biointerfaces Unit, Institute of Innovative Research, Tokyo Institute of Technology, Yokohama, Japan
Department of Functional Brain Research, National Institute of Neuroscience, National Center of Neurology and Psychiatry, Kodaira, Japan

Akihiko Ozaki
Social Welfare Organization Saiseikai Imperial Gift Foundation, Inc., Osaka Saiseikai Nakatsu Hospital, Osaka, Japan

Miho Ota
Department of Advanced Neuroimaging, Integrative Brain Imaging Center, National Center of Neurology and Psychiatry, Kodaira, Japan
Department of Mental Disorder Research, National Institute of Neuroscience, National Center of Neurology and Psychiatry, Kodaira, Japan

Yurie Oka
Department of Advanced Neuroimaging, Integrative Brain Imaging Center, National Center of Neurology and Psychiatry, Kodaira, Japan

Namiko Nishida and Hayato Tabu
Kitano Hospital, Tazuke Kofukai Medical Research Institute, Osaka, Japan

Noriko Sato
Department of Radiology, National Center of Neurology and Psychiatry Hospital, Kodaira, Japan
Department of Clinical Neuroimaging, Integrative Brain Imaging Center, National Center of Neurology and Psychiatry, Kodaira, Japan

Takashi Hanakawa
Department of Advanced Neuroimaging, Integrative Brain Imaging Center, National Center of Neurology and Psychiatry, Kodaira, Japan
Department of Functional Brain Research, National Institute of Neuroscience, National Center of Neurology and Psychiatry, Kodaira, Japan

Sara Marceglia
Fondazione IRCCS Ca' Granda Ospedale Maggiore Policlinico, Milan, Italy
Dipartimento di Ingegneria e Architettura, Università degli Studi di Trieste, Trieste, Italy

Simona Mrakic-Sposta
Fondazione IRCCS Ca' Granda Ospedale Maggiore Policlinico, Milan, Italy
Istituto di Bioimmagini e di Fisiologia Molecolare, Consiglio Nazionale delle Ricerche, Segrate, Italy

Manuela Fumagalli, Francesca Mameli and Maurizio Vergari
Fondazione IRCCS Ca' Granda Ospedale Maggiore Policlinico, Milan, Italy

Roberta Ferrucci and Sergio Barbieri
Fondazione IRCCS Ca' Granda Ospedale Maggiore Policlinico, Milan, Italy
"Aldo Ravelli" Center for Neurotechnology and Experimental Brain Therapeutics, University of Milan, Milan, Italy

Alberto Priori
Fondazione IRCCS Ca' Granda Ospedale Maggiore Policlinico, Milan, Italy
"Aldo Ravelli" Center for Neurotechnology and Experimental Brain Therapeutics, University of Milan, Milan, Italy
Department of Health Sciences, University of Milan and ASST Santi Paolo e Carlo, Milan, Italy

Nang T. T. Htike, Haruka Soutome and Kyaw H. Aung
Area of Regulatory Biology, Division of Life Science, Graduate School of Science and Engineering, Saitama University, Saitama, Japan

Sho Maejima
Area of Life-NanoBio, Division of Strategy Research, Graduate School of Science and Engineering, Saitama University, Saitama, Japan

Masaaki Tokuda
Department of Cell Physiology, Faculty of Medicine/ Graduate School of Medicine, Kagawa University, Kagawa, Japan

Andrea Cancelli, Carlo Cottone and Giampiero Asta
Laboratory of Electrophysiology for Translational Neuroscience, Istituto di scienze e tecnologie della cognizione (ISTC), Consiglio Nazionale Delle Ricerche (CNR), Rome, Italy

Alessandro Giordani and Domenico Lupoi
AFaR Division, Fatebenefratelli Foundation for Health Research and Education, Rome, Italy

Vittorio Pizzella
Department of Neuroscience, Imaging and Clinical Sciences, Università degli Studi G. d'Annunzio Chieti e Pescara, Chieti, Italy
Institute for Advanced Biomedical Technologies, Università degli Studi G. d'Annunzio Chieti e Pescara, Chieti, Italy

Franca Tecchio
Institute of Neurology, Catholic University of the Sacred Heart, Rome, Italy
Laboratory of Electrophysiology for Translational Neuroscience, Istituto di scienze e tecnologie della cognizione (ISTC), Consiglio Nazionale Delle Ricerche (CNR), Rome, Italy
Adel Derghal, Jérôme Trouslard and Lourdes Mounien
Aix Marseille University, PPSN, Marseille, France

Mehdi Djelloul
Aix Marseille University, PPSN, Marseille, France
Department of Cell and Molecular Biology, Karolinska Institute, Stockholm, Sweden

Takeo Fujiwara
Department of Social Medicine, National Research Institute for Child Health and Development, Okura, Setagaya-ku, Tokyo, Japan
Department of Global Health Promotion, Tokyo Medical and Dental University, Tokyo, Japan

Naho Morisaki and Makiko Sampei
Department of Social Medicine, National Research Institute for Child Health and Development, Okura, Setagaya-ku, Tokyo, Japan

Yukiko Honda
Department of Social Medicine, National Research Institute for Child Health and Development, Okura, Setagaya-ku, Tokyo, Japan
Global Cooperation Institute for Sustainable Cities, Yokohama City University, Yokohama, Japan

Yukako Tani
Department of Social Medicine, National Research Institute for Child Health and Development, Okura, Setagaya-ku, Tokyo, Japan
Department of Global Health Promotion, Tokyo Medical and Dental University, Tokyo, Japan
Department of Health Education and Health Sociology, School of Public Health, The University of Tokyo, Tokyo, Japan

Mario Stampanoni Bassi, Luana Gilio, Fabio Buttari and Diego Centonze
Unit of Neurology & Unit of Neurorehabilitation, IRCCS Istituto Neurologico Mediterraneo Neuromed, Pozzilli, Italy
Multiple Sclerosis Research Unit, Department of Systems Medicine, Tor Vergata University, Rome, Italy

Pierpaolo Maffei and Ennio Iezzi
Unit of Neurology & Unit of Neurorehabilitation, IRCCS Istituto Neurologico Mediterraneo Neuromed, Pozzilli, Italy

Girolama A. Marfia
Multiple Sclerosis Research Unit, Department of Systems Medicine, Tor Vergata University, Rome, Italy
Domenico A. Restivo
Department of Neurology, Nuovo Garibaldi Hospital, Catania, Italy

Chaw Kyi-Tha-Thu, Yadanar Moe and Shinji Tsukahara
Division of Life Science, Graduate School of Science and Engineering, Saitama University, Saitama City, Japan

Yuji Fujitani and Seishiro Hirano
Center for Environmental Risk Research, National Institute for Environmental Studies, Tsukuba, Japan

Jiayue Cai and Z. Jane Wang
Department of Electrical and Computer Engineering, University of British Columbia, Vancouver, BC, Canada

Soojin Lee
School of Biomedical Engineering, University of British Columbia, Vancouver, BC, Canada,
Pacific Parkinson's Research Centre, Vancouver, BC, Canada

Fang Ba
Division of Neurology, Department of Medicine, University of Alberta, Edmonton, AB, Canada
Saurabh Garg and Laura J. Kim
Pacific Parkinson's Research Centre, Vancouver, BC, Canada

Aiping Liu
Pacific Parkinson's Research Centre, Vancouver, BC, Canada
School of Electronics and Applied Physics, Hefei University of Technology, Hefei, China

Diana Kim
Department of Medicine (Neurology), University of British Columbia, Vancouver, BC, Canada

Martin J. McKeown
Department of Electrical and Computer Engineering, University of British Columbia, Vancouver, BC, Canada
Department of Medicine (Neurology), University of British Columbia, Vancouver, BC, Canada

Kazuhiro Sano, Tomohiko Isobe, Jiaxin Yang, Tin-Tin Win-Shwe, Mitsuha Yoshikane, Shoji F. Nakayama, Fumihiko Maekawa and Keiko Nohara
Center for Health and Environmental Risk Research, National Institute for Environmental Studies, Tsukuba, Japan

Takaharu Kawashima
Center for Environmental Biology and Ecosystem Studies, National Institute for Environmental Studies, Tsukuba, Japan

Go Suzuki
Center for Health and Environmental Risk Research, National Institute for Environmental Studies, Tsukuba, Japan
Center for Material Cycles and Waste Management Research, National Institute for Environmental Studies, Tsukuba, Japan

Shunji Hashimoto
Center for Environmental Measurement and Analysis, National Institute for Environmental Studies, Tsukuba, Japan

Kazuki Harada, Taichi Kamiya and Takashi Tsuboi
Department of Life Sciences, Graduate School of Arts and Sciences, The University of Tokyo, Tokyo, Japan

Laura Marchal-Crespo and Robert Riener
Sensory-Motor Systems Lab, Department of Health Sciences and Technology, Institute of Robotics and Intelligent Systems, ETH Zurich, Zurich, Switzerland
Reharobotics Group, Spinal Cord Injury Center, Balgrist University Hospital, Medical Faculty, University of Zurich, Zurich, Switzerland

Lars Michels
Clinic of Neuroradiology, University Hospital Zurich, Zurich, Switzerland,
MR-Center, University Children's Hospital Zurich, Zurich, Switzerland

Lukas Jaeger
Sensory-Motor Systems Lab, Department of Health Sciences and Technology, Institute of Robotics and Intelligent Systems, ETH Zurich, Zurich, Switzerland
Clinic of Neuroradiology, University Hospital Zurich, Zurich, Switzerland

Jorge López-Olóriz
Sensory-Motor Systems Lab, Department of Health Sciences and Technology, Institute of Robotics and Intelligent Systems, ETH Zurich, Zurich, Switzerland

Joel Cano-Nicolau, Colette Vaillant, Elisabeth Pellegrini, Thierry D. Charlier, Olivier Kah and Pascal Coumailleau
Research Institute in Health, Environment and Occupation, Institut National de la Santé et de la Recherche Médicale U1085, SFR Biosite, Université de Rennes 1, Rennes, France

Jin-Fang Ge, Ya-Yun Xu, Gan Qin, Jiang-Qun Cheng and Fei-Hu Chen
Anhui Key Laboratory of Bioactivity of Natural Products, School of Pharmacy, Anhui Medical University, Hefei, Anhui, China

Wenting Ling and Toshihiro Endo
Laboratory of Environmental Health Sciences, Center for Disease Biology and Integrative Medicine, Graduate School of Medicine, The University of Tokyo, Tokyo, Japan

Ken-ichiro Kubo and Kazunori Nakajima
Department of Anatomy, Keio University School of Medicine, Tokyo, Japan

Angelo Quartarone and Demetrio Milardi
Department of Biomedical, Dental Sciences and Morphological and Functional Images, University of Messina, Messina, Italy
Centro Neurolesi Bonino Pulejo (IRCCS), Messina, Italy

Vincenzo Rizzo, Carmen Terranova, Gaetana Chillemi and Paolo Girlanda
Department of Clinical and Experimental Medicine, University of Messina, Messina, Italy

Alberto Cacciola
Centro Neurolesi Bonino Pulejo (IRCCS), Messina, Italy

Alessandro Calamuneri
Department of Biomedical, Dental Sciences and Morphological and Functional Images, University of Messina, Messina, Italy

Walaa M. S. Ahmed
Center for Environmental Health Sciences, National Institute for Environmental Studies, Tsukuba Japan,
Department of Clinical Pathology, Faculty of Veterinary Medicine, Beni-Suef University, Beni-Suef, Egypt

Koki Nagino
Center for Environmental Biology and Ecosystem Studies, National Institute for Environmental Studies, Tsukuba, Japan
Laboratory of Integrative Brain Sciences, Department of Biology and Center for Medical Life Science, Waseda University, Tokyo, Japan

Takayoshi Ubuka
Laboratory of Integrative Brain Sciences, Department of Biology and Center for Medical Life Science, Waseda University, Tokyo, Japan
Jeffrey Cheah School of Medicine and Health Sciences, Brain Research Institute Monash Sunway, Monash University Malaysia, Bandar Sunway, Malaysia

Kazuyoshi Tsutsui
Laboratory of Integrative Brain Sciences, Department of Biology and Center for Medical Life Science, Waseda University, Tokyo, Japan

Yusuke Furukawa
Division of Cellular and Molecular Toxicology, Biological Safety Research Center, National Institute of Health Sciences, Tokyo, Japan
Department of Comprehensive Pathology, Graduate School, Tokyo Medical and Dental University, Tokyo, Japan

Kentaro Tanemura
Laboratory of Animal Reproduction and Development, Graduate School of Agricultural Science, Tohoku University, Sendai, Japan

Katsuhide Igarashi and Maky Ideta-Otsuka
Life Science Tokyo Advanced Research Center, Hoshi University School of Pharmacy and Pharmaceutical Sciences, Tokyo, Japan

Ken-Ichi Aisaki and Satoshi Kitajima
Division of Cellular and Molecular Toxicology, Biological Safety Research Center, National Institute of Health Sciences, Tokyo, Japan

Masanobu Kitagawa
Department of Comprehensive Pathology, Graduate School, Tokyo Medical and Dental University, Tokyo, Japan

Jun Kanno
Division of Cellular and Molecular Toxicology, Biological Safety Research Center, National Institute of Health Sciences, Tokyo, Japan
Japan Bioassay Research Center, Japan Organization of Occupational Health and Safety, Hadano, Japan

Anna Steinberg and Tiago P. Moreira
Department of Neurology, Karolinska University Hospital, Stockholm, Sweden
Stroke Research Unit, Department of Clinical Neuroscience, Karolinska Institutet, Stockholm, Sweden

Shozo Tomonaga
Graduate School of Agriculture, Kyoto University, Kyoto, Japan

Camila B. Pinto
Laboratory of Neuromodulation and Center for Clinical Research Learning, Department of Physical Medicine and Rehabilitation, Harvard Medical School, Spaulding Rehabilitation Hospital, Harvard University, Boston, MA, United States
Department of Neuroscience and Behavior, Psychology Institute, University of São Paulo, São Paulo, Brazil

Faddi G. Saleh Velez and Fernanda Lopes
Laboratory of Neuromodulation and Center for Clinical Research Learning, Department of Physical Medicine and Rehabilitation, Harvard Medical School, Spaulding Rehabilitation Hospital, Harvard University, Boston, MA, United States

Polyana V. de Toledo Piza
Laboratory of Neuromodulation and Center for Clinical Research Learning, Department of Physical Medicine and Rehabilitation, Harvard Medical School, Spaulding Rehabilitation Hospital, Harvard University, Boston, MA, United States
Department of Severe Patients, Hospital Israelita Albert Einstein, São Paulo, Brazil

Qing M. Wang
Stroke Biological Recovery Laboratory, Department of Physical Medicine and Rehabilitation, Harvard Medical School, Spaulding Rehabilitation Hospital, Harvard University, Boston, MA, United States

Nicole L. Mazwi and Randie Black-Schaffer
Department of Physical Medicine and Rehabilitation, Harvard Medical School, Spaulding Rehabilitation Hospital, Harvard University, Boston, MA, United States

Erica C. Camargo
Department of Neurology, Harvard Medical School, Massachusetts General Hospital , Harvard University, Boston, MA, United States

Felipe Fregni
Laboratory of Neuromodulation and Center for Clinical Research Learning, Department of Physical Medicine and Rehabilitation, Harvard Medical School, Spaulding Rehabilitation Hospital, Harvard University, Boston, MA, United States

Tsuyoshi Okayama and Atsushi Toyoda
Department of Biological Production Science, College of Agriculture, Ibaraki University, Ami, Ibaraki, Japan
Department of Biological Production Science, Ibaraki University Cooperation between Agriculture and Medical Science, Ami, Ibaraki, Japan
Department of Biological Production Science, United Graduate School of Agricultural Science, Tokyo University of Agriculture and Technology, Fuchu, Japan

Laura Dipietro
Highland Instruments, Cambridge, MA, United States

Tatsuhiko Goto
Department of Biological Production Science, College of Agriculture, Ibaraki University, Ami, Ibaraki, Japan
Department of Biological Production Science, Ibaraki University Cooperation between Agriculture and Medical Science, Ami, Ibaraki, Japan

Index

www.ingramcontent.com/pod-product-compliance
Lightning Source LLC
LaVergne TN
LVHW080928210926
848485LV00004B/755